LIFETIME
Physical Fitness and Wellness
SEVENTH EDITION

LIFETIME
Physical Fitness and Wellness
A PERSONALIZED PROGRAM SEVENTH EDITION

Werner W. K. Hoeger
Boise State University

Sharon A. Hoeger
Fitness & Wellness, Inc.

Australia • Canada • Mexico • Singapore • Spain
United Kingdom • United States

THOMSON
WADSWORTH

THOMSON
WADSWORTH

PUBLISHER Peter Marshall

ASSOCIATE EDITOR April Lemons

ASSISTANT EDITOR John Boyd

EDITORIAL ASSISTANT Andrea Kesterke

EXECUTIVE TECHNOLOGY PROJECT MANAGER Donna M. Kelley

MARKETING MANAGER Jennifer Somerville

MARKETING ASSISTANT Mona Weltmer

ADVERTISING PROJECT MANAGER Shemika Britt

Sandra Craig PROJECT MANAGER, EDITORIAL PRODUCTION

Judy Inouye PRINT/MEDIA BUYER

Stephanie Keough-Hedges PERMISSIONS EDITOR

Ash Street Typecrafters PRODUCTION AND COMPOSITION

Baugher Design Inc. TEXT AND COVER DESIGNER

Carol Lombardi COPY EDITOR

© Lisette Le Bon/SuperStock COVER IMAGE

Courier/Kendallville PRINTER

Printed in the United States of America
1 2 3 4 5 6 7   06 05 04 03 02

For more information about our products, contact us at:
Thomson Learning Academic Resource Center
1-800-423-0563
For permission to use material from this text, contact us by:
Phone: 1-800-730-2214
Fax: 1-800-730-2215
Web: http://www.thomsonrights.com

ExamView® and ExamView Pro® are registered trademarks of FSCreations, Inc. Windows is a registered trademark of the Microsoft Corporation used herein under license. Macintosh and Power Macintosh are registered trademarks of Apple Computer, Inc. Used herein under license.

Library of Congress Cataloging-in-Publication Data
Hoeger, Werner W. K.
  Lifetime physical fitness and wellness: a personalized program / Werner W. K. Hoeger, Sharon A. Hoeger.—7th ed.
    p. cm.
  Includes bibliographical references and index.
  ISBN 0-534-58257-5
  1. Health promotion. 2. Physical fitness. 3. Health behavior.
4. Exercise. I. Hoeger, Sharon A. II. Title.

RA781 .H6 2003
613—dc21   2001057453

WADSWORTH/THOMSON LEARNING
10 Davis Drive
Belmont, CA 94002-3098
USA

ASIA
Thomson Learning
60 Albert Street, #15-01
Albert Complex
Singapore 189969

AUSTRALIA
Nelson Thomson Learning
102 Dodds Street
South Melbourne, Victoria 3205
Australia

CANADA
Nelson Thomson Learning
1120 Birchmount Road
Toronto, Ontario M1K 5G4
Canada

EUROPE/MIDDLE EAST/AFRICA
Thomson Learning
Berkshire House
168-173 High Holborn
London WC1 V7AA
United Kingdom

LATIN AMERICA
Thomson Learning
Seneca, 53
Colonia Polanco
11560 Mexico D.F.
Mexico

SPAIN
Paraninfo Thomson Learning
Calle/Magallanes, 25
28015 Madrid, Spain

Brief Contents

Table of Contents

Chapter 3

Chapter 4

Chapter 5

Muscular Strength Assessment and Prescription   111

Chapter 6

Muscular Flexibility Assessment and Prescription   149

Chapter 12   Stress Assessment and Management Techniques   327

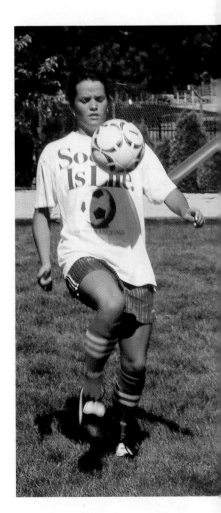

Chapter 13   Freedom from Addictive Behavior   355

THE CURRENT American way of life does not provide the human body with sufficient physical activity to enhance or maintain adequate health. Further, many present lifestyle patterns are such a serious threat to our health that they actually increase the deterioration rate of the human body and often lead to premature illness and mortality.

Although people in the United States are firm believers in the benefits of physical activity and positive lifestyle habits as a means to promote better health, most do not reap these benefits because they simply do not know how to implement a sound physical fitness and wellness program that will indeed yield the desired results. According to the Surgeon General, more than 60 percent of U.S. adults do not achieve the recommended amount of physical activity, and 25 percent are not physically active at all.

Scientific evidence has clearly shown that improving the quality and most likely the longevity of our lives is a matter of personal choice. The biggest challenge that we face in the twenty-first century is to teach individuals how to take control of their personal health habits to ensure a healthier, happier, and more productive life. The information presented in this book has been written with this objective in mind, providing you with the opportunity to initiate your own healthy lifestyle program.

Lifetime Physical Fitness and Wellness: A Personalized Approach contains 15 chapters and more than 40 fitness and wellness tests that serve as a guide to implement a complete lifetime of fitness and wellness. As you work through the different chapters in this book, you will be able to develop and regularly update your own lifetime program to improve the various components of physical fitness and wellness. The emphasis is on teaching you how to take control of your personal health and lifestyle habits, so that you can make a deliberate effort to stay healthy and realize your highest potential for well-being.

NEW AND ENHANCED FEATURES OF THE SEVENTH EDITION

All chapters in this edition of *Lifetime Physical Fitness and Wellness* have been revised and updated to conform with advances and recommendations made since the publication of the Sixth Edition. The most significant changes in this new edition are:

● **Chapter 1** has been extensively revised and now includes a much broader discussion of each dimension of wellness. Also, a new section on occupational wellness has been added. The information on spirituality and accident prevention and personal safety has been moved to this chapter from Chapter 15. The concept of "healthy life expectancy," as opposed to just life expectancy, with year 2000 statistics, is introduced in this chapter. An update on health care costs throughout the world and the lack of preventive approaches is also discussed in Chapter 1. A wellness questionnaire that includes questions on all dimensions of wellness has been incorporated at the end of the chapter.

● In **Chapter 2** corrections were made to the sixth stage of the Transtheoretical Model of behavioral change. Instead of the termination stage, it is now referred to as the termination/adoption stage. The word *termination* is used for undesirable behaviors that are permanently eliminated, while *adoption* is used for positive behaviors that have been successfully implemented.

● A discussion of the physiological principles that govern oxygen uptake and determine changes in aerobic fitness has been added to **Chapter 3**.

● In **Chapter 4** the list of suggestions to help motivate individuals to start and adhere to exercise has been expanded. New questions were added to the Specific Exercise Considerations section, including the 2000 American College of Sports Medicine (ACSM) exercise guidelines for diabetics. The section on Exercise and Aging was also updated and moved from Chapter 15 to this chapter, and spinning was added to the list of aerobic activity choices.

- The concepts of positive and negative resistance, concentric and eccentric muscle contractions, and guidelines for strength-training exercises were added to **Chapter 5**. Other additions include differences in strength training between free weights and machines, new free weight strength-training exercises, and graphic illustration of muscles exercised with each exercise. A worksheet to help students develop their personalized strength-training program has been incorporated into this chapter.

- In **Chapter 6** the benefits of flexibility training have been revised, along with an enhanced section on the prevention and treatment of low-back pain. A new worksheet to help students develop a flexibility fitness and back conditioning program has been added to the chapter.

- Statistical updates on mortality rates based on Body Mass Index (BMI) and the ever-growing obesity epidemic are discussed in **Chapter 7**. An introduction to the air displacement technique for body composition analysis is also included in this chapter.

- The content of **Chapter 8**, nutrition, has been extensively updated. New nutrient composition guidelines for the American diet based on 2001 recommendations by National Cholesterol Education Program (NCEP) Expert Panel have been included. The sections on antioxidant nutrients and osteoporosis were updated, and new information has been added regarding the Dietary Reference Intakes (DRIs), the 2000 Dietary Guidelines for Americans, creatine supplementation, vegetarian diets, ethnic diets, dietary benefits of nuts and soy, and FDA-approved health claims that link foods and disease.

- A new section, The Diet Craze, that discusses myths and detrimental effects of popular diets on the market today is included in **Chapter 9**. The glycemic index, effects of high-intensity versus low-intensity exercise in weight loss, and additional tips for behavior modification have all been added to this chapter.

- In **Chapter 10** revisions include information on strokes, diabetes, the treatment of high blood lipids, the metabolic syndrome (Syndrome X), the effects of soy foods on cardiovascular disease risk, the benefits of strength training on heart health and hypertension, new blood pressure classification guidelines, and the healthy lifestyle approach to the treatment of high blood pressure. The chapter also includes statistical updates from the American Heart Association and new graphs on the incidence of cardiovascular diseases and high blood pressure in the United States.

- All cancer statistics were updated in **Chapter 11**. The general guidelines for cancer prevention were revised along with risk factors, prevention, and warning signals for each specific cancer site. A new cancer prevention questionnaire and a section on skin self-examination was also added to this chapter

- **Chapter 12** includes information on the effects of hostile behaviors on health. Mental visualization (imagery) and introduction to yoga as stress management techniques are now also included. A new activity has been included for students to participate in a stress management session and report their feelings about the experience.

- The contents on substance abuse previously found in Chapter 14 were combined with the information on freedom from tobacco to form **Chapter 13**. This chapter is now entitled Addictive Behavior and Wellness. Information on heroin, methamphetamine, and MDMA (ecstasy) was also added to the chapter.

- **Chapter 14** is now fully devoted to the topic of sexually transmitted diseases.

- Two new sections on life expectancy and physiological age and on complementary and alternative medicine were added to **Chapter 15**. A thorough 46-item questionnaire that can be used to predict life expectancy and physiological age, based on lifestyle factors discussed throughout the book, is introduced at the end of this chapter. This figure provides a good summary to many of the fitness and wellness concepts learned by the students throughout the course.

- New color photography and graphs have been added throughout the book.

ANCILLARIES

- **ExamView®—Computerized Testing.** Create, deliver, and customize tests and study guides (both print and online) in minutes with this easy-to-use assessment and tutorial system. ExamView offers both a Quick Test Wizard and an Online Test Wizard that guide you step-by-step through the process of creating tests, while its unique "WYSIWYG" capability allows you to see the test you are creating on the screen exactly as it will print or display online.

- **Multimedia Manager for Health, Fitness, and Wellness: A Microsoft PowerPoint® Link Tool.** This link tool includes a wide array of PowerPoint slides and images from Wadsworth health, fitness, and wellness texts, plus digital videos.

CNN Today: Fitness and Wellness Video.
Launch your lectures with riveting footage from CNN, the world's leading 24-hour global news television network. The CNN Today: Fitness and Wellness Video allows you to integrate the news gathering and programming power of CNN into the classroom to show students the relevance of course topics to their everyday lives. Organized by topics introduced in the text, the clips are presented in short 2–5 minute segments, and a new video is available each year.

Relaxation Video. Explores techniques to decrease vulnerability to stress, enhance sports performance, and manage time more effectively.

Wadsworth Video Library for Health, Fitness, and Wellness. A comprehensive library of videos is available to adopters of this textbook. Topics include weight control and fitness, AIDS, sexual communication, peer pressure, compulsive and addictive behaviors and the relationship between alcohol and violence. Contact your local Wadsworth/Thomson representative for a detailed list of video options.

Personal Daily Log. This log contains an exercise pyramid, ethnic foods pyramid, tips for achieving test success, a body composition record form, body mass index chart, cardiorespiratory exercise record forms, strength training record forms, and much more.

Instructor's Manual with Test Bank. The Instructor's Manual with Test Bank helps instructors plan and coordinate their lectures by offering detailed outlines of each chapter with specific transparency and PowerPoint references. Instructor's Activities are included for each chapter. These activities offer instructors ideas for incorporating the material into classroom activities and discussions. A set of Key Point Transparencies is provided. Each chapter contains a description of relevant Web sites for resources to aid instructors and offer health activities. The full test bank contains approximately 30 multiple-choice, true/false, matching, fill-in-the-blank, and essay questions per chapter.

Instructor's Resource CD-ROM. This CD-ROM includes Instructor's Manual and Test Bank resources.

Transparencies. Approximately 80 color transparency acetates of graphs, tables, and illustrations from the text can be used to enhance lectures. The transparencies will also be available on the Web and on Multimedia Manager. Also provided is a set of Key Point Transparencies—text-only transparencies that list important terms from each chapter.

Profile Plus 2003. This interactive CD-ROM includes study guides, quizzes, lecture outlines, and digital video clips. The CD allows students to generate personalized fitness and wellness programs, conduct self-assessments, analyze their diets, and keep an exercise log.

Diet Analysis Plus 6.0 CD-ROM. This interactive nutrition learning tool allows students to create personal profiles and determine the nutritional value of their diet. The program calculates nutrition intakes, goal percentages, and actual percentages of nutrients, vitamins, and minerals, customized according to the student's profile. The information is displayed in colorful, easy-to-read graphs, charts, and spreadsheets.

Wellness Worksheets. Forty detachable self-assessments and a complete wellness inventory are included.

Integrative Medicine: The Mind-Body Prescription. This interesting supplement, written by Dr. John Janowiak from Appalachian State University, explains the relationship between Western medical practice and more traditional therapies. The supplement explains the evolution of integrative medicine, provides a detailed list of Internet resources, a comprehensive list of herbs and their interactions, and more.

Trigger Video Series. Exclusive to Wadsworth/Thomson! This video is designed to promote classroom discussion on a variety of important topics related to physical fitness and stress. Each 60-minute video contains five 8–10 minute clips, followed by questions for answer or discussion and material appropriate to the chapters in this text.

InfoTrac® College Edition. This extensive online library gives professors and students access to the latest news and research articles online—updated daily and spanning four years! Conveniently accessible from students' own computers or the campus library, InfoTrac College Edition opens the door to the full text of articles from hundreds of scholarly and popular journals and publications.

InfoTrac® College Edition Student Guide for Health/Wellness. This handy booklet assists students using InfoTrac College Edition for research. It includes 15 pages of keyword search terms to help find results related to subject searches.

Health, Fitness, and Wellness Internet Explorer. This handy trifold brochure contains Web sites relevant to health, fitness, and wellness. Topics include stress, nutrition, alternative medicine, and much more.

● **The Wadsworth Health, Fitness, and Wellness Resource Center Web Site:**

http://health.wadsworth.com

When you adopt *Lifetime Physical Fitness and Wellness*, you and your students will have access to a rich array of teaching and learning resources you won't find anywhere else. This outstanding site features both student and instructor resources for this text, including self-quizzes, Web links, suggested online readings, and discussion forums for students—as well as downloadable supplementary resources, PowerPoint® presentations, and more for instructors.

● **Thomson Learning WebTutor**™. Available on WebCT or Blackboard! This content-rich, Web-based teaching and learning tool is rich with study and mastery tools, communication tools, and course content. WebTutor is filled with pre-loaded content and is ready to use as soon as you and your students log on. At the same time, you can customize the content in any way you choose, from uploading images and other resources, to adding Web links, to creating your own practice materials.

ACKNOWLEDGMENTS

The authors wish to extend special gratitude to Ambe Lee Fawson for her valuable editorial comments and assistance with the revisions of Chapters 12, 13, and 15. Thanks are also expressed to Chuck Scheer, Brent Fawson, Michelle Wiens, and Annalyn Harper for their help with new photography in this edition.

Finally, we would like to thank the reviewers for their valuable comments and contributions to the Seventh Edition:

Lewis Bowling, North Carolina Central University
Barb Coleman, Northern Michigan University
Ronnie Carda, University of Wisconsin-Madison
Paul Smith, Huntington College

CNN Today: Fitness and Wellness Video. Launch your lectures with riveting footage from CNN, the world's leading 24-hour global news television network. The CNN Today: Fitness and Wellness Video allows you to integrate the news gathering and programming power of CNN into the classroom to show students the relevance of course topics to their everyday lives. Organized by topics introduced in the text, the clips are presented in short 2–5 minute segments, and a new video is available each year.

Relaxation Video. Explores techniques to decrease vulnerability to stress, enhance sports performance, and manage time more effectively.

Wadsworth Video Library for Health, Fitness, and Wellness. A comprehensive library of videos is available to adopters of this textbook. Topics include weight control and fitness, AIDS, sexual communication, peer pressure, compulsive and addictive behaviors and the relationship between alcohol and violence. Contact your local Wadsworth/Thomson representative for a detailed list of video options.

Personal Daily Log. This log contains an exercise pyramid, ethnic foods pyramid, tips for achieving test success, a body composition record form, body mass index chart, cardiorespiratory exercise record forms, strength training record forms, and much more.

Instructor's Manual with Test Bank. The Instructor's Manual with Test Bank helps instructors plan and coordinate their lectures by offering detailed outlines of each chapter with specific transparency and PowerPoint references. Instructor's Activities are included for each chapter. These activities offer instructors ideas for incorporating the material into classroom activities and discussions. A set of Key Point Transparencies is provided. Each chapter contains a description of relevant Web sites for resources to aid instructors and offer health activities. The full test bank contains approximately 30 multiple-choice, true/false, matching, fill-in-the-blank, and essay questions per chapter.

Instructor's Resource CD-ROM. This CD-ROM includes Instructor's Manual and Test Bank resources.

Transparencies. Approximately 80 color transparency acetates of graphs, tables, and illustrations from the text can be used to enhance lectures. The transparencies will also be available on the Web and on Multimedia Manager. Also provided is a set of Key Point Transparencies—text-only transparencies that list important terms from each chapter.

Profile Plus 2003. This interactive CD-ROM includes study guides, quizzes, lecture outlines, and digital video clips. The CD allows students to generate personalized fitness and wellness programs, conduct self-assessments, analyze their diets, and keep an exercise log.

Diet Analysis Plus 6.0 CD-ROM. This interactive nutrition learning tool allows students to create personal profiles and determine the nutritional value of their diet. The program calculates nutrition intakes, goal percentages, and actual percentages of nutrients, vitamins, and minerals, customized according to the student's profile. The information is displayed in colorful, easy-to-read graphs, charts, and spreadsheets.

Wellness Worksheets. Forty detachable self-assessments and a complete wellness inventory are included.

Integrative Medicine: The Mind-Body Prescription. This interesting supplement, written by Dr. John Janowiak from Appalachian State University, explains the relationship between Western medical practice and more traditional therapies. The supplement explains the evolution of integrative medicine, provides a detailed list of Internet resources, a comprehensive list of herbs and their interactions, and more.

Trigger Video Series. Exclusive to Wadsworth/Thomson! This video is designed to promote classroom discussion on a variety of important topics related to physical fitness and stress. Each 60-minute video contains five 8–10 minute clips, followed by questions for answer or discussion and material appropriate to the chapters in this text.

InfoTrac® College Edition. This extensive online library gives professors and students access to the latest news and research articles online—updated daily and spanning four years! Conveniently accessible from students' own computers or the campus library, InfoTrac College Edition opens the door to the full text of articles from hundreds of scholarly and popular journals and publications.

InfoTrac® College Edition Student Guide for Health/Wellness. This handy booklet assists students using InfoTrac College Edition for research. It includes 15 pages of keyword search terms to help find results related to subject searches.

Health, Fitness, and Wellness Internet Explorer. This handy trifold brochure contains Web sites relevant to health, fitness, and wellness. Topics include stress, nutrition, alternative medicine, and much more.

● **The Wadsworth Health, Fitness, and Wellness Resource Center Web Site:**

http://health.wadsworth.com

When you adopt *Lifetime Physical Fitness and Wellness*, you and your students will have access to a rich array of teaching and learning resources you won't find anywhere else. This outstanding site features both student and instructor resources for this text, including self-quizzes, Web links, suggested online readings, and discussion forums for students—as well as downloadable supplementary resources, PowerPoint® presentations, and more for instructors.

● **Thomson Learning WebTutor™.** Available on WebCT or Blackboard! This content-rich, Web-based teaching and learning tool is rich with study and mastery tools, communication tools, and course content. WebTutor is filled with pre-loaded content and is ready to use as soon as you and your students log on. At the same time, you can customize the content in any way you choose, from uploading images and other resources, to adding Web links, to creating your own practice materials.

ACKNOWLEDGMENTS

The authors wish to extend special gratitude to Amber Lee Fawson for her valuable editorial comments and assistance with the revisions of Chapters 12, 13, and 15. Thanks are also expressed to Chuck Scheer, Brent Fawson, Michelle Wiens, and Annalyn Harper for their help with new photography in this edition.

Finally, we would like to thank the reviewers for their valuable comments and contributions to the Seventh Edition:

Lewis Bowling, North Carolina Central University
Barb Coleman, Northern Michigan University
Ronnie Carda, University of Wisconsin-Madison
Paul Smith, Huntington College

Introduction to Physical Fitness and Wellness

Objectives

Define wellness and list its dimensions.

Define physical fitness and list health-related and skill-related fitness components.

State the differences between physical fitness and wellness.

Distinguish between health fitness standards and physical fitness standards.

Identify the major health problems in the United States.

Understand the benefits and the significance of participating in a lifetime fitness and wellness program.

Identify lifestyle factors that improve health and longevity.

Identify risk factors that may interfere with safe participation in exercise.

Movement and physical activity are basic functions for which the human organism was created. Advances in modern technology, however, have almost completely eliminated physical activity from almost everyone's daily life. Physical activity is no longer a natural part of our existence. We live in an automated society, where most of the activities that used to require strenuous exertion can be accomplished by machines with the simple pull of a handle or push of a button.

Available scientific evidence shows that physical inactivity and sedentary lifestyle are a serious threat to our health and rapidly increase the deterioration rate of the human body. Physically active people live longer than their inactive counterparts, even if activity is started later in life. United States estimates indicate that more than 250,000 yearly deaths are attributed to lack of regular physical activity.[1] Similar trends are found in most industrialized nations throughout the world.

At the beginning of the 20th century, **life expectancy** for a child born in the United States was only 47 years. The most common health problems in the Western world were infectious diseases, such as tuberculosis, diphtheria, influenza, kidney disease, polio, and other diseases of infancy. Progress in the medical field largely eliminated these diseases. Then, as more North American people started to enjoy the "good life" (sedentary living, alcohol, fatty foods, excessive sweets, tobacco, drugs), we saw a parallel increase in the incidence of **chronic diseases**, such as hypertension, coronary heart disease, atherosclerosis, stroke, diabetes, cancer, emphysema, and cirrhosis of the liver (see Figure 1.1).

As the incidence of chronic diseases climbed, we recognized that prevention is the best medicine. Consequently, a fitness and wellness movement developed gradually at the end of the 20th century. From an initial fitness fad in the early 1970s, physical activity and wellness programs became a trend that now is very much a part of the North American way of life. People have begun to realize that good **health** is mostly self-controlled and that the leading causes of premature death and illness can be prevented by adhering to positive lifestyle habits. Whereas we all desire to live a long life, following a wellness program helps us focus on enhancing our overall quality of life—for as long as we live.

Presently, the average life expectancy in the United States is 76.8 years (73.8 for men and 79.5 for

> **Daily lifestyle habits have a lot more to do with what makes a person sick and when the person dies than all of the influence of medicine.**

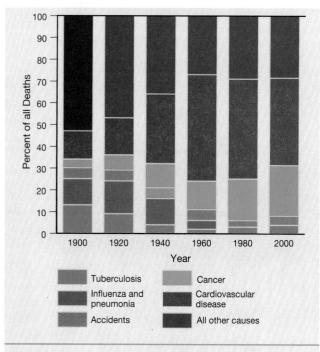

FIGURE 1.1 Causes of death in the United States for selected years.

Percent of all Deaths (y-axis)

Year (x-axis): 1900, 1920, 1940, 1960, 1980, 2000

Tuberculosis · Cancer · Influenza and pneumonia · Cardiovascular disease · Accidents · All other causes

SOURCE: National Center for Health Statistics, Division of Vital Statistics.

women). In a break with tradition, however, for the first time in the year 2000, the World Health Organization (WHO) calculated **healthy life expectancy (HLE)** estimates for 191 nations. (This figure is obtained by subtracting the years of ill health from total life expectancy.) The United States ranked 24th in this report with a HLE of 70 years; Japan was first with a HLE of 74.5 years (see Figure 1.2). The U.S. ranking was a major surprise, given its status as a developed country with one of the best medical care systems in the world. The rating indicates that Americans die earlier and spend more time disabled than people in most other advanced countries. The WHO report points to several factors that may account for this unexpected finding:

1. The extremely poor health of some groups, such as Native Americans, rural African Americans, and the inner-city poor. Their health status is more characteristic of poor developing nations rather than of a rich industrialized country.

2. The HIV epidemic, which causes more U.S. deaths and disability than in other developed nations.

FIGURE 1.2 Life expectancy (top values) and healthy life expectancy (bottom values) for selected countries.

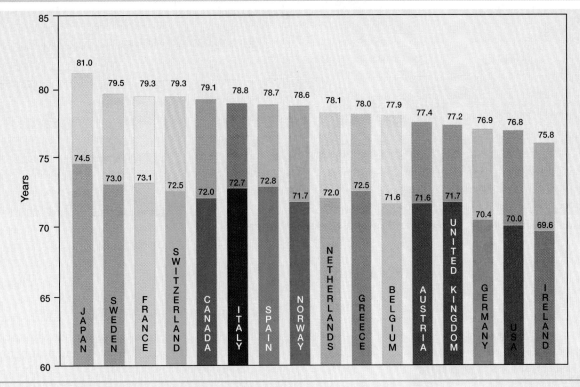

SOURCE: World Health Organization, http://www.who.int/inf-pr-2000/en/pr2000-life.html. Retrieved June 4, 2000.

3. The high incidence of tobacco use.
4. The high incidence of coronary heart disease.
5. Fairly high levels of violence, notably homicides, compared with other developed countries.

PHYSICAL ACTIVITY VERSUS EXERCISE

The abundance of scientific research on physical activity and exercise over the last three decades has established a clear distinction between physical activity and exercise. **Physical activity** is bodily movement produced by skeletal muscles. It requires energy expenditure and produces progressive health benefits.[2] Typical examples of physical activity include walking to and from work, taking the stairs instead of elevators and escalators, gardening, doing household chores, dancing,

> **Physical inactivity and a sedentary lifestyle seriously threaten our health and hasten the deterioration rate of our bodies.**

and washing the car by hand. Physical inactivity, on the other hand, implies a level of activity that is lower than that required to maintain good health.

Exercise is a type of physical activity that requires "planned, structured, and repetitive bodily movement

Photos © Fitness & Wellness, Inc.

Exercise and an active lifestyle increase health, quality of life, and longevity.

to improve or maintain one or more components of physical fitness."[3] Examples of exercise are walking, running, cycling, aerobics, swimming, and strength training.

SURGEON GENERAL'S REPORT ON PHYSICAL ACTIVITY AND HEALTH

In 1996, the U.S. Surgeon General released a landmark report on the influence of regular physical activity on health.[4] The significance of this historic document cannot be underestimated. Until 1996, the Surgeon General had released only two other such reports—one on smoking and health in 1964, and a second one on nutrition and health in 1988. The 1996 document on physical activity and health summarized more than 1,000 scientific studies from the fields of epidemiology, exercise physiology, medicine, and the behavioral sciences.

According to the 1996 report, poor health because of the lack of physical activity is a serious public health problem that we must meet head-on at once. More than 60 percent of adults do not achieve the recommended amount of physical activity (see Table 1.1), and 25 percent are not physically active at all. Further, almost half of all people between 12 and 21 years of age are not vigorously active on a regular basis. The report also stated that physical inactivity is more prevalent in

1. Women than men
2. African Americans and Hispanic Americans than whites
3. Older than younger adults
4. Less affluent than more affluent people
5. More educated than less educated adults

Furthermore, the number of people who are not physically active is more than twice the number of people who suffer from hypertension, have high cholesterol, or smoke cigarettes. This report became a nationwide call to action.

The report states that regular **moderate physical activity** can prevent premature death, unnecessary

TABLE 1.1	Percent of Total U.S. Adult Population that Regularly Participates in Physical Activity	
	Moderate Intensity*	High Intensity**
Overall	20%	14%
By Gender		
Men	21	13
Women	19	16
By Ethnicity		
White	21	15
African American	15	9
Hispanic American	20	12

SOURCE: U.S. Department of Health and Human Services, *Physical Activity and Health: A Report of the Surgeon General* (Atlanta: Centers for Disease Control and Prevention, National Center for Chronic Disease Prevention and Health Promotion, 1996).

* A minimum of 5 days per week for at least 30 minutes per session.

** A minimum of 3 days per week for a minimum of 20 minutes.

illness, and disability. It could provide substantial benefits in health and well-being for the vast majority of people who are not physically active. Among these benefits are significantly reduced risks of developing or dying from heart disease, diabetes, colon cancer, and high blood pressure. Regular physical activity also is important for the health of muscles, bones, and joints, and it seems to reduce symptoms of depression and anxiety, improve mood, and enhance the ability to perform daily tasks throughout life. Individuals who are already moderately active can achieve greater health benefits by increasing their amount of physical activity. It also can help control health care costs and help to maintain a high quality of life into old age.

> **Only 4 in 10 U.S. adults currently perform the recommended amount of weekly physical activity as established by the U.S. Surgeon General.**

The report defined moderate physical activity as using 150 calories of energy per day, or 1,000 calories per week. It recommended that people strive to achieve at least 30 minutes of physical activity per day most days of the week. Examples of moderate physical activity (generally more strenuous than the typical examples previously listed) are walking, cycling, playing basketball or volleyball, swimming, doing water aerobics, dancing fast, pushing a stroller, raking leaves, shoveling snow, washing or waxing a car, washing windows or floors, and even gardening.

A WELLNESS LIFESTYLE

Most people recognize that participating in fitness programs improves their quality of life. In recent years, however, we came to realize that improving physical fitness alone was not always sufficient to lower the risk for disease and ensure better health. For example, individuals who run 3 miles (about 5 km) a day, lift weights regularly, participate in stretching exercises, and watch their body weight might be easily classified as having good or excellent fitness. Offsetting these good habits, however, might be **risk factors**, including high blood pressure, smoking, constant stress, drinking excessive alcohol, and eating too many fatty foods. These factors place people at risk for cardiovascular disease and other chronic diseases of which they may not be aware.

One of the best examples that good fitness does not always provide a guarantee of a healthy and productive life was the tragic death in 1984 of Jim Fixx, author of the best-seller *The Complete Book of Running*.

More than one million copies of this book were sold. At the time of his death by heart attack, Fixx was 52 years old. He had been running between 60 and 80 miles a week and believed that his high level of fitness would prevent dying from heart disease.

At age 36, Jim Fixx smoked two packs of cigarettes per day, weighed about 215 pounds, did not participate in regular physical activity, and had a family history of heart disease. His father, having had a first heart attack at age 35, later died at age 43. Perhaps in an effort to lessen his risk for heart disease, Fixx began to raise his level of fitness. He started to jog, lost 50 pounds, and quit smoking. On several occasions, though, Fixx declined to have an exercise electrocardiogram (ECG) test, which likely would have revealed his cardiovascular problem. His unfortunate death illustrates that an exercise program by itself will not make high-risk people immune to heart disease, though it may delay the onset of a serious or fatal problem.

Wellness

Even though most people are aware of their unhealthy behaviors (smoking, inactivity, high-fat diets, excessive stress), they seem satisfied with life as long as they are free from symptoms of disease or illness. They do not contemplate change until they suffer a major health problem. Present lifestyle habits, however, dictate the health and well-being of tomorrow.

Good health is no longer viewed as simply the absence of illness. The definition of good health has evolved notably in the last few decades and continues to change as scientists learn more about lifestyle factors that bring on illness and affect wellness. Furthermore, once the idea took hold that fitness by itself would not always decrease the risk for disease and ensure better health, the wellness concept developed in the 1980s.

The term "**wellness**" covers several components that are conducive to health. Wellness living requires implementing positive programs to change behavior

KeyTerms

Moderate physical activity Activity that uses 150 calories of energy per day, or 1,000 calories per week.

Risk factors Characteristics that predict the development of certain diseases.

Wellness The constant and deliberate effort to stay healthy and achieve the highest potential for well-being. It encompasses seven dimensions—physical, emotional, mental, social, environmental, occupational, and spiritual—and integrates them all into a quality life.

to improve health and quality of life, prolong life, and achieve total well-being.

Wellness has seven dimensions: physical, emotional, mental, social, environmental, occupational, and spiritual (see Figure 1.3). These dimensions are interrelated: One frequently affects the others. For example, a person who is emotionally down often has no desire to exercise, study, socialize with friends, or attend church, and may be more susceptible to illness and disease.

The seven dimensions of wellness show how the concept clearly goes beyond the absence of disease. Wellness incorporates factors such as adequate fitness, proper nutrition, stress management, disease prevention, spirituality, not smoking or abusing drugs, personal safety, regular physical examinations, health education, and environmental support (see Figure 1.4).

To achieve a wellness way of life, individuals must not only be physically fit and manifest no signs of disease, but they must also be free of risk factors for disease (such as hypertension, hyperlipidemia, cigarette smoking, negative stress, faulty nutrition, careless sex). The relationship between adequate fitness and wellness is illustrated in the continuum in Figure 1.5. Even though an individual tested in a fitness center may demonstrate adequate or even excellent fitness, indulgence in

> **Wellness living requires implementing positive programs to change behavior to improve health and quality of life, prolong life, and achieve total well-being.**

FIGURE 1.3 Dimensions of wellness.

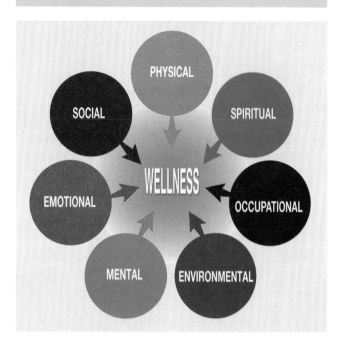

FIGURE 1.4 Selected wellness components.

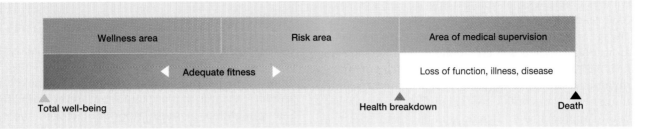

FIGURE 1.5 Wellness continuum.

unhealthy lifestyle behaviors will still increase the risk for chronic diseases and diminish the person's well-being.

THE SEVEN DIMENSIONS OF WELLNESS*

Physical

Physical wellness is the dimension most commonly associated with being healthy. Physically well individuals are physically active, exercise regularly, eat a well-balanced diet, maintain recommended body weight, get sufficient sleep, practice safe sex, minimize exposure to environmental contaminants, avoid harmful drugs (including tobacco and excessive alcohol), and seek medical care and exams as needed. Physically well people also exhibit good cardiorespiratory endurance, adequate muscular strength and flexibility, proper body composition, and the ability to carry out ordinary and unusual demands of daily life safely and effectively.

Emotional

Emotional wellness is the ability to understand your own feelings, accept your limitations, and achieve emotional stability. Furthermore, it implies the ability to express emotions appropriately, adjust to change, cope with stress in a healthy way, and enjoy life despite its occasional disappointments and frustrations.

Emotional wellness brings with it a certain stability, an ability to look both success and failure squarely in the face and to keep moving along your chosen course. When success is evident, the emotionally well person radiates the expected joy and

confidence. When failure seems imminent, the emotionally well person responds by making the best of circumstances and moving beyond the failure. Wellness enables you to move ahead with optimism and energy instead of spending time and talent worrying about failure. You learn from it, identify ways to avoid it in the future, and then go on with the business at hand.

Emotional wellness also involves happiness—an emotional anchor that gives meaning and joy to life. Happiness is a long-term state of mind that permeates the various facets of life and influences our outlook. Although there is no simple recipe for creating happiness, researchers agree that happy people are usually part of a family; they are partners, parents, or children; they love others, and they feel loved themselves. Healthy, happy people enjoy friends, work hard at something fulfilling, get plenty of exercise, and enjoy play and leisure time. They know how to laugh, and they laugh often. They give of themselves freely to others and seem to have found deep meaning in life.

An attitude of true happiness signals freedom from the tension and depression that many people endure. Emotionally well people are obviously subject to the same kinds of depression and unhappiness that occasionally plague us all, but the difference lies in their ability to bounce back. Well people take minor setbacks in stride and have the ability to enjoy life despite it all. They don't waste energy or time recounting the situation, wondering how they could have changed it, or dwelling on the past.

---

* Adapted from W.W.K. Hoeger, L.W. Turner, and B.Q. Hafen, *Wellness: Guidelines for a Healthy Lifestyle* (Belmont, CA: Wadsworth/Thomson Learning, 2002).

Key Terms

Physical wellness Good physical fitness and confidence in one's personal ability to take care of health problems.

Emotional wellness The ability to understand your own feelings, accept your limitations, and achieve emotional stability.

Mental

Mental wellness, also referred to as "intellectual wellness," implies that you can apply the things you have learned, create opportunities to learn more, and engage your mind in lively interaction with the world around you. When you are mentally well, you are not intimidated by facts and figures with which you are unfamiliar, but you embrace the chance to learn something new. Your confidence and enthusiasm enables you to approach any learning situation with eagerness that leads to success.

Mental wellness brings with it vision and promise. More than anything else, mentally well people are open-minded and accepting of others. Instead of being threatened by people different from themselves, they show respect and curiosity without feeling they have to conform. They are faithful to their own ideas and philosophies and allow others the same privilege. Their self-confidence guarantees that they can take their place among others in the world without having to give up part of themselves and without requiring others to do the same.

Social

Social wellness, with its accompanying positive self-image, endows you with the ease and confidence to be outgoing, friendly, and affectionate toward others. Social wellness involves not only a concern for oneself, but also an interest in humanity and the environment as a whole.

One of the hallmarks of social wellness is the ability to relate to others and to reach out to other people, both within one's family and outside it. Similar to emotional wellness, it involves being comfortable with your emotions and thus helps you understand and accept the emotions of others. Your own balance and sense of self allows you to extend respect and tolerance to others. Healthy people are honest and loyal. This dimension of wellness leads to the ability to maintain close relationships with other people.

Environmental

The toxicity of the environment, whether natural or synthetic, has a direct effect on personal wellness. To enjoy health, we require clean air, pure water, quality food, adequate shelter, satisfactory work conditions, personal safety, and healthy relationships. Health is negatively affected when we live in a polluted, toxic, unkind, and unsafe environment. To enjoy **environmental wellness**, it is our personal responsibility not only to educate and protect ourselves against environmental hazards, but also to protect the environment so that we, our children, and future generations can enjoy a safe and clean environment.

Occupational

Occupational wellness is not tied to high salary, prestigious position, or extravagant working conditions. Any job can bring occupational wellness if it provides rewards that are important to the individual. Salary might be the most important factor to one person, whereas another might place a much greater value on creativity. A person who is occupationally well has his or her own "ideal" job, which allows them to thrive.

People with occupational wellness face demands on the job, but they also have some say over demands that are placed on them. Any job has routine demands, but occupational wellness means that routine demands are mixed with new, unpredictable challenges that keep a job exciting. Occupationally well people are able to maximize their skills, and they have the opportunity to broaden existing skills or gain new ones. Their occupation offers opportunity for advancement and recognition for achievement. Occupational wellness encourages collaboration and interaction among co-workers, which foster a sense of teamwork and support.

Spiritual

Spiritual wellness provides a unifying power that integrates all dimensions of wellness. Basic characteristics of spiritual people include a sense of meaning and direction in life and a relationship to a higher being. Pursuing these may lead to personal freedom, prayer, faith, love, closeness to others, peace, joy, fulfillment, and altruism.

Several studies have reported positive relationships among spiritual well-being, emotional well-being, and satisfaction with life. People who attend church regularly and participate in religious organizations enjoy better health, have a lower incidence of chronic diseases, handle stress more effectively, and seem to live longer.

Although the ways that religious affiliation enhances wellness are difficult to determine, possible reasons include the promotion of healthy lifestyle behaviors, social support, assistance in times of crisis and need, and counseling to overcome one's weaknesses. Spiritual beliefs also seem to help people overcome crises and aid them in developing better coping techniques to deal with future trauma.

Prayer is a signpost of our spirituality, at the core of most spiritual experiences. As communication with

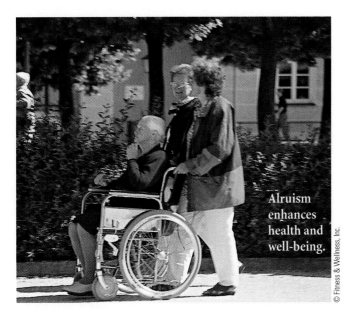

Altruism enhances health and well-being.

© Fitness & Wellness, Inc.

a higher power, prayer is offered for a multiplicity of reasons, from thanksgiving to requests for guidance, wisdom, strength, protection, and health.

Research has shown that for prayers to be effective, a person needs to accept the efficacy of prayer and pray with sincerity, humility, and love. Approximately 200 studies have been conducted on the effects of prayer on health. About two-thirds of these studies have linked prayer to positive health outcomes as long as the prayers are offered with love, empathy, and compassion. Some studies have shown faster healing time and fewer complications in patients that didn't even know that they were being prayed for as compared with patients that were not prayed for.[5]

Altruism, a key attribute of spiritual people, seems to enhance health and longevity. Studies indicate that people who perform regular volunteer work live longer. Doing good for others is good for oneself, especially for the immune system. Research has found that health benefits of altruism to be so powerful that simply watching films of altruistic endeavors enhances the formation of an immune system chemical that helps fight disease.

Wellness requires a balance among all of its seven dimensions. The relationship between spirituality and wellness, therefore, is meaningful in our quest for a better quality of life. As with other parameters listed above, optimum wellness requires development of the spiritual dimension to its fullest potential.

WELLNESS, FITNESS, AND LONGEVITY

During the 1960s and 1970s, scientists began to realize the importance of good fitness and improved

lifestyle in the fight against chronic diseases, particularly those of the cardiovascular system. Because of more participation in wellness programs, cardiovascular mortality rates dropped: The decline began in about 1963 and, between 1960 and 2000, the incidence of cardiovascular disease dropped by 26 percent. This decrease is credited to higher levels of wellness and better health care in the United States. More than half of the decline is specifically attributed to improved diet and reduction in smoking.

Furthermore, several studies have shown an inverse relationship between physical activity and premature cardiovascular mortality rates. The first of these studies was conducted among 16,936 Harvard alumni. The researchers linked physical activity habits and mortality rates and found that as the amount of weekly physical activity increased, the risk of cardiovascular death decreased. The largest decrease in cardiovascular deaths was observed among individuals who used more than 2,000 calories per week through physical activity.[6] Figure 1.6 graphically illustrates the study results.

A second major study conducted at the Aerobics Research Institute in Dallas upheld the findings of the Harvard alumni study.[7] Based on data from 13,344 people followed over an average of 8 years, the results confirmed that the level of physical activity is related to mortality from all causes. The study revealed a graded and consistent inverse relationship between physical activity levels and mortality, regardless of age and other risk factors. As illustrated in Figure 1.7, the higher the level of physical activity, the longer the lifespan. The death rate during the 8-year study from

KeyTerms

Mental wellness A state in which your mind is engaged in lively interaction with the world around you.

Social wellness The ability to relate well to others, both within and outside the family unit.

Environmental wellness The capability to live in a clean and safe environment that is not detrimental to health.

Occupational wellness The ability to perform one's job skillfully and effectively under conditions that provide personal and team satisfaction and adequately reward each individual.

Spiritual wellness The sense that life is meaningful, that life has purpose, and that some power brings all humanity together; the ethics, values, and morals that guide us and give meaning and direction to life.

Prayer Sincere and humble communication with a higher power.

Altruism True concern for the welfare of others.

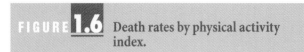

FIGURE 1.6 Death rates by physical activity index.

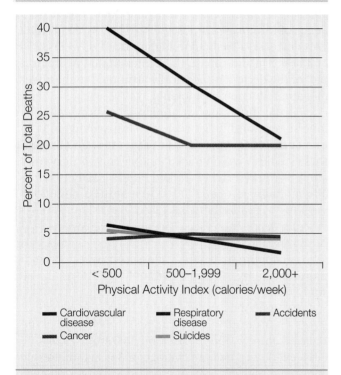

Note: The graph represents cause-specific death rates per 10,000 man-years of observation among 16,936 Harvard alumni, 1962–1978, by physical activity index; adjusted for differences in age, cigarette smoking, and hypertension.

SOURCE: Data from R. S. Paffenbarger, R. T. Hyde, A. L. Wing, and C. H. Steinmetz, "A Natural History of Athleticism on Cardiovascular Health," *Journal of the American Medical Association*, 252 (1989): 491–495. Used by permission.

all causes for the least-fit (group 1) men was 3.4 times higher than that of the most-fit men. For the least-fit women, the death rate was 4.6 times higher than that of the most-fit women.

This study also reported a greatly reduced rate of premature death, even at moderate fitness levels that most adults can achieve easily. Greater protection is attained by combining higher fitness levels with reduction in other risk factors such as hypertension, serum cholesterol, cigarette smoking, and excessive body fat.

A follow-up 5-year research study on fitness and mortality found a substantial (44 percent) reduction in mortality risk when people abandoned a **sedentary** lifestyle and become moderately fit.[8] The lowest death rate was found in people who were fit at the start of the study and remained fit; the highest death rate was found in men who were unfit at the beginning of the study and remained unfit (see Figure 1.8).

Subsequent research published in 1995 substantiated previous findings and indicated that primarily **vigorous activity** is associated with greater longevity.[9] Vigorous activity was defined as any activity that requires a MET level equal to or greater than 6 METs (21 ml/kg/min—see "Health Fitness Standards" on page 13) or, briefly, an activity that provides a substantial challenge to the cardiorespiratory system. One MET is the energy expenditure at rest, or approximately 3.5 ml/kg/min. Six or more METs represents exercising at an oxygen uptake (VO_2) equal to or greater than 6 times the resting energy requirement. Examples of vigorous activities in this study include brisk walking, jogging, swimming laps, shoveling snow, and playing squash, racquetball, or tennis. Also, vigorous exercise was found to be as important as maintaining recommended weight and not smoking. (See also the discussion of MET and oxygen uptake in Chapter 4.)

In another major research study, a healthy lifestyle was shown to contribute to some of the lowest mortality rates ever reported in the literature.[10] The investigators in this study looked at three general health habits among the participants: regular physical activity, sufficient sleep, and lifetime abstinence from smoking. Additionally, study participants abstained from alcohol, caffeine, drugs, and all forms of tobacco.

Compared with the general white population, this group of over 10,000 people had much lower cancer, cardiovascular, and overall death rates. Men in the study had one-third the death rate from cancer, one-seventh the death rate from cardiovascular disease, and one-fifth the rate of overall mortality. Women had about half the rate of cancer and overall mortality and one-third the death rate from cardiovascular disease. Life expectancies for 25-year-olds who adhered to the three health habits were 85 and 86 years, respectively, compared with 74 and 80 for the average U. S. white man and woman. The additional 6 to 11 "golden years" are precious—and more enjoyable—for those who maintain a lifetime wellness program.

If you don't make time to be physically active, sooner or later you will need to make time to treat illness.

The results of these studies clearly indicate that fitness improves wellness, quality of life, and longevity. Vigorous exercise is preferable to the extent of one's capabilities because it is most clearly associated with longer life, although moderate-intensity activities provide substantial health benefits to the vast majority of people who are not physically active.

FIGURE **1.7** Death rates by physical fitness groups.*

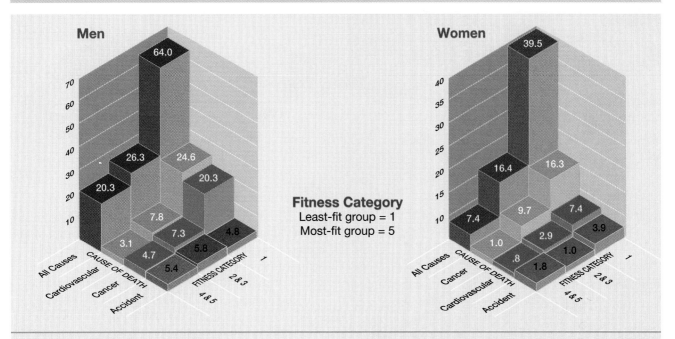

*Death rate per 10,000 man-years observation.

SOURCE: Based on data from S. N. Blair, H. W. Kohl III, R. S. Paffenbarger, Jr., D. G. Clark, K. H. Cooper, and L. W. Gibbons, "Physical Fitness and All-Cause Mortality: A Prospective Study of Healthy Men and Women," *Journal of the American Medical Association* 262 (1989): 2395–2401.

FIGURE **1.8** Five-year follow-up in mortality rates associated with maintenance and improvements in fitness.

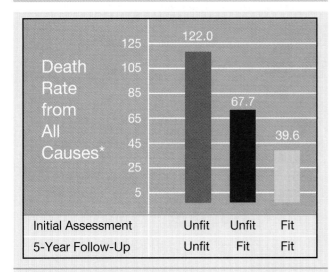

	Unfit	Unfit	Fit
Initial Assessment	Unfit	Unfit	Fit
5-Year Follow-Up	Unfit	Fit	Fit

*Death rate per 10,000 man-years observation.

SOURCE: Based on data from S. N. Blair, H. W. Kohl III, C. E. Barlow, R. S. Paffenbarger, Jr., L. W. Gibbons, and C. A. Macera, "Changes in Physical Fitness and All-Cause Mortality: A Prospective Study of Healthy and Unhealthy Men," *Journal of the American Medical Association* 273 (1995): 1193–1198.

TYPES OF PHYSICAL FITNESS

As the fitness concept grew during the 1970s, it became clear that a battery of tests was necessary to assess physical fitness, because several specific components contribute to an individual's overall level of fitness.

Physical fitness can be classified into health-related and motor skill–related fitness. The four **health-related fitness** components are cardio-respiratory (aerobic) endurance, muscular strength

Key Terms

Sedentary A lifestyle characterized by inactivity and a lot of sitting.

Vigorous activity Any activity that requires a MET level equal to or greater than 6 METs (21 ml/kg/min); 1 MET = energy expenditure at rest, 3.5 ml/kg/min.

Physical fitness The ability to meet the ordinary as well as the unusual demands of daily life safely and effectively without being overly fatigued and still have energy left for leisure and recreational activities.

Health-related fitness Fitness programs that are pre-scribed to improve the overall health of the individual.

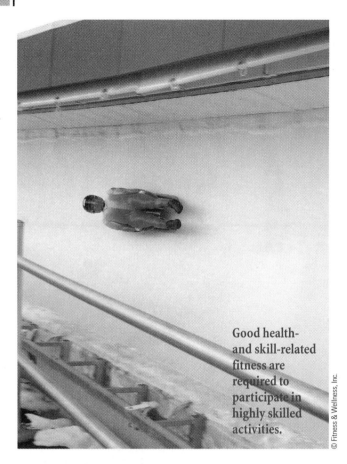

Good health- and skill-related fitness are required to participate in highly skilled activities.

© Fitness & Wellness, Inc.

FIGURE **1.10** Motor skill–related components of physical fitness.

and endurance, muscular flexibility, and body composition (Figure 1.9). **Skill-related fitness** components consist of agility, balance, coordination, power, reaction time, and speed (Figure 1.10). The latter are aimed primarily at succeeding in sports and athletics and may not be as crucial to better health. In terms of preventive medicine, the main emphasis of fitness programs should be on the health-related components. Nevertheless, total fitness is achieved by taking part in specific programs to improve both health-related and skill-related components.

FIGURE **1.9** Health-related components of physical fitness.

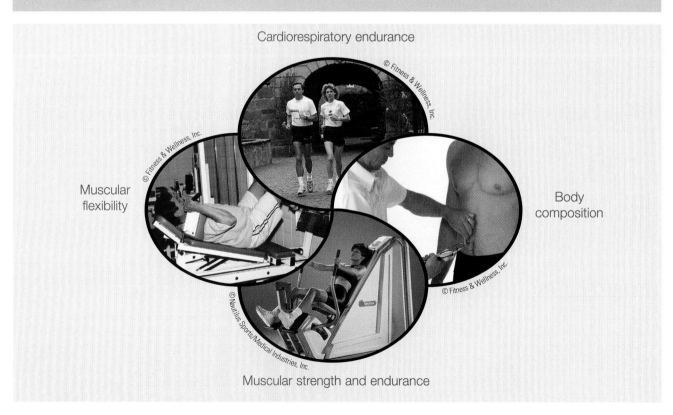

Cardiorespiratory endurance

Muscular flexibility

Body composition

Muscular strength and endurance

FIGURE **1.11** Health and fitness benefits based on the type of lifestyle and physical activity program.

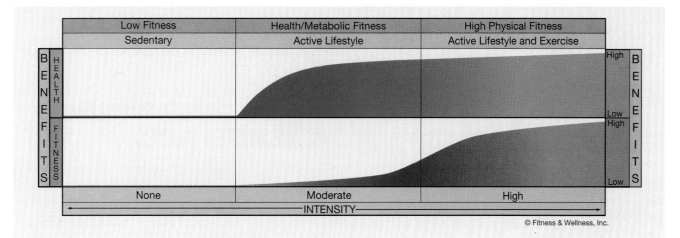

© Fitness & Wellness, Inc.

FITNESS STANDARDS: HEALTH VERSUS PHYSICAL FITNESS

A meaningful debate regarding age- and gender-related fitness standards for the general population has resulted in the two standards: a health fitness standard (also referred to as "criterion-referenced") and a physical fitness standard. The discussions of health-related fitness assessment in Chapters 3, 4, 5, 6, and 7 describe several tests to assess fitness.

Health Fitness Standards

The **health fitness standards** proposed here are based on data linking minimum fitness values to disease prevention and health. Attaining the health fitness standard requires only moderate physical activity. For example, a 2-mile walk in less than 30 minutes, 5 to 6 times per week, seems to be sufficient to achieve the health-fitness standard for cardiorespiratory endurance.

As illustrated in the center column of Figure 1.11, significant health benefits can be reaped with such a program, although fitness (expressed in terms of oxygen uptake, VO_{2max}—see discussion on cardio-respiratory endurance) improvements are not as notable. The health improvements are quite striking, and only slightly greater benefits are obtained with a more intense exercise program. These benefits include reduction in blood lipids, lower blood pressure, weight loss, stress release, decreased risk for

diabetes, and lower risk for disease and premature mortality.

More specifically, improvements in the **metabolic profile** (better insulin sensitivity and glucose tolerance and improved cholesterol levels) can be notable despite little or no improvement in aerobic capacity or weight loss. **Metabolic fitness** can be attained through an active lifestyle and moderate physical activity.

Another assessment of health-related fitness uses **cardiorespiratory endurance**, measured in terms of the maximal amount of oxygen the body is able to utilize per minute of physical activity (maximal oxygen uptake, or VO_{2max})—essentially, a measure of how efficiently your heart, lungs, and muscles can operate

Skill-related fitness Fitness programs that are used to improve athletic ability.

Health fitness standards The lowest fitness requirements for maintaining good health, decreasing the risk for chronic diseases, and lowering the incidence of muscular-skeletal injuries.

Metabolic profile A measurement to assess risk for diabetes and cardiovascular disease through plasma insulin, glucose, lipid, and lipoprotein levels.

Metabolic fitness Denotes improvements in the metabolic profile through a moderate-intensity exercise program in spite of little or no improvement in physical fitness standards.

Cardiorespiratory endurance The ability of the lungs, heart, and blood vessels to deliver adequate amounts of oxygen to the cells to meet the demands of prolonged physical activity.

during maximal exertion (see Chapter 3). VO_{2max} is commonly expressed in milliliters (ml) of oxygen (volume of oxygen) per kilogram (kg) of body weight per minute (ml/kg/min). Individual values can range from about 10 ml/kg/min in cardiac patients to over 80 ml/kg/min in world-class runners, cyclists, and cross-country skiers.

Research data from the study presented in Figure 1.7 reported that achieving VO_{2max} values of 35 and 32.5 ml/kg/min for men and women, respectively, may be sufficient to lower the risk for all-cause mortality significantly. Although greater improvements in fitness yield a slightly lower risk for premature death, the largest drop is seen between the least fit (group 1) and the moderately fit (groups 2 and 3). Therefore, the 35 and 32.5 ml/kg/min values could be selected as the health fitness standards.

Physical Fitness Standards

Physical fitness standards are set higher than the health fitness standards and require a more vigorous exercise program. Physically fit people of all ages have the freedom to enjoy most of life's daily and recreational activities to their fullest potential. Current health fitness standards may not be enough to achieve these objectives.

Sound physical fitness gives the individual a degree of independence throughout life that many people in the United States no longer enjoy. Most older people should be able to carry out activities similar to those they conducted in their youth, though not with the same intensity. These standards do not require being a championship athlete, but activities such as changing a tire, chopping wood, climbing several flights of stairs, playing basketball, mountain biking, playing soccer with grandchildren, walking several miles around a lake, and hiking through a national park do require more than the current U.S. "average fitness" level.

> **Current health fitness standards in the United States may not be enough to allow people of all ages the freedom to enjoy most of life's daily and recreational activities to their fullest potential.**

Which Program Is Best?

If the main objective of one's fitness program is to lower the risk of disease, attaining the health fitness standards may be enough to ensure better health. If, however, the individual wants to participate in moderate-to-vigorous fitness activities, achieving a high physical fitness standard is recommended. This book gives both health fitness and physical fitness standards for each fitness test. Your own personal objectives will determine the fitness program you use.

LEADING HEALTH PROBLEMS IN THE UNITED STATES

The leading causes of death in the United States today are largely lifestyle-related. Nearly 62 percent of all deaths in the United States are caused by cardiovascular disease and cancer (see Figure 1.12).[11] Nearly 80 percent of these deaths could be prevented through a healthy lifestyle program. The third and fourth leading causes of death are chronic and obstructive pulmonary disease (COPD) and accidents.

The most prevalent degenerative diseases in the United States are those of the cardiovascular system. About 40 percent of all deaths in this country are attributed to diseases of the heart and blood vessels. According to the American Heart Association, 58.8 million people in the United States were afflicted with diseases of the cardiovascular system in 1999, including 50 million with hypertension (high blood pressure) and 12 million with coronary heart disease (many of these people have more than one type of cardiovascular disease). About 1.1 million people have heart attacks each year, and more than 350,000 of them die as a result. The estimated cost of heart and blood vessel disease in 2000 exceeded $326 billion.[12] A complete cardiovascular disease prevention program is outlined in Chapter 10.

The second leading cause of death in the United States is cancer. Unlike cardiovascular disease, the mortality rate for cancer has increased steadily over the last few decades (see Figure 1.1). In 1996, the cancer rate declined slightly for the first time. Even though cancer is not the number-one killer, it is the number-one health fear of the American people.

Twenty-three percent of all deaths in the United States are attributable to cancer. More than 550,000 people died from this disease in 2000, and an estimated 1,220,100 new cases were reported the same year.[13] The major contributor to the increase in the incidence of cancer during the last five decades is lung cancer. Without lung cancer, cancer mortality rates would have decreased by 14 percent between 1950 and 1990.

The American Cancer Society maintains that the most influential factor in fighting cancer today is

Snell from Sandy, Utah. At age 45, Snell weighed approximately 400 pounds, his blood pressure was 220/180, he was blind because of undiagnosed diabetes, and his blood glucose level was 487.

Snell had determined to do something about his physical and medical condition, so he started a walking/jogging program. After about 8 months of conditioning, Snell had lost almost 200 pounds, his eyesight had returned, his glucose level was down to 67, and he was taken off medication. Just 2 months later, less than 10 months after beginning his personal exercise program, he completed his first marathon, a running course of 26.2 miles!

Health Benefits

Most people exercise because it improves their personal appearance and makes them feel good about themselves. Although many benefits accrue from participating in a regular fitness and wellness program and active people generally live longer, the greatest benefit of all is that physically fit individuals enjoy a better quality of life. These people live life to its fullest, with fewer health problems than inactive individuals (who may also indulge in other negative lifestyle behaviors). Although compiling an all-inclusive list of the benefits reaped from participating in a fitness and wellness program is difficult, the following list summarizes many of them:

- Improves and strengthens the cardiorespiratory system.
- Maintains better muscle tone, muscular strength, and endurance.
- Improves muscular flexibility.
- Enhances athletic performance.
- Helps maintain recommended body weight.
- Helps preserve lean body tissue.
- Increases resting metabolic rate.
- Improves the body's ability to use fat during physical activity.
- Improves posture and physical appearance.
- Improves functioning of the immune system.
- Lowers the risk for chronic diseases and illness (such as cardiovascular diseases and cancer).
- Decreases the mortality rate from chronic diseases.
- Thins the blood so it doesn't clot as readily (thereby decreasing the risk for coronary heart disease and strokes).
- Helps the body manage cholesterol levels more effectively.

- Prevents or delays the development of high blood pressure and lowers blood pressure in people with hypertension.
- Helps prevent and control diabetes.
- Helps achieve peak bone mass in young adults and maintain bone mass later in life, thereby decreasing the risk for osteoporosis.
- Helps people sleep better.
- Helps prevent chronic back pain.
- Relieves tension and helps cope with life stresses.
- Raises levels of energy and job productivity.
- Extends longevity and slows the aging process.
- Promotes psychological well-being and better morale, self-image, and self-esteem.
- Reduces depression and anxiety.
- Motivates a person to make positive lifestyle changes (improving nutrition, quitting smoking, controlling alcohol and drug use).
- Speeds recovery time following physical exertion.
- Speeds recovery following injury or disease.
- Regulates and improves overall body functions.
- Improves physical stamina and counteracts chronic fatigue.
- Helps maintain independent living, especially in older adults.
- Enhances quality of life: People feel better and live a healthier and happier life.

Economic Benefits

Sedentary living can have a strong impression on a nation's economy. As the need for physical exertion in Western countries decreased steadily during the last century, health care expenditures increased dramatically. In the United States, health care costs have risen from $12 billion in 1950 to $1.3 trillion in 2000 (Figure 1.15). At the present rate of escalation, health care expenditures will more than double to $2.64 trillion by the year 2010. The 2000 figure represents 13.1 percent of the gross national product (GNP), and it is projected to reach 15.9 percent by the year 2010.

In terms of yearly health care costs per person, as illustrated in Figure 1.16, the United States spends more per person ($3,724) than any other industrialized nation—yet, overall, the health care system ranks only 37th in the world. One of the reasons for the low overall ranking is the overemphasis on state-of-the art cures instead of prevention programs. The United States is the best place in the world to treat someone once they are sick, but the system does a poor job of

FIGURE **1.15** U.S. health care cost increments since 1950.

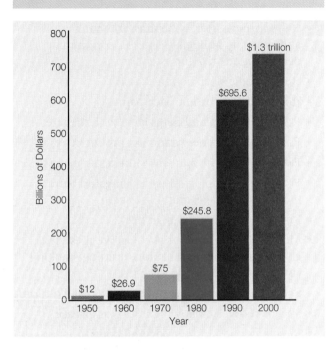

> **The cost of preventing illness is much lower than the cost of treating illness.**

keeping people healthy in the first place. The United States also fails to provide good health care for all: Some 44 million residents do not have health insurance.

Unhealthy behaviors are contributing to the staggering U.S. health care costs. Risk factors for disease carry a heavy price tag (see Figure 1.17). According to estimates, 1 percent of the people account for 30 percent of these costs.[15] Half of the people use up about 97 percent of health care dollars. Furthermore, the average health care cost per person in the United States is almost twice as high as for most other industrialized nations.[16]

Strong scientific evidence now links participation in fitness and wellness programs not only to better health but also to lower medical costs and higher job productivity. Most of this research is being conducted and reported by organizations that already have implemented fitness or wellness programs.

FIGURE **1.16** Estimated 1997 (top values) and 1989 (bottom values) health care costs per person for selected countries.

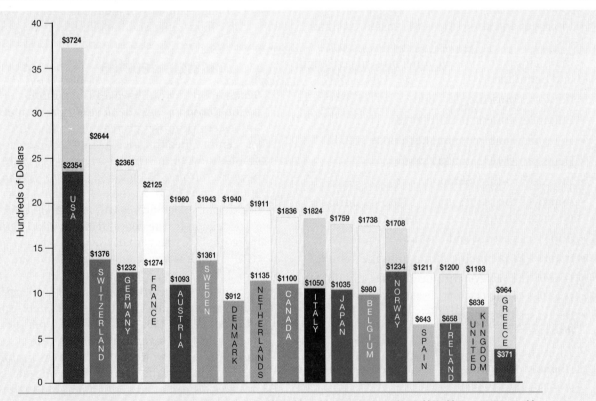

SOURCES: "Daten Der Woche," *Welt am Sonntag* 25 (1991), 35 and World Health Organization, *The World Health Report 2000—Health Systems: Improving Performance* (2000): Annex Table 8.

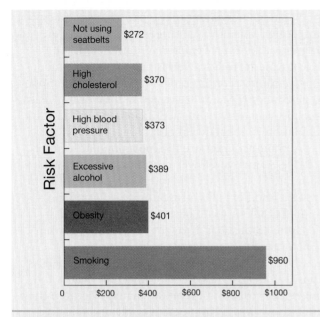

FIGURE 1.17 Average annual health care costs for leading risk factors.

SOURCE: *Journal of Occupational Medicine* (November 1991).

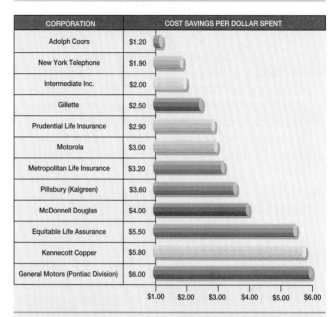

FIGURE 1.18 Health care cost savings by selected corporations per dollar spent on health promotion programs.

CORPORATION	COST SAVINGS PER DOLLAR SPENT
Adolph Coors	$1.20
New York Telephone	$1.90
Intermediate Inc.	$2.00
Gillette	$2.50
Prudential Life Insurance	$2.90
Motorola	$3.00
Metropolitan Life Insurance	$3.20
Pillsbury (Kalgreen)	$3.60
McDonnell Douglas	$4.00
Equitable Life Assurance	$5.50
Kennecott Copper	$5.80
General Motors (Pontiac Division)	$6.00

SOURCE: 1991 survey by the American Institute for Preventive Medicine, Southfield, Michigan.

As a result of the recent staggering rise in medical costs, many organizations now realize that keeping employees healthy costs less than treating them once they are sick. A survey by the American Institute for Preventive Medicine found that large corporations are reaping health-cost savings by implementing health promotion programs.[17] A sample return on investment per dollar spent is provided in Figure 1.18. Containing the costs of health care through fitness and wellness programs has become a major issue for many organizations around the United States.

Another reason some organizations are offering wellness programs to their employees—overlooked by many because it does not seem to affect the bottom line directly—is simply concern by top management for employees' physical well-being. The main issue for top management is not that wellness programs lower medical costs, but that they help individuals feel better about themselves and improve their quality of life.

In addition to the financial and physical benefits, some corporations are offering health promotion programs as an incentive to attract, hire, and retain employees. Many executives believe that an on-site health promotion program is the best fringe benefit they can offer at their company. Young executives are looking for organizations such as these, not only because of the added health benefits but also because of the corporate officers' attitude of concern and care.

THE WELLNESS CHALLENGE OF THE 21ST CENTURY

Because a better and healthier life is something every person should strive for, our biggest challenge, as we begin the new century, is to teach people how to take control of their personal health habits and adhere to a positive lifestyle. Considering the wealth of information available on the benefits of fitness and wellness programs, improving the quality and possible length of our lives is a matter of personal choice.

Research indicates that accomplishing the following changes will significantly improve health and extend life:

1. Participate in a lifetime physical activity program. Exercise regularly at least 3 times per week and try to accumulate a minimum of 30 minutes of physical activity each day of your life. The exercise program should consist of 20 to 30 minutes of aerobic exercise, along with some strengthening and stretching exercises.

2. Do not smoke cigarettes. Cigarette smoking is the largest preventable cause of illness and premature death in the United States. If we include all related

deaths, smoking is responsible for more than 400,000 unnecessary deaths each year.

3. Eat right. Eat a good breakfast and two additional well-balanced meals every day. Avoid eating too many calories and foods with a lot of sugar, fat, and salt. Increase your daily consumption of fruits, vegetables, and whole-grain products.

4. Avoid snacking. Researchers have found that, every time a person eats, insulin is released to remove sugar from the blood. There seems to be a relationship between these frequent spikes in insulin and the development heart disease. Fewer daily increases of insulin—that is, eating fewer times per day—may be more conducive to good health.

5. Maintain recommended body weight through adequate nutrition and exercise. This is important in preventing chronic diseases and in developing a higher level of fitness.

6. Get enough rest. Sleep 7 to 8 hours each night.

7. Lower your stress levels. Reduce your vulnerability to stress and practice stress management techniques as needed.

8. Be wary of alcohol. Drink alcohol moderately or not at all. Alcohol abuse leads to mental, emotional, physical, and social problems.

9. Surround yourself with healthy friendships. Unhealthy friendships contribute to destructive behaviors and low self-esteem. Associating with people who strive to maintain good fitness and health reinforces a positive outlook in life and encourages positive behaviors. Constructive social interactions enhance well-being. Researchers have also found that mortality rates are much higher among people who are not socially connected. People who aren't socially integrated are more likely to give up. Giving up accelerates dying.

10. Be informed about the environment. Seek clean air, clean water, and a clean environment. Be aware of pollutants and occupational hazards: asbestos fibers, nickel dust, chromate, uranium dust, and so on. Take precautions when using pesticides and insecticides.

11. Increase education. Data indicates that people who are more educated live longer. The theory is that as education increases, so do the number of connections between nerve cells. The increased number of connections in turn help the individual make better survival (healthy lifestyle) choices.

12. Take personal safety measures. Although not all accidents are preventable, many are. Taking simple precautionary measures, such as using seat belts and keeping electrical appliances away from water, lessens the risk of avoidable accidents.

Thanks to current scientific data and the fitness and wellness movement of the past three decades, most Americans now see a need to participate in programs that improve and maintain health. The typical American, however, is not a good role model when cardiorespiratory fitness is concerned. Almost 60 percent of U.S. adults engage in little or no leisure-time physical activity. In fact, 25 percent of the adult population is not active at all.

Aerobic activities are the most popular form of exercise, so an even lower percentage of the population probably engages in and derives benefits from strength and flexibility programs. In addition, an estimated half or more of the adult population in the United States has a weight problem, and a third of all adults are considered obese.

Even though people in the United States believe a positive lifestyle has a great impact on health and longevity, most do not reap the benefits because they don't know how to implement a safe and effective fitness and wellness program. Others are exercising incorrectly and, therefore, are not reaping the full benefits of their program.

NATIONAL HEALTH OBJECTIVES FOR THE YEAR 2010

Every 10 years, the U.S. Department of Health and Human Services releases a list of objectives for preventing disease and promoting health. Since its initiation in 1980, this 10-year plan has helped instill a new sense of purpose and focus for public health and preventive medicine. These national health objectives are intended to be realistic goals to improve the health of all Americans. Two unique goals of the new 2010 objectives emphasize increased quality and length of healthy life and seek to eliminate health disparities among all groups of people (see Figure 1.19). The objectives address three important points:[18]

1. Personal responsibility for health behavior. Individuals need to become ever more health-conscious. Responsible and informed behaviors are the key to good health.

2. Health benefits for all people and all communities. Lower socioeconomic conditions and poor health often are interrelated. Extending the benefits of good health to all people is crucial to the health of the nation.

FIGURE 1.19 National Health Objectives 2010: Healthy People in Healthy Communities.

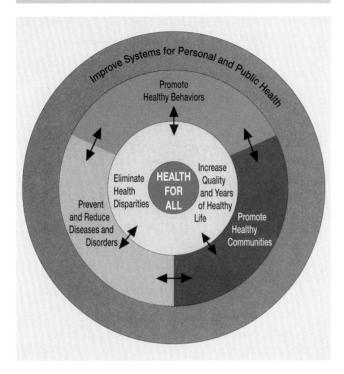

3. Health promotion and disease prevention. A shift from treatment to preventive techniques will drastically cut health care costs and help all Americans achieve a better quality of life.

Development of these health objectives usually involves more than 10,000 people representing 300 national organizations, including the Institute of Medicine of the National Academy of Sciences, all state health departments, and the federal Office of Disease Prevention and Health Promotion. A summary of key 2010 objectives is provided in Figure 1.20. Living the fitness and wellness principles provided in this book not only will enhance the quality of your life but also will allow you to be an active participant in achieving the Healthy People 2010 Objectives.

> **The nation's top health goals as we begin the new millennium are exercise, increased consumption of fruits and vegetables, smoking cessation, and the practice of safe sex.**
> —David Satcher, U. S. Surgeon General

Wellness Education

Most people go to college to learn how to make a living, but a fitness and wellness course will teach you how to live—how to truly live life to its fullest potential. Some people seem to think that success is measured by how much money they make. Making a good living will not help you unless you live a wellness lifestyle that will allow you to enjoy what you have.

Although everyone would like to enjoy good health and wellness, most people don't know how to reach this objective. Lifestyle is the most important factor affecting personal well-being. Granted, some people live long because of genetic factors, but quality of life during middle age and the "golden years" is more often related to wise choices initiated during youth and continued throughout life.

> **Your wellness lifestyle today will determine the health and quality of your life tomorrow.**

In a few short years, lack of wellness leads to a loss of vitality and gusto for life, as well as premature morbidity and mortality. The Wellness Lifestyle Questionnaire given in Figure 1.21 will provide an initial rating of your current efforts to stay healthy and well. The components of a wellness lifestyle are discussed in subsequent chapters of this book.

Because fitness and wellness needs vary significantly from one individual to another, all exercise and wellness prescriptions must be personalized to obtain best results. The information and worksheets in the following chapters set forth the necessary guidelines that will allow you to develop a personal lifetime program to improve fitness and promote preventive health care and personal wellness.

The worksheets have been prepared on tear-out pages so they can be turned in to instructors. As you study this book and complete the worksheets, you will learn to do the following:

- Implement motivational and behavior modification techniques to help you adhere to a lifetime fitness and wellness program.

- Determine whether medical clearance is needed for your safe participation in exercise.

- Conduct nutritional analyses and follow the recommendations for adequate nutrition.

- Write sound diet and weight-control programs.

- Assess the health-related components of fitness (cardiorespiratory endurance, muscular strength and endurance, muscular flexibility, and body composition).

FIGURE 1.20 Selected Health Objectives for the Year 2010.

1. Increase quality and years of healthy life.

2. Eliminate health disparities.

3. Improve the health, fitness, and quality of life of all Americans through the adoption and maintenance of regular, daily physical activity.

4. Promote health and reduce chronic disease risk, disease progression, debilitation, and premature death associated with dietary factors and nutritional status among all people in the United States.

5. Reduce disease, disability, and death related to tobacco use and exposure to secondhand smoke.

6. Increase the quality, availability, and effectiveness of educational and community-based programs designed to prevent disease and improve the health and quality of life of the American people.

7. Promote health for all people through a healthy environment.

8. Reduce the incidence and severity of injuries from unintentional causes, as well as violence and abuse.

9. Promote worker health and safety through prevention.

10. Improve access to comprehensive, high quality health care.

11. Ensure that every pregnancy in the United States is intended.

12. Improve maternal and pregnancy outcomes and reduce rates of disability in infants.

13. Improve the quality of health-related decisions through effective communication.

14. Decrease the incidence of functional limitations due to arthritis, osteoporosis, and chronic back conditions.

15. Decrease cancer incidence, morbidity, and mortality.

16. Promote health and prevent secondary conditions among persons with disabilities.

17. Enhance the cardiovascular health and quality of life of all Americans through prevention and control of risk factors, and promotion of healthy lifestyle behaviors.

18. Prevent HIV transmission and associated morbidity and mortality.

19. Improve the mental health of all Americans.

20. Raise the public's awareness of the signs and symptoms of lung disease.

21. Increase awareness of healthy sexual relationships and prevent all forms of sexually transmitted diseases.

22. Reduce the incidence of substance abuse by all people, especially children.

U.S. Department of Health and Human Services, *Healthy People 2010* (Washington DC: U.S. Government Printing Office, November 2000).

- Write exercise prescriptions for cardiorespiratory endurance, muscular strength and endurance, and muscular flexibility.

- Determine your levels of tension and stress, lessen your vulnerability to stress, and implement a stress management program if necessary.

- Determine your potential risk for cardiovascular disease and implement a risk reduction program.

- Follow a cancer risk reduction program.

- Implement a smoking cessation program, if applicable.

- Avoid chemical dependency and know where to find assistance if needed.

- Learn the health consequences of sexually transmitted diseases, including HIV/AIDS, and guidelines for preventing STDs.

- Discover the relationship between fitness and aging.

- Write objectives to improve your fitness and wellness and learn how to chart a wellness program for the future.

- Differentiate myths and facts of exercise and health-related concepts.

Exercise Safety

Even though testing and participation in exercise are relatively safe for most apparently healthy individuals under age 45, the reaction of the cardiovascular system to higher levels of physical activity cannot be totally predicted.[19] Consequently, a small but real risk exists for exercise-induced abnormalities in people with a history of cardiovascular problems and those who are at higher risk for disease. These include abnormal blood pressure, irregular heart rhythm, fainting, and, in rare instances, a heart attack or cardiac arrest.

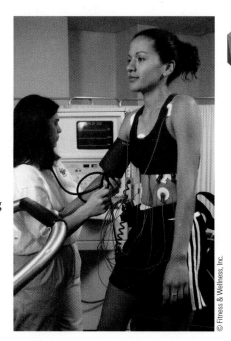

An exercise tolerance test (stress test) with 12-lead electrocardiographic monitoring may be required of some individuals prior to initiating an exercise program.

© Fitness & Wellness, Inc.

WEB INTERACTIVE

Healthy People 2010

Healthy People is a health promotion and disease prevention initiative that lists national goals for improving the health of all Americans by the year 2010.

http://www.health.gov/healthypeople

National Wellness Institute

The premier site for college and university wellness programs and assessment tools.

http://www.nationalwellness.org

CDC's National Physical Activity Initiative

The Centers for Disease Control and Prevention provide scientific and technical leadership and assistance to promote physical activity through the National Physical Activity Initiative. This reflects the CDC's continuing commitment to reducing the major risk factors for chronic disease in the United States.

http://www.cdc.gov/nccdphp/sgr/npai.htm

INTERACTIVE SITES

Lifescan Health Risk Appraisal

This site (created by Bill Hettler, M.D., of the National Wellness Institute) helps you identify specific lifestyle factors that can impair your health and longevity.

http://www.wellness.uwsp.edu/Health_Service/
Services/lifescan/lifescan.shtml

Your Personalized Health Portrait

Take this confidential health questionnaire to determine your personal lifestyle score and receive a list of health habits to change, in order of importance. You will also receive a list of screening tests and immunizations to ask your doctor about.

http://www.thriveonline.com/cgi-bin/hmi/
healthportrait.cgi

Live Well Personal Wellness Assessment

This comprehensive site features 100 multiple-choice self-assessment questions encompassing ten dimensions of wellness.

http://www.wellness.uwsp.edu/Health_Service/

Before you start to engage in an exercise program or participate in any exercise testing, you should fill out the questionnaire in Figure 1.22. If your answer to any of the questions is yes, you should see a physician before participating in a fitness program. Exercise testing and participation is not wise under some of the conditions listed in this questionnaire and may require a stress electrocardiogram (ECG) test. If you have any questions regarding your current health status, consult your doctor before initiating, continuing, or increasing your level of physical activity.

Now that you are about to embark in a wellness lifestyle program, sit down and subjectively determine where you are on each of the seven dimensions of wellness. Use Figure 1.23 to help you with this exercise. As you continue to study the content of this book, use this same form to monitor your progress. At least once a month, make adjustments in your specific objectives so you may reach the desired goals. Modifying unhealthy behaviors and developing new positive habits take time. The plan of action that you are about to develop will help you achieve your desired outcomes.

n*tes

1. U.S. Centers for Disease Control and Prevention and American College of Sports Medicine, "Summary Statement: Workshop on Physical Activity and Public Health," *Sports Medicine Bulletin* 28, no. 4 (1993): 7.

2. National Institutes of Health, Consensus Development Conference Statement, "Physical Activity and Cardiovascular Health" (Washington, DC: NIH, December 18–20, 1995).

3. See note 2.

4. U.S. Department of Health and Human Services, Physical Activity and Health, *A Report of the Surgeon General* (Atlanta: Centers for Disease Control and Prevention, National Center for Chronic Disease Prevention and Health Promotion, 1996).

5. L. Dossey, "Can Spirituality Improve Your Health," *Bottom Line/ Personal Health* 15 (July 2001): 11–13.

6. R. S. Paffenbarger, Jr., R. T. Hyde, A. L. Wing, and C. H. Steinmetz, "A Natural History of Athleticism and Cardiovascular Health," *Journal of the American Medical Association* 252 (1984): 491–495.

7. S. N. Blair, H. W. Kohl III, R. S. Paffenbarger, Jr., D. G. Clark, K. H. Cooper, and L. W. Gibbons, "Physical Fitness and All-Cause Mortality: A Prospective Study of Healthy Men and Women," *Journal of the American Medical Association* 262 (1989): 2395–2401.

8. S. N. Blair, H. W. Kohl III, C. E. Barlow, R. S. Paffenbarger, Jr., L. W. Gibbons, and C. A. Macera, "Changes in Physical Fitness and All-Cause Mortality: A Prospective Study of Healthy and Unhealthy Men," *Journal of the American Medical Association* 273 (1995): 1193–1198.

9. I. Lee, C. Hsieh, and R. S. Paffenbarger, Jr., "Exercise Intensity and Longevity in Men: The Harvard Alumni Health Study," *Journal of the American Medical Association* 273 (1995): 1179–1184.

10. J. E. Enstrom, "Health Practices and Cancer Mortality Among Active California Mormons," *Journal of the National Cancer Institute* 81 (1989): 1807–1814.

11. U.S. Department of Health and Human Services, Centers for Disease Control and Prevention, National Center for Health Statistics, National Vital Statistics System, *Deaths: Preliminary Data for 2000* 49, no. 12 (October 10, 2001).

12. *2000 Heart and Stroke Statistical Update* (Dallas: American Heart Association, 2000).

13. American Cancer Society, *2000 Cancer Facts and Figures* (New York: ACS, 2000).

14. T. A. Murphy and D. Murphy, *The Wellness for Life Workbook* (San Diego: Fitness Publications, 1987).

15. "Wellness Facts," *University of California at Berkeley Wellness Letter* (Palm Coast, FL: The Editors, April 1995).

16. "Daten Der Woche," *Welt am Sonntag* 25, no. 35 (1991).

17. Robert C. Chadbourne, "Fit for Hire," *Fitness Management* 12, no. 2 (1996): 28–30.

18. U.S. Department of Health and Human Services, *Healthy People 2010* (Washington DC: U.S. Government Printing Office, November 2000).

19. American College of Sports Medicine, *Guidelines for Exercise Testing and Prescription* (Baltimore: Williams & Wilkins, 2000).

 Suggested Readings

■ American College of Sports Medicine. "Position Stand: The Recommended Quantity and Quality of Exercise for Developing and Maintaining Cardiorespiratory and Muscular Fitness, and Flexibility in Healthy Adults." *Medicine and Science in Sports and Exercise* 30 (1998): 975–991.

■ Blair, S. N. "C. H. McCloy Research Lecture: Physical Activity, Physical Fitness, and Health." *Research Quarterly for Exercise and Sport* 64 (1993): 365–376.

■ Blair, S. N., et al. "Influences of Cardiorespiratory Fitness and Other Precursors on Cardiovascular Disease and All-Cause Mortality in Men and Women." *Journal of the American Medical Association* 276 (1996): 205–210.

■ Booth, F. W., and B. S. Tseng. "America Needs to Exercise for Health." *Medicine and Science in Sports and Exercise* 27 (1995): 462–465.

■ Hoeger, W. W. K., L. W. Turner, and B. Q. Hafen. *Wellness: Guidelines for a Healthy Lifestyle* (Belmont, CA: Wadsworth/Thomson Learning, 2002).

■ Nieman, D. C. *The Exercise-Health Connection.* (Champaign, IL: Human Kinetics, 1998).

■ Pate, R., et al. "Physical Activity and Public Health." *Journal of the American Medical Association* 273 (1995): 402–407.

■ U.S. Department of Health and Human Services, Physical Activity and Health. *A Report of the Surgeon General.* (Atlanta: Centers for Disease Control and Prevention, National Center for Chronic Disease Prevention and Health Promotion, 1996).

■ U.S. Department of Health and Human Services, Public Health Service, *Healthy People 2010: Conference Edition.* (http://www.health.gov/healthypeople/Document/tableofcontents.htm).

FIGURE 1.21 Wellness lifestyle questionnaire.

Name: _Duncan Brown_   Date: _1-24-03_

Course: _LF117_   Section: _02_   Gender: _male_   Age: _19_

The purpose of this questionnaire is to analyze current lifestyle habits and help determine changes necessary for future health and wellness. Check the appropriate answer to each question and obtain a final score according to the guidelines provided at the end of the questionnaire.

	Always	Nearly always	Often	Seldom	Never
1. I participate in vigorous aerobic activity for 20 minutes on 3 or more days per week, and I accumulate at least 30 minutes of moderate-intensity physical activity on a minimum of 3 additional days per week.	5	4	3	2	1 ✓
2. I participate in strength training exercises, using a minimum of eight different exercises, 2 or more days per week.	5	4	3	2 ✓	1
3. I perform flexibility exercises a minimum of 3 days per week.	5	4	3	2	1 ✓
4. I maintain recommended body weight and I avoid excessive body fat, excessive thinness, or frequent fluctuations in body weight.	5	4	3 ✓	2	1
5. Every day, I eat three regular meals that include a wide variety of foods.	5	4 ✓	3	2	1
6. I limit the amount of fat and saturated fat in my diet on most days of the week.	5	4	3	2 ✓	1
7. I eat a minimum of five servings of fruits and vegetables and six servings from grain products on a daily basis.	5	4	3	2	1 ✓
8. I regularly avoid snacks, especially those that are high in calories and fat and low in nutrients and fiber.	5	4	3	2 ✓	1
9. I do not smoke cigarettes or use tobacco in any other form.	5 ✓	4	3	2	1
10. I do not drink alcoholic beverages. If I drink, I do so in moderation (one daily drink for women and two for men), and I do not combine alcohol with other drugs.	5 ✓	4	3	2	1
11. I do not use addictive drugs or needles used by others.	5 ✓	4	3	2	1
12. I use prescription drugs and over-the-counter drugs sparingly, only when needed, and I follow all directions for their proper use.	5 ✓	4	3	2	1
13. I readily recognize when I am under excessive tension and stress (distress).	5 ✓	4	3	2	1
14. I am able to perform effective stress management techniques.	5	4	3 ✓	2	1
15. I have close friends and relatives that I can discuss personal problems with and approach for help when needed, and with whom I can express my feelings freely.	5 ✓	4	3	2	1
16. I spend most of my daily leisure time in wholesome recreational activities.	5	4	3	2 ✓	1
17. I sleep 7 to 8 hours each night.	5	4	3 ✓	2	1
18. I floss my teeth every day and brush them at least twice daily.	5 ✓	4	3	2	1
19. I avoid overexposure to the sun, and I use sunscreen and appropriate clothing when I am out in the sun for extended periods of time.	5 ✓	4	3	2	1
20. I avoid using products that have not been shown by science to be safe and effective (this includes anabolic steroids and unproven nutrient or weight loss supplements).	5 ✓	4	3	2	1
21. I know the warning signs for heart attack, stroke, and cancer.	5	4	3	2 ✓	1
22. I practice monthly breast/testicle self-exams, get recommended screening tests (blood lipids, blood pressure, Pap tests), and seek a medical evaluation when I am not well or disease symptoms arise.	5	4	3	2	1 ✓
23. I have a dental checkup at least once a year, and I get regular medical exams according to age recommendations.	5 ✓	4	3	2	1

(continued)

(Figure 1.21 Wellness lifestyle questionnaire—continued)

	Always	Nearly always	Often	Seldom	Never
24. I am not sexually active/I always practice safe sex.	5	4	3	2	1
25. I can effectively deal with disappointments and temporary feelings of sadness, loneliness, and depression. If I am unable to deal with these feelings, I seek professional help.	5	4	3	2	1
26. I can work out emotional problems without turning to alcohol or other drugs.	5	4	3	2	1
27. I associate with people who have a positive attitude about life.	5	4	3	2	1
28. I respond to temporary setbacks by making the best of the circumstances and by moving ahead with optimism and energy. I do not spend time and talent worrying about failures.	5	4	3	2	1
29. I wear a seatbelt whenever I am in a car, I ask others in my vehicle to do the same, and I make sure that children are in an infant seat or wear a shoulder harness.	5	4	3	2	1
30. I do not drive under the influence of alcohol or other drugs, and I make an effort to keep others from doing the same.	5	4	3	2	1
31. I avoid being alone in public places, especially after dark; I seek escorts when I visit or exercise in unfamiliar places.	5	4	3	2	1
32. I seek to make my living quarters accident-free, and I keep doors and windows locked, especially when home alone.	5	4	3	2	1
33. I try to minimize environmental pollutants, and I support community efforts to minimize pollution.	5	4	3	2	1
34. I keep my living quarters clean and organized.	5	4	3	2	1
35. I study and/or work in a clean environment (including avoidance of second-hand smoke).	5	4	3	2	1
36. I participate in recycling programs for paper, cardboard, glass, plastic, and aluminum.	5	4	3	2	1

How to Score

Enter the score you have circled for each question in the spaces provided below. Next, total the score for each specific wellness lifestyle category and obtain a rating for each category according to the criteria provided below.

	Health-Related Fitness	Nutrition	Avoiding Chemical Dependency	Stress Management	Personal Hygiene/ Health	Disease Prevention	Emotional Well-Being	Personal Safety	Environmental Health & Protection
	1. 1	5. 4	9. 5	13. 5	17. 3	21. 2	25. 4	29. 5	33. 1
	2. 2	6. 2	10. 5	14. 3	18. 5	22. 1	26. 5	30. 5	34. 2
	3. 1	7. 1	11. 5	15. 5	19. 5	23. 5	27. 5	31. 3	35. 3
	4. 3	8. 2	12. 5	16. 2	20. 5	24. 5	28. 2	32. 2	36. 3
Total:	7	9	20	15	18	13	16	15	10
Rating:	NI	NI	E	G	E	G	G	G	NI

Category Rating

Excellent (E) = ≥17 Your answers show that you are aware of the importance of this category to your health and wellness. You are putting your knowledge to work for you by practicing good habits. As long as you continue to do so, this category should not pose a health risk. You are also setting a good example for family and friends to follow. Because you got a very high test score on this part of the test, you may want to consider other categories where your score indicates room for improvement.

Good (G) = 13–16 Your health practices in this area are good, but there is room for improvement. Look again at the items you answered with a 4 or below and identify changes that you can make to improve your lifestyle. Even small changes can often help you achieve better health.

Needs Improvement (NI) = ≤12 Your health risks are showing. You may be taking serious and unnecessary risks with your health. Perhaps you are not aware of the risks and what to do about them. Most likely you need additional information and help in deciding how to successfully make the changes you desire. You can easily get the information that you need to improve, if you wish. The next step is up to you.

Please note that no final overall rating is provided for the entire questionnaire, because it may not be indicative of overall wellness. For example, an excellent rating in most categories will not offset the immediate health risks and life-threatening consequences of using addictive drugs and not wearing a seatbelt.

FIGURE 1.22 Health history questionnaire

Name: _Duncan Brown_ Date: _1-24-03_

Course: _Lf 117_ Section: _02_ Gender: _M_ Age: _19_

Although exercise testing and exercise participation are relatively safe for most apparently healthy individuals, the reaction of the cardiovascular system to increased physical activity cannot always be totally predicted. Consequently, a person takes a small but real risk of certain changes occurring during exercise testing or participation. These changes may include abnormal blood pressure, irregular heart rhythm, fainting, and, in rare instances, a heart attack or cardiac arrest.

Therefore, it is imperative that you provide honest answers to this questionnaire. Exercise may be ill-advised under some of the conditions listed below; others simply may require special consideration. If any of the conditions apply, consult your physician before you participate in an exercise program. Also, promptly report to your instructor any exercise-related abnormalities that you may experience during exercise participation.

A. Have you ever had or do you now have any of the following conditions?

☐ 1. Myocardial infarction

☐ 2. Coronary artery disease

☐ 3. Congestive heart failure

☐ 4. Elevated blood lipids (cholesterol and triglycerides)

☐ 5. Chest pain at rest or during exertion

☐ 6. Shortness of breath

☐ 7. Abnormal resting or stress electrocardiogram

☐ 8. Uneven, irregular, or skipped heartbeats (including racing or fluttering heart)

☐ 9. Blood embolism

☐ 10. Thrombophlebitis

☐ 11. Rheumatic heart fever

☐ 12. Elevated blood pressure

☐ 13. Stroke

☐ 14. Diabetes

☐ 15. Family history of coronary heart disease, syncope, or sudden death before age 60

☐ 16. Any other heart problem that makes exercise unsafe

B. Do you have any of the following conditions?

☐ 1. Arthritis, rheumatism, or gout

☐ 2. Chronic low back pain

☐ 3. Any other joint, bone, or muscle problems

☐ 4. Any respiratory problems

☐ 5. Obesity (more than 30% overweight)

☐ 6. Anorexia

☐ 7. Bulimia

☐ 8. Mononucleosis

☐ 9. Any physical disability that could interfere with safe participation in exercise

C. Do any of the following conditions apply?

☐ 1. Do you smoke cigarettes?

☐ 2. Are you taking any prescription drug?

☐ 3. Are you 45 years or older?

D. Do you have any other concern regarding your ability to safely participate in an exercise program? If so, explain:

Student's Signature: _Duncan Brown_

FIGURE 1.23 Dimensions of wellness scale.

Name: _____ Date: _____

Course: _____ Section: _____ Gender: _____ Age: _____

Instructions

1. Record the date at the top of the first column, then fill in that column using the following scale to indicate your wellness rating for each dimension:

   poor = 5, fair = 4, average = 3, good = 2, excellent = 1

2. Next, write a goal that you want to accomplish prior to the end of this course for each wellness dimension and list three specific objectives that will help you accomplish each goal.

3. Once a month, review this form, fill in another column of self-evaluation, and adjust your objectives as necessary.

Here's an example:

Social goal: _To improve my social life at school._

Specific objectives

1. _Find study buddies. Ask each instructor and counselor about study groups._

2. _Attend Friday night discussion groups in Student Center._

3. _Locate activities I enjoy–basketball, chess, dancing–and start a conversation._

Dates

Wellness Dimension					
Physical					
Emotional					
Social					
Environmental					
Mental					
Spiritual					
Occupational					

Goals and Objectives

Physical goal: _____
Specific objectives

1. _____
2. _____
3. _____

Emotional goal: _____
Specific objectives

1. _____
2. _____
3. _____

Mental goal: _____
Specific objectives

1. _____
2. _____
3. _____

Social goal: _____
Specific objectives

1. _____
2. _____
3. _____

Spiritual goal: _____
Specific objectives

1. _____
2. _____
3. _____

Environmental goal: _____
Specific objectives

1. _____
2. _____
3. _____

Occupational goal: _____
Specific objectives

1. _____
2. _____
3. _____

Behavior Modification

Learn the effects of environment on human behavior.

Understand obstacles that hinder our ability to change behavior.

Understand the concepts of motivation and locus of control.

Identify the stages of change.

Become familiar with the processes of change.

Learn techniques that will facilitate the process of change.

Learn the role of goal setting in the process of change.

Be able to write your own specific objectives for behavioral change.

Research studies during the last three decades have convincingly documented the benefits of physical activity and healthy lifestyles. Although the scientific evidence continues to mount each day and the data are impressive, most people are still unable to implement or adhere to a healthy lifestyle program.

The information in this book will be of little value to you if you are unable to abandon negative habits and adopt new, healthy behaviors. Before looking at physical fitness and wellness guidelines, you will need to take a critical look at your behaviors and lifestyle—and most likely make some permanent changes to promote overall health and wellness.

The science of behavioral therapy has established that most of the behaviors we adopt are a product of our environment—the forces of social influences and the thought processes we go through. This environment includes family, friends, peers, homes, schools, workplaces, television, radio, and movies, as well as our communities, country, and culture in general.

Unfortunately, when it comes to fitness and wellness, we live in a "toxic environment." Healthy children are often driven to places they could easily and safely walk or bicycle. From a young age, parents, relatives, and friends influence our behaviors. Children watch adults drive short distances to run errands. We see them take escalators and elevators and ride moving sidewalks at malls and airports. We notice that they use remote controls, pagers, and cellular phones. We observe as they stop at fast-food restaurants and pick up super-sized, calorie-dense, high-fat meals. They watch television and surf the Net for hours at a time. Some smoke, some drink heavily, and some have hard-drug addictions. Others engage in risky behaviors by not wearing seat belts, drinking and driving, and having unprotected sex. All of these unhealthy habits can be passed along, unquestioned, to the next generation.

Even architecture can reinforce unhealthy behavior. Elevators and escalators are often of the finest workmanship and located in convenient places. Many of our best and finest shopping centers and convention centers don't provide accessible stairwells, so people are all but forced to ride escalators. If they want to walk up the escalator, they can't because the people in front of them obstruct the way. Entrances to buildings provide electric sensors and automatic door openers. Without a second thought, people walk through automatic doors instead of taking the time to push a door open.

Walking, jogging, and bicycle trails are too sparse in our cities, further discouraging physical activity. Lack of places for safe exercise is a problem in many metropolitan areas. Many people remain indoors during leisure hours for fear for their personal safety and well-being.

In recent years the food portion sizes have substantially increased at restaurants. Patrons consume huge amounts of food, almost as if it were the last meal they will ever have. They drink entire pitchers of soda pop or beer instead of the traditional 8-ounce cup size. Most restaurants are colorful, well-lit, and nicely decorated to enhance comfort and appetite and increase the length of stay to entice more eating.

All of the these examples influence our thought processes and hinder our ability to be physically active and adopt healthy behaviors. From childhood through young adulthood, we observe, we learn, we emulate, and gradually, without realizing it, we incorporate many of these unhealthy behaviors into our personal lifestyle.

> **We have very few inferior people in the world. We have lots of inferior environments. Try to enrich your environments.**
>
> —Frank Lloyd Wright

Our environment is not conducive to a healthy, physically active lifestyle.

Photos © Fitness & Wellness, Inc.

Let's look at weight gain. Most people do not start life with a weight problem. By age 20, a man may weigh 160 pounds. A few years later, the weight starts to climb and may reach 170 pounds. He now adapts and accepts 170 pounds as his weight. He may "go on a diet" but not make the necessary lifestyle changes to make it work. Gradually the weight continues to climb to 180, 190, 210 pounds. Although he may not like it and would like to weigh less, once again he adapts and accepts 210 pounds as his stable weight.

The time comes, usually around middle age, when most people want to make changes in their lives but find it difficult to accomplish—providing personal proof that "old habits die hard." Acquiring positive behaviors that will lead to better health and well-being is a long-lasting process and requires continual effort. Understanding why most people are unsuccessful at changing their behaviors and are unable to live a healthy lifestyle may increase your readiness and motivation for change. The next sections will examine barriers to change, what motivates people to change, the various stages of change, the process of change, techniques for change, and actions required to make permanent changes in behavior.

Salzburg, Austria: Bicycles are the preferred mode of transportation in this European city.

Photos © Fitness & Wellness, Inc.

BARRIERS TO CHANGE

In spite of the best intentions, people make unhealthy choices daily. The most common reasons are

1. Procrastination. People seem to think that tomorrow, next week, or after the holiday is the best time to start change.

   Tip to initiate change. Ask yourself: Why wait until tomorrow when you can start changing today? Lack of motivation is a key factor in procrastination (motivation is discussed on page 32).

2. Preconditioned cultural beliefs. If we accept the principle that we are a product of our environment, our cultural beliefs and our physical surroundings pose significant barriers to change. In Salzburg, Austria, people of both genders and all ages use bicycles as a primary mode of transportation. In the United States, few people other than children ride bicycles.

   Tip to initiate change. In the pre-Columbian era, people thought the world was flat. Few dared to sail long distances for fear that they would fall off the edge. If your health and fitness are at stake, preconditioned cultural beliefs shouldn't keep you from making changes. Finding people who are willing to "sail" with you will help overcome this barrier.

3. Gratification. People prefer instant gratification to long-term benefits. Therefore, they will overeat (instant pleasure) instead of using self-restraint to eat moderately to prevent weight gain (long-term satisfaction). We love tanning (instant gratification) and avoid paying much attention to skin cancer (long-term consequence).

   Tip to initiate change. Think ahead and ask yourself the following questions: How did you feel the last time you engaged in this behavior? How did it affect you? Did you really feel good about yourself or about the results? In retrospect, was it worth it?

4. Risk complacency. Consequences of unhealthy behaviors often don't manifest themselves until years later. People will tell themselves, "If I get heart disease, I'll deal with it then. For now, let me eat, drink, and be merry."

   Tip to initiate change. Ask yourself these questions: How long do you want to live? How do you want to live the rest of your life and what type of health do you want to have? What do you want to be able to do when you are 60, 70, or 80 years old?

5. Complexity. People think the world is too complicated, with too much to think about. If you

are living the typical lifestyle, you may feel over-whelmed by everything that seems to be required to lead a healthy lifestyle, for example:

- Getting exercise
- Eating low-fat/high-fiber meals and cutting total calories
- Controlling use of substances
- Managing stress
- Wearing seat belts
- Practicing safe sex
- Getting annual physicals, including blood tests, Pap smears, and so on
- Taking nutrient supplements if indicated
- Fostering spirituality

Tip to initiate change. Take it one step at a time. Work only on one or two behaviors at a time so the task at hand won't feel insurmountable.

6. Indifference and helplessness. A defeatist thought process often takes over, and we may believe that the way we live won't really affect our health, that we have no control over our health, or that our destiny is all in our genes (also see discussion of locus of control, page 33).

Tip to initiate change. As much as 84 percent of the leading causes of death in the United States are preventable. Realize that only you can take control over your personal health and lifestyle habits and affect the quality of your life. Implementing many of the behavioral modification strategies and programs outlined in this book will get you started on a wellness way of life.

7. Rationalization. Even though people are not prac-ticing healthy behaviors, they often tell themselves that they do get sufficient exercise, that their diet is fine, that they have good solid relationships, or that they really don't smoke/drink/get high enough to affect their health.

Tip to initiate change. Rationalizing in this manner will not right the wrong. You need to face up to the fact that you have a problem and commit to change. Your health and your life are at stake. Monitoring lifestyle habits through daily logs and then analyzing the results can help you make necessary changes in self-defeating behaviors.

8. Illusions of invincibility. At times people believe that unhealthy behaviors will not harm them. Young adults often have the attitude that, "I can smoke now, and in a few years I'll quit before it causes any damage." When it comes to cigarettes, nicotine is one of the most addictive drugs known to us. Quitting smoking is not an easy task (see

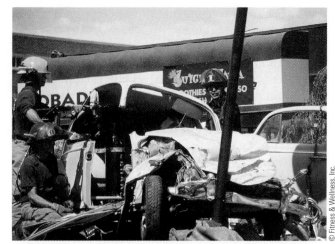

Feelings of invincibility are a strong barrier to change that can bring about life-threatening consequences.

Chapter 13). Health problems may arise before you quit, and the risk of lung cancer lingers for years after you quit. Drinking and driving is another example. The feeling of "I'm in control" or "I can handle it" while under the influence is a deadly combination.

Others perceive low risk when engaging in negative behaviors with people they like (for example, sex with someone you've recently met and feel attracted to), but perceive themselves at risk just by being in the same classroom with an HIV-infected person.

Tip to initiate change. No one is immune to sickness, disease, and tragedy. The younger you are when you implement a healthy lifestyle, the better your odds for a long and healthy life. Thus, initiating change right now will help you enjoy the best possible quality of life for as long as you live.

When health and appearance begin to deteriorate —usually around middle age—people seek out health care professionals in search of a "magic pill" to reverse and cure the many ills accumulated during years of abuse and overindulgence. The sooner we implement a healthy lifestyle program, the greater will be the health benefits and quality of life that lie ahead.

MOTIVATION AND LOCUS OF CONTROL

Motivation is often the explanation given for why some people succeed and others do not. Although motivation comes from within, external factors trigger the inner desire to accomplish a given task. These external factors, then, control behavior.

When you study motivation, understanding **locus of control** is helpful. People who believe they have control over events in their lives are said to have an internal locus of control. People with an external locus of control believe that what happens to them is a result of chance or the environment and is unrelated to their behavior. People with an internal locus of control generally are healthier and have an easier time initiating and adhering to a wellness program than those who perceive that they have no control and think of themselves as powerless and vulnerable. The latter people also are at greater risk for illness. When illness does strike a person, establishing a sense of control is vital to the recovery.

Few people have either a completely external or a completely internal locus of control. They fall somewhere along a continuum. The more external one's locus of control, the greater will be the challenge to change and adhere to exercise and other healthy lifestyle behaviors. Fortunately, developing a more internal locus of control can be accomplished. Understanding that most events in life are not determined genetically or environmentally helps people pursue goals and gain control over their lives. Three impediments, however, can keep people from taking action: lack of competence, confidence, and motivation.[1]

1. Problems of competence. Lacking the skills to get a given task done leads to feelings of less competence. If your friends play basketball regularly but you don't know how to play, you might not be inclined to participate. The solution to this problem of competence is to master the skills you need to participate. Most people are not born with all-inclusive natural abilities, including playing sports.

   Another alternative is to select an activity in which you are already skilled. It may not be basketball, but it well could be aerobics. Don't be afraid to try new activities, though. Similarly, if your body weight is a problem, you could learn to cook low-fat meals. Try different recipes until you find foods that you like.

2. Problems of confidence. Problems with confidence arise when you have the skill but don't believe you can get it done. Fear and feelings of inadequacy often interfere with ability to perform the task. You shouldn't talk yourself out of something until you have given it a fair try. If the skills are there, the sky is the limit. Initially, try to visualize yourself doing the task and getting it done. Repeat this several times, then actually try it. You will surprise yourself.

   Sometimes lack of confidence arises when the task seems insurmountable. In these situations, dividing a goal into smaller, more realistic

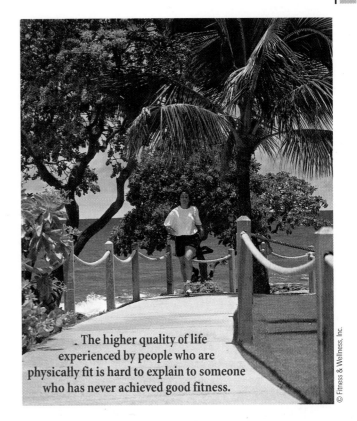

The higher quality of life experienced by people who are physically fit is hard to explain to someone who has never achieved good fitness.

© Fitness & Wellness, Inc.

objectives helps to accomplish the task. You may know how to swim, but building endurance to swim a continuous mile may take several weeks. Set up your training program so you swim a little farther each day until you are able to swim the entire mile. If you don't meet your objective on a given day, try it again, reevaluate, cut back a little—and, most important, don't give up.

3. Problems of motivation. In problems of motivation, both the competence and the confidence are there, but individuals are unwilling to change because the reasons to change are not important to them. For example, people begin contemplating a smoking cessation program only when the reasons for quitting outweigh the reasons for smoking. The primary causes of this unwillingness to change are lack of knowledge and lack of goals. Knowledge often determines goals, and goals determine motivation. How badly you want something dictates how hard you'll work at it. Many people are unaware of the magnitude of the benefits of a wellness program. When it comes to a healthy lifestyle, however, you may not get a second

KeyTerms

Motivation The desire and will to do something.

Locus of control The extent to which a person believes he or she can influence the external environment.

chance. A stroke, a heart attack, or cancer can have irreparable or fatal consequences. Greater understanding of what leads to disease may be all that is needed to initiate change.

Also, feeling physically fit is difficult to explain unless you have experienced it yourself. Feelings of fitness, self-esteem, confidence, health, and quality of life cannot be conveyed to someone who is constrained by sedentary living. In a way, achieving wellness is like reaching the top of a mountain. The quiet, the clean air, the lush vegetation, the flowing water in the river, the wildlife, and the majestic valley below are difficult to explain to someone who has spent a lifetime within city limits.

CHANGING BEHAVIOR

Psychotherapy has been used successfully to help change behavior. The great majority of people, however, do not seek professional help. They usually attempt change by themselves with limited or no knowledge of the process itself.

The simplest model of change is the two-stage model of unhealthy behavior and healthy behavior. This model states that either you do it or you don't. Most people who use this model attempt self-change but end up asking themselves why they're unsuccessful: They just can't do it (exercise, perhaps, or quitting cigarettes). Their intention to change may be good, but to accomplish it, they need knowledge about how to achieve change.

THE TRANSTHEORETICAL MODEL

For most people, changing chronic/unhealthy behaviors to stable/healthy behaviors is a challenging process. Change usually does not happen all at once. It is a gradual process that involves several stages. To aid with the process of self-change, psychologists James Prochaska, John Norcross, and Carlo DiClemente developed the Transtheoretical Model of Stages of Change.[2]

The Transtheoretical Model identifies six stages in the process of willful change. These stages describe underlying processes that people go through to change most problem behaviors and adopt healthy behaviors, and understanding the six stages will help you use this process. Most frequently, the model is used to change health-related behaviors such as physical inactivity, smoking, poor nutrition, weight problems, stress, and alcohol abuse.

The six stages of change in the Transtheoretical Model are precontemplation, contemplation, preparation, action, maintenance, and termination/adoption (see Figure 2.1). After years of study, researchers

FIGURE 2.1 Stages of change model.

Precontemplation

Contemplation

Preparation

Termination/Adoption

Maintenance

Action

found that applying specific behavioral-change processes during each stage of the model increases the success rate for change (specific processes for each stage are shown in Table 2.1, page 38). Understanding each stage of this model will help you determine where you are in relation to your personal healthy-lifestyle behaviors. It will also help you identify processes to make successful changes.

Precontemplation

People in the **precontemplation stage** are not considering change or do not want to change a given behavior. They typically deny having a problem and have no intention of changing in the immediate future. These people are usually unaware or under-aware of the problem. Other people around them, including family, friends, health care practitioners, and co-workers, however, identify the problem clearly. Precontemplators do not care about the problem behavior and may even avoid information and materials that address the issue. They tend to avoid free screenings and workshops that might help identify and change the problem, even if they receive financial compensation for attendance. These people frequently have an active resistance to change and seem resigned to accepting the unhealthy behavior as their "fate."

> **People don't contemplate change until they begin to feel uncomfortable with their lifestyle habits.**

Precontemplators are the most difficult people to inspire toward behavioral change. Many think that change isn't even a possibility. At this stage, knowledge is power. Educating them about the problem behavior is critical to help them start contemplating the process of change. The challenge is to find ways to help them realize that they are ultimately responsible for the consequences of their behavior. Typically, they initiate change only when people they respect or job requirements pressure them to do so.

Contemplation

In the **contemplation stage**, people acknowledge that they have a problem and begin to seriously think about overcoming it. Although they are not quite ready for change, they are weighing the pros and cons of changing. Even though people may remain in this stage for years, in their minds they are planning to take some action within the next 6 months. Education and peer support remain valuable during this stage.

Preparation

In the **preparation stage**, people are seriously considering and planning to change a behavior within the next month. They are taking initial steps for change and may even try the new behavior for a short while, such as stopping smoking for a day or exercising a few times during the month. During this stage, people define a general goal for behavioral change (to quit smoking by the last day of the month) and write specific objectives to accomplish this goal (see the section on "Goal Setting" later in this chapter). Continued peer and environmental support are helpful during the preparation phase.

> **Self-defeating behaviors can be defeated.**
> —David J. Lieberman

Action

This stage requires the greatest commitment of time and energy on the part of the individual. Here people are actively doing things to change or modify the problem behavior or to adopt a new health behavior. The **action stage** requires that the person follow the specific guidelines set forth for that behavior. For example, a person has actually stopped smoking completely, is exercising aerobically 3 times per week according to exercise prescription guidelines, or is maintaining a diet that derives less than 30 percent of its calories from fat. Relapse is common during this stage, and the individual may regress to previous stages. Once people maintain the action stage for 6 consecutive months, they move into the maintenance stage.

Maintenance

During the **maintenance stage**, the person continues the new behavior for up to 5 years. The

Key Terms

Precontemplation stage Stage of change in which people are unwilling to change behavior.

Contemplation stage Stage of change in which people are considering changing behavior in the next 6 months.

Preparation stage Stage of change in which people are getting ready to make a change within the next month.

Action stage Stage of change in which people are actively changing a negative behavior or adopting a new, healthy behavior.

Maintenance stage Stage of change in which people maintain behavioral change for up to 5 years.

maintenance phase requires continued adherence to the specific guidelines that govern the behavior (such as complete smoking cessation, exercising aerobically 3 times per week, practicing proper stress management techniques). At this time the person works to reinforce the gains made through the various stages of change and strives to prevent lapses and relapse.

Termination/Adoption

Once a behavior has been maintained for more than 5 years, a person is said to be in the **termination** or **adoption** phase and exits from the cycle of change without fear of relapse. In the case of negative behaviors that are terminated, the stage of change is referred to as termination. If a positive behavior has been successfully adopted for over 5 years, this stage is designated as the adoption stage. Some researchers have also labeled this stage the "transformed" stage of change because the word literally means "to have changed."[3]

Many experts believe that, once an individual enters the termination/adoption stage, former addictions, problems, or lack of compliance with healthy behaviors no longer present an obstacle in the quest for wellness. The change has now become a part of one's lifestyle. This phase is the ultimate goal for all people searching for a healthier lifestyle.

However, for addictive behaviors like alcoholism and hard drug use, many health care practitioners believe that the individual never enters the termination stage. Chemical dependency is so strong that most former alcoholics and hard-drug users must make a lifetime effort to prevent relapse. Similarly, some behavioral scientists suggest that the adoption stage may not be applicable to health behaviors like exercise and weight control, because the likelihood for relapse is always high.[4]

Using the guidelines provided in Figure 2.2 you can determine where you stand in respect to behaviors you want to change or new ones you wish to adopt. As you follow the guidelines, you will realize that you might be at different stages for different behaviors. For instance, you may be in the preparation stage for aerobic exercise and smoking, in the action stage for strength training, but only in the contemplation stage for a healthy diet. Realizing where you are with respect to different behaviors will help you design a better action plan for a healthy lifestyle.

FIGURE 2.2 Stage of change identification.

Please indicate which response most accurately describes your current _____ behavior (in the blank space identify the behavior: smoking, physical activity, stress, nutrition, weight control). Next, select the statement below (select only one) that best represents your current behavior pattern. To select the most appropriate statement, fill in the blank for one of the first three statements if your current behavior is a problem behavior. (For example, you may say, "I currently smoke and I do *not* intend to change in the foreseeable future," or "I currently *do not exercise* but I am contemplating changing in the next 6 months.") If you have already started to make changes, fill in the blank in one of the last three statements. (In this case, you may say: "I currently *eat a low-fat diet* but I have only done so within the last 6 months," or "I currently *practice adequate stress management techniques* and I have done so for over 6 months.") As you can see, you may use this form to identify your stage of change for any type of health-related behavior.

1. I currently _____ , and I do not intend to change in the foreseeable future.

2. I currently _____ , but I am contemplating changing in the next 6 months.

3. I currently _____ regularly, but I intend to change in the next month.

4. I currently _____ , but I have done so only within the last 6 months.

5. I currently _____ , and I have done so for more than 6 months.

6. I currently _____ , and I have done so for more than 5 years.

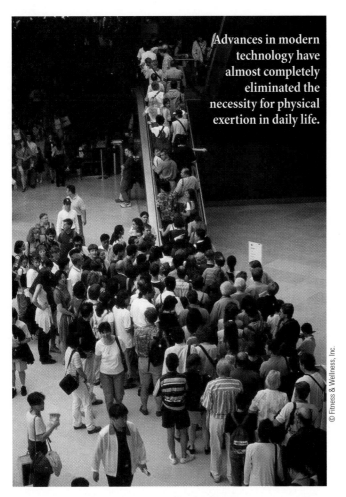

Advances in modern technology have almost completely eliminated the necessity for physical exertion in daily life.

© Fitness & Wellness, Inc.

Relapse

After getting out of the precontemplation stage, **relapse** may occur at any level of the model. Even individuals in the maintenance and termination/ adoption stages may regress to any of the first three stages of the model (see Figure 2.3). Relapse, how- ever, does not mean failure. Failure comes only to those who give up and don't use prior experiences as a building block for future success. The chances of moving back up to a higher stage of the model are far better for someone who has previously made it into one of those stages.

Key Terms

Termination/adoption stage Stage of change in which people have eliminated an undesirable behavior or main- tained a positive behavior for over 5 years.

Relapse To slip or fall back into unhealthy behavior(s); failure to maintain healthy behaviors.

FIGURE 2.3 Model of progression and relapse.

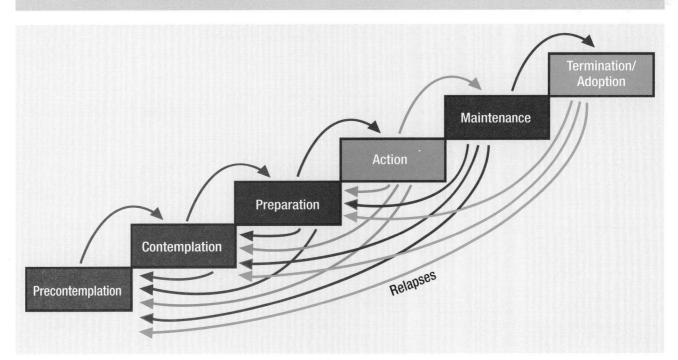

THE PROCESS OF CHANGE

Using the same plan for every individual who wishes to change a behavior will not work. For instance, the same exercise prescription would not provide optimal results for a person who has been inactive for 20 years, compared with one who walks regularly 3 times each week. (We provide customized prescriptions to people of varying fitness levels [see Chapters, 4, 5, 6, and 7]). This principle also holds true for people who are attempting to change other behaviors.

Timing is important in the process of willful change. People respond more effectively to selected **processes of change** according to the stage of change they have reached at any given time.[5] Thus, applying specific processes at each stage of change enhances the likelihood of changing behavior permanently. The following description of 14 of the most common processes of change will help you develop a personal plan for change. The respective stages of change where each process works best are summarized in Table 2.1.

Consciousness-Raising

The first step in a **behavior modification** program is consciousness-raising. This process involves obtaining information so you can make a better decision about the problem behavior. For example, the problem could be physical inactivity. Learning about the benefits of exercise or the difference in benefits between physical activity and exercise (see Chapter 1) can help you decide the type of fitness program (health or physical) that you want to pursue. It is also possible that you don't even know that a certain behavior is a problem, such as unawareness of fat content in many fast-food items. This is part of the precontemplation stage.

Social Liberation

Social liberation stresses external alternatives that make you aware of problem behaviors and contemplate change. Examples of social liberation include finding and using pedestrian-only traffic areas,

TABLE 2.1 Applicable Processes of Change During Each Stage of Change

Precontemplation	Contemplation	Preparation	Action	Maintenance	Termination/Adoption
Consciousness-raising	Consciousness-raising	Consciousness-raising			
Social liberation	Social liberation	Social liberation	Social liberation		
	Self-analysis	Self-analysis			
	Emotional arousal	Emotional arousal			
	Positive outlook	Positive outlook	Positive outlook		
		Commitment	Commitment	Commitment	Commitment
		Behavior analysis			
		Goal setting	Goal setting	Goal setting	
		Self-reevaluation	Self-reevaluation	Self-reevaluation	
			Countering	Countering	
			Monitoring	Monitoring	Monitoring
			Environment control	Environment control	Environment control
			Helping relationships	Helping relationships	Helping relationships
			Rewards	Rewards	Rewards

SOURCE: Adapted from J. O. Prochaska, J. C. Norcross, and C. C. DiClemente, *Changing for Good*, (New York: William Morrow, 1994); and W. W. K. Hoeger and S. A. Hoeger, *Principles and Labs for Fitness and Wellness* (Belmont, CA: Wadsworth/Thomson Learning, 2002).

nonsmoking areas, and health-oriented cafeterias and restaurants or joining advocacy groups, civic organizations, policy interventions, and self-help groups. Social liberation often provides opportunities to get involved, stir up emotions, and enhance self-esteem—helping you gain confidence in your ability to change.

Self-Analysis

The second step in modifying behavior is developing a decisive desire to do so, called "self-analysis." If you have no interest in changing a behavior, you won't do it. You will remain a precontemplator or a contemplator. A person who has no intention of quitting smoking will not quit, regardless of what anyone may say or how strong the evidence in favor of quitting may be. In your self-analysis, you may want to prepare a list of reasons for continuing or discontinuing the behavior. When the reasons for changing outweigh the reasons for not changing, you are ready for either the contemplation or preparation stage.

Emotional Arousal

In emotional arousal, a person experiences and expresses feelings about the problem and its solutions. Also referred to as "dramatic release," this process often involves deep emotional experiences. Watching a loved one die from lung cancer caused by cigarette smoking may be all that is needed to make a person quit smoking. Other examples of emotional arousal are dramatizations of the consequences of drug use and abuse, a film about a person undergoing open-heart surgery, or books illustrating damage to body systems as a result of unhealthy behaviors.

Positive Outlook

Having a positive outlook means taking an optimistic approach from the beginning and believing in yourself. Following the guidelines in this chapter will help you design a plan so you can work toward change and remain enthused about your progress. Also, you may become motivated by looking at the outcome—how much healthier you will be, how much better you will look, or how far you will be able to jog.

Commitment

Upon making a decision to change, you now accept the responsibility to change and believe in your ability to do so—you've begun the preparation stage. During this process, you may draw up a specific plan of action.

Write down your goals and, preferably, share them with others. In essence, you are signing a behavioral contract for change. You will be more likely to adhere to your program if others know you are committed to change.

Behavior Analysis

Now determine the frequency, circumstances, and consequences of the behavior to be altered or implemented. If the desired outcome is to consume less fat, you must first find out what foods in your diet are high in fat, when you eat them, and when you don't eat them—all part of the preparation stage. Knowing when you don't eat them points to circumstances under which you exert control of your diet and will help as you set goals.

Goal Setting

Goals motivate change in behavior. The stronger the goal or desire, the more motivated you'll be either to change unwanted behaviors or to implement new, healthy behaviors. The section titled "Goal Setting" (page 41) will help you write goals and prepare an action plan to achieve them. This will aid with behavior modification.

Self-Reevaluation

During this process, individuals analyze their feelings about a problem behavior. The pros and cons or advantages and disadvantages of a certain behavior can be reevaluated at this time. For example, you may decide that strength training will help you tone up and boost your metabolism, but implementing this change will require you to stop watching an hour of TV 3 times per week. If you presently have a weight problem and you are unable to lift certain objects around the house, you may feel good about weight loss and enhanced physical capacity as a result of a strength-training program. You may also visualize what it would be like if you were successful at changing.

KeyTerms

Processes of change Actions that help you achieve change in behavior.

Behavior modification The process to permanently change negative behaviors in favor of positive behaviors that will lead to better health and well-being.

Countering: Replacing problem behaviors with healthy behaviors facilitates change.

© Fitness & Wellness, Inc.

Countering

This is the process whereby you substitute healthy behaviors for a problem behavior. This step is critical in changing behaviors as part of the action and maintenance stages. You need to replace unhealthy behaviors with new, healthy ones. You can use exercise to combat sedentary living, smoking, stress, or overeating. You may also use exercise, diet, yardwork, volunteer work, or reading to prevent overeating and achieve recommended body weight.

Monitoring

During the action and maintenance stages, continuous behavior monitoring increases awareness of the desired outcome. Sometimes this process in itself is sufficient to cause change. For example, keeping track of daily food intake reveals sources of fat in the diet. This can help you cut down gradually or completely eliminate high-fat foods. If the goal is to increase daily intake of fruit and vegetables, keeping track of the number of servings consumed each day raises awareness and may help increase intake.

Environment Control

In environment control, the person restructures the physical surroundings to avoid problem behaviors and decrease temptations. If you don't buy alcohol, you can't drink any. If you shop on a full stomach, you can reduce impulse-buying of junk food.

Similarly, you can create an environment where exceptions become the norm and then the norm can flourish. Instead of bringing home cookies for snacks, bring fruit. Place notes to yourself on the refrigerator and pantry to avoid unnecessary snacking. Place baby carrots or sugarless gum where you used to place cigarettes. Post notes around the house to remind you of your exercise time. Leave exercise shoes and clothing by the entry way so they are visible as you walk into your home. Put an electric timer on the TV so it will shut off automatically at 7:00 PM. All of these tactics will be helpful throughout the action, maintenance, and termination/adoption stages.

Helping Relationships

Surrounding yourself with people who will work toward a common goal with you or those who care about and will encourage you along the way will be helpful during the action, maintenance, and termination/adoption stages.

Attempting to quit smoking, for instance, is easier when a person is around others who are trying as well. The person could also get help from friends who have quit already. Losing weight is difficult if meal planning and cooking is shared with roommates who enjoy foods that are high in fat and sweets. It can be even worse if roommates also have a weight problem and do not desire to lose weight.

Peer support is a strong incentive for behavioral change. During this process, the individual should avoid people who will not be supportive. Friends who have no desire to quit smoking or lose weight may tempt one to smoke or overeat and encourage relapse into unwanted behaviors. People who have achieved the same goal already may not be supportive either. For instance, someone may say, "I can do six consecutive miles." The response should be, "I'm proud that I can jog three consecutive miles."

Rewards

People tend to repeat behaviors that are rewarded and disregard those that are not rewarded or are punished. Rewarding oneself or being rewarded by others is a powerful tool during the process of change in all stages. If you have successfully cut down your fat intake during the week, reward yourself by going to a show or buying a new pair of shoes. Do not reinforce yourself with destructive behaviors such as eating a high-fat dinner. If you fail to change a desired behavior (or to implement a new one), you may want to put off buying the new shoes you had planned for that week. When a positive behavior becomes habitual, give yourself an even better reward. Treat yourself to a weekend away from home or buy a new bicycle.

TECHNIQUES OF CHANGE

Not to be confused with the processes of change, within each process you can apply any number of **techniques of change** that help you through that particular process (see Table 2.2). For example, following dinner, people with a weight problem often can't resist continuous snacking during the rest of the evening until it is time to retire for the night. Using the process of countering, you can use various techniques to avoid unnecessary snacking. Examples include: going for a walk, flossing and brushing your teeth right after dinner, going for a drive, playing the piano, going to a show, or going to bed earlier.

As you develop your behavior modification plan, you need to identify specific techniques that may work for you within each process of change. A list of techniques for each process is provided in Table 2.2. This is only a sample list; dozens of other techniques may be used as well. For example, Behavior Modification and Adherence to a Weight Management Program is found on page 263, Getting Started and Adhering to a Lifetime Exercise Program is presented on page 106, stress management techniques are provided throughout Chapter 12, and tips to help stop smoking on pages 383–384. Some of the techniques can also be used with more than one process, such as visualization in emotional arousal and self-reevaluation.

Goal Setting

To initiate change, **goals** are essential. Goals motivate behavioral change and provide a plan of action. Goals are most effective when they are

1. Well planned. Only a well-conceived action plan will help you attain your goal. The items below (as well as others discussed in following chapters) will help you design your plan of action. You also should write specific **objectives** to help you reach each goal.

    The specific objectives are the steps required to reach a goal. For example, a goal might be to

achieve recommended body weight. Several specific objectives could be to (a) lose an average of 1 pound (or 1 fat percentage point) per week (b) monitor body weight before breakfast every morning (c) assess body composition every 2 weeks (d) limit fat intake to less than 25 percent of total calories (e) eliminate all pastries from the diet during this time, and (f) exercise in the proper target zone for 45 minutes, 5 times per week.

2. Personalized. Goals that you set for yourself are more motivational than goals that someone else sets for you.

3. Written. An unwritten goal is simply a wish. A written goal, in essence, becomes a contract with yourself. Show this goal to a friend or an instructor and have him or her witness the contract you made with yourself by signing alongside your signature.

4. Realistic. Goals should be within reach. If you currently weigh 190 pounds and your target weight (at 22 percent body fat) is 140 pounds, setting a goal to lose 50 pounds in 2 months would be unsound, if not impossible. This program would not allow implementation of adequate behavior modification techniques or ensure weight maintenance at the target weight. Unattainable goals lead to discouragement and loss of interest.

    At times problems arise even with realistic goals. Try to anticipate potential difficulties as much as possible and plan for ways to deal with them. If your goal is to jog for 30 minutes on 6 consecutive days, what are the alternatives if the weather turns bad? Possible solutions are to jog in the rain, find an indoor track, jog at a different time of day when the weather improves, or participate in a different aerobic activity such as stationary cycling, swimming, or step aerobics.

5. Embraced with positive thoughts. As difficult as some tasks may seem, where there's a will, there's a way. A plan of action, prepared according to the guidelines in this chapter, will help you achieve your goals.

6. Short-term and long-term. If the long-term goal is to attain recommended body weight and you are 50 pounds overweight, you might set a short-term

TABLE 2.2 Sample Techniques for Use With Processes of Change

Process	Techniques
Consciousness-Raising	Become aware that there is a problem, read educational materials about the problem behavior or about people who have overcome this same problem, find out about the benefits of changing the behavior, watch an instructional program on television, visit a therapist, talk and listen to others, ask questions, take a class.
Social Liberation	Seek out advocacy groups (Overeaters Anonymous, Alcoholics Anonymous), join a health club, buy a bike, join a neighborhood walking group, work in nonsmoking areas.
Self-Analysis	Question yourself on the problem behavior, express your feelings about it, become aware that there is a problem, analyze your values, list advantages and disadvantages of continuing (smoking) or not implementing a behavior (exercise), take a fitness test, do a nutrient analysis.
Emotional Arousal	Practice mental imagery of yourself going through the process of change, visualize yourself overcoming the problem behavior, do some role-playing in overcoming the behavior or practicing a new one, watch dramatizations (a movie) of the consequences or benefits of your actions, visit an auto salvage yard or a drug rehabilitation center.
Positive Outlook	Believe in yourself, know that you are capable, know that you are special, draw from previous personal successes.
Commitment	Just do it, set New Year's resolutions, sign a behavioral contract, set start and completion dates, tell others about your goals, work on your action plan.
Behavior Analysis	Prepare logs of circumstances that trigger or prevent a given behavior and look for patterns that prompt the behavior or cause you to relapse.
Goal Setting	Write goals, objectives, and design a specific action plan.
Self-Reevaluation	Determine accomplishments and evaluate progress, rewrite goals and objectives, list pros and cons, weigh sacrifices (can't eat out with others) versus benefits (weight loss), visualize continued change, think before you act, learn from mistakes, and prepare new action plans accordingly.
Countering	Seek out alternatives: Stay busy, walk (don't drive), read a book (instead of snacking), attend alcohol-free socials, carry your own groceries, mow your yard, dance (don't eat), go to a movie (instead of smoking), practice stress management.
Monitoring	Use exercise logs (days exercised, sets and resistance used in strength training), keep journals, conduct nutrient analyses; count grams of fat, number of consecutive days without smoking, days and type of relaxation technique(s) used.
Environment Control	Rearrange your home (no TVs, ashtrays, large-sized cups), get rid of unhealthy items (cigarettes, junk food, alcohol), then avoid unhealthy places (bars, happy hour), avoid relationships that encourage problem behaviors, use reminders to control problem behaviors (post notes indicating "don't snack after dinner" or "lift weights at 8:00 P.M."). Frequent healthy environments (a clean park, a health club, restaurants with low-fat/low-calorie/nutrient-dense menus, friends with goals similar to yours).
Helping Relationships	Associate with people who have and want to overcome the same problem, form or join self-help groups, join community programs specifically designed to deal with your problem.
Rewards	Go to a movie, buy a new outfit or shoes, buy a new bike, go on a weekend get-away, reassess your fitness level, use positive self-talk ("good job," "that felt good," "I did it," "I knew I'd make it," "I'm good at this").

goal of losing 10 pounds and write specific objectives to accomplish this goal. Then the task will not seem as overwhelming and will be easier.

7. Measurable. Whenever possible, goals and objectives should be measurable. For example, "to lose weight" is not measurable. If the goal is to achieve recommended body weight, this implies lowering your body weight (fat) to the recommended

percent body fat standard given in Table 7.9 (page 184). For a 19-year-old female, the high fitness recommended fat percent would be in the range of 17 to 27 percent.

To be more descriptive, the goal could be reworded to read "Reduce body weight to 22 percent body fat." Also note that all of the sample specific objectives (a) through (f) given in Item 1

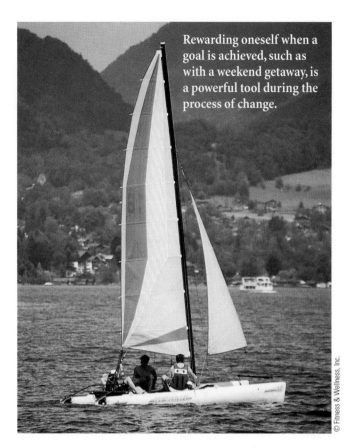

Rewarding oneself when a goal is achieved, such as with a weekend getaway, is a powerful tool during the process of change.

© Fitness & Wellness, Inc.

exercise log or doing a body composition assessment periodically enables you to determine your progress at any given time.

10. Evaluated. Periodic reevaluations are vital for success. You may find that a goal is unreachable. If so, reassess the goal. On the other hand, if a goal is too easy, you may lose interest and stop working toward it. Once you achieve a goal, set a new one to improve upon or maintain what you have achieved. Goals keep you motivated.

Recognize that you will face obstacles, and you will not always meet your goals. Making mistakes is human and does not mean failure. Failure comes only to those who give up. Use your setbacks and learn from them. Rewrite your goal and create a plan that will help you get around self-defeating behaviors in the future.

Now that you have read this chapter, use Figure 2.4 to identify two problem behaviors in your life. In this worksheet you will be asked to determine your stage of change for each behavior according to six standard statements. Based on your selection, determine the stage of change classification according to the ratings provided in Table 2.3. Identification of stages of change for other fitness and wellness behaviors are also provided in subsequent worksheets in this book.

on page 41 are measurable. For instance, you can figure out easily whether you are losing a pound or a percentage point per week; you can conduct a nutrient analysis to assess your average fat intake; or you can monitor your weekly exercise sessions to make sure you are meeting this specific objective.

8. Time-specific. A goal always should have a specific date set for completion. Simply stating, "I will decrease body fat to 22 percent" is not time-specific. The chosen date should be realistic but not too distant in the future. With a deadline, a task is much easier to work toward.

9. Monitored. Monitoring your progress as you move toward a goal reinforces behavior. Keeping an

TABLE 2.3 Stage of Change Classification

Selected Statement (see Figure 2.4, page 45)	Classification
1	Precontemplation
2	Contemplation
3	Preparation
4	Action
5	Maintenance
6	Termination/Adoption

WEB INTERACTIVE

Transtheoretical Model

This site, from the University of South Florida Community and Department of Family Health describes the development of the Transtheoretical Model and features several useful print references.

http://www.med.usf.edu/~kmbrown/Stages_of_Change_Overview.htm

Behavior Change Theories

This very comprehensive site, by the Department of Health Promotion and California Polytechnic University at Pomona, describes various theories of behavioral change, including learning theories, Transtheoretical Model, health belief model, relapse prevention model, reasoned action and planned behavior, social learning/social cognitive theory and social support.

http://www.csupomona.edu/~jvgrizzell/best_practices/bctheory.html

A User-Friendly Model of Change

This site, written by Robert Westermeyer, describes a cycle model for behavioral change similar to the Transtheoretical Model. This model views change as flexible in response to individual needs and the site describes relapses and backslides.

http://www.harbistamart.com/motivate.htm

INTERACTIVE SITES

Personalized Fitness Planner

This visually appealing site has five interactive assessments, each of which allows you to set your personal fitness goals. The assessments include flexibility and balance, strength, cardiovascular, body composition, and total fitness. The site also features a glossary and an index of exercises.

http://thriveonline.oxygen.com/fitness/planner/

The Transtheoretical Model

This excellent site features self-assessment tools to help you determine what stage of change you are in, based on the Transtheoretical Model, for the following behaviors: smoking, exercise, eating and diet, alcohol and drug usage, and practice of safe sex (including condom use and HIV prevention).

http://www2.msstage.edu/~bhunt/Stages_of_Change_Theory/transtheoretical.html

n*tes

1. G. S. Howard, D. W. Nance, and P. Myers, *Adaptive Counseling and Therapy* (San Francisco: Jossey-Bass, 1987).

2. J. O. Prochaska, J. C. Norcross, and C. C. DiClemente, *Changing for Good* (New York: William Morrow, 1994).

3. B. J. Cardinal, "Extended Stage Model of Physical Activity Behavior," *Journal of Human Movement Studies* 37 (1999): 37–54.

4. See note 3.

5. See note 2. Also in B. H. Marcus et al., "Evaluation of Motivationally Tailored vs. Standard Self-help Physical Activity Interventions at the Workplace," *American Journal of Health Promotion* 12 (1998): 246–253.

Suggested Readings

- Annesi, J. J. *Enhancing Exercise Motivation: A Guide to Increasing Fitness Center Member Retention.* Los Angeles: Leisure Publications, 1996.

- Bouchard, C., et al. *Exercise, Fitness, and Health: A Consensus of Current Knowledge.* Champaign, IL: Human Kinetics, 1990.

- Bouchard, C., et al. *Physical Activity, Fitness, and Health.* Champaign, IL: Human Kinetics, 1994.

- Cardinal, B. J., and S. S. Levy. "Are Sedentary Behaviors Terminable?" *Journal of Human Movement Studies* 38 (2000): 137–150.

- Dishman, R. *Exercise Adherence.* Champaign, IL: Human Kinetics, 1988.

- Dishman, R. "Increasing and Maintaining Exercise and Physical Activity." *Behavioral Therapy* 22 (1991): 345–378.

- Guttman, M. "The New Science of Risky Behavior." *USA Weekend* (March 6–8, 1998): 4–5.

- Marcus, B., and L. Simkin. "The Stages of Exercise Behavior." *Journal of Sports Medicine and Physical Fitness* 33 (1993): 83–88.

- Marcus, B., et al. "The Stages and Processes of Exercise Adoption and Maintenance in a Worksite Sample." *Health Psychology* 11 (1992): 386–395.

- Prochaska, J. O., and B. H. Marcus. "The Transtheoretical Model: Applications to Exercise." In *Advances in Exercise Adherence*, edited by R. K. Dishman, 161–180. Champaign, IL: Human Kinetics, 1994.

- Prochaska, J. O., J. C. Norcross, and C. C. DiClemente. *Changing for Good.* New York: William Morrow, 1994.

- Prochaska, J. O., and W. F. Velcier. "The Transtheoretical Model of Health Behavior Change." *American Journal of Health Promotion* 12 (1997): 38–48.

- Samuelson, M. "Stages of Change: From Theory to Practice." *The Art of Health Promotion* 2 (1998): 1–7

FIGURE 2.4 Behavior modification.

Name: _____ Date: _____

Course: _____ Section: _____ Gender: _____ Age: _____

I. Stages of Change Instructions

Please indicate which response most accurately describes your current [   ] behavior (in the blank space identify the behavior: smoking, physical activity, stress, nutrition, weight control). Next, select one of the six statements below (select only one) that best represents your current behavior pattern. To select the most appropriate statement, fill in the blank for one of the first three statements if your current behavior is a problem behavior. For example, you may say:

"I currently <u>smoke</u> and I do not intend to change in the foreseeable future" OR

"I currently <u>do not exercise</u> but I am contemplating changing in the next 6 months."

If you have already started to make changes, fill in the blank in one of the last three statements. In this case you may say:

"I currently <u>eat a low-fat diet</u> but I have done so only within the last 6 months" OR

"I currently <u>practice adequate stress management techniques</u> and I have done so for over 6 months."

You may use this form to identify your stage of change for any type of health-related behavior. After identifying two problem behaviors, look up your stage of change for each one of these behaviors using the ratings provided in Table 2.3.

Behavior #1

☐ 1. I currently [   ], and do not intend to change in the foreseeable future.

☐ 2. I currently [   ], but I am contemplating changing in the next 6 months.

☐ 3. I currently [   ] regularly, but I intend to change in the next month.

☐ 4. I currently [   ], but I have done so only within the last 6 months.

☐ 5. I currently [   ], and I have done so for more than 6 months.

☐ 6. I currently [   ], and I have done so for more than 5 years.

Stage of change: [   ] (*see stages listed in Table 2.3, page 43*).

Behavior #2

☐ 1. I currently [   ], and I do not intend to change in the foreseeable future.

☐ 2. I currently [   ], but I am contemplating changing in the next 6 months.

☐ 3. I currently [   ] regularly, but I intend to change in the next month.

☐ 4. I currently [   ], but I have done so only within the last 6 months.

☐ 5. I currently [   ], and I have done so for more than 6 months.

☐ 6. I currently [   ], and I have done so for more than 5 years.

Stage of change: [   ] (*see stages listed in Table 2.3, page 43*).

(continued)

(Figure 2.4 Behavior modification—continued)

II. Processes of Change

According to your stage of change for the two behaviors identified above, list the processes of change that apply to each behavior (see Table 2.1, page 38).

Behavior #1:

_____

_____

_____

Behavior #2:

_____

_____

_____

III. Techniques for Change

List a minimum of three techniques that you will use with each process of change (see Table 2.2, page 42).

Behavior #1:

_____

_____

_____

_____

Behavior #2:

_____

_____

_____

_____

conclusion   Will you continue to use these techniques as a process of behavior modification in the future? Briefly, discuss the techniques that were most beneficial to you.

_____

_____

_____

_____

_____

_____

_____

_____

_____

_____

Today's date: _____ Completion Date: _____

Signature: _____

Exercise is the closest thing we'll ever get to the miracle pill that everyone is seeking. It brings weight loss, appetite control, improved mood and self-esteem, an energy kick, and longer life by decreasing the risk of heart disease, diabetes, stroke, osteoporosis, and chronic disabilities.[1]

Cardiorespiratory Endurance Assessment

Objectives

Define cardiorespiratory endurance and understand the benefits of cardiorespiratory endurance training.

Explain the importance of adequate cardiorespiratory endurance in maintaining good health and well-being.

Define aerobic and anaerobic exercise.

Understand the purposes of fitness testing.

Learn the underlying principles that determine oxygen uptake.

Be able to assess cardiorespiratory fitness through five different test protocols (1.5-Mile Run Test, 1.0-Mile Walk Test, Step Test, Astrand-Ryhming Test, and 12-Minute Swim Test).

Learn to interpret cardiorespiratory endurance assessment test results according to health fitness and physical fitness standards.

47

The most important component of physical fitness and best indicator of overall health—**cardiorespiratory endurance**—is being eroded by our lifestyle. Physical activity is no longer a natural part of our existence. Current technological developments have driven most people in developed countries into sedentary lifestyles. For instance, to go to a store only a couple of blocks away, most people drive their automobiles and then spend several minutes driving around the parking lot to find a spot 20 yards closer to the store's entrance. They do not even have to carry out the groceries any more: A youngster working at the store usually takes them out in a cart and places them in the vehicle.

Similarly, during a visit to a multilevel shopping mall, almost everyone chooses to ride the escalators instead of taking the stairs (which tend to be inaccessible). Automobiles, elevators, escalators, telephones, intercoms, remote controls, electric garage door openers—all are modern-day conveniences that minimize the amount of movement and effort required of the human body.

> **Modern-day commodities have reduced the amount of daily physical activity, thus enhancing the deterioration rate of the human body.**

One of the most harmful effects of modern-day technology is an increase in chronic conditions related to a lack of physical activity. These include hypertension, heart disease, chronic low-back pain, and obesity. They are referred to as **hypokinetic diseases**. The term "hypo" means low or little, and "kinetic" implies motion. Lack of adequate physical activity is a fact of modern life that most people can avoid no longer. If we want to enjoy modern-day commodities and still expect to live life to its fullest, however, we must adopt a personalized lifetime exercise program as a part of daily living.

The epitome of physical inactivity is driving around a parking lot for several minutes in search of a parking spot 20 yards closer to the store's entrance.

Advances in modern technology have almost completely eliminated the need for physical activity, significantly enhancing deterioration rate of the human body.

BASIC CARDIORESPIRATORY PHYSIOLOGY: A QUICK SURVEY

Before we begin to overhaul our bodies with an exercise program, we should understand the mechanisms that we propose to alter and survey the ways their performance can be measured.

Cardiorespiratory endurance is a measure of how efficiently our bodies work. The pulmonary (lungs), cardiovascular (heart and blood vessels), and muscular systems work together during cardiorespiratory activities.

As a person breathes, part of the oxygen in the air is taken up by the **alveoli** in the lungs. As blood passes through the alveoli, oxygen is picked up by **hemoglobin** and transported in the blood to the heart. The heart then is responsible for pumping the oxygenated blood through the circulatory system to all organs and tissues of the body.

At the cellular level, oxygen is used to convert food substrates (primarily carbohydrates and fats) through aerobic metabolism into **adenosine triphosphate (ATP)**. This compound provides the energy for physical activity, body functions, and maintenance of a constant internal equilibrium. During physical exertion, more ATP is needed to perform the activity. As a result, the lungs, heart, and blood vessels have to deliver more oxygen to the muscles to supply the required energy.

During prolonged exercise, an individual with a high level of cardiorespiratory endurance is able to deliver the required amount of oxygen to the tissues with relative ease. The cardiorespiratory system of a

Astrand-Ryhming Test

Because of its simplicity and practicality, the Astrand-Ryhming is one of the most popular tests used to estimate maximal oxygen uptake in the laboratory setting. The test is conducted on a bicycle ergometer, and, similar to the Step Test, it requires only submaximal workloads and little time to administer.

The cautions given for the Step Test also apply to the Astrand-Ryhming Test. Nevertheless, because the participant does not have to support his or her own body weight while riding the bicycle, overweight individuals and those with limited joint problems in the lower extremities can take this test.

The bicycle ergometer to be used for this test should allow for the regulation of workloads (see the test procedure in Figure 3.4). Besides the bicycle ergometer, a stopwatch and an additional technician to monitor the heart rate are needed to conduct the test.

The heart rate is taken every minute for 6 minutes. At the end of the test, the heart rate should be in the range given for each workload in Table 3.5, generally between 120 and 170 beats per minute. Table 3.6 contains correction factors for this test.

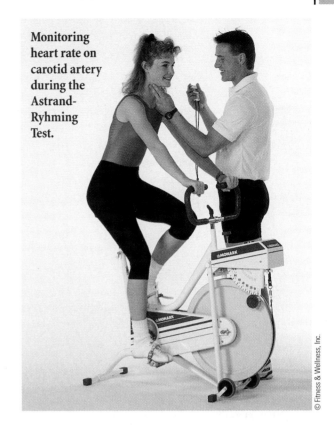

Monitoring heart rate on carotid artery during the Astrand-Ryhming Test.

© Fitness & Wellness, Inc.

FIGURE 3.4   Procedure for the Astrand-Ryhming Test.

1. Adjust the bike seat so the knees are almost completely extended as the foot moves through the bottom of the pedaling stroke.
2. During the test, keep the speed constant at 50 revolutions per minute. Test duration is 6 minutes.
3. Select the appropriate workload for the bike based on age, weight, health, and estimated fitness level. For unconditioned individuals: women, use 300 kpm (kilopounds per meter) or 450 kpm; men, 300 kpm or 600 kpm. For conditioned adults: women, 450 kpm or 600 kpm; men, 600 kpm or 900 kpm.*
4. Ride the bike for 6 minutes and check the heart rate every minute, during the last 10 seconds of each minute. Determine heart rate by recording the time it takes to count 30 pulse beats, and then converting to beats per minute using Table 3.4.
5. Average the final two heart rates (5th and 6th minutes). If these two heart rates are not within 5 beats per minute of each other, continue the test for another few minutes until this is accomplished. If the heart rate continues to climb significantly after the 6th minute, stop the test and rest for 15 to 20 minutes. You then may retest, preferably at a lower workload. The final average heart rate should also fall between the ranges given for each workload in Table 3.5 (for example, men using 300 kpm should average 120 to 140 beats per minute; 600 kpm, 120 to 170).
6. Based on the average heart rate of the final 2 minutes and your workload, look up the maximal oxygen uptake (VO_{2max}) in Table 3.5 (for example, in men at 600 kpm with average heart rate of 145, VO_{2max} = 2.4 liters/minute).
7. Correct VO_{2max} using the correction factors found in Table 3.6 (if VO_{2max} = 2.4 and age 35, correction factor = .870. Multiply 2.4 × .870 and final corrected VO_{2max} = 2.09 liters/minute).
8. To obtain VO_{2max} in ml/kg/min, multiply the VO_{2max} by 1,000 (to convert liters to milliliters) and divide by body weight in kilograms (to obtain kilograms, divide your body weight in pounds by 2.2046).

     Example: Corrected VO_{2max} = 2.09 liters/minute
                 Body weight = 132 pounds or 60 kilograms (132 ÷ 2.2046 = 60)

$$VO_{2max} \text{ in ml/kg/min} = \frac{2.09 \times 1,000}{60} = \frac{2,090}{60} = 34.8 \text{ ml/kg/min}$$

*On the Monarch bicycle ergometer, when riding at a speed of 50 revolutions per minute, a load of 1 kp = 300 kpm, 1.5 kp = 450, 2 kp = 600 kpm, and so forth, with increases of 150 kpm to each half kp.

TABLE 3.4 Conversion of the Time for 30 Heart Beats to Heart Rate Per Minute

Sec.	bpm	Sec.	bpm	Sec.	bpm	Sec.	bpm	Sec.	bpm	Sec.	bpm	Sec.	bpm
22.0	82	19.9	90	17.8	101	15.7	115	13.6	132	11.5	157	9.4	191
21.9	82	19.8	91	17.7	102	15.6	115	13.5	133	11.4	158	9.3	194
21.8	83	19.7	91	17.6	102	15.5	116	13.4	134	11.3	159	9.2	196
21.7	83	19.6	92	17.5	103	15.4	117	13.3	135	11.2	161	9.1	198
21.6	83	19.5	92	17.4	103	15.3	118	13.2	136	11.1	162	9.0	200
21.5	84	19.4	93	17.3	104	15.2	118	13.1	137	11.0	164	8.9	202
21.4	84	19.3	93	17.2	105	15.1	119	13.0	138	10.9	165	8.8	205
21.3	85	19.2	94	17.1	105	15.0	120	12.9	140	10.8	167	8.7	207
21.2	85	19.1	94	17.0	106	14.9	121	12.8	141	10.7	168	8.6	209
21.1	85	19.0	95	16.9	107	14.8	122	12.7	142	10.6	170	8.5	212
21.0	86	18.9	95	16.8	107	14.7	122	12.6	143	10.5	171	8.4	214
20.9	86	18.8	96	16.7	108	14.6	123	12.5	144	10.4	173	8.3	217
20.8	87	18.7	96	16.6	108	14.5	124	12.4	145	10.3	175	8.2	220
20.7	87	18.6	97	16.5	109	14.4	125	12.3	146	10.2	176	8.1	222
20.6	87	18.5	97	16.4	110	14.3	126	12.2	148	10.1	178	8.0	225
20.5	88	18.4	98	16.3	110	14.2	127	12.1	149	10.0	180		
20.4	88	18.3	98	16.2	111	14.1	128	12.0	150	9.9	182		
20.3	89	18.2	99	16.1	112	14.0	129	11.9	151	9.8	184		
20.2	89	18.1	99	16.0	113	13.9	129	11.8	153	9.7	186		
20.1	90	18.0	100	15.9	113	13.8	130	11.7	154	9.6	188		
20.0	90	17.9	101	15.8	114	13.7	131	11.6	155	9.5	189		

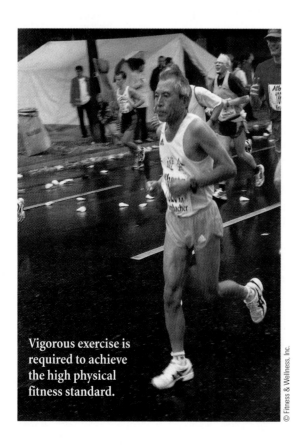

Vigorous exercise is required to achieve the high physical fitness standard.

© Fitness & Wellness, Inc.

© Fitness & Wellness, Inc.

Maximal oxygen uptake can be improved with aerobic exercise.

Photos © Fitness & Wellness, Inc.

TABLE 3.5 Maximal Oxygen Uptake (VO_{2max}) Estimates in l/min for Astrand-Ryhming Test

Heart Rate	MEN kpm						WOMEN kpm				
	300	600	900	1200	1500		300	450	600	750	900
120	2.2	3.4	4.8				2.6	3.4	4.1	4.8	
121	2.2	3.4	4.7				2.5	3.3	4.0	4.8	
122	2.2	3.4	4.6				2.5	3.2	3.9	4.7	
123	2.1	3.4	4.6				2.4	3.1	3.9	4.6	
124	2.1	3.3	4.5	6.0			2.4	3.1	3.8	4.5	
125	2.0	3.2	4.4	5.9			2.3	3.0	3.7	4.4	
126	2.0	3.2	4.4	5.8			2.3	3.0	3.6	4.3	
127	2.0	3.1	4.3	5.7			2.2	2.9	3.5	4.2	
128	2.0	3.1	4.2	5.6			2.2	2.8	3.5	4.2	4.8
129	1.9	3.0	4.2	5.6			2.2	2.8	3.4	4.1	4.8
130	1.9	3.0	4.1	5.5			2.1	2.7	3.4	4.0	4.7
131	1.9	2.9	4.0	5.4			2.1	2.7	3.4	4.0	4.6
132	1.8	2.9	4.0	5.3			2.0	2.7	3.3	3.9	4.5
133	1.8	2.8	3.9	5.3			2.0	2.6	3.2	3.8	4.4
134	1.8	2.8	3.9	5.2			2.0	2.6	3.2	3.8	4.4
135	1.7	2.8	3.8	5.1			2.0	2.6	3.1	3.7	4.3
136	1.7	2.7	3.8	5.0			1.9	2.5	3.1	3.6	4.2
137	1.7	2.7	3.7	5.0			1.9	2.5	3.0	3.6	4.2
138	1.6	2.7	3.7	4.9			1.8	2.4	3.0	3.5	4.1
139	1.6	2.6	3.6	4.8			1.8	2.4	2.9	3.5	4.0
140	1.6	2.6	3.6	4.8	6.0		1.8	2.4	2.8	3.4	4.0
141		2.6	3.5	4.7	5.9		1.8	2.3	2.8	3.4	3.9
142		2.5	3.5	4.6	5.8		1.7	2.3	2.8	3.3	3.9
143		2.5	3.4	4.6	5.7		1.7	2.2	2.7	3.3	3.8
144		2.5	3.4	4.5	5.7		1.7	2.2	2.7	3.2	3.8
145		2.4	3.4	4.5	5.6		1.6	2.2	2.7	3.2	3.7
146		2.4	3.3	4.4	5.6		1.6	2.2	2.6	3.2	3.7
147		2.4	3.3	4.4	5.5		1.6	2.1	2.6	3.1	3.6
148		2.4	3.2	4.3	5.4		1.6	2.1	2.6	3.1	3.6
149		2.3	3.2	4.3	5.4			2.1	2.6	3.0	3.5
150		2.3	3.2	4.2	5.3			2.0	2.5	3.0	3.5
151		2.3	3.1	4.2	5.2			2.0	2.5	3.0	3.4
152		2.3	3.1	4.1	5.2			2.0	2.5	2.9	3.4
153		2.2	3.0	4.1	5.1			2.0	2.4	2.9	3.3
154		2.2	3.0	4.0	5.1			2.0	2.4	2.8	3.3
155		2.2	3.0	4.0	5.0			1.9	2.4	2.8	3.2
156		2.2	2.9	4.0	5.0			1.9	2.3	2.8	3.2
157		2.1	2.9	3.9	4.9			1.9	2.3	2.7	3.2
158		2.1	2.9	3.9	4.9			1.8	2.3	2.7	3.1
159		2.1	2.8	3.8	4.8			1.8	2.2	2.7	3.1
160		2.1	2.8	3.8	4.8			1.8	2.2	2.6	3.0
161		2.0	2.8	3.7	4.7			1.8	2.2	2.6	3.0
162		2.0	2.8	3.7	4.6			1.8	2.2	2.6	3.0
163		2.0	2.8	3.7	4.6			1.7	2.2	2.6	2.9
164		2.0	2.7	3.6	4.5			1.7	2.1	2.5	2.9
165		2.0	2.7	3.6	4.5			1.7	2.1	2.5	2.9
166		1.9	2.7	3.6	4.5			1.7	2.1	2.5	2.8
167		1.9	2.6	3.5	4.4			1.6	2.1	2.4	2.8
168		1.9	2.6	3.5	4.4			1.6	2.0	2.4	2.8
169		1.9	2.6	3.5	4.3			1.6	2.0	2.4	2.8
170		1.8	2.6	3.4	4.3			1.6	2.0	2.4	2.7

SOURCE: From I. Astrand, *Acta Physiologica Scandinavica* 49 (1960). Supplementum 169:45–60.

l/min = liters per minute

TABLE 3.6 Age-Based Correction Factors for Maximal Oxygen Uptake

Age	Correction Factor	Age	Correction Factor	Age	Correction Factor	Age	Correction Factor
14	1.11	27	.974	40	.830	53	.726
15	1.10	28	.961	41	.820	54	.718
16	1.09	29	.948	42	.810	55	.710
17	1.08	30	.935	43	.800	56	.704
18	1.07	31	.922	44	.790	57	.698
19	1.06	32	.909	45	.780	58	.692
20	1.05	33	.896	46	.774	59	.686
21	1.04	34	.883	47	.768	60	.680
22	1.03	35	.870	48	.762	61	.674
23	1.02	36	.862	49	.756	62	.668
24	1.01	37	.854	50	.750	63	.662
25	1.00	38	.846	51	.742	64	.656
26	.987	39	.838	52	.734	65	.650

SOURCE: Adapted from I. Astrand, *Acta Physiologica Scandinavica* 49 (1960). Supplementum 169:45–60.

If you administer the test to older people, good judgment is essential. Low workloads should be used, because if the higher heart rates are reached (around 150 to 170 bpm), these individuals could be working near or at their maximal capacity, making it an unsafe test without adequate medical supervision. When choosing workloads for older people, be sure that final exercise heart rates do not exceed 130 to 140 bpm.

12-Minute Swim Test

Similar to the 1.5-Mile Run test, the 12-Minute Swim Test is considered a maximal exercise test, and the same precautions apply. The objective is to swim as far as possible during the 12-minute test.

A swimming test (Figure 3.5) is practical only for those who are planning to take part in a swimming program. Unlike land-based tests, predicting maximal oxygen uptake through a swimming test is difficult. Differences in skill level, swimming conditioning, and body composition greatly affect the energy requirements (oxygen uptake) of swimming.

SWIMMING TEST LIMITATIONS

Note that results of this test may be affected by several factors: A skilled swimmer is able to swim more efficiently and expend much less energy than an unskilled swimmer. Improper breathing patterns cause premature fatigue. Overweight individuals are more buoyant in the water, and the larger surface area (body size) produces greater friction against movement in the water medium—both affect test

Swimming efficiency requires skill and proper conditioning.

© Fitness & Wellness, Inc.

FIGURE 3.5 Procedure for the 12-Minute Swim Test.

1. Enlist a friend to time the test. The only other requisites are a stopwatch and a swimming pool. Do not attempt to do this test in an unsupervised pool.
2. Warm up by swimming slowly and doing a few mild stretching exercises before taking the test.
3. Start the test and swim as many laps as possible in 12 minutes. Pace yourself throughout the test and do not swim to the point of complete exhaustion.
4. After completing the test, cool down by swimming another 2 or 3 minutes at a slower pace.
5. Determine the total distance you swam during the test, and look up your fitness category in Table 3.7.

results. Lack of specific, appropriate conditioning affects swimming test results as well. A skilled but unconditioned swimmer who is in good cardiorespiratory shape because of a regular jogging program will not perform as effectively in a swimming test. Swimming conditioning is important for adequate performance on this test.

Because of these limitations, maximal oxygen uptake cannot be estimated

> Good cardiorespiratory fitness leads to better health, improved quality of life, and increased longevity.

for a swimming test and the fitness categories given in Table 3.7 are only estimated ratings. This test should be limited to people who cannot perform any of the other tests and whose primary aerobic exercise will be a swimming program. Unskilled and unconditioned swimmers can expect lower cardiorespiratory fitness ratings than those obtained with a land-based test.

TABLE **3.7** 12-Minute Swim Test Fitness Categories

Distance (yards)	Fitness Category
≥700	Excellent
500–700	Good
400–500	Average
200–400	Fair
≤200	Poor

SOURCE: Adapted from K. H. Cooper, *The Aerobics Program for Total Well-Being* (New York: Bantam Books, 1982).

Interpreting Your Maximal Oxygen Uptake Results

After obtaining your maximal oxygen uptake, you can determine your current level of cardiorespiratory fitness by consulting Table 3.8. Locate the maximal oxygen uptake in your age category, and on the top row you will find your present level of cardiorespiratory fitness. For example, a 19-year-old male with a maximal oxygen uptake of 35 ml/kg/min would be classified in the average cardiorespiratory fitness category. Table 3.8 also shows ratings according to health versus physical fitness standards, discussed in Chapter 1, pages 13 and 14. After you initiate your personal cardiorespiratory exercise program (see

TABLE **3.8** Cardiorespiratory Fitness Classification According to Maximal Oxygen Uptake (VO$_{2max}$)

Gender	Age	FITNESS CLASSIFICATION (based on VO$_{2max}$ in ml/kg/min)				
		Poor	Fair	Average	Good	Excellent
Men	<29	<24.9	25–33.9	34–43.9	44–52.9	>53
	30–39	<22.9	23–30.9	31–41.9	42–49.9	>50
	40–49	<19.9	20–26.9	27–38.9	39–44.9	>45
	50–59	<17.9	18–24.9	25–37.9	38–42.9	>43
	60–69	<15.9	16–22.9	23–35.9	36–40.9	>41
	≥70	≤12.9	13–20.9	21–32.9	33–37.9	≥38
Women	<29	<23.9	24–30.9	31–38.9	39–48.9	>49
	30–39	<19.9	20–27.9	28–36.9	37–44.9	>45
	40–49	<16.9	17–24.9	25–34.9	35–41.9	>42
	50–59	<14.9	15–21.9	22–33.9	34–39.9	>40
	60–69	<12.9	13–20.9	21–32.9	33–36.9	>37
	≥70	≤11.9	12–19.9	20–30.9	31–34.9	≥35

High physical fitness standard
Health fitness standard

See the Chapter 1 discussion on health fitness versus physical fitness.

Chapter 4), you may wish to retest yourself periodically to evaluate your progress.

RESTING HEART RATE AND BLOOD PRESSURE ASSESSMENT

Resting Heart Rate

As mentioned previously, heart rate can be obtained by counting your pulse either on the wrist (using the radial artery) or on the neck (using the carotid artery). You may count your pulse for 30 seconds and multiply by 2 or take it for a full minute. The heart rate usually is at its lowest point (resting heart rate) late in the evening after you have been sitting quietly for about half an hour watching a relaxing TV show or reading in bed, or early in the morning just before you get out of bed.

Unless you have a pathological condition, a lower resting heart rate indicates a stronger heart. To adapt to cardiorespiratory or aerobic exercise, the heart enlarges and the muscle gets stronger. A bigger and stronger heart can pump more blood with fewer strokes.

Resting heart rate ratings are given in Table 3.9. Although resting heart rate decreases with training, the extent of **bradycardia** also depends on genetic factors. Although most highly trained athletes have a resting heart rate around 40 beats per minute, occasionally, an aerobic endurance trained athlete exhibits a resting heart rate in the 60s or 70s—even during peak training months of the season. For most individuals, however, the resting heart rate decreases as the level of cardiorespiratory endurance increases.

Resting Blood Pressure

Blood pressure is assessed using a **sphygmomanometer** and a stethoscope. A cuff of the appropriate size

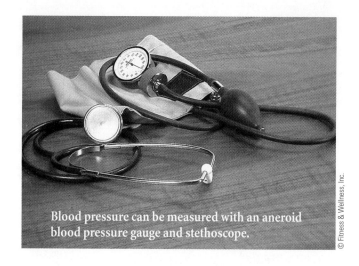

Blood pressure can be measured with an aneroid blood pressure gauge and stethoscope.

© Fitness & Wellness, Inc.

must be used to get accurate readings. Size is determined by the width of the inflatable bladder, which should be about 40% of the circumference of the midpoint of the arm.

Blood pressure usually is measured while the subject is in the sitting position, with the forearm and the manometer at the same level as the heart. At first, the pressure is recorded from each arm, and after that from the arm with the highest reading.

The cuff should be applied approximately an inch above the antecubital space (natural crease of the elbow), with the center of the bladder directly over the medial (inner) surface of the arm. The stethoscope head should be applied firmly, but with little pressure, over the brachial artery in the antecubital space. The subject's arm should be flexed slightly and placed on a flat surface.

The person recording the blood pressure inflates the bladder while feeling the radial pulse to about 30 to 40 mm Hg above the point at which the pulse disappears. This procedure will give the person taking the blood pressure a good indication of how high the bladder should be inflated. The pressure should then be released, the stethoscope applied to the antecubital space, and after a minute the bladder can be reinflated to the pre-determined pressure. The cuff should not be overinflated, because this may cause blood vessel spasm, resulting in higher blood pressure readings. The pressure should then be released at a rate of 2 to 4 mm Hg per second.

As the pressure is released, the recorder listens for the heartbeat and watches the mercury manometer, noting (1) the point at which the pulse becomes audible (**systolic pressure**) and (2) the point at which the sound of the pulse disappears (**diastolic pressure**). The recordings should be expressed as systolic over diastolic pressure—for example, 124/80.

If you take more than one reading, allow the bladder to deflate completely and wait at least one

TABLE **3.9** Resting Heart Rate Ratings	
Heart Rate (beats/minute)	Rating
≤59	Excellent
60–69	Good
70–79	Average
80–89	Fair
≥90	Poor

A mercury gravity manometer can be used to measure blood pressure.

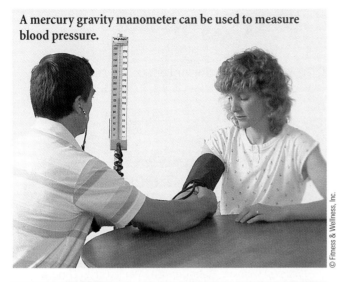

© Fitness & Wellness, Inc.

TABLE **3.10** Blood Pressure Guidelines		
Rating	Systolic	Diastolic
Optimal	≤120	≤80
Normal	121–129	81–84
High Normal	130–139	85–89
Stage 1 Hypertension	140–159	90–99
Stage 2 Hypertension	160–179	100–109
Stage 3 Hypertension	≥180	≥110

SOURCE: National Heart, Lung and Blood Institute.

minute before making the next recording. The recorder should also note whether the pressure was recorded from the left or the right arm. Resting blood pressure risk levels are given in Table 3.10.

In some cases the pulse sounds do not disappear abruptly, but simply become less intense (point of muffling sounds) and still can be heard at a lower pressure (50 or 40 mm Hg)—perhaps all the way down to 0 mm Hg. In this situation, the diastolic pressure is recorded at the point of a clear, definite change in the loudness of the sound (also referred to as "fourth phase"), and at complete disappearance of the sound ("fifth phase") (for example, 120/78/60 or 120/82/0).

Mean Blood Pressure

During a normal resting contraction/relaxation cycle of the heart, the heart spends more time in the relaxation (diastolic) phase than in the contraction (systolic) phase. Accordingly, mean blood pressure (MBP) cannot be computed by taking an average of the systolic (SBP) and diastolic (DBP) blood pressures. The equations used to determine MBP are shown in Figure 3.7.

You can record the results of your resting heart rate and your systolic, diastolic, and mean blood pressure assessments in Figure 3.7. When measuring blood pressure, be aware that a single reading may not be an accurate value because of the various factors (rest, stress, physical activity, food) that can affect blood pressure. Thus, if you are able, ask different people to take several readings at different times of the day, to establish the real values. In Figure 3.8 you can calculate the effects of aerobic activity on resting heart rate; in Figure 3.9, you can interpret the results of your cardiovascular test results.

Key Terms

Bradycardia Slower heart rate than normal.

Sphygmomanometer Device to measure blood pressure; consists of inflatable bladder contained within a cuff and a manometer (either mercury gravity or aneroid) from which the pressure is read.

Systolic blood pressure Pressure exerted by blood against walls of arteries during forceful contraction (systole) of the heart.

Diastolic blood pressure Pressure exerted by the blood against the walls of the arteries during the relaxation phase (diastole) of the heart.

WEB INTERACTIVE

American Council of Exercise Cardiovascular Fitness Facts

This site features information about cardiovascular forms of exercise, including walking, running, jumping rope, swimming, spinning, cross-training, interval training, and others.

http://www.acefitness.org/fitfacts/fitfacts_list.cfm#1

Improving Cardiovascular Health in African Americans

This document, written by the National Heart, Lung, and Blood Institute, provides information on the value of cardiovascular exercise to improving health.

http://www.nhlbi.nih.gov/health/public/heart/other/chdblack/energize.htm

The Cooper Institute for Aerobics Research

The Cooper Institute for Aerobics Research—founded on June 22, 1970 by Kenneth H. Cooper, M.D., M.P.H.—has become widely acclaimed as a leader in preventive medicine research and education. A nonprofit research organization, the Cooper Institute is dedicated to advancing the understanding of the relationship between living habits and health and to providing leadership in implementing these concepts to enhance people's physical and emotional well-being.

http://www.cooperinst.org

INTERACTIVE SITES

Check Your Physical Activity and Heart IQ

This site, sponsored by the National Heart, Lung, and Blood Institute, provides a true/false quiz to allow you to assess what you know about how physical activity affects your heart. The answers provided will uncover exercise myths and give you information on ways to improve your heart health.

http://www.nhlbi.nih.gov/health/public/heart/obesity/pa_iq_ab.htm

Universal Fitness Tester

This site provides a quick and easy 300-second test to determine aerobic fitness and prescribes exercise based on your fitness level.

http://www.aerobictest.com/

n*tes

1. H. Atkinson, "Exercise for Longer Life: The Physician's Perspective," *HealthNews* 7, no. 3 (1997): 3.

Suggested Readings

- American College of Sports Medicine. *Guidelines for Exercise Testing and Prescription*. Philadelphia: Lippincott Williams & Wilkins, 2000.

- Hoeger, W. W. K., and S. A. Hoeger. *Principles and Labs for Fitness & Wellness*. Belmont, CA: Wadsworth/Thomson Learning, 2002.

- McArdle, W. D., F. I. Katch, and V. L. Katch. *Essentials of Exercise Physiology*. Philadelphia: Lippincott Williams & Wilkins, 2000.

- Wilmore, J. H., and D. L. Costill. *Physiology of Sport and Exercise*. Champaign, IL: Human Kinetics, 1999.

FIGURE 3.6 Cardiorespiratory endurance report.

Name: _____ Date: _____

Course: _____ Section: _____ Gender: _____ Age: _____

Date	Test Used	VO$_{2max}$	Fitness Classification

FIGURE 3.7 Resting heart rate and blood pressure results.

Name:_____ Date: _____

Course: _____ Section: _____ Gender:_____ Age:_____

Resting Heart Rate: [   ] Rating: [   ] (see Table 3.9, page 62)

Blood Pressure (see Table 3.10, page 63, for ratings)

	Right arm	Rating	Left arm	Rating
Systolic				
Diastolic				

Mean Blood Pressure Computation

The following equation is used to determine MBP:

$$MBP = DBP + \tfrac{1}{3} PP$$

Where PP = pulse pressure, or the difference between the systolic and diastolic pressures.

1. Compute your MBP using your own blood pressure results:

   PP = [   ] (systolic) − [   ] (diastolic) = [   ] mm Hg

   MBP = [   ] (DBP) + $\dfrac{[\quad] \ (PP)}{3}$ = [   ] mm Hg

2. Determine the MBP for a person with a BP of 130/80 and a second person with a BP of 120/90.

   130/80   120/90

Which subject has the lower MBP?

FIGURE 3.8 Effects of aerobic activity on resting heart rate.

Name:_____ Date: _____

Course: _____ Section: _____ Gender:_____ Age: _____

Using your actual resting heart rate (RHR), compute the total number of times your heart beats each day and each year:

A. Beats per day = RHR (bpm) × 60 (min per hour) × 24 (hours per day) = [____] × 60 × 24 = [____] beats per day

B. Beats per year = heart rate in beats per day (use Item A) × 365 = [____] × 365 = [____] beats per year

If your RHR dropped 20 bpm through an aerobic exercise program, determine the number of beats that your heart would save each year at that lower RHR:

C. Beats per day = RHR (use your current RHR) − 20 × 60 × 24 = ([____] − 20) × 60 × 24 = [____] beats per day

D. Beats per year = heart rate in beats per day (use Item C) × 365 = [____] × 365 = [____] beats per year

E. Number of beats saved per year (B − D) = [____] − [____] = [____] beats saved per year

Assuming that you will reach the average U.S. life expectancy of 80 years for women or 74 for men, determine the additional number of "heart rate life years" available to you if your RHR was 20 bpm lower:

F. Years of life ahead = 80 or 74 − current age = [____] − [____] = [____] years

G. Number of beats saved during the next [____] (use Item F) years of life (E × F) = [____] (E) × [____] (F) = [____] beats saved.

H. Number of heart rate life years based on the lower RHR = [____] (G) ÷ [____] (D) = [____] years

conclusion

Draw conclusions based on your observed resting and activity heart rates and blood pressures. Discuss the importance of a lower resting heart rate to your health and comment on the effects of a higher systolic versus diastolic blood pressure on the mean arterial blood pressure.

_____

_____

_____

_____

_____

FIGURE 3.9   Interpretation of cardiovascular test results.

Name:_____ Date: _____

Course: _____ Section: _____ Gender:_____ Age: _____

In the next few lines, discuss the results of your cardiorespiratory fitness, resting heart rate, and blood pressure assessments. Next, indicate how these results may affect your health, longevity, quality of life, and future lifestyle habits.

© 2002 Steve Satushek/Image Bank/Getty Images

Cardiorespiratory Exercise Prescription

No drug in current or prospective use holds as much promise for sustained health as a lifetime program of physical exercise.[1]

Objectives

Determine readiness to start an exercise program.

Learn the principles that govern cardiorespiratory exercise prescription: intensity, mode, duration, and frequency.

Identify some popular cardiorespiratory activities and their specific benefits.

Learn concepts for preventing and treating injuries.

Learn some ways to foster adherence to exercise.

Describe the relationship between fitness and aging.

Learn to predict oxygen uptake and caloric expenditure from exercise heart rate.

For most people, cardiorespiratory endurance is the single most important of the four components of health-related physical fitness (shown in Figure 1.9, page 12). The exception occurs among older adults, for whom muscular strength is particularly important. A person does need a certain amount of muscular strength and flexibility to engage in normal daily activities. Nevertheless, one can get by without a lot of strength and flexibility, but cannot do without a good cardiorespiratory system.

Aerobic exercise is especially important in preventing coronary heart disease. A poorly conditioned heart, which has to pump more often just to keep a person alive, is subject to more wear and tear than a well-conditioned heart. In situations that place strenuous demands on the heart, such as doing yardwork, lifting heavy objects or weights, or running to catch a bus, the unconditioned heart may not be able to sustain the strain.

Regular participation in cardiorespiratory endurance activities also helps a person achieve and maintain recommended body weight, the fourth component of health-related physical fitness.

> **Cardiorespiratory endurance is the most important component of health-related physical fitness.**

willing to give exercise a try. A low percentage of the U. S. population is truly committed to exercise. Further, surveys indicate that more than half of the people who start exercising drop out during the first 3 to 6 months of the program.[2] Sports psychologists are trying to find out why some people exercise habitually and many do not. All of the benefits of exercise cannot help unless people commit to a lifetime program of physical activity.

The first step is to answer the question Am I ready to start an exercise program? The information provided in Figure 4.1 can help you answer this question. You are evaluated in four categories: mastery (self-control), attitude, health, and commitment. The higher you score in any category—mastery, for example—the more important that reason is for you to exercise.

Scores can vary from 4 to 16. A score of 12 and above is a strong indicator that that factor is important to you, whereas 8 and below is low. If you score below 8 in any category, you might benefit from the tips on how you can become committed to exercise (provided in the section "Getting Started and Adhering to a Lifetime Exercise Program," page 106).

Next, you will have to decide positively that you will try. Using Figure 4.2, you can list the advantages and disadvantages of incorporating exercise into your lifestyle. Your list of advantages may include things such as the following:

- It will make me feel better.
- I will lose weight.
- I will have more energy.
- It will lower my risk for chronic diseases.

READINESS FOR EXERCISE

Before proceeding with the principles of exercise prescription, you should ask yourself if you are

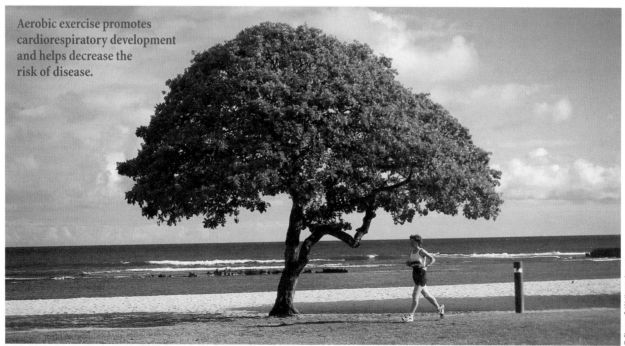

Aerobic exercise promotes cardiorespiratory development and helps decrease the risk of disease.

FIGURE 4.1 Exercise readiness questionnaire.

Name: _Duncan Brown_   Date: _1-24-03_

Course: _LF 117_ Section: _02_ Gender: _M_ Age: _19_

Carefully read each statement and circle the number that best describes your feelings in each statement.
Please be completely honest with your answers.

	Strongly Agree	Mildly Agree	Mildly Disagree	Strongly Disagree
1. I can walk, ride a bike (or a wheelchair), swim, or walk in a shallow pool.	(4)	3	2	1
2. I enjoy exercise.	4	(3)	2	1
3. I believe exercise can lower the risk for disease and premature mortality.	(4)	3	2	1
4. I believe exercise contributes to better health.	(4)	3	2	1
5. I have participated previously in an exercise program.	(4)	3	2	1
6. I have experienced the feeling of being physically fit.	(4)	3	2	1
7. I can envision myself exercising.	(4)	3	2	1
8. I am contemplating an exercise program.	(4)	3	2	1
9. I am willing to stop contemplating and give exercise a try for a few weeks.	(4)	3	2	1
10. I am willing to set aside time at least three times a week for exercise.	(4)	3	2	1
11. I can find a place to exercise (the streets, a park, a YMCA, a health club).	(4)	3	2	1
12. I can find other people who would like to exercise with me.	4	(3)	2	1
13. I will exercise when I am moody, fatigued, and even when the weather is bad.	(4)	3	2	1
14. I am willing to spend a small amount of money for adequate exercise clothing (shoes, shorts, leotards, or swimsuit).	(4)	3	2	1
15. If I have any doubts about my present state of health, I will see a physician before beginning an exercise program.	(4)	3	2	1
16. Exercise will make me feel better and improve my quality of life.	(4)	3	2	1

Scoring Your Test:

This questionnaire allows you to examine your readiness for exercise. You have been evaluated in four categories: mastery (self-control), attitude, health, and commitment. Mastery indicates that you can be in control of your exercise program. Attitude examines your mental disposition toward exercise. Health measures the strength of your convictions about the wellness benefits of exercise. Commitment shows dedication and resolution to carry out the exercise program. Write the number you circled after each statement in the corresponding spaces below. Add the scores on each line to get your totals. Scores can vary from 4 to 16. A score of 12 and above is a strong indicator that that factor is important to you, and 8 and below is low. If you score 12 or more points in each category, your chances of initiating and adhering to an exercise program are good. If you fail to score at least 12 points in three categories, your chances of succeeding at exercise may be slim. You need to be better informed about the benefits of exercise, and a retraining process may be required.

Mastery: 1. _4_ + 5. _4_ + 6. _4_ + 9. _4_ = _16_
Attitude: 2. _3_ + 7. _4_ + 8. _4_ + 13. _4_ = _15_
Health: 3. _4_ + 4. _4_ + 15. _4_ + 16. _4_ = _16_
Commitment: 10. _4_ + 11. _4_ + 12. _3_ + 14. _4_ = _15_

From W. W. K. Hoeger and S. A. Hoeger, *Fitness & Wellness* (Belmont, CA: Wadsworth/Thomson Learning, 2002).

FIGURE 4.2 Behavior modification plan for cardiorespiratory endurance exercise.

Name: _____ Date: _____

Course: _____ Section: _____ Gender: _____ Age: _____

I. Advantages and disadvantages of starting an exercise program

Advantages _____

_____

_____

_____

_____

Disadvantages _____

_____

_____

_____

_____

II. Stage of change for cardiorespiratory exercise

Use Figure 2.4 (page 45) and Table 2.3 (page 43) to identify your current stage of change in regard to participation in a cardiorespiratory endurance exercise program: _____

III. Processes and techniques for change

Identify the processes of change (Table 2.1, page 38) that may help you implement a cardiorespiratory endurance exercise program and list a minimum of three techniques (Table 2.2, page 42) that you will use with each process of change.

Processes for change _____

_____

_____

_____

Techniques for change to be used with each process _____

_____

_____

_____

_____

_____

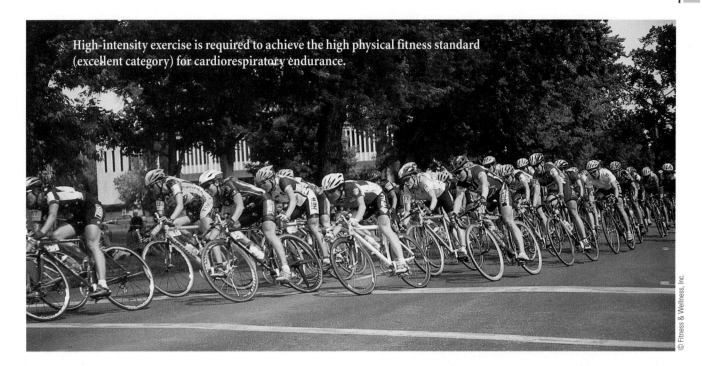

High-intensity exercise is required to achieve the high physical fitness standard (excellent category) for cardiorespiratory endurance.

rate will remain at the same level for about 15 seconds following the aerobic phase of exercise. After 15 seconds, your heart rate will drop rapidly. Do not hesitate to stop during your exercise bout to check your pulse. If the rate is too low, increase the intensity of exercise. If the rate is too high, slow down.

To develop the cardiorespiratory system, you do not have to exercise above the 85 percent rate. From a fitness standpoint, training above this percentage will not give extra benefits and actually may be unsafe for some individuals. Unconditioned people and older adults should train at around the 50 percent rate to discourage potential problems associated with high-intensity exercise.

When determining the training intensity for your own program, you need to consider your personal fitness goals. Individuals who exercise at around the 50 percent training intensity will reap significant health benefits—in particular, improvements in the metabolic profile (see "Health Fitness Standards," page 13). Training at this lower percentage, however, may place you in only the "average" category (see Table 3.8, page 61). Exercising at this lower intensity does lower the risk for cardiovascular mortality (the health fitness standard), but will not allow you to achieve a "good" or "excellent" cardiorespiratory fitness rating (the physical

> **Maintain your heart rate between the 40 and 85 percent training intensities to obtain adequate cardiorespiratory development.**

fitness standard). The latter ratings are obtained by exercising closer to the 85 percent threshold.

Rate of Perceived Exertion

Because many people do not check their heart rate during exercise, an alternative method of prescribing intensity of exercise is according to the **rate of perceived exertion (RPE)** scale. Using the scale in Figure 4.4, a person subjectively rates the perceived exertion or difficulty of exercise when training in the appropriate target zone. The exercise heart rate then is associated with the corresponding RPE value.

For example, if the training intensity requires a heart rate between 150 and 170 bpm, the person may associate this with training between "hard" and "very hard." Some individuals perceive less exertion than others when training in the correct zone. Therefore, you have to associate your own inner perception of the task with the phrases given on the scale. You then may proceed to exercise at that rate of perceived exertion.

The numbers on the scale can also be used in reference to exercise heart rates. If you multiply each number by 10, it will approximate the exercise heart rate at the perceived exertion phase. For example, when you are exercising "somewhat hard," your heart rate will be around 130 bpm (13 × 10). When

KeyTerms

Rate of perceived exertion (RPE) A perception scale to monitor or interpret the intensity of aerobic exercise.

FIGURE 4.4 Rate of perceived exertion (RPE) scale.

6	
7	Very, very light
8	
9	Very light
10	
11	Fairly light
12	
13	Somewhat hard
14	
15	Hard
16	
17	Very Hard
18	
19	Very, very hard
20	

SOURCE: From G. Borg, "Perceived Exertion: A Note on History and Methods," *Medicine and Science in Sports and Exercise*, 5 (1983): 90–93.

you exercise "hard," the heart rate will be about 150 bpm.

You must be sure to cross-check your target zone with your perceived exertion during the first weeks of your exercise program. To help you develop this association, you should regularly keep a record of your activities using the form provided in Figure 4.11 (page 109). After several weeks of training, you should be able to predict your exercise heart rate just by your own perceived exertion of the intensity of exercise.

Whether you monitor the intensity of exercise by checking your pulse or through rate of perceived exertion, you should be aware that changes in normal exercise conditions will affect the training zone. For example, exercising on a hot, humid day or at high altitude increases the heart rate response to a given task, requiring adjustments in the intensity of your exercise.

Mode of Exercise

The **mode** of exercise that develops the cardiorespiratory system has to be aerobic in nature. Once you have established your cardiorespiratory training zone, any activity or combination of activities that will get your heart rate up to that training zone and keep it there for as long as you exercise will give you adequate

development. Examples of these activities are walking, jogging, aerobics, swimming, water aerobics, cross-country skiing, rope skipping, cycling, racquetball, stair climbing, and stationary running or cycling.

The activity you choose should be based on your personal preferences, what you most enjoy doing, and your physical limitations. Low-impact activities greatly reduce the risk for injuries. Most injuries to beginners result from high-impact activities. General strength conditioning (see Chapter 5) is also recommended prior to initiating an aerobic exercise program for individuals who have been inactive. Strength conditioning can significantly reduce the incidence of injuries. The amount of strength or flexibility you develop through various activities differs, so your goals should help determine your choice of activity.

Whatever exercise you choose, the heart doesn't know whether you are walking, swimming, or cycling. All the heart knows is that it has to pump at a certain rate, and as long as that rate is in the desired range, your cardiorespiratory fitness will improve. From a health fitness point of view, training in the lower end of the cardiorespiratory zone will yield optimal health benefits. The closer the heart rate is to the higher end of the cardiorespiratory training zone, however, the greater will be the improvements in maximal oxygen uptake (high physical fitness).

Aerobic exercise has to involve the major muscle groups of the body, and it has to be rhythmic and continuous. As the amount of muscle mass involved during exercise increases, so does the resulting cardiorespiratory development.

© Aero-belt Aerobics

Combined upper-/lower-body exercise is designed to provide resistance to the arms during lower-body physical activity, thereby increasing the person's oxygen consumption, energy expenditure, and development of upper-body strength and endurance during aerobic exercise.

Cross-country skiing is regarded as the prime exercise modality for aerobic development. This activity uses several major muscle groups, because it requires both upper- and lower-body work and therefore uses more oxygen and energy (calories) than most other aerobic activities do. Limitations of this activity, of course, are the lack of year-round conditions for skiing and the cost of cross-country skiing simulation equipment.

A modality of aerobic activity that has gained popularity in recent years is combined upper-lower-body exercise. The objective of this type of activity is to add resistance to the arms during lower-body aerobic exercise, thereby increasing the person's oxygen consumption, energy expenditure, and upper-body strength and endurance development. Examples of these activities are walking and jogging with dumbbells, wrist weights, poles, and resistive belts (belts with elastic or retractable cords that are either handheld or attached to the wrists—these belts can also be used during aerobics routines).

The physiological responses of combined upper/lower-body activity while wearing a belt with an elastic cord that slides freely through the belt have been investigated.[7] Increases in heart rate, oxygen uptake, and caloric expenditure ranged from 32 to 54

> The more muscle mass that is involved during aerobic activity, the higher the oxygen and energy demands of the activity.

percent in regular walking (4.0 and 4.2 mph), jogging (6.0 mph), and step aerobics versus walking, jogging, and step aerobics using the belt (see Figure 4.5).

People who already exercise at high intensities need to realize that adding upper-body activity may require them to decrease the rate of lower-body work. For example, a runner who already trains at 85 percent intensity may have to decrease the pace when running with an exercise belt, because few people are able to sustain prolonged aerobic exercise at an intensity above 85 percent.

Combined upper-/lower-body exercise is particularly useful for people who have functional limitations or injuries that keep them from doing a high-impact activity such as jogging. By adding upper-body resistance, they can achieve high training intensities during a low-impact activity such as walking and low-impact aerobics. A word of caution: Combined upper-/lower-body activity may cause a slight increase in blood pressure during exercise. Although this increase in blood pressure usually does not pose

KeyTerms

Mode Form of exercise.

FIGURE 4.5 Oxygen uptake, heart rate, and energy expenditure response to walking, jogging, and step aerobics with and without an exercise belt with elastic cords providing resistance to the arms.

- Walking (4.0 mph) → Walking with exercise belt (4.0 mph)
- Jogging (6.0 mph) → Jogging with exercise belt (6.0 mph)
- Step aerobics → Step aerobics with exercise belt

a problem in people with normal blood pressure, individuals with elevated pressure should seek the advice of a physician before they participate in combined upper- /lower-body exercise.

Duration of Exercise

The general recommendation is that a person train between 20 and 60 minutes per session. The duration is based on how intensely a person trains. If the training is done at around 85 percent, 20 minutes are sufficient. At 50 percent intensity, the person should train between 30 and 60 minutes. As mentioned under "Intensity of Exercise" above, unconditioned people and older adults should train at lower percentages; therefore, the activity should be carried out over a longer time.

Although most experts recommend 20 to 30 minutes of aerobic exercise per session, accumulating 30 minutes or more of moderate-intensity physical activity throughout the day can provide substantial health benefits.[8] Three 10-minute exercise sessions per day (separated by at least 4 hours), at approximately 70 percent of maximal heart rate, also produce training benefits.[9] Although the increases in maximal oxygen uptake with the latter program were not as large (57 percent) as those found in a group performing a single continuous 30-minute bout of exercise per day, the researchers concluded that moderate-intensity exercise training, conducted for 10 minutes, three times per day, benefits the cardiorespiratory system significantly.

Results of this study are meaningful because people often mention lack of time as the reason for not taking part in an exercise program. Many think they have to exercise at least 20 continuous minutes to get any benefits at all. Even though 20 to 30 minutes are ideal, short, intermittent exercise bouts also benefit the cardiorespiratory system.

Exercise sessions should always be preceded by a 5-minute **warm-up** and followed by a 5-minute **cool-down** period (see Figure 4.3). The warm-up should consist of general calisthenics, stretching exercises, or exercising at a lower intensity level than the actual target zone. In the cool-down, the intensity of exercise is decreased gradually. Stopping abruptly causes blood to pool in the exercised body parts, diminishing the return of blood to the heart. Less blood return can cause dizziness and faintness or even bring on cardiac abnormalities.

Frequency of Exercise

When you start an exercise program, a **frequency** of three to five 20- to 30-minute training sessions per

week is recommended to improve maximal oxygen uptake. When training is conducted more than 5 days a week, further improvements are minimal.

For individuals on a weight-loss program, 45- to 60-minute exercise sessions of low-to-moderate intensity, conducted 5 to 6 days per week, are recommended. Longer exercise sessions increase caloric expenditure for faster weight reduction (see "Exercise: The Key to Weight Loss and Weight Maintenance," page 248). Three 20- to 30-minute training sessions per week, on nonconsecutive days, will maintain cardiorespiratory fitness as long as the heart rate is in the appropriate target zone. A summary of the cardiorespiratory exercise prescription guidelines according to the American College of Sports Medicine is provided in Figure 4.6.

Although three exercise sessions per week will maintain cardiorespiratory fitness, the importance of regular physical activity in preventing disease and enhancing quality of life was pointed out clearly in 1993 at a news briefing held at the National Press Club in Washington, DC. At this briefing, the American College of Sports Medicine and the U.S. Centers for Disease Control and Prevention, in conjunction with the President's Council on Physical Fitness and Sports, set forth recommendations on the types of physical activity needed to maintain and promote health.[10] This summary statement advocates at least 30 minutes of moderate-intensity physical activity almost daily.

FIGURE 4.6 Cardiorespiratory exercise prescription guidelines.

Activity:	Aerobic (examples: walking, jogging, cycling, swimming, aerobics, racquetball, soccer, stair climbing)
Intensity:	40/50%–85% of heart rate reserve
Duration:	20–60 minutes of continuous aerobic activity
Frequency:	3 to 5 days per week

Based on the recommended quantity and quality of exercise for developing and maintaining cardiorespiratory and muscular fitness and flexibility in healthy adults by the American College of Sports Medicine, *Medical Science Sports Exercise*, 30 (1998): 975–991.

Key Terms

Warm-up Starting a workout slowly.

Cool-down Tapering off an exercise session slowly.

Frequency How often a person engages in an exercise session.

FIGURE 4.7 Cardiorespiratory exercise prescription form.

Name: _____ Date: _____

Course: _____ Section: _____ Gender:_____ Age: _____

I. Intensity of Exercise

1. Estimate your own maximal heart rate (MHR)

MHR = 220 minus age (220 − age)

MHR = 220 − [   ] = [   ] bpm

2. Resting Heart Rate (RHR) = [   ] bpm

3. Heart Rate Reserve (HRR) = MHR − RHR

HRR = [   ] − [   ] = [   ] beats

4. Training Intensities (TI) = HRR × TI + RHR

40 Percent TI = [   ] × .40 + [   ] = [   ] bpm

50 Percent TI = [   ] × .50 + [   ] = [   ] bpm

60 percent TI = [   ] × .60 + [   ] = [   ] bpm

85 Percent TI = [   ] × .85 + [   ] = [   ] bpm

5. Cardiorespiratory Training Zone. The optimum cardiorespiratory training zone is found between the 60% and 85% training intensities. Older adults, individuals who have been physically inactive, or people in the poor or fair cardiorespiratory fitness categories, however, should follow a 40% to 50% training intensity during the first few weeks of the exercise program.

Cardiorespiratory Training Zone: [   ] (60% TI) to [   ] (85% TI)

Rate of Perceived Exertion (see Figure 4.4, page 76): [   ] to [   ]

II. Mode of Exercise

Select any activity or combination of activities that you enjoy doing. The activity has to be continuous in nature and must get your heart rate up to the cardiorespiratory training zone and keep it there for as long as you exercise. Indicate your preferred mode(s) of exercise:

1. [   ]   2. [   ]   3. [   ]

4. [   ]   5. [   ]   6. [   ]

(continued)

(Figure 4.7 Cardiorespiratory exercise prescription form—continued)

III. Cardiorespiratory Exercise Program

The following is your weekly program for development of cardiorespiratory endurance. If you are in the average, good, or excellent fitness category, you may start at week 5. After completing this 12-week program, for you to maintain your fitness level, you should exercise in the 60% to 85% training zone for about 20 to 30 minutes, a minimum of three times per week, on nonconsecutive days. You should also recompute your target zone periodically, because you will experience a significant reduction in resting heart rate with aerobic training (approximately 10 to 20 beats in about 8 to 12 weeks).

Week	Duration (min)	Frequency	Training Intensity	10-Sec Pulse Count*
1	15	3	Between 40% and 50%	
2	15	4	Between 40% and 50%	
3	20	4	Between 40% and 50%	▢ beats
4	20	5	Between 40% and 50%	
5	20	4	Between 50% and 60%	
6	20	5	Between 50% and 60%	
7	30	4	Between 50% and 60%	▢ beats
8	30	5	Between 50% and 60%	
9	30	4	Between 60% and 85%	
10	30	5	Between 60% and 85%	
11	30–40	5	Between 60% and 85%	▢ to ▢ beats
12	30–40	5	Between 60% and 85%	

*Fill out your own 10-second pulse count under this column.

conclusion

Briefly state your experiences regarding aerobic activities. Which activities do you prefer and how will you use these activities to reach and maintain your fitness goals?

_____

_____

_____

_____

_____

_____

_____

_____

_____

_____

_____

_____

FIGURE **4.8** Sample computerized exercise prescription.

Personalized Cardiorespiratory Exercise Prescription
Fitness & Wellness Series
Wadsworth Group / Thomson Learning

Jane Doe   August 14, 2001
Maximal heart rate: 170 bpm   Resting heart rate: 68 bpm
Present cardiorespiratory fitness level: Fair   Age: 50

The following is your personal program for cardiorespiratory fitness development and maintenance. If you have been exercising regularly and you are in the average or good category, you may start at week five. If you are in the excellent category, you can start at week ten.

Week	Time (min.)	Frequency (per week)	Training Intensity (beats per minute)	Pulse (10 sec. count)
1	15	3	109 - 119	18 - 20 beats
2	15	4	109 - 119	18 - 20 beats
3	20	4	109 - 119	18 - 20 beats
4	25	4	109 - 119	18 - 20 beats
5	30	4	109 - 119	18 - 20 beats
6	20	4	119 - 129	20 - 22 beats
7	25	4	119 - 129	20 - 22 beats
8	30	4	119 - 129	20 - 22 beats
9	20	5	119 - 129	20 - 22 beats
10	25	5	119 - 129	20 - 22 beats
11	30	5	119 - 129	20 - 22 beats
12	20	4	129 - 155	22 - 26 beats
13	25	4	129 - 155	22 - 26 beats
14	30	4	129 - 155	22 - 26 beats
15	30	5	129 - 155	22 - 26 beats
16	30-40	5	129 - 155	22 - 26 beats

You may participate in any combination of activities which are aerobic and continuous in nature such as walking, jogging, swimming, cross country skiing, aerobelt exercise, rope skipping, cycling, aerobic dancing, racquetball, stair climbing, stationary running or cycling, etc. As long as the heart rate reaches the desired rate, and it stays at that level for the period of time indicated, the cardiorespiratory system will improve.

Following the sixteen week program, in order to maintain your fitness level, you should exercise between 129 and 155 bpm for about 30 minutes, a minimum of three times per week on non-consecutive days. When you exercise, allow about 5 minutes for a gradual warm-up period and another 5 for gradual cool-down. Also, when you check your exercise heart rate, only count your pulse for 10 seconds (start counting with 0) and then refer to the above 10 second pulse count. You may also multiply by 6 to obtain your rate in beats per minute.

Good cardiorespiratory fitness will greatly contribute toward the enhancement and maintenance of good health. It is especially important in the prevention of cardiovascular disease. We encourage you to be persistent in your exercise program and to participate regularly.

FIGURE **4.9**   Sample exercise record using the exercise log (EXLOG) computer software option.

Exercise Log
Fitness & Wellness Series
Wadsworth Group / Thomson Learning

Jim R. Johnson

Date	Exercise	Body Weight (lbs)	Heart Rate (bpm)	Duration (min)	Distance (miles)	Calories Burned
10/01/2001	Walking (4.5 mph)	179.5	120	30	2.0	242
	Running (11 min/mile)	179.5	156	34	3.0	427
10/03/2001	Running (11 min/mile)	179.0	156	33	3.0	413
10/05/2001	Tennis/Moderate	179.0	126	60		483
	Running (11 min/mile)	179.0	162	38	3.5	476
10/07/2001	Running (8.5 min/mile)	178.5	180	12	1.5	193
10/09/2001	Water Aerobics/Vigorous	178.0	156	45		561
10/11/2001	Running (8.5 min/mile)	177.5	174	28	3.0	447
10/12/2001	Racquetball	177.0	144	60		690
	Swimming (25 yds/min)	177.0	138	25	0.5	177
10/14/2001	Running (8.5 min/mile)	176.0	174	29	3.0	459
10/16/2001	Aero-belt Step-Aerobics	176.0	144	45		832
	Calisthenics	176.0	102	15		87
10/18/2001	Running (8.5 min/mile)	175.5	174	26	3.0	411
10/19/2001	Soccer	175.0	136	60		620
	Golf	175.0	102	90		473
10/21/2001	Running (7 min/mile)	175.0	172	18	2.5	321
10/23/2001	Step-Aerobics	174.5	144	60		733
10/24/2001	Bowling	175.0	102	90		473
10/25/2001	Basketball/Moderate	174.5	150	60		482
	Dance/Moderate	174.5	102	120		628
10/26/2001	Running (7 min/mile)	174.0	168	30	4.0	532
	Skiing/Downhill	174.0	114	60		626
10/28/2001	Running (7 min/mile)	174.0	168	30	4.0	532
	Strength Training	174.0	138	60		522
10/30/2001	Stationary Cycling/Vig.	173.5	156	60		729

Totals

				Duration	Distance	Calories
Totals				20 hr 18 min	33.0	12569

Average per exercise session
Number of exercise sessions: 26

Body Weight	Heart Rate	Duration	Distance	Calories
176.2	145	47	2.8	483

Average per day exercised
Number of days exercised: 18

Duration	Calories
68	698

Distance summary

Total miles run:	30.5
Total miles walked:	2.0
Total miles swum:	0.5

This routine has been promoted as an effective way to improve health.

These recommendations were subsequently upheld by the U.S. Surgeon General's 1996 Report on Physical Activity and Health[11] and later in the 2000 Dietary Guidelines for Americans.[12] The Surgeon General's report states that people can improve their health and quality of life substantially by including moderate amounts of physical activity on most, preferably all, days of the week. Further, it states that no one, including older adults, is too old to enjoy the benefits of regular physical activity.

If you want to enjoy better health and fitness, physical activity must be pursued on a regular basis. Many of the benefits of exercise and activity diminish within 2 weeks of substantially decreased physical activity. These benefits are completely lost within 2 to 8 months of inactivity.[13]

Ideally, a person should engage in physical activity six to seven times per week. Based on the above discussion, to reap both the physical-fitness and health-fitness benefits of exercise, a person needs to exercise a minimum of three times per week in the appropriate target zone for high fitness maintenance and three to four additional times per week in moderate-intensity activities. All exercise/activity sessions should last about 30 minutes.

> **Most of the health-related benefits of exercise are relatively short-term, so people should think of exercise as medication and take it on a daily basis.**
> —Dr. William Haskell
> Stanford University

CHOICES OF AEROBIC ACTIVITIES

One of the fun aspects of exercise is that you can choose from many different activities to promote fitness. You may select one or a combination of activities for your program. The choice should be based on personal enjoyment, convenience, and availability.

Most people who exercise pick and adhere to a single mode, such as walking, swimming, or jogging. No single activity develops total fitness. Many activities contribute to cardiorespiratory development. The extent of contribution to other fitness components is limited, though, and varies among the activities. For total fitness, aerobic activities should be supplemented with strength and flexibility exercises. **Cross-training**

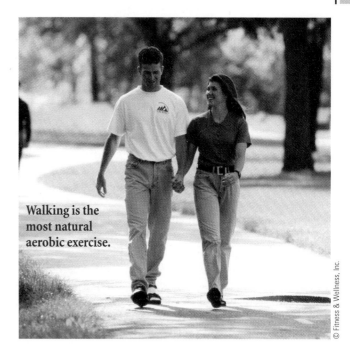

Walking is the most natural aerobic exercise.

© Fitness & Wellness, Inc.

can add enjoyment to the program, decrease the risk of incurring injuries from overuse, and keep exercise from becoming monotonous.

Exercise sessions should be convenient. To enjoy exercise, be sure to select a time when you will not be rushed. A nearby location is recommended. People do not enjoy driving across town to get to the gym, health club, track, or pool. If parking is a problem, you may get discouraged quickly and quit. All of these factors are used as excuses not to stick to an exercise program.

Walking

The most natural, easiest, safest, and least expensive form of aerobic exercise is walking. For years many fitness practitioners believed that walking was not vigorous enough to improve cardiorespiratory functioning. Now studies have established that brisk walking at speeds of 4 miles per hour or faster improves cardiorespiratory fitness. From a health-fitness viewpoint, a regular walking program can prolong life significantly (see the discussion of cardiovascular disease in Chapter 10). Although walking takes longer than jogging, the caloric cost of brisk walking is only about 10 percent lower than jogging the same distance.

Walking is perhaps the best activity to start a conditioning program for the cardiorespiratory system. Inactive people should start with 1-mile walks four

KeyTerms

Cross-training A combination of aerobic activities that contribute to overall fitness.

or five times per week. Walk times can be increased gradually by 5 minutes each week. Following 3 to 4 weeks of conditioning, a person should be able to walk 2 miles at a 4-mile-per-hour pace, five times per week. Greater aerobic benefits accrue from walking longer and swinging the arms faster than normal. Light hand weights, a backpack (4 to 6 pounds), or the use of an upper-arm resistive belt add to the intensity of walking. Because of the additional load on the cardiorespiratory system, extra weights or loads are not recommended for people who have cardiovascular disease.

Walking in water (chest-deep level) is another excellent form of aerobic activity, particularly for people with leg and back problems. Because of the buoyancy that water provides, individuals submerged in water to armpit level weigh only about 10 to 20 percent of their weight outside the water. The resistance the water creates as a person walks in the pool makes the intensity quite high, providing an excellent cardiorespiratory workout.

Hiking

Hiking is an excellent activity for the entire family, especially during the summer and on summer vacations. Many people feel guilty if they are unable to continue their exercise routine during vacations. The intensity of hiking over uneven terrain is greater than walking. An 8-hour hike can burn as many calories as a 20-mile walk or jog.

Another benefit of hiking is the relaxing effects of beautiful scenery. This is an ideal activity for highly stressed people who live near woods and hills. A rough day at the office can be forgotten quickly in the peacefulness and beauty of the outdoors.

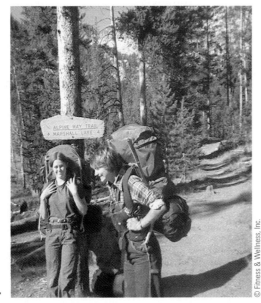

An 8-hour hike can burn as many calories as a 20-mile walk or jog.

Jogging

Jogging is the most popular form of aerobic exercise. Next to walking, it is one of the most accessible forms of exercise. A person can find places to jog almost everywhere. The lone requirement to prevent injuries is a good pair of jogging shoes.

The popularity of jogging in the United States started shortly after publication of Dr. Kenneth Cooper's first aerobics book in 1968. Jim Fixx's *Complete Book of Running* in the mid-1970s further contributed to the phenomenal growth of jogging as the predominant fitness activity in the United States.

Jogging three to five times a week is one of the fastest ways to improve cardiorespiratory fitness. The risk of injury, however, especially in beginners, is greater with jogging than walking. For proper conditioning, jogging programs should start with 1 to 2 weeks of walking. As fitness improves, walking and jogging can be combined, gradually increasing the jogging segment until it composes the full 20 to 30 minutes.

Many people abuse this activity. People run too fast and too long. Some joggers think that if a little is good, more is better. Not so with cardiorespiratory endurance. As indicated under "Frequency of Exercise" earlier in this chapter, the aerobic benefit of training more than 30 minutes five times per week is minimal. Furthermore, the risk of injury increases greatly as speed (running instead of jogging) and mileage go up. Jogging approximately 15 miles per week is sufficient to reach an excellent level of cardiorespiratory fitness.

A good pair of shoes is a must for joggers. Many foot, knee, and leg problems originate from improperly fitting or worn-out shoes. A good pair of shoes should offer good lateral stability and not lean to either side when placed on a flat surface. The shoe also should bend at the ball of the foot, not at midfoot. Worn-out shoes should be replaced. After 500 miles of use, jogging shoes lose about a third of their shock absorption capabilities. If you suddenly have problems, check your shoes first. It may be time for a new pair. Guidelines for choosing the right jogging shoe are provided in Figure 4.10.

For safety reasons, joggers should stay away from high-speed roads, not wear headphones, and always run (or walk) against the traffic so they will be able to see all oncoming traffic. At night, reflective clothing or fluorescent material should be worn on different parts of the body. Carrying a flashlight is even better,

The aerobic benefit of training more than 30 minutes five times per week is minimal.

FIGURE 4.10 What to look for in a good pair of shoes.

CHOOSING THE RIGHT SHOE

TONGUE
Should be well-padded to prevent irritation of the top of the foot.

COLLAR
About an inch-high rim of soft material to protect the heel cord.

ACHILLES PAD
Should be low and soft enough to prevent irritation to the tendon or blistering of the skin.

UPPER
Leather, nylon mesh or other breatheable materials are best for ventilation.

FIRM HEEL COUNTER
Durable plastic cup placed in the heel of the shoe to help stability.

FLARED HEEL
Added for support.

EXTERNAL STABILIZER
Supports the heel counter and offers extra stability.

TOE BOX
Allow enough space for the toes to fit comfortably.

Flexibility under forefoot.

OUTSOLE
Solid or carbon rubber outsoles are best for running, walking, and cross-training traction.

MIDSOLE
Principal shock-absorbing feature of the shoe. Usually becomes worn out after 500 miles of use. Multi-density EVA or polyurethane midsoles offer best support and durability.

because motorists can see the light from a greater distance than they can see the reflective material.

DEEP-WATER RUNNING

An alternative form of jogging, especially for injured people, those with chronic back problems, and overweight individuals, is deep-water running—running in place while treading water. Deep-water running is almost as strenuous as jogging on land. In deep-water running, the running motions used on land are accentuated by pumping the arms and legs hard through a full range of motion. The participant usually wears a flotation vest to help maintain the body in an upright position. Many elite athletes train frequently in water to lessen the wear and tear on the body caused by long-distance running. These athletes have been able to maintain high oxygen uptake values through rigorous water running programs.

Aerobics

Aerobics, formerly known as **aerobic dance**, is thought to be the most common fitness activity for women in the United States. Routines consist of a combination of stepping, walking, jogging, skipping, kicking, and arm-swinging movements performed to

music. It is a fun way to exercise and promote cardiorespiratory development at the same time.

Aerobics was developed initially in the early 1970s by Jacki Sorenson as a fitness program for Air Force wives in Puerto Rico. At first considered a fad, it now is a legitimate fitness activity with more than 20 million participants of all ages. Aerobics programs now regularly appear in school curricula, health clubs, and recreational facilities.

High-impact aerobics (HIA) is the traditional form of aerobics. The movements exert a great amount of vertical force on the feet as they contact the floor. Proper leg conditioning through other forms of weight-bearing aerobic exercises (brisk walking and jogging), as well as strength training, are recommended prior to participating in high-impact aerobics.

High-impact aerobics is an intense activity, and it produces the highest rate of aerobics injuries. Shin splints, stress fractures, low-back pain, and tendinitis

Key Terms

Aerobic dance A series of exercise routines performed to music.

High-impact aerobics Exercises incorporating movements in which both feet are off the ground at the same time momentarily.

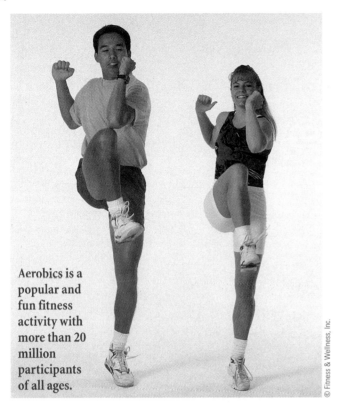

Aerobics is a popular and fun fitness activity with more than 20 million participants of all ages.

© Fitness & Wellness, Inc.

are all too common in HIA enthusiasts. These injuries are caused by the constant impact of the feet on firm surfaces. As a result, several alternative forms of aerobics have been developed.

In **low-impact aerobics** (LIA) the impact is less because one foot always remains in contact with the floor. The recommended exercise intensity is therefore more difficult to maintain than HIA. To help elevate the exercise heart rate, all arm movements and weight-bearing actions that lower the center of gravity should be accentuated. Sustained movement throughout the program is also crucial to keep the heart rate in the target cardiorespiratory zone.

Step aerobics (SA) is an activity in which participants step up and down from a bench, which ranges in height from 2 to 10 inches. Step aerobics adds another dimension to the aerobics program. As noted previously, variety adds enjoyment to aerobic workouts.

Step aerobics is viewed as a high-intensity but low-impact activity. The intensity of the activity can be controlled easily by the height of the bench. Aerobic benches or plates, commercially available, can be stacked together safely to adjust the height of the steps. Beginners are encouraged to use the lowest step height and then advance gradually to a higher bench to decrease the risk of injury. Even though one foot is always in contact with the floor or bench during step aerobics, this activity is not recommended for individuals with ankle, knee, or hip problems.

Other forms of aerobics include a combination of HIA and LIA, as well as moderate-impact aerobics (MIA). The latter incorporates **plyometric training**, a type of training frequently used by jumpers (high, long, and triple jumpers) and athletes in sports that require quick jumping ability, such as basketball and gymnastics. With moderate-impact aerobics, one foot is in contact with the ground most of the time. Plyometric training participants, however, focus on quick, forceful recovery from all lower-body flexion actions. This is done by extending the hip, knee, and ankle joints quickly without allowing the foot (or feet) to leave the ground. These quick movements make the exercise intensity of moderate-impact aerobics quite high.

Swimming

Swimming is another excellent form of aerobic exercise because it uses almost all of the major muscle groups in the body, thereby providing a good training stimulus for the heart and lungs. Swimming is a great exercise option for individuals who cannot jog or walk for extended periods.

Compared with other activities, the risk of injuries from swimming is low. The aquatic medium helps to support the body, taking pressure off bones and joints in the lower extremities and the back.

Maximal heart rates during swimming are approximately 10 to 13 beats per minute (bpm) lower than during running.[14] The horizontal position of the body is thought to aid blood flow distribution throughout the body, decreasing the demand on the cardiorespiratory system. Cool water temperatures and direct contact with the water seem to help dissipate body heat more efficiently, further decreasing the strain on the heart.

Some exercise specialists recommend that this difference in maximal heart rate (10 to 13 bpm) be subtracted prior to determining cardiorespiratory training intensities. For example, the estimated maximal swimming heart rate for a 20-year old would be approximately 187 bpm ($220 - 20 = 200$; $200 - 13 = 187$).

Studies are inconclusive as to whether this decrease in heart rate in water also occurs at submaximal intensities below 70 percent of maximal heart rate.[15] Further, research comparing physiologic differences between self-paced treadmill running and self-paced water aerobics exercise showed that individuals work at lower intensities in water.[16] One can argue, therefore, that apparently healthy people are able to achieve higher work capacities during land-based activities; therefore, the same exercise intensity can be given for water activities. If a lower intensity is used, training benefits of swimming may be less.

To produce better training benefits during swimming, the swimmer should minimize gliding periods such as those in the breast stroke and side stroke. Achieving proper training intensities with these strokes is difficult. The forward crawl is recommended for better aerobic results.

Overweight individuals need to swim fast enough to achieve an adequate training intensity. Excessive body fat makes the body more buoyant, and often the tendency is to just float along. This may be good for reducing stress and relaxing, but it does not greatly increase caloric expenditure to aid with weight loss. Walking or jogging in waist- or armpit-deep water are better choices for overweight individuals who cannot walk or jog on land for a long time.

Swimming participants need to remember the principle of specificity of training, which dictates that cardiorespiratory improvements cannot be measured adequately with a land-based walk/jog test. Most of the work with swimming is done by the upper body musculature. Although the heart's ability to pump more blood improves significantly with any type of aerobic activity, the primary increase in the cells' ability to utilize oxygen (VO_2 or oxygen uptake) with swimming occurs in the upper body, and not the lower extremities. Therefore, fitness improvements with swimming are best measured by comparing changes in distances a person swims in a given time, say, 10 minutes.

Water Aerobics

Water aerobics is a relatively new form of exercise that is fun and safe for people of all ages. Besides developing fitness, it provides an opportunity for socialization and fun in a comfortable and refreshing setting.

Water aerobics incorporates a combination of rhythmic arm and leg actions performed in a vertical position while submerged in waist- to armpit-deep water. The vigorous limb movements against the water's resistance during water aerobics provide the training stimuli for cardiorespiratory development.

The popularity of water aerobics as an exercise modality to develop the cardiorespiratory system has been on the rise in recent years. Its increase in popularity can be attributed to several factors:

1. Water buoyancy reduces weight-bearing stress on joints and thereby lessens the risk for injuries.

2. Water aerobics is a more feasible type of exercise for overweight individuals and those with arthritic conditions who may not be able to participate in

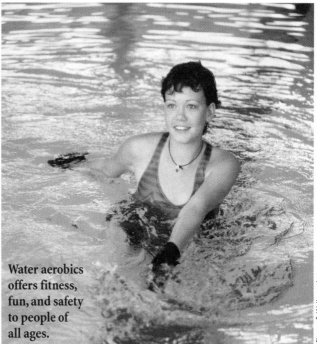

Water aerobics offers fitness, fun, and safety to people of all ages.

© Fitness & Wellness, Inc.

land-based weight-bearing activities such as walking, jogging, and aerobics.

3. Water aerobics is an excellent exercise modality to improve functional fitness in older adults (see section titled "Exercise and Aging" later in this chapter).

4. Heat dissipation in water is beneficial to obese participants, who seem to undergo a higher heat strain than average-weight individuals.

5. Water aerobics is available to swimmers and non-swimmers alike.

The exercises used during water aerobics are designed to elevate the heart rate, which contributes to cardiorespiratory development. In addition, the aquatic medium provides increased resistance for strength improvement with virtually no impact. Because of this resistance to movement, strength gains with water aerobics seem to be better than with land-based aerobic activities. Water exercises also help the joints move through a fuller range of motion, promoting flexibility.

Key Terms

Low-impact aerobics Exercises in which at least one foot is in contact with the ground or floor at all times.

Step aerobics A form of exercise that combines stepping up and down from a bench with arm movements.

Plyometric training A form of aerobic exercise that requires forceful jumps or springing off the ground immediately after landing from a previous jump.

Another benefit is the reduction of pain and fear of injuries common to many people who initiate exercise programs. Water aerobics provides a relatively safe environment for injury-free participation in exercise. The cushioned environment of the water allows patients recovering from leg and back injuries, individuals with joint problems, injured athletes, pregnant women, and obese people to benefit from water aerobics. In water, these people can exercise to develop and maintain cardiorespiratory endurance or to lose weight while limiting or eliminating the potential for further injury.

As observed with swimming, maximal heart rates achieved during water aerobics are lower than during running. The difference between water aerobics and running is about 10 bpm.[17] Apparently healthy people, nonetheless, can sustain land-based exercise intensities during a water aerobics workout and experience similar or greater fitness benefits than during land aerobics.[18] As with swimming, land-based exercise intensities, therefore, are recommended for water aerobics.

> Water aerobics provides a relatively safe environment for injury-free participation in exercise.

Cycling

Most people learn cycling in their youth. Because it is a non-weight–bearing activity, cycling is a good exercise modality for people with lower body or lower-back injuries. Cycling helps to develop the cardiorespiratory system as well as muscular strength and endurance in the lower extremities. With the advent of stationary bicycles, this activity can be performed year-round.

Raising the heart rate to the proper training intensity is more difficult with cycling. As the amount of muscle mass involved during aerobic exercise decreases, so does the demand placed on the cardiorespiratory system. The thigh muscles do most of the work in cycling, making it harder to achieve and maintain a high cardiorespiratory training intensity.

Maintaining a continuous pedaling motion and eliminating coasting periods helps the participant achieve a faster heart rate. Exercising for longer periods also helps to compensate for the lower heart rate intensity during cycling. Comparing cycling with jogging, similar aerobic benefits take roughly three times the distance at twice the speed of jogging. Cycling, however, puts less stress on muscles and joints than jogging does, making the former a good exercise modality for people who cannot walk or jog.

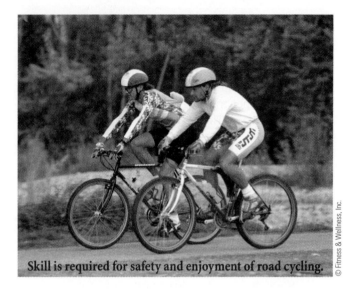

Skill is required for safety and enjoyment of road cycling.

© Fitness & Wellness, Inc.

To increase riding efficiency, the height of the bike seat should be adjusted so the legs are almost completely extended when the heels are placed on the pedals. The body should not sway from side to side as the person rides. The cycling cadence also is important for maximal efficiency. Bike tension or gears should be set at a moderate level so the rider can achieve about 60 to 100 revolutions per minute.

Skill is important in road cycling. Cyclists must be in control of the bicycle at all times. They have to be able to maneuver the bike in traffic, maintain balance at slow speeds, switch gears, apply the brakes, watch for pedestrians and stoplights, and ride through congested areas. Stationary cycling, in contrast, does not require special skills. Nearly everyone can do it.

Safety is a key issue in road cycling. More than a million bicycle injuries occur each year. Proper equipment and common sense are necessary. A well-designed and -maintained bike is easier to maneuver. Toe clips are recommended to keep feet from sliding and to maintain equal upward and downward force on the pedals.

Bike riders must follow the same rules as motorists. Many accidents happen because cyclists run traffic lights and stop signs. Some further suggestions are

- Use bike hand signals to let the traffic around you know of your intended actions.
- Don't ride side by side with another rider.
- Be aware of turning vehicles and cars backing out of alleys and parking lots; always yield to motorists in these situations.
- Avoid storm drains, which can cause unpleasant surprises: If you do not cross them at the proper angle, front wheels can get caught and riders may be thrown from the bike.

- Wear a good helmet that is certified by the Snell Memorial Foundation or the American National Standards Institute. Many serious accidents and even deaths have been prevented by use of helmets. Fashion, aesthetics, comfort, or price should not be a factor when selecting and using a helmet for road cycling. Health and life are too precious to give up because of vanity and thriftiness.

- Wear appropriate clothes and shoes. Special clothing for cycling is not required. Clothing should be lightweight and not restrict movement. Shorts should be long enough to keep the skin from rubbing against the seat. For greater comfort, cycling shorts have extra padding sewn into the seat and crotch areas. Experienced cyclists often wear special shoes with a cleat that snaps directly onto the pedal.

The stationary bike is the most popular piece of equipment that sporting goods stores sell. Before buying a stationary bike, though, be sure to try the activity for a few days. If you enjoy it, you may want to purchase one. Invest with caution. If you opt to buy a lower-priced model, you may be disappointed. Good stationary bikes have comfortable seats, are stable, and provide a smooth and uniform pedaling motion. A sticky bike that is hard to pedal leads to discouragement and ends up stored in the corner of a basement.

Spinning

Spinning is a low-impact activity typically performed under the direction of a certified instructor in a room or studio with dim lights, motivational music, and the noise of many bikes working together. This exercise modality gained immediate popularity upon its introduction in the mid-1990s.

Spinning, sometimes referred to as "studio" or "indoor cycling," is performed on stationary bicycles, initially developed by Johnny Goldberg. To bring his rigorous workouts indoors, Mr. Goldberg modified his stationary bike into the first Spinner bike. Participants now use specially designed Spinner bikes that include racing handlebars, pedals with clips, adjustable seats, and a resistance knob to control the intensity of the workout. Use of an exercise heart rate monitor is also encouraged to monitor the intensity of the various stages of the workout.

As presently designed, the Spinning program combines five basic movements and five workout stages with the understanding that participants' exercise needs and goals vary. The five exercise movements are

- **Seated flat** The basic seated bike-riding position.

- **Seated hill climb** The basic seated position but with increased resistance on the bike.
- **Standing running** Pedaling while standing up.
- **Standing hill climb** Pedaling standing up but with a challenging resistance level.
- **Jumping** Surging out of the saddle using either controlled movements and a constant speed or at a fast pace, as during a breakaway in a bike race.

The five workout stages, also known as "energy zones," are used to simulate actual cycling training and racing. The workouts are divided into endurance, all-terrain, strength, recovery, and advanced training. Cadence, exercise movements, and exercise heart rate dictate the differences among the various zones. Workouts are planned according to each person's fitness level and selected percentages of maximal heart rate during each stage. These workouts provide a challenging program for people of all ages and fitness levels. The social aspect of this activity makes Spinning appealing to many exercisers.

Cross-Training

Cross-training combines two or more activities in an exercise program. This type of training is designed to enhance fitness, provide needed rest to tired muscles, decrease injuries, and eliminate the monotony and burnout of single-activity programs. Cross-training may combine aerobic and nonaerobic activities such as moderate jogging, speed training, and strength training.

Cross-training can produce better workouts than a single activity. For example, jogging develops the lower body and swimming builds the upper body. Rowing contributes to upper-body development and cycling builds the legs. Combining activities such as these provides good overall conditioning and at the same time helps to improve or maintain fitness. Cross-training also offers an opportunity to develop new skills and have fun with different activities.

Speed training is often coupled with cross-training. Faster performance times in aerobic activities (running, cycling) are generated with speed or **interval training**. People who want to improve their running times often run shorter intervals at faster speeds than the actual racing pace. For example, a person wanting to run a 6-minute mile may run four 440-yard intervals at a speed of 1 minute and 20 seconds per interval. A 440-yard walk/jog can become a recovery interval between fast runs.

Interval training A series of exercise work bouts (intervals) interspersed with low-intensity or rest intervals.

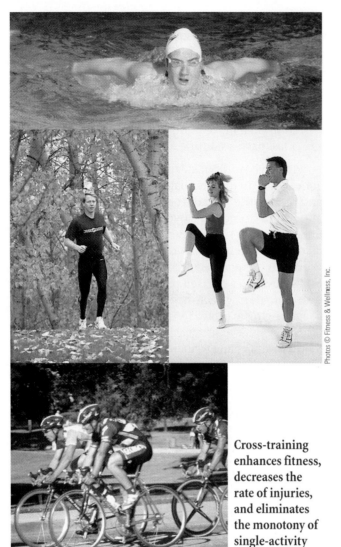

Photos © Fitness & Wellness, Inc.

Cross-training enhances fitness, decreases the rate of injuries, and eliminates the monotony of single-activity programs.

Strength training is also used commonly with cross-training. It helps to condition muscles, tendons, and ligaments. Improved strength enhances overall performance in many activities and sports. For example, although road cyclists in one study who trained with weights showed no improvement in aerobic capacity, the cyclists had a 33 percent improvement in riding time to exhaustion when exercising at 75 percent of their maximal capacity.[19]

Rope Skipping

Rope skipping not only contributes to cardiorespiratory fitness, but it also helps to increase reaction time, coordination, agility, dynamic balance, and muscular strength in the lower extremities. At first, rope skipping may appear to be a highly strenuous form of aerobic exercise. Beginners often reach maximal heart rates after only 2 or 3 minutes of jumping. As skill

improves, however, the energy demands decrease considerably.

Some people have claimed training benefits equal to a 30-minute jog in only 10 minutes of skipping. Although differences in strength and flexibility development are observed in different activities, 10 minutes at a certain heart rate provide similar cardiorespiratory benefits regardless of the nature of the activity. To obtain an adequate aerobic workout, the duration of exercise must be at least 20 minutes.

As with high-impact aerobics, a major concern of rope skipping is the stress placed on the lower extremities. Skipping with one foot at a time decreases the impact somewhat, but it does not eliminate the risk of injuries. Fitness experts recommend that skipping be used sparingly, primarily as a supplement to an aerobic exercise program.

Cross-Country Skiing

Many consider cross-country skiing to be the ultimate aerobic exercise because it requires vigorous lower and upper body movements. The large amount of muscle mass involved in cross-country skiing makes the intensity of the activity high, yet it places little strain on muscles and joints. One of the highest maximal oxygen uptakes ever measured (85 ml/kg/min) was found in an elite cross-country skier.

In addition to being an excellent aerobic activity, cross-country skiing is soothing. Skiing through the beauty of the snow-covered countryside can be highly enjoyable. Although the need for snow is an obvious limitation, simulation equipment for year-round cross-country training is available at many sporting goods stores.

Cross-country skiing is considered by many to be the ultimate aerobic exercise because it requires vigorous lower- and upper-body movements.

Some skill is necessary to be proficient at cross-country skiing. Poorly skilled individuals are not able to elevate their heart rate enough to cause adequate aerobic development. Individuals contemplating this activity should seek out instruction to fully enjoy and reap the rewards of cross-country skiing.

In-Line Skating

Frequently referred to as "blading," in-line skating has become a highly popular fitness activity in recent years. Suddenly millions of children and adults are

In-line skating is a low-impact fitness activity.

trying this activity. In the early 1990s, stores could not keep up with the demand for in-line skates.

In-line skating has its origin in ice skating. Because warm-weather ice skating was not feasible, blades were replaced by wheels for summertime participation. Although four-wheel roller skates were invented in the mid-1700s, the activity did not really catch on until the late 1800s. The first in-line skate, with five wheels in a row attached to the bottom of a shoe, was developed in 1823. The in-line concept took hold in the United States in 1980, when hockey skates were adapted for road-skating.

In-line skating is an excellent activity to develop cardiorespiratory fitness and lower-body strength. Intensity of the activity is regulated by how hard you blade. The key to effective cardiorespiratory training is to maintain a constant and rhythmic pattern, using arms and legs, and minimizing the gliding phase. Because this is a weight-bearing activity, in-line bladers also develop superior leg strength.

Instruction is necessary to achieve a minimum level of proficiency in this sport. Bladers commonly encounter hazards—potholes, cracks, rocks, gravel, sticks, oil, street curbs, and driveways. Unskilled bladers are more prone to falls and injuries.

Good equipment will make the activity safer and more enjoyable. Blades range in price from $40 to $500. Recreational participants need not purchase the more costly competitive skates. An adequate blade should provide strong ankle support; soft and flexible boots do not provide enough support. Small wheels offer more stability, and larger wheels enable greater speed. Blades should be purchased from stores that understand the sport and can provide sound advice according to your skill level and needs.

Protective equipment is a must for in-line skating. Similar to road cycling, a good helmet that meets the safety standards set by the Snell Memorial Foundation or the American National Standards Institute is important to protect yourself in case of a fall. Wrist guards and knee and elbow pads also are recommended, because the kneecaps and the elbows are easily injured in a fall. Nighttime bladers should wear light-colored clothing and reflective tape.

Rowing

Rowing is a low-impact activity that provides a complete body workout. It mobilizes most major muscle groups, including those in the arms, legs, hips, abdomen, trunk, and shoulders. Rowing is a good form of aerobic exercise and, because of the nature of the activity (constant pushing and pulling against resistance), also promotes total strength development.

To accommodate different fitness levels, workloads can be regulated on most rowing machines. Stationary rowing, however, is not among the most popular forms of aerobic exercise. Similar to stationary bicycles, people should try the activity for a few weeks before purchasing a unit.

Stair Climbing

If sustained for at least 20 minutes, stair climbing is a very efficient form of aerobic exercise. Precisely because of the high intensity of stair climbing, many people stay away from stairs and instead take escalators and elevators. Many people dislike living in two-story homes because they have to climb the stairs frequently.

Stair climbing provides a rigorous aerobic workout.

Not too many places have enough flights of stairs to climb continuously for 20 minutes. Stair-climbing machines offer an alternative. Stair climbing has become so popular that fitness enthusiasts often wait in line at health clubs to use the machines. In terms of injuries, stair climbing seems to be a relatively safe exercise modality. Because the feet never leave the climbing surface, it is considered a low-impact activity. Joints and ligaments are not strained during climbing. The intensity of exercise is controlled easily, because most stair climbing equipment can be programmed to regulate the workload.

Racquet Sports

In racquet sports such as tennis, racquetball, squash, and badminton, the aerobic benefits are dictated by players' skill, intensity of the game, and how long a given game lasts. Skill is necessary to participate effectively in these sports and also is crucial to sustain continuous play. Frequent pauses during play do not allow people to maintain the heart rate in the appropriate target zone to stimulate cardiorespiratory development.

Many people who participate in racquet sports do so for enjoyment, social fulfillment, and relaxation. For cardiorespiratory fitness development, these people supplement the sport with other forms of aerobic exercise such as jogging, cycling, or swimming.

If a racquet sport is the main form of aerobic exercise, participants need to try to run hard, fast, and as constantly as possible during play. They should not have to spend much time retrieving balls (or, in

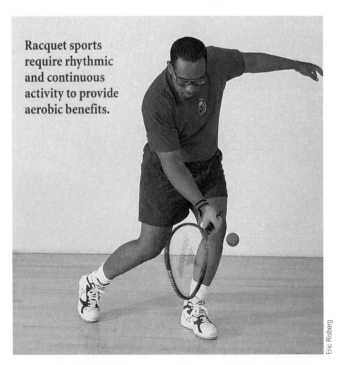

Racquet sports require rhythmic and continuous activity to provide aerobic benefits.

Eric Risberg

badminton, the bird or shuttlecock). Similar to low-impact aerobics, all movements should be accentuated by reaching out and bending more than usual, for better cardiorespiratory development.

FITNESS BENEFITS OF AEROBIC ACTIVITIES

The contributions of different aerobic activities to the health-related components of fitness vary. Although an accurate assessment of the contributions to each fitness component is difficult to establish, a summary of likely benefits of several activities is provided in Table 4.1. Instead of a single rating or number, ranges are given for some of the categories. The benefits derived are based on the person's effort while participating in the activity.

The nature of the activity often dictates the potential aerobic development. For example, jogging is much more strenuous than walking. The effort during exercise also has an impact on the amount of physiological development. The training benefits of just going through the motions of a low-impact aerobics routine, as compared with accentuating all motions, are much reduced. Accentuating all motions increases training benefits by orders of magnitude.

Table 4.1 indicates a starting fitness level for each aerobic activity. Attempting to participate in high-intensity activities without proper conditioning often leads to injuries and discouragement. Beginners should start with low-intensity activities that carry a minimum risk for injuries.

In some cases, such as high-impact aerobics and rope skipping, the risk for injuries remains high even if the participants are adequately conditioned. These activities should be supplemental only and are not recommended as the sole mode of exercise. Most exercise-related injuries occur as a result of high-impact activities, not high intensity of exercise.

Physicians who work with cardiac patients frequently use **METs** as an alternative method of prescribing exercise intensity. One MET represents the rate of energy expenditure at rest. The MET range for the various activities is included in Table 4.1. A 10-MET activity requires a tenfold increase in the resting energy requirement, or approximately 35 ml/kg/min. MET levels for a given activity vary according to the effort expended. The harder a person exercises, the higher the MET level.

The effectiveness of various aerobic activities in weight management also is provided in Table 4.1. As a general rule, the greater the muscle mass involved in exercise, the better the results. Rhythmic and

TABLE 4.1 Ratings for Selected Aerobic Activities

Activity	Recommended Starting Fitness Level[1]	Risk of Injury[2]	Potential Cardiovascular Endurance Development (VO_{2max})[3,4]	Upper Body Strength Development[3]	Lower Body Strength Development[3]	Upper Body Flexibility Development[3]	Lower Body Flexibility Development[3]	Weight Control[3]	MET Level[4,5,6]	Caloric Expenditure (cal/hour)[4,6]
Walking	B	L	1–2	1	2	1	1	3	4–6	300–450
Walking/water, chest-deep	I	L	2–4	2	3	1	1	3	6–10	450–750
Hiking	B	L	2–4	1	3	1	1	3	6–10	450–750
Jogging	I	M	3–5	1	3	1	1	5	6–15	450–1125
Jogging, deep water	A	L	3–5	2	2	1	1	5	8–15	600–1125
High-impact aerobics	A	H	3–4	2	4	3	2	4	6–12	450–900
Low-impact aerobics	B	L	2–4	2	3	3	2	3	5–10	375–750
Step aerobics	I	M	2–4	2	3–4	3	2	3–4	5–12	375–900
Moderate-impact aerobics	I	M	2–4	2	3	3	2	3	6–12	450–900
Swimming (front crawl)	B	L	3–5	4	2	3	1	3	6–12	450–900
Water aerobics	B	L	2–4	3	3	3	2	3	6–12	450–900
Stationary cycling	B	L	2–4	1	4	1	1	3	6–10	450–750
Road cycling	I	M	2–5	1	4	1	1	3	6–12	450–900
Cross-training	I	M	3–5	2–3	3–4	2–3	1–2	3–5	6–15	450–1125
Rope skipping	I	H	3–5	2	4	1	2	3–5	8–15	600–1125
Cross-country skiing	B	M	4–5	4	4	2	2	4–5	10–16	750–1200
Aero-belt exercise	B	M	4–5	4	4	3	2	4–5	10–16	750–1200
In-line skating	I	M	2–4	2	4	2	2	3	6–10	450–750
Rowing	B	L	3–5	4	2	3	1	4	8–14	600–1050
Stair climbing	B	L	3–5	1	4	1	1	4–5	8–15	600–1125
Racquet sports	I	M	2–4	3	3	3	2	3	6–10	450–750

[1] B = Beginner, I = Intermediate, A = Advanced

[2] L = Low, M = Moderate, H = High

[3] 1 = Low, 2 = Fair, 3 = Average, 4 = Good, 5 = Excellent

[4] Varies according to the person's effort (exercise intensity) during exercise.

[5] One MET represents the rate of energy expenditure at rest (3.5 ml/kg/min). Each additional MET is a multiple of the resting value. For example, 5 METs represents an energy expenditure equivalent to five times the resting value, or about 17.5 ml/kg/min.

[6] Varies according to body weight.

continuous activities that involve large amounts of muscle mass are most effective in burning calories.

Higher-intensity activities increase caloric expenditure as well. Exercising longer, however, compensates for lower intensities. If carried out long enough (45 to 60 minutes five to six times per week), even

Key Terms

MET The rate of resting energy expenditure at rest; MET is the equivalent of 3.5 ml/kg/min.

walking can be an excellent exercise mode for weight loss. Additional information on a comprehensive weight management program is given in Chapter 9.

Specific Considerations

In addition to the exercise-related issues discussed previously, many concerns require clarification or are somewhat controversial. Let's examine some of these issues.

1. Does aerobic exercise make a person immune to heart and blood vessel disease? Although aerobically fit individuals as a whole have a lower incidence of cardiovascular disease, a regular aerobic exercise program by itself does not offer an absolute guarantee against cardiovascular disease. Overall management of the risk factors is the best way to minimize the risk for cardiovascular disease. Many factors, including a genetic predisposition, can increase the person's risk. In any case, experts believe that a regular aerobic exercise program not only will delay the onset of cardiovascular problems, but also will improve the chances of surviving a heart attack.

Even moderate increases in aerobic fitness significantly lower the incidence of premature cardiovascular deaths. Data from the research study illustrated in Chapter 1, Figure 1.7, indicate that the decrease in cardiovascular mortality is greatest between the unfit (group 1) and the moderately fit (2 and 3) groups. A further decrease in cardiovascular mortality is observed between the moderately fit and the highly fit groups (4 and 5), although the difference is not as pronounced as that between the unfit and moderately fit groups.

> A regular aerobic exercise program by itself does not offer an absolute guarantee against cardiovascular disease. Overall management of the risk factors is the best way to minimize the risk for cardiovascular disease.

2. How much aerobic exercise is required to decrease the risk for cardiovascular disease? Even though research has not yet indicated the exact amount of aerobic exercise required to lower the risk for cardiovascular disease, some general recommendations have been set forth. In their study, Dr. Ralph Paffenbarger and his co-researchers showed that expending 2,000 calories per week as a result of physical activity yielded the lowest risk for cardiovascular disease among a group of almost 17,000 Harvard alumni.[20] Two thousand calories per week represents about 300 calories per daily exercise session.

3. Do people get a "physical high" during aerobic exercise? During vigorous exercise, **endorphins** are released from the pituitary gland in the brain. They can create feelings of euphoria and natural well-being. Higher levels of endorphins are often a result of aerobic endurance activities and may remain elevated for as long as 30 to 60 minutes following exercise. Many experts believe these higher levels explain the physical high some people get during and after prolonged exercise.

Endorphin levels have also been shown to increase during pregnancy and childbirth. Endorphins act as pain killers. The higher levels could explain a woman's greater tolerance for the pain and discomfort of natural childbirth and her pleasant feelings shortly after the baby's birth. Several reports have indicated that well-conditioned women have shorter and easier labor. These women may attain higher endorphin levels during delivery, making childbirth less traumatic than it is for untrained women.

4. Can people with asthma exercise? Asthma, a condition that causes difficulty breathing, is characterized by coughing, wheezing, and shortness of breath induced by narrowing of the airway passages because of contraction (bronchospasm) of the airway muscles, swelling of the mucous membrane, and excessive secretion of mucus. In a few people, asthma can be triggered by exercise itself, particularly in cool and dry environments. This type of condition is referred to as exercise-induced asthma (EIA).

People with asthma need to obtain proper medication from a physician prior to initiating an exercise program. A regular program is best, because random exercise bouts are more likely to trigger asthma attacks. In the initial stages of exercise, an intermittent program (frequent rest periods during the exercise session) is recommended. Gradual warm-up and cool-down are also essential to reduce the risk of an acute attack. Furthermore, exercise in warm and humid conditions (swimming) is better because it helps to moisten the airways and minimizes the asthmatic response. For land-based activities (walking, aerobics), drinking water before, during, and after exercise helps to keep the airways moist, thus decreasing the risk of an attack. During the winter months, wearing an exercise mask is recommended to increase warmth and humidity of inhaled air. People with asthma should not exercise alone and should always carry their medication with them during workouts.

5. What types of activities are recommended for people with arthritis? Individuals who suffer swimming, or water aerobics—that minimize the risk of injury and may allow continuation of exercise throughout pregnancy.

- Avoid activities that could precipitate a loss of balance or cause even mild trauma to the abdomen.
- Get proper nourishment (pregnancy requires approximately 300 extra calories per day).
- During the first 3 months in particular, avoid exercising in the heat. Wear clothing that allows for proper dissipation of heat and drink plenty of water.

8. Does exercise help relieve dysmenorrhea? Although exercise has not been shown to either cure or aggravate **dysmenorrhea**, it has been shown to relieve menstrual cramps because it improves circulation to the uterus. Less severe menstrual cramps also could be related to higher levels of endorphins produced during prolonged physical activity, which may counteract pain. Particularly, stretching exercises of the muscles in the pelvic region seem to reduce and prevent painful menstruation that is not the result of disease.[22]

9. Does participation in exercise hinder menstruation? In some instances, highly trained athletes develop **amenorrhea** during training and competition. This condition is seen most often in extremely lean women who also engage in sports that require strenuous physical effort over a sustained time. It is by no means irreversible. At present, we do not know whether the condition is caused by physical or emotional stress related to high-intensity training, excessively low body fat, or other factors.

Although, on the average, women have a lower physical capacity during menstruation, medical surveys at the Olympic games have shown that women have broken Olympic and world records at all stages of the menstrual cycle. Menstruation should not keep a woman from participating in athletics, and it will not necessarily have a negative impact on performance.

10. Does exercise offset the detrimental effects of cigarette smoking? Physical exercise often motivates smoking cessation, but it does not offset any ill effects of smoking. Smoking greatly decreases the ability of the blood to transport oxygen to working muscles.

Oxygen is carried in the circulatory system by hemoglobin, the iron-containing pigment of the red blood cells. Carbon monoxide, a byproduct of cigarette smoke, has 210 to 250 times greater affinity for hemoglobin over oxygen. Consequently, carbon monoxide combines much faster with hemoglobin, decreasing the oxygen-carrying capacity of the blood.

Chronic smoking also increases airway resistance, requiring the respiratory muscles to work much harder and consume more oxygen just to ventilate a given amount of air. If a person quits smoking, exercise does help increase the functional capacity of the pulmonary system.

A regular exercise program seems to be a powerful incentive to quit smoking. A random survey of 1,250 runners conducted at the 6.2-mile Peachtree Road Race in Atlanta provided impressive results. The survey indicated that 81 percent and 75 percent of the men and women, respectively, who smoked cigarettes when they started running had quit before the race date.

11. How long should a person wait after a meal before exercising strenuously? The length of time to wait before exercising after a meal depends on the amount of food eaten. On the average, after a regular meal, you should wait about 2 hours before participating in strenuous physical activity. A walk or some other light physical activity is fine following a meal, though. If anything, it helps burn extra calories and may help the body metabolize fats more efficiently.

12. What type of clothing should I wear when I exercise? The type of clothing you wear during exercise is important. In general, clothing should fit comfortably and allow free movement of the various body parts. Select clothing according to air temperature, humidity, and exercise intensity. Avoid nylon and rubberized materials and tight clothes that interfere with the cooling mechanism of the human body or obstruct normal blood flow. Choose fabrics made from polypropylene, Capilene, Thermax, or any synthetic that draws moisture away from the skin, enhancing evaporation and cooling of the body. It's also important to consider your exercise intensity, because the harder you exercise, the more heat your body produces.

When exercising in the heat, avoid the hottest time of the day—between 11:00 A.M. and 5:00 P.M. Surfaces such as asphalt, concrete, and artificial turf absorb heat, which then radiates to the body. Therefore, these surfaces are not recommended. (Also see the discussion about heat and humidity that follows.)

Only a minimal amount of clothing is necessary during exercise in the heat, to allow for maximal evaporation. Clothing should be lightweight, light-colored, loose-fitting, airy, and absorbent. Examples

KeyTerms

Dysmenorrhea Painful menstruation.

Amenorrhea Cessation of regular menstrual flow.

© Fitness & Wellness, Inc.

Activity-specific shoes are recommended to prevent lower-extremity injuries.

of commercially available products that can be used during exercise in the heat are Asci's Perma Plus, Cool-max, and Nike's Dri-F.I.T. Double-layer acrylic socks are more absorbent than cotton and help to prevent blistering and chafing of the feet. A straw-type hat can be worn to protect the eyes and head from the sun. (Clothing for exercise in the cold is discussed on page 100.)

A good pair of shoes is vital to prevent injuries to lower limbs. Shoes manufactured specifically for your choice of activity are a must. When selecting proper footwear, you should consider body type, tendency toward pronation (rotating foot outward) or supination (rotating foot inward), and exercise surfaces. Shoes should have good stability, motion control, and comfortable fit. Purchase shoes in the middle of the day when your feet have expanded and might be one-half size larger. For increased breathability, choose shoes with nylon or mesh uppers. Generally, salespeople at reputable athletic shoe stores are knowledgeable and can help you select a good shoe that fits your needs. After 300 to 500 miles or 6 months, examine your shoes and obtain a new pair if they are worn out. Old shoes frequently are responsible for lower-limb injuries.

13. What time of the day is best for exercise? You can do intense exercise almost any time of the day, with the exception of about 2 hours following a heavy meal or the midday and early afternoon hours on hot, humid days. Moderate exercise seems to be beneficial shortly after a meal, because exercise enhances the **thermogenic response**. A walk shortly after a meal burns more calories than a walk several hours after a meal.

Many people enjoy exercising early in the morning because it gives them a boost to start the day. People who exercise in the morning also seem to stick with it more than others. Some prefer the lunch hour for weight-control reasons. By exercising at noon, they do not eat as big a lunch, which helps keep down the daily caloric intake. Highly stressed people seem to like the evening hours because of the relaxing effects of exercise.

14. Why is exercising in hot and humid conditions unsafe? When a person exercises, only 30 to 40 percent of the energy the body produces is used for mechanical work or movement. The rest of the energy (60 to 70 percent) is converted into heat. If this heat cannot be dissipated properly because either the weather is too hot or the relative humidity is too high, body temperature increases and, in extreme cases, can result in death.

The specific heat of body tissue (the heat required to raise the temperature of the body by 1 degree C) is .38 calories per pound of body weight (.38 cal/lb). This indicates that if no body heat is dissipated, a 150-pound person has to burn only 57 calories (150 × .38) to increase total body temperature by 1 degree C. If this person were to conduct an exercise session requiring 300 calories (e.g., running about 3 miles) without any heat dissipation, the inner body temperature would increase by 5.3 degrees C, which is the equivalent of going from 98.6 degrees F to 108.1 degrees F.

This example illustrates clearly the need for caution when exercising in hot or humid weather. If the relative humidity is too high, body heat cannot be lost through evaporation because the atmosphere already is saturated with water vapor. In one instance, a football casualty occurred when the temperature was only 64 degrees F—but the relative humidity was 100 percent. People must be cautious when air temperature is above 90 degrees F and the relative humidity is above 60 percent.

The American College of Sports Medicine recommends avoiding strenuous physical activity when the readings of a wet-bulb globe thermometer exceed 82.4 degrees F. With this type of thermometer, the wet bulb is cooled by evaporation, and on dry days it shows a lower temperature than the regular (dry) thermometer. On humid days, the cooling effect is less because of less evaporation; hence, the difference between the wet and dry readings is not as great.

Following are descriptions of and first-aid measures for the three major signs of trouble when exercising in the heat:

- **Heat cramps**. Symptoms include cramps, spasms, and muscle twitching in the legs, arms, and abdomen. To relieve heat cramps, stop exercising, get out of the heat, massage the painful area, stretch slowly, and drink plenty of fluids (water, fruit drinks, or electrolyte beverages).

- **Heat exhaustion.** Symptoms include fainting; dizziness; profuse sweating; cold, clammy skin; weakness; headache; and a rapid, weak pulse. If you incur any of these symptoms, stop and find a cool place to rest. If conscious, drink cool water. Do not give water to an unconscious person. Loosen or remove clothing, and rub your body with a cool, wet towel or ice packs. Place yourself in a supine position with the legs elevated 8 to 12 inches. If you are not fully recovered in 30 minutes, seek immediate medical attention.

- **Heat stroke.**
Symptoms include serious disorientation; warm, dry skin; no sweating; rapid, full pulse; vomiting; diarrhea; unconsciousness; and high body temperature. As the body temperature climbs, unexplained anxiety sets in. When the body temperature reaches 104 to 105 degrees F, the individual may feel a cold sensation in the trunk of the body, goose bumps, nausea, throbbing in the temples, and numbness in the extremities. Most people become incoherent after this stage. When body temperature reaches 105 to 107 degrees F, disorientation, loss of fine-motor control, and muscular weakness set in. If the temperature exceeds 106 degrees F, serious neurologic injury and death may be imminent.

> **Heat stroke is a medical emergency. Request help, get the person into a cool, humidity-controlled environment, spray the body with cool water, and rub with cool towels. If possible, place cold packs in areas with abundant blood supply, such as the head, neck, armpits, and groin.**

Heat stroke requires immediate emergency medical attention. Request help and get out of the sun and into a cool, humidity-controlled environment. While you are waiting to be taken to the hospital emergency room, you should be placed in a semi-seated position, and your body should be sprayed with cool water and rubbed with cool towels. If possible, cold packs should be placed in areas with abundant blood supply, such as the head, neck, armpits, and groin. Fluids should not be given if you are unconscious. In any case of

heat-related illness, if the person refuses water, vomits, or starts to lose consciousness, call for an ambulance immediately. Proper initial treatment of heat stroke is critical.

15. What should a person do to replace fluids lost during prolonged aerobic exercise?

> **The main objective of fluid replacement during prolonged aerobic exercise is to maintain the blood volume so circulation and sweating can continue at normal levels.**

The main objective of fluid replacement during prolonged aerobic exercise is to maintain the blood volume so circulation and sweating can continue at normal levels. Adequate water replacement is the most important factor in preventing heat disorders. Drinking about 6 to 8 ounces of cool water every 15 to 20 minutes during exercise seems to be ideal to prevent dehydration. Cold fluids seem to be absorbed more rapidly from the stomach.

Other relevant points are the following:

- Commercial fluid-replacement solutions (such as Powerade® and Gatorade®) contain about 6 to 8 percent glucose, which seems to be optimal for fluid absorption and performance. Sugar does not become available to the muscles until about 30 minutes after a glucose solution is consumed.

  Commercially prepared sports drinks are recommended when exercise will be strenuous and carried out for more than an hour. For exercise lasting less than an hour, water is just as effective in replacing lost fluid. The sports drinks you select should be based on your personal preference. Try different drinks at 6 to 8 percent glucose concentration to see which drink you tolerate best and suits your tastes as well.

- Drinks high in fructose or with a glucose concentration above 8 percent are not recommended because they slow down water absorption when exercising in the heat.

KeyTerms

Thermogenic response Amount of energy required to digest food.

Heat cramps Muscle spasms caused by heat-induced changes in electrolyte balance in muscle cells.

Heat exhaustion Heat-related fatigue.

Heat stroke Emergency situation resulting from the body being subjected to high atmospheric temperatures.

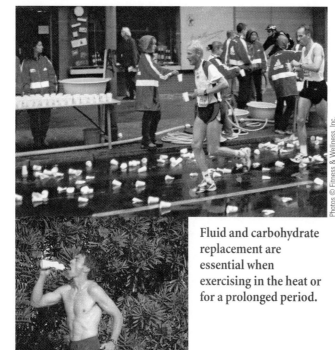

Photos © Fitness & Wellness, Inc.

Fluid and carbohydrate replacement are essential when exercising in the heat or for a prolonged period.

- Most sodas (cola, non-cola) contain between 10 and 12 percent glucose, an amount that is too high for proper rehydration during exercise in the heat.

16. What precautions must a person take when exercising in the cold? When exercising in the cold, the two factors to consider are frostbite and **hypothermia**. In contrast to hot and humid conditions, cold weather usually does not threaten health because clothing can be selected for heat conservation, and exercise itself increases the production of body heat.

Most people actually overdress for exercise in the cold. Because exercise increases body temperature, a moderate workout on a cold day makes a person feel that the temperature is 20 to 30 degrees warmer than it actually is. Overdressing for exercise can make the clothes damp from excessive perspiration. The risk for hypothermia increases when a person is wet or not moving around sufficiently to increase body heat.

Initial warning signs of hypothermia include shivering, loss of coordination, and difficulty speaking. With a continued drop in body temperature, shivering stops, the muscles weaken and stiffen, and the person has feelings of elation or intoxication and eventually loses consciousness. To prevent hypothermia, use common sense, dress properly, and be aware of environmental conditions.

The popular belief that exercising in cold temperatures (32 degrees F and lower) freezes the lungs is false, because the air is warmed properly in the air passages before it reaches the lungs. Cold is not what poses a threat. Rather, wind velocity is what affects the chill factor greatly.

For example, exercising at a temperature of 25 degrees F with adequate clothing is not too cold, but if the wind is blowing at 25 miles per hour, the chill factor lowers the actual temperature to 15 degrees F. This effect is even worse if a person is wet and exhausted. When the weather is windy, exercise (jog or cycle) against the wind on the way out and with the wind when you return.

Even though the lungs are under no risk when you exercise in the cold, your face, head, hands, and feet should be protected, because they are subject to frostbite. Watch for signs of frostbite—numbness and discoloration. In cold temperatures, as much as half of the body's heat can be lost through an unprotected head and neck. A wool or synthetic cap, hood, or hat will help to hold in body heat. Mittens are better than gloves, because they keep the fingers together so the surface area from which to lose heat is less. Inner linings of synthetic material to wick (draw) moisture away from the skin are recommended. Avoid cotton next to the skin, because once cotton gets wet— whether from perspiration, rain, or snow—it loses its insulating properties.

Wearing several layers of lightweight clothing is preferable to wearing one single, thick layer because warm air is trapped between layers of clothes, enabling greater heat conservation. As body temperature increases, you can remove layers as necessary. For lengthy or long-distance workouts (cross-country skiing or long runs), take a small backpack to carry the clothing that is removed. You also can carry extra warm and dry clothes in case you stop exercising away from shelter. If you remain outdoors following exercise, added clothing and continuous body movement are essential.

The first layer of clothes should wick moisture away from

> When exercising in cold weather, several layers of lightweight clothing is preferable to wearing one single, thick layer. Warm air is trapped between layers of clothes, enabling greater heat conservation.

the skin. Polypropylene, Capilene, and Thermax are recommended materials. Next, a layer of wool, dacron, or polyester fleece insulates well even when wet. Lycra tights or sweatpants help protect the legs. The outer layer should be waterproof, wind-resistant, and breathable. A synthetic material such as Gortex is best, so moisture can still escape from the body. A ski mask or face mask helps protect the face. In extremely cold conditions, exposed skin, such as the nose, cheeks, or around the eyes, can be insulated with petroleum jelly.

17. Can I exercise when I have a cold or the flu? The most important consideration is to use common sense and pay attention to your symptoms. Typically, you may continue to exercise if your symptoms include a runny nose, sneezing, or a scratchy throat. However, if you are running a fever or your muscles ache or if you are vomiting, have diarrhea, or have a hacking cough, you should avoid exercise. Following an illness, be sure to ease back gradually into your program. Do not attempt to return at the same intensity and duration that you were used to prior to your illness.

EXERCISE-RELATED INJURIES

To enjoy and maintain physical fitness, preventing injury during a conditioning program is essential. Exercise-related injuries, nonetheless, are common in individuals who participate in exercise programs. Surveys indicate that more than half of all new participants incur injuries during the first 6 months of the conditioning program.

The four most common causes of injuries are

1. High-impact activities,
2. Rapid conditioning programs—doing too much too quickly,
3. Improper shoes or training surfaces, and
4. Anatomical predisposition (body propensity).

High-impact activities and a significant increase in quantity, intensity, and duration of activities are by far the most common causes of injuries. The body requires time to adapt to more intense activities. Most of these injuries can be prevented through a more gradual and correct conditioning (low-impact) program.

Proper shoes for specific activities are essential. Shoes should be replaced when they show a lot of wear and tear. Softer training surfaces, such as grass and dirt, produce less trauma than asphalt and concrete.

Because few people have perfect body alignment, injuries associated with overtraining may occur eventually. In case of injury, proper treatment can avert a lengthy recovery process. A summary of common exercise-related injuries and how to manage them follows.

Acute Sports Injuries

The best treatment always has been prevention itself. If an activity causes unusual discomfort or chronic irritation, you need to treat the cause by decreasing the intensity, switching activities, substituting equipment, or upgrading clothing (such as buying proper-fitting shoes).

In cases of acute injury, the standard treatment is rest, cold application, compression or splinting (or both), and elevation of the affected body part. This commonly is referred to as "RICE":

R = rest
I = ice application
C = compression
E = elevation

Cold should be applied three to five times a day for 15 to 20 minutes at a time during the first 24 to 36 hours, by submerging the injured area in cold water, using an icebag, or applying ice massage to the affected part. An elastic bandage or wrap can be used for compression. Elevating the body part decreases blood flow (and therefore swelling) in that body part.

The purpose of these treatment modalities is to minimize swelling in the area, which hastens recovery time. After the first 36 to 48 hours, heat can be used if the injury shows no further swelling or inflammation. If you have doubts regarding the nature or seriousness of the injury (such as suspected fracture), you should seek a medical evaluation.

Obvious deformities (such as exhibited by fractures, dislocations, or partial dislocations) call for splinting, cold application with an icebag, and medical attention. Do not try to reset any of these conditions by yourself, because you could further damage muscles, ligaments, and nerves. Treatment of these injuries always should be in the hands of specialized medical personnel. A quick reference guide for the signs or symptoms and treatment of exercise-related problems is provided in Table 4.2.

KeyTerms

Hypothermia A breakdown in the body's ability to generate heat; a drop in body temperature below 95 degrees F.

TABLE 4.2 Reference Guide for Exercise-Related Problems

Injury	Signs/Symptoms	Treatment*
Bruise (contusion)	Pain, swelling, discoloration	Cold application, compression, rest
Dislocations Fractures	Pain, swelling, deformity	Splinting, cold application, seek medical attention
Heat cramps	Cramps, spasms, and muscle twitching in the legs, arms, and abdomen	Stop activity, get out of the heat, stretch, massage the painful area, drink plenty of fluids
Heat exhaustion	Fainting, profuse sweating, cold/clammy skin, weak/rapid pulse, weakness, headache	Stop activity, rest in a cool place, loosen clothing, rub body with cool, wet towel, drink plenty of fluids, stay out of heat for 2–3 days
Heat stroke	Hot/dry skin, no sweating, serious disorientation, rapid/full pulse, vomiting, diarrhea, unconsciousness, high body temperature	*Seek immediate medical attention*, request help and get out of the sun, bathe in cold water/spray with cold water/rub body with cold towels, drink plenty of cold fluids
Joint sprains	Pain, tenderness, swelling, loss of use, discoloration	Cold application, compression, elevation, rest, heat after 36 to 48 hours (if no further swelling)
Muscle cramps	Pain, spasm	Stretch muscle(s), use mild exercises for involved area
Muscle soreness and stiffness	Tenderness, pain	Mild stretching, low-intensity exercise, warm bath
Muscle strains	Pain, tenderness, swelling, loss of use	Cold application, compression, elevation, rest, heat after 36 to 48 hours (if no further swelling)
Shin splints	Pain, tenderness	Cold application prior to and following any physical activity, rest, heat (if no activity is carried out)
Side stitch	Pain on the side of the abdomen below the rib cage	Decrease level of physical activity or stop altogether, gradually increase level of fitness
Tendinitis	Pain, tenderness, loss of use	Rest, cold application, heat after 48 hours

*Cold should be applied three to four times a day for 15 minutes. Heat can be applied three times a day for 15 to 20 minutes.

Muscle Soreness and Stiffness

Individuals who begin an exercise program or participate after a long layoff from exercise often develop muscle soreness and stiffness. The acute soreness that sets in the first few hours after exercise is thought to be related to a lack of blood (oxygen) flow and general fatigue of the exercised muscles.

Delayed muscle soreness that appears several hours after exercise (usually about 12 hours later) and lasts 2 to 4 days may be related to actual tiny tears in muscle tissue, muscle spasms that increase fluid retention (stimulating the pain nerve endings), and overstretching or tearing of connective tissue in and around muscles and joints.

Mild stretching before and adequate stretching after exercise help to prevent soreness and stiffness.

Gradually progressing into an exercise program is important, too. A person should not attempt to do too much too quickly. To relieve pain, mild stretching, low-intensity exercise to stimulate blood flow, and a warm bath might help.

Exercise Intolerance

When starting an exercise program, participants should stay within the safe limits. The best method to determine whether you are exercising too strenuously —**exercise intolerance**—is to check your heart rate and make sure it does not exceed the limits of your target zone. Exercising above this target zone may not be safe for unconditioned or high-risk individuals. You do not have to exercise beyond your target zone to gain the desired cardiorespiratory benefits.

Several physical signs will tell you when you are exceeding your functional limitations. Signs of intolerance include rapid or irregular heart rate, difficult breathing, nausea, vomiting, lightheadedness, headache, dizziness, unusually flushed or pale skin, extreme weakness, lack of energy, shakiness, sore muscles, cramps, and tightness in the chest. Learn to listen to your body. If you notice any of these symptoms, seek medical attention before continuing your exercise program.

Recovery heart rate is another indicator of overexertion. To a certain extent, recovery heart rate is related to fitness level. The higher your cardiorespiratory fitness level, the faster your heart rate will decrease following exercise. As a rule of thumb, heart rate should be below 120 beats per minute 5 minutes into recovery. If your heart rate is above 120, you most likely have overexerted yourself or possibly could have some other cardiac abnormality. If you lower the intensity or duration of exercise, or both, and you still have a fast heart rate 5 minutes into recovery, you should consult your physician.

Side Stitch

Side stitch happens primarily in the early stages of participation in exercise. The exact cause is unknown. Some experts suggest that it could relate to a lack of blood flow to the respiratory muscles during strenuous physical exertion. Side stitch occurs primarily in unconditioned beginners and in trained individuals when they exercise at higher intensities than usual. As one's physical condition improves, this condition tends to disappear unless training is intensified. Some people encounter side stitch during downhill running. If side stitch is a problem for you, slow down, and if it persists, stop altogether. Lying down on your back and gently bringing both knees to the chest and holding that position for 30 to 60 seconds also helps.

Some people get side stitch if they eat or drink juice shortly before exercise. Drinking only water an hour to two prior to exercise sometimes prevents side stitch. Other individuals have problems with commercially available carbohydrate solutions during high-intensity exercise. Unless carbohydrate replacement is crucial to complete an event (such as a marathon or a triathlon), drink cool water for fluid replacement or try a different carbohydrate solution.

Shin Splints

Shin splints, one of the most common injuries to the lower limbs, usually results from one or more of the following: (a) lack of proper and gradual conditioning, (b) doing physical activities on hard surfaces (wooden floors, hard tracks, cement, or asphalt), (c) fallen arches, (d) chronic overuse, (e) muscle fatigue, (f) faulty posture, (g) improper shoes, and (h) participating in weight-bearing activities when excessively overweight.

To manage shin splints,

1. Remove or reduce the cause (exercise on softer surfaces, wear better shoes or arch supports, or completely stop exercise until the shin splints heal);
2. Do stretching exercises before and after physical activity;
3. Use ice massage for 10 to 20 minutes before and after exercise;
4. Apply active heat (whirlpool and hot baths) for 15 minutes, two to three times a day; or
5. Use supportive taping during physical activity (a qualified athletic trainer can teach you the proper taping technique).

Muscle Cramps

Muscle cramps are caused by the body's depletion of essential electrolytes or a breakdown in the coordination between opposing muscle groups. If you have a muscle cramp, you should first attempt to stretch the muscles involved. In the case of the calf muscle, for example, pull your toes up toward the knees. After stretching the muscle, rub it down gently, and finally, do some mild exercises requiring the use of that muscle.

In pregnant and lactating women, muscle cramps often are related to a lack of calcium. If women get cramps during these times, calcium supplements usually relieve the problem. Tight clothing also can cause cramps by decreasing blood flow to active muscle tissue.

Leisure-Time Physical Activity

Although individuals have notable differences, the average person in developed countries has about 3.5 hours of "free" or leisure time daily. In our current automated society, most of this time is spent in sedentary living. People would be better off doing some

KeyTerms

Exercise intolerance Inability to function during exercise because of excessive fatigue or extreme feelings of discomfort.

Side stitch A sharp pain in the side of the abdomen.

Shin splints Injury to the lower leg characterized by pain and irritation in the shin region of the leg.

physical activities based on personal interests. Motivational factors include health, aesthetics, weight control, competition and challenge, fun, social interaction, mental arousal, relaxation, and stress management.

Frequently, leisure-time physical activity does not include exercise performed during a regular exercise program. It consists of activities such as walking, hiking, gardening, yardwork, occupational work and chores, and moderate sports such as tennis, table tennis, badminton, golf, or croquet.

Every small increase in daily physical activity contributes to better health and wellness. Small increases in physical activity have a large impact in decreasing early risks for disease and premature death. Therefore, a new, concerted effort must be made to spend leisure time in activities that will promote the expenditure of energy, provide a break from daily tasks, and contribute to health-related fitness.

EXERCISE AND AGING

Unlike any prior time in U. S. history, the elderly population constitutes the fastest-growing segment. In 1880, less than 3 percent of the total population, or fewer than 2 million people, was older than 65. By 1980 the elderly population had reached approximately 25 million, more than 11.3 percent of the population. By the year 2030, more than 70 million people in the United States are expected to be older than age 65.

Historically, older adults have been neglected when developing fitness programs. Nevertheless, fitness is just as important for older people as it is for young people. Although much research remains to be done in this area, studies indicate that older individuals who are physically fit also enjoy better health and a higher quality of life.

The main objective of fitness programs for older adults should be to help them improve their functional status and contribute to healthy aging. This implies the ability to maintain independent living status and to avoid disability. The American Alliance of Health, Physical Education, Recreation and Dance (AAHPERD) has defined functional fitness for older adults as the physical capacity of the individual to meet ordinary and unexpected demands of daily life safely and effectively.[23] This definition clearly indicates the need for fitness programs that closely relate to activities this population normally encounters. Older adults are encouraged to participate in programs that will help develop cardiorespiratory endurance, muscular strength and endurance, muscular flexibility, agility and balance, and motor coordination.

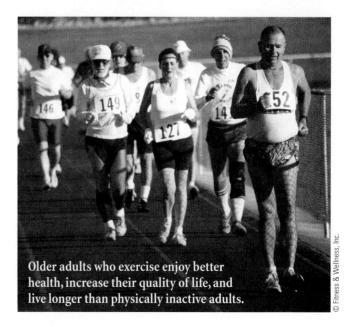

Older adults who exercise enjoy better health, increase their quality of life, and live longer than physically inactive adults.

Physical Training in the Older Adult

Regular participation in physical activity provides both physiological and physical benefits to older adults.[24] Cardiorespiratory endurance training helps to increase functional capacity, decrease the risk for disease, improve health status, and increase life expectancy. Strength training decreases the rate at which strength and muscle mass are lost. Among the psychological benefits are preserved cognitive function, reduced symptoms and behaviors related to depression, and improved self-confidence and self-esteem.

The trainability of older men and women alike and the effectiveness of physical activity in enhancing health have been demonstrated in prior research. Older adults who increase their physical activity experience significant changes in cardiorespiratory endurance, strength, and flexibility. The extent of the changes depends on their initial fitness level and the types of activities they select for their training (walking, cycling, strength training, and so on).

Improvements in maximal oxygen uptake in older adults are similar to those of younger people, although older people seem to require a longer training period to achieve these changes. Declines in maximal oxygen uptake average about 1 percent per year between age 25 and 75.[25] A slower rate of decline is seen in people who maintain a lifetime aerobic exercise program.

Results of research on the effects of aging on the cardiorespiratory system of male exercisers versus nonexercisers showed that the maximal oxygen uptake of regular exercisers was almost twice that of the nonexercisers (see Table 4.3).[26] The study revealed a

TABLE **4.3** Effects of Physical Activity and Inactivity on Older Men	Exercisers	Non-exercisers
Age (yrs)	68.0	69.8
Weight (lbs)	160.3	186.3
Resting heart rate (bpm)	55.8	66.0
Maximal heart rate (bpm)	157.0	146.0
Heart rate reserve* (bpm)	101.2	80.0
Blood pressure (mm Hg)	120/78	150/90
Maximal oxygen uptake (ml/kg/min)	38.6	20.3

SOURCE: Data from F. W. Kash, J. L. Boyer, S. P. Van Camp, L. S. Verity, and J. P. Wallace, "The Effect of Physical Activity on Aerobic Power in Older Men (A Longitudinal Study)," *The Physician and Sports Medicine* 18, no. 4 (1990): 73–83.

*Heart rate reserve = maximal heart rate − resting heart rate.

A high level of physical fitness can be maintained throughout the life span.

© Fitness & Wellness, Inc.

decline in maximal oxygen uptake between ages 50 and 68 of only 13 percent in the active group, compared with 41 percent in the inactive group. These changes indicate that about one-third of the loss in maximal oxygen uptake results from aging and two-thirds of the loss comes from inactivity. Blood pressure, heart rate, and body weight also were remarkably better in the exercising group. Furthermore, aerobic training seems to decrease high blood pressure in the older patients at the same rate as in young hypertensive people.[27]

In terms of aging, muscle strength declines by 10 to 20 percent between the ages of 20 and 50, but between ages 50 and 70, it drops by another 25 to 30 percent. Through strength training, frail adults in their 80s or 90s can double or triple their strength in just a few months. The amount of muscle hypertrophy achieved, however, decreases with age. Strength gains close to 200 percent have been found in previously inactive adults over age 90.[28] In fact, research has shown that regular strength training improves balance, gait, speed, **functional independence**, morale, depression symptoms, and energy intake.[29] (The health-related components of strength and flexibility fitness are addressed in Chapters 5 and 6 respectively.)

Although muscle flexibility drops by about 5 percent per decade of life, 10 minutes of stretching every other day can prevent most of this loss as a person ages.[30] Improved flexibility enhances mobility skills.[31] The latter promotes independence because it helps

> Older adults require a longer training period to achieve similar oxygen uptake improvements as those seen in younger people.

older adults successfully perform activities of daily living.

In terms of body composition, inactive adults continue to gain body fat after age 60 despite the tendency toward lower body weight. The increase in body fatness is most likely related to a decrease in basal metabolic rate and physical activity along with increased caloric intake above that required to maintain daily energy requirements.[32]

Older adults who wish to initiate or continue an exercise program are strongly encouraged to have a complete medical exam, including a stress electrocardiogram test (see Chapter 10). Recommended activities for older adults include calisthenics, walking, jogging, swimming, cycling, and water aerobics.

Older people should avoid isometric and very high intensity weight-training exercises (see Chapter 5). Activities that require all-out effort or require participants to hold their breath (e.g., the valsalva maneuver) tend to lessen blood flow to the heart and cause a significant increase in blood pressure and increases the load placed on the heart. Older adults should participate in activities that require continuous and rhythmic muscular activity (about 40 to 60

KeyTerms

Functional independence Ability to carry out activities of daily living without assistance from other individuals.

percent of HHR). These activities do not cause large increases in blood pressure or place an intense overload on the heart.

GETTING STARTED AND ADHERING TO A LIFETIME EXERCISE PROGRAM

Following the guidelines provided in Figure 4.7 (page 79), you may proceed to initiate your cardiorespiratory endurance program. If you have not been exercising regularly, you might begin by attempting to train five or six times a week for 30 minutes at a time. You may find this discouraging, however, and may drop out before getting too far because you will probably develop some muscle soreness and stiffness and possibly incur minor injuries.

Muscle soreness and stiffness and the risk for injuries can be lessened or eliminated by increasing the intensity, duration, and frequency of exercise progressively, as outlined in Figure 4.7. Once you have determined your exercise prescription, the difficult part begins: starting and sticking to a lifetime exercise program. Although you may be motivated after reading the benefits to be gained from physical activity, lifelong dedication and perseverance are necessary to reap and maintain good fitness.

The first few weeks probably will be the most difficult, but where there's a will, there's a way. Once you begin to see positive changes, it won't be as hard. Soon you will develop a habit for exercise that will be deeply satisfying and will bring about a sense of self-accomplishment. The following suggestions have been used successfully to help change behavior and adhere to a lifetime exercise program.

1. Set aside a regular time for exercise. If you don't plan ahead, it is a lot easier to skip. On a weekly basis, using red ink, schedule your exercise time into your day planner. Next, hold your exercise hour "sacred." Give exercise priority equal to the most important school or business activity of the day.

   If you are too busy, attempt to accumulate 30 minutes of activity by doing three separate 10-minute sessions throughout the day. Try reading the mail while you walk, take stairs instead of elevators, walk the dog, or ride the stationary bike as you watch the evening news.

2. Exercise early in the day, when you will be less tired and the chances of something interfering with your workout are minimal; thus you will be less likely to skip your exercise session.

3. Select aerobic activities you enjoy. Exercise should be as much fun as your favorite hobby. If you pick an activity you don't enjoy, you will be unmotivated and less likely to keep exercising. Don't be afraid to try out a new activity, even if that means learning new skills.

4. Combine different activities. You can train by doing two or three different activities the same week. This cross-training may deter the monotony of repeating the same activity every day. Try lifetime sports. Many endurance sports, such as racquetball, basketball, soccer, badminton, roller skating, cross-country skiing, and body surfing (paddling the board), provide a nice break from regular workouts.

5. Use the proper clothing and equipment for exercise. A poor pair of shoes, for example, can make you more prone to injury and discourage you at the outset.

6. Find a friend or group of friends to exercise with. Social interaction will make exercise more fulfilling. Besides, it's harder to skip if someone is waiting to go with you.

7. Set goals and share them with others. Quitting is tougher when someone else knows what you are trying to accomplish. When you reach a targeted goal, reward yourself with a new pair of shoes or a jogging suit.

8. Don't become a chronic exerciser. Learn to listen to your body. Overexercising can lead to chronic fatigue and injuries. Exercise should be enjoyable, and in the process you should stop and smell the roses.

9. Exercise in different places and facilities. This will add variety to your workouts.

10. Exercise to music. People who listen to fast-tempo music tend to exercise more vigorously and longer. Using headphones when exercising outdoors, however, can be dangerous. Even indoors, it is preferable not to use headphones, so that you can still be aware of your surroundings.

11. Keep a regular record of your activities. Keeping a record allows you to monitor your progress and compare it against previous months and years (see Figures 4.9 and 4.11, pages 82 and 109).

12. Conduct periodic assessments. Improving to a higher fitness category is a reward in itself.

13. Listen to your body. Stop exercise if you experience pain or unusual discomfort. Pain and aches are an indication of potential injury. If you do suffer an injury, do not return to your regular workouts until you are fully recovered. You may cross-train using activities that do not aggravate

your injury (for instance, swimming instead of jogging).

14. If a health problem arises, see a physician. When in doubt, it's better to be safe than sorry.

A LIFETIME COMMITMENT TO FITNESS

The benefits of fitness can be maintained only through a regular lifetime program. Exercise is not like putting money in the bank. It does not help much to exercise 4 or 5 hours on Saturday and not do anything else the rest of the week. If anything, exercising only once a week is unsafe for unconditioned adults.

Even the greatest athletes on earth, if they were to stop exercising, would be, after just a few years, at a risk for disease similar to someone who never has done any physical activity. Staying with a physical fitness program long enough brings about positive physiological and psychological changes. Once you are there, you will not want to have it any other way.

The time involved in losing the benefits of exercise varies among the different components of physical fitness and also depends on the person's condition before the interruption. In regard to cardiorespiratory endurance, it has been estimated that 4 weeks of aerobic training are completely reversed in 2 consecutive weeks of physical inactivity. On the other hand, if you have been exercising regularly for months or years, 2 weeks of inactivity will not hurt you as much as it will someone who has exercised only a few weeks. As a rule of thumb, after 48 to 72 hours of

aerobic inactivity, the cardiorespiratory system starts to lose some of its capacity.

To maintain fitness, you should keep up a regular exercise program, even during vacations. If you have to interrupt your program for reasons beyond your control, you should not attempt to resume training at the same level you left off, but rather build up gradually again.

WEB INTERACTIVE

Running: Preventing Over-Use Injuries
Site features excellent information from the *American Family Physician* journal.

http://familydoctor.org/handouts/147.html

Aerobic Exercises
This site features tips on aerobic exercises, answering questions like How often? How long? and How intense?

http://www.hom.net

Exercise and the Elderly
This site provides research, guidelines, and exercise benefits for the elderly.

http://www.drkoop.com/family/seniors/fitness/

INTERACTIVE SITES

Aerobics and Fitness Association of America
This interactive site features "Exercise Gets Personal," where you can create a customized exercise program that includes activities you select geared to your current level of fitness activity. Exercises include aerobics, muscular conditioning, and flexibility with descriptions and precautions for each activity.

http://www.afaa.com

n*tes

1. W. M. Bortz II, "Disuse and Aging," *Journal of the American Medical Association* 248 (1982): 1203–1208.
2. R. K. Dishman, "Compliance/ Adherence in Health-Related Exercise," *Health Psychology* 1 (1982): 237–267.
3. U. S. Department of Health and Human Services, *Physical Activity and Health: A Report of the Surgeon General* (Atlanta: U. S. Department of Health and Human Services, Centers for Disease Control and Prevention, National Center for Chronic Disease Prevention and Health Promotion, 1996).
4. American College of Sports Medicine, "Position Stand: The Recommended Quantity and

Quality of Exercise for Developing and Maintaining Cardiorespiratory and Muscular Fitness, and Flexibility in Healthy Adults," *Medicine and Science in Sports and Exercise* 30 (1998): 975–991.
5. American College of Sports Medicine, *Guidelines for Exercise Testing and Prescription* (Baltimore: Williams & Wilkins, 2000).
6. See note 4.
7. W. W. K. Hoeger, C. Harris, W. L. Nurge, and M. L. Jensen, "Physiologic Responses to Step Aerobics Combined with Upper Work in Trained Subjects," *Journal for the International Council for Health Physical Education, Recreation, Sport, and Dance* 27 (2001): 9–10.

D. R. Hopkins, W. W. K. Hoeger, D. E. Van Zee, and W. J. Nurge, "Physiologic Responses to Aerobelt Walking," *Medicine and Science*

in Sports and Exercise 26 (1994): 243–245.

W. J. Nurge, D. E. Van Zee, and W. W. K. Hoeger. "Physiologic Responses to Aero-belt Walking and Jogging," *Medicine and Science in Sports and Exercise* 26 (1994): 243–247.
8. S. Blair, "Surgeon General's Report on Physical Fitness: The Inside Story," *ACSM's Health & Fitness Journal* 1 (1997): 14–18.
9. R. F. DeBusk, U. Stenestrand, M. Sheehan, and W. L. Haskell, "Training Effects of Long Versus Short Bouts of Exercise in Healthy Subjects," *American Journal of Cardiology* 65 (1990): 1010–1013.
10. "Summary Statement: Workshop on Physical Activity and Public Health," *Sports Medicine Bulletin* 28 (1993): 7.
11. See note 3.

12. U. S. Department of Agriculture and U. S. Department of Health and Human Services, "Nutrition and Your Health: Dietary Guidelines for Americans," *Home and Garden Bulletin* 232 (2000).

13. See note 4.

14. W. D. McArdle, F. I. Katch, and V. L. Katch, *Essentials of Exercise Physiology* (Philadelphia: Lippincott Williams & Wilkins, 2000).

15. J. L. Christi, L. M. Sheldahl, F. E. Tristani, L. S. Wann, K. B. Sagar, S. G. Levandoski, M. J. Ptacin, K. A. Sobocinski, and R. D. Morris, "Cardiovascular Regulation During Head-out Water Immersion Exercise," *Journal of Applied Physiology* 69 (1990): 657–664.

    L. M. Sheldahl, F. E. Tristani, P. S. Clifford, C. V. Hughes, K. A. Sobocinski, and R. D. Morris, "Effect of Head-out Water Immersion on Cardiorespiratory Response to Dynamic Exercise," *Journal of American College of Cardiology* 10 (1987): 1254–1258.

    J. Svedenhang and J. Seger, "Running on Land and in Water: Comparative Exercise Physiology," *Medicine and Science in Sports and Exercise* 24 (1992): 1155–1160.

16. W. W. K. Hoeger, "Is Water Aerobics Aerobic?" *Fitness Management* 11 (April 1995): 29–30, 43.

17. W. W. K. Hoeger, D. Hopkins, and D. Barber, "Physiologic Responses to Maximal Treadmill Running and Water Aerobic Exercise," *National Aquatics Journal* 11 (1995): 4–7.

18. W. W. K. Hoeger, T. S. Gibson, J. Moore, and D. R. Hopkins, "A Comparison of Selected Training Responses to Low Impact Aerobics and Water Aerobics," *National Aquatics Journal* 9 (1993): 13–16.

19. E. J. Marcinick, J. Potts, G. Schlabach, S. Will, P. Dawson, and B. F. Hurley, "Effects of Strength Training on Lactate Threshold and Endurance Performance," *Medicine and Science in Sports and Exercise* 23 (1991): 739–743.

20. R. S. Paffenbarger, Jr., R. T. Hyde, A. L. Wing, and C. H. Steinmetz, "A Natural History of Athleticism and Cardiovascular Health," *Journal of the American Medical Association* 252 (1984): 491–495.

21. American College of Sports Medicine, "Position Stand: Exercise and Type 2 Diabetes," *Medicine and Science in Sports and Exercise* 32 (2000): 1345–1360.

22. University of California at Berkeley, *The Wellness Guide to Lifelong Fitness* (New York: Random House, 1993): 198.

23. W. Osness, M. Adrian, B. Clark, W. W. K. Hoeger, D. Raab, and R. Wiswell, "The AAHPERD Fitness Task Force: History and Philosophy," *Journal of Physical Education, Recreation and Dance* 60, no. 3 (1989): 64–65.

24. American College of Sports Medicine, "Position Stand: Exercise and Physical Activity for Older Adults," *Medicine and Science in Sports and Exercise* 30 (1998): 992–1008.

25. R. J. Shephard, "Exercise and Aging: Extending Independence in Older Adult," *Geriatrics* 48 (1993): 61–64.

26. F. W. Kash, J. L. Boyer, S. P. Van Camp, L. S. Verity, and J. P. Wallace, "The Effect of Physical Activity on Aerobic Power in Older Men (A Longitudinal Study)," *Physician and Sports Medicine* 18, no. 4 (1990): 73–83.

27. J. Hagberg, S. Blair, A. Ehsani, N. Gordon, N. Kaplan, C. Tipton, and E. Zambraski, "Position Stand: Physical Activity, Physical Fitness, and Hypertension," *Medicine and Science in Sports and Exercise* 25 (1993): i–x.

28. W. S. Evans, "Exercise, Nutrition and Aging," *Journal of Nutrition* 122 (1992): 796–801.

29. See note 19.

30. The Editors, "Exercise for the Ages," *Consumer Reports on Health* (Yonkers, NY: July, 1996).

31. J. M. Walker, D. Sue, N. Miles-Elkousy, G. Ford, and H. Trevelyan, "Active Mobility of the Extremities in Older Subjects," *Physical Therapy* 64 (1994): 919–923.

32. S. B. Roberts, et al., "What are the Dietary Needs of Adults?" *International Journal of Obesity* 16 (1992): 969–976.

Suggested Readings

- *ACSM's Resource Manual for Guidelines for Exercise Testing and Prescription*. Baltimore: Williams & Wilkins, 1998.

- American College of Sports Medicine. *Guidelines for Exercise Testing and Prescription*. Baltimore: Williams & Wilkins, 2000.

- Arnheim, D. D., and W. Prentice. *Principles of Athletic Training*. Dubuque, IA: Brown & Benchmark, 1996.

- Borg, G. "Perceived Exertion: A Note on History and Methods." *Medicine and Science in Sports and Exercise* 5 (1993): 90–93.

- Clark, B., W. Osness, W. W. K. Hoeger, M. Adrian, D. Raab, and R. Wiswell. "Tests for Fitness in Older Adults: AAHPERD Fitness Task Force." *Journal of Physical Education, Recreation and Dance* 60, no. 3 (1989): 66–71.

- Coleman, E. *Eating for Endurance*. Palo Alto, CA: Bull Publishing, 1997.

- Fox, E. L., R. W. Bowers, and M. L. Foss. *The Physiological Basis for Exercise and Sport*. Madison, WI: Brown & Benchmark, 1993.

- Heyward, V. H. *Advanced Fitness Assessment & Exercise Prescription*. Champaign, IL: Human Kinetics, 1998.

- Karvonen, M. J., E. Kentala, and O. Mustala. "The Effects of Training on the Heart Rate: A Longitudinal Study." *Annales Medicinae Experimetalis et Biologiae Fenniae* 35 (1957): 307–315.

- Kushi, L. H. "Physical Activity and Mortality in Postmenopausal Women." *Journal of the American Medical Association* 277 (1997): 1287–1292.

- McArdle, W. D., F. I. Katch, and V. L. Katch. *Exercise Physiology*. Baltimore: Williams & Wilkins, 1996.

- Metcalf, J. A. "Exercising During Pregnancy." *Certified News* 5, no. 2 (1995): 10–11.

- Pfeiffer, R. P, and B. C. Mangus. *Concepts of Athletic Training*. Boston: Jones and Bartlett, 1998.

- Teitz, C. C. "Overuse Injuries." In *Scientific Foundations of Sports Medicine*, edited by C. C. Teitz, 299–328. Philadelphia: B. C. Decker, 1989.

FIGURE 4.11 Cardiorespiratory exercise record form.

Name _____   Month _____

Date	Body Weight	Exercise Heart Rate	Type of Exercise	Distance In Miles	Time Hrs/Min	RPE*
1						
2						
3						
4						
5						
6						
7						
8						
9						
10						
11						
12						
13						
14						
15						
16						
17						
18						
19						
20						
21						
22						
23						
24						
25						
26						
27						
28						
29						
30						
31						
			Total			

*Rate of perceived exertion.

Name _____   Month _____

Date	Body Weight	Exercise Heart Rate	Type of Exercise	Distance In Miles	Time Hrs/Min	RPE*
1						
2						
3						
4						
5						
6						
7						
8						
9						
10						
11						
12						
13						
14						
15						
16						
17						
18						
19						
20						
21						
22						
23						
24						
25						
26						
27						
28						
29						
30						
31						
			Total			

*Rate of perceived exertion.

FIGURE **4.11** Cardiorespiratory exercise record form.

Name _____ Month _____

Date	Body Weight	Exercise Heart Rate	Type of Exercise	Distance In Miles	Time Hrs/Min	RPE*
1						
2						
3						
4						
5						
6						
7						
8						
9						
10						
11						
12						
13						
14						
15						
16						
17						
18						
19						
20						
21						
22						
23						
24						
25						
26						
27						
28						
29						
30						
31						
			Total			

*Rate of perceived exertion.

Name _____ Month _____

Date	Body Weight	Exercise Heart Rate	Type of Exercise	Distance In Miles	Time Hrs/Min	RPE*
1						
2						
3						
4						
5						
6						
7						
8						
9						
10						
11						
12						
13						
14						
15						
16						
17						
18						
19						
20						
21						
22						
23						
24						
25						
26						
27						
28						
29						
30						
31						
			Total			

*Rate of perceived exertion.

Muscular Strength Assessment and Prescription

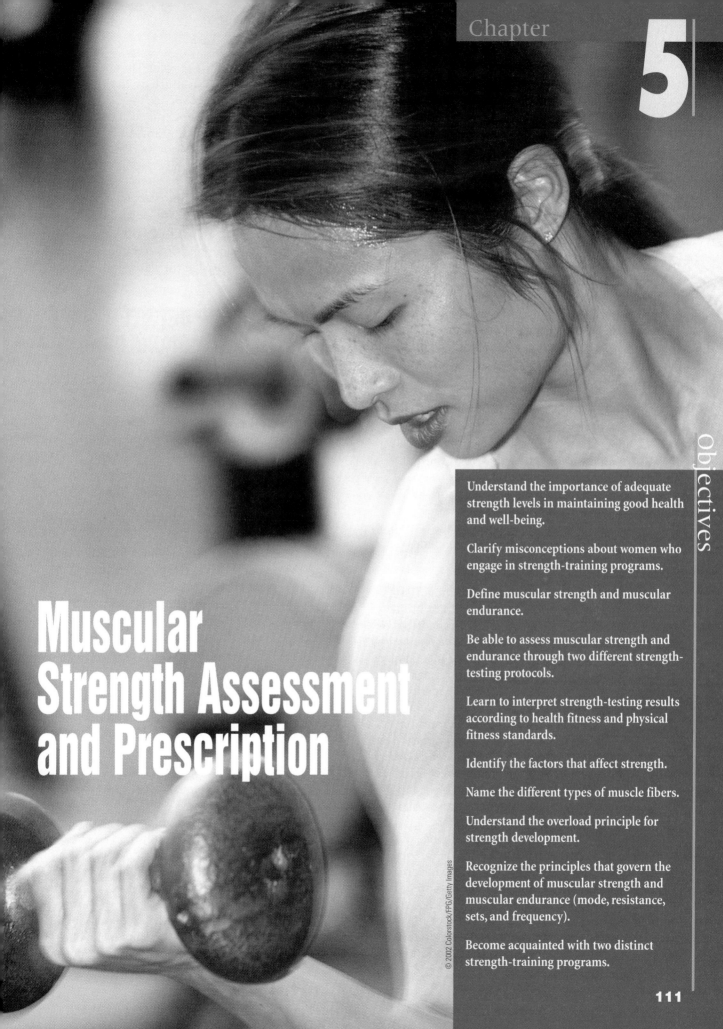

© 2002 Colorstock/FPG/Getty Images

Understand the importance of adequate strength levels in maintaining good health and well-being.

Clarify misconceptions about women who engage in strength-training programs.

Define muscular strength and muscular endurance.

Be able to assess muscular strength and endurance through two different strength-testing protocols.

Learn to interpret strength-testing results according to health fitness and physical fitness standards.

Identify the factors that affect strength.

Name the different types of muscle fibers.

Understand the overload principle for strength development.

Recognize the principles that govern the development of muscular strength and muscular endurance (mode, resistance, sets, and frequency).

Become acquainted with two distinct strength-training programs.

The benefits of strength training in enhancing health and well-being are well documented. Many people, nonetheless, still have the impression that strength is necessary only for highly trained athletes, fitness enthusiasts, and individuals who hold jobs that require heavy muscular work. In fact, a well-planned strength-training program increases muscle strength and endurance, muscle tone, tendon and ligament strength, and bone density—all of which improve functional physical capacity.

Strength is a basic component of fitness and wellness and is crucial for optimal performance in daily activities such as sitting, walking, running, lifting and carrying objects, doing housework, and enjoying recreational activities. Strength is also of great value in improving posture, personal appearance, and self-image; developing sports skills; promoting joint stability; and meeting certain emergencies in life. From a health standpoint, increasing strength helps to increase or maintain muscle and a higher resting metabolic rate, lessens the risk for injury, helps to reduce chronic low-back pain, reduces arthritic pain, aids in childbearing, improves cholesterol levels, and may also help lower blood pressure and control blood sugar.

An important adaptation to strength training is that, with time, the heart rate and blood pressure response to lifting a heavy resistance (that is, a weight) decreases. This adaptation reduces the demands on the cardiovascular system during activities such as carrying the groceries, a child, or a suitcase.

Muscular strength may be the most important health-related component of physical fitness in the older adult population. Though proper cardiorespiratory endurance is necessary to help maintain a healthy heart, good strength contributes more to independent living than any other fitness component. Older adults with good strength levels can successfully perform most **activities of daily living**. Strength training also slows the age-related loss of muscle function.

More than anything else, older adults want to enjoy good health and function independently. Many of them, however, are confined to nursing homes because they lack sufficient strength to move about. They cannot walk very far, and many have to be helped in and out of beds, chairs, and tubs.

A strength-training program can enhance quality of life tremendously, and nearly everyone can benefit from it. In fact, only people with advanced heart disease are advised to refrain from strength training. Inactive adults between the ages of 56 and 86 who participated in a 12-week strength-training program increased lean body mass by about 3 pounds, lost about 4 pounds of fat, and increased their resting metabolic rate by almost 7 percent.[1] In other research, leg strength improved by as much as 200 percent in previously inactive adults over age 90.[2] As strength improves, so does the ability to move about, the capacity for independent living, and enjoyment of life during the "golden years." More specifically, good strength enhances quality of life in the following ways:

- It improves balance and restores mobility.
- It makes lifting and reaching easier.
- It decreases the risk for injuries and falls.
- It stresses the bones and preserves bone mineral density, thus decreasing the risk for osteoporosis.

RELATIONSHIP BETWEEN STRENGTH AND METABOLISM

Perhaps one of the most significant benefits of maintaining a good strength level is its relationship to human **metabolism**. A primary outcome of a strength-training program is an increase in muscle mass or size (lean body mass), known as "muscle **hypertrophy**."

Muscle tissue uses energy even at rest. In contrast, fatty tissue uses little energy and may be considered metabolically inert from the standpoint of caloric use (that is, your body expends X calories to maintain muscle and very few calories to maintain fat). As muscle size increases, so does **resting metabolism**. Even small increases in muscle mass may improve resting metabolism.

Each additional pound of muscle tissue increases resting metabolism by 35 calories per day.[3] All other factors being equal, if two individuals both weigh 150 pounds but have different amounts of muscle mass, the one with more muscle mass will have a higher resting metabolic rate, allowing this person to ingest more calories (which will be used to maintain the muscle tissue, not to create fat). Briefly, the higher your metabolic rate, the more you can eat without gaining fat.

Effect on Aging Metabolism

Loss of lean tissue is also thought to be the main reason for the decrease in metabolism as people grow older. Contrary to some beliefs, metabolism does not have to slow down significantly with aging. It is not so much that metabolism slows down. It's that we slow down.

Lean body mass decreases with sedentary living, which, in turn, slows down the resting metabolic rate. If people continue eating at the same rate, body fat increases. The average decrease in resting metabolism from age 26 to age 60 is about 360 calories per day.[4] Hence, participating in a strength-training program is important in maintaining lean body mass and in preventing and reducing excess body fat.

GENDER DIFFERENCES

One of the most common misconceptions about physical fitness concerns women in strength training. Because of the increase in muscle mass typically seen in men, some women think that a strength-training program will have adverse effects because they, too, will develop large musculature. Even though the quality of muscle in men and women is the same, endocrinological differences do not allow women to achieve the same amount of muscle hypertrophy (size) as men. Men also have more muscle fibers and, because of sex-specific male hormones, each individual fiber has more potential for hypertrophy.

The idea that strength training allows women to develop muscle hypertrophy to the same extent as men do is as false as the notion that playing basketball will turn women into giants. Masculinity and femininity are established by genetic inheritance, not by the amount of physical activity. Variations in the extent of masculinity and femininity are determined by individual differences in hormonal secretions of androgen, testosterone, estrogen, and progesterone. Women with a bigger-than-average build often are inclined to participate in sports because of their natural physical advantage. As a result, many women have associated participation in sports and strength training with large muscle size.

As the number of females who participate in sports has increased steadily during the last few years, the myth that strength training in women leads to large increases in muscle size has abated somewhat. For example, per pound of body weight, female gymnasts are considered among the strongest athletes in the world. These athletes engage regularly in serious strength-training programs. Yet, female gymnasts have some of the most well-toned and graceful figures of all women.

In recent years, improved body appearance has become the rule rather than the exception for women who participate in strength-training programs. Some of the most attractive female movie stars also train with weights to further improve their personal image.

Nonetheless, you may ask, "If weight training does not masculinize women, why do so many women

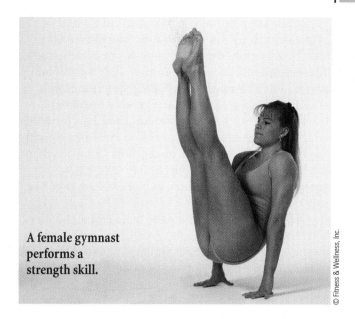

A female gymnast performs a strength skill.

© Fitness & Wellness, Inc.

> Improved body appearance is the rule rather than the exception for women who participate in strength-training programs.

body builders develop such heavy musculature?" In the sport of body building, the athletes follow intense training routines consisting of two or more hours of constant weight lifting with short rest intervals between sets. Many body-building training routines call for back-to-back exercises using the same muscle groups. The objective of this type of training is to pump extra blood into the muscles. This additional fluid makes the muscles appear much bigger than they do in a resting condition. Based on the intensity and the length of the training session, the muscles can remain filled with blood, appearing measurably larger for several hours after completing the training session. Performing such routines is a common practice before competitions. Therefore, in real life, these women are not as muscular as they seem when they are participating in a contest.

Key Terms

Activities of daily living Everyday behaviors that people normally do to function in life (cross the street, carry groceries, lift objects, do laundry, sweep floors).

Metabolism All energy and material transformations that occur within living cells; necessary to sustain life.

Hypertrophy An increase in the size of the cell (for example, muscle hypertrophy).

Resting metabolism Amount of energy (expressed in milliliters of oxygen per minute or in total calories per day) an individual requires during resting conditions to sustain proper body function.

In the sport of body building, another point of controversy is the use of **anabolic steroids** and human growth hormones among women participants. These hormones, however, produce detrimental and undesirable side effects (such as hypertension, fluid retention, decreased breast size, deepening of the voice, whiskers, and other atypical body hair growth), which some women deem tolerable. Anabolic steroid use in general—except for medical reasons and when carefully monitored by a physician—can lead to serious health consequences in both male and female users.

Anabolic steroid use among female body builders is widespread. According to several sports medicine physicians and female body builders, about 80 percent of female body builders have used steroids. Furthermore, according to several female track-and-field coaches, as many as 95 percent of female athletes around the world in this sport have used anabolic steroids to remain competitive at the international level.

Women who take steroids undoubtedly will build heavy musculature and, if taken long enough, the steroids will produce masculinizing effects. As a result, the International Federation of Body Building instituted a mandatory steroid-testing program for females participating in the Miss Olympia contest. When drugs are not used to promote development, improved body image is the rule rather than the exception among females who participate in body building, strength training, or sports in general.

CHANGES IN BODY COMPOSITION

Another benefit of strength training, accentuated even more when combined with aerobic exercise, is a decrease in adipose or fatty tissue around muscle fibers themselves. The decrease in fatty tissue often is greater than the amount of muscle hypertrophy (see

Selected detrimental effects of using anabolic steroids

- Liver tumors
- Hepatitis
- Hypertension
- Reduction of high density lipoprotein (HDL)
- Elevation of low density lipoprotein (LDL)
- Hyperinsulinism
- Impaired pituitary function
- Impaired thyroid function
- Mood swings
- Aggressive behavior
- Increased irritability
- Acne
- Fluid retention
- Decreased libido
- HIV infection (via injection apparatus)
- Prostate problems (men)
- Testicular atrophy (men)
- Reduced sperm count (men)
- Clitoral enlargement (women)
- Decreased breast size (women)
- Increased body and facial hair (irreversible in women)
- Deepening of the voice (irreversible in women)

Figure 5.1). Therefore, losing inches but not body weight is common.

Because muscle tissue is more dense than fatty tissue (and despite the fact that inches are lost during a combined strength-training and aerobic program), people, especially women, often become discouraged because they cannot see the results readily on the scale. They can offset this discouragement by determining body composition regularly to monitor changes in percent body fat rather than simply measuring changes in total body weight (see Chapter 7).

FIGURE 5.1 Changes in body composition as a result of a combined aerobic and strength-training program.

Pre-Training **Post-Training**

Skin
Adipose tissue (fat)
Muscle tissue

ASSESSMENT OF MUSCULAR STRENGTH AND ENDURANCE

Although muscular strength and endurance are interrelated, they do differ. **Muscular strength** is the ability to exert maximum force against resistance. **Muscular endurance** is the ability of a muscle to exert submaximal force repeatedly over time.

Muscular endurance (also referred to as "localized muscular endurance") depends to a large extent on muscular strength. Weak muscles cannot repeat an action several times or sustain it. Based upon these principles, strength tests and training programs have been designed to measure and develop absolute muscular strength, muscular endurance, or a combination of the two.

Muscular strength is usually determined by the maximal amount of resistance (weight)—**one repetition maximum**, or **1 RM**—an individual is able to lift in a single effort. Although this assessment yields a good measure of absolute strength, it does require a considerable amount of time, because the 1 RM is determined through trial and error. For example, strength of the chest muscles is frequently measured through the bench press exercise. If an individual has not trained with weights, he may try 100 pounds and lift this resistance quite easily. After adding 50 pounds, he fails to lift the resistance. The resistance then is decreased by 10 or 20 pounds. Finally, after several trials, the 1 RM is established.

Using this method, a true 1 RM might be difficult to obtain the first time an individual is tested, because fatigue becomes a factor. By the time the 1 RM is established, the person has already made several maximal or near-maximal attempts.

Muscular endurance is typically established by the number of repetitions an individual can perform against a submaximal resistance or by the length of time a given contraction can be sustained. For example: How many push-ups can an individual do? Or how many times can she lift 30 pounds? Or how long can a person hold a chin-up?

If time is a factor and only one test item can be done, the hand grip test, described in Figure 5.2, is commonly used to assess strength. This test, though, provides only a weak correlation with overall body strength. For the most accurate assessment, use procedures in Figures 5.2, 5.3, and 5.4. You may take one or more of these tests according to your time and the facilities available.

Muscular strength and endurance are both highly specific. A high degree of strength or endurance in one body part does not necessarily indicate this is the case in other parts. Accordingly, exercises for the strength tests were selected to obtain a profile including the upper body, lower body, and abdominal regions.

Before taking the strength test, you should become familiar with the procedures for the respective tests. For safety reasons, always take a friend or group of friends with you whenever you train with weights or conduct any type of strength assessment. Also, these are different tests, so to make valid comparisons, the same test should be used for pre- and post-training assessments. The following are your options.

Muscular Strength: Hand Grip Test

As indicated earlier, when time is a factor, the hand grip test can be used to provide a rough estimate of strength. Unlike the next two tests, this is an isometric (static contraction) test. If the proper grip is used, no finger or body movement is visible during the test. The test procedure is given in Figure 5.2, and percentile ranks based on your results are provided in Table 5.1. The results of this test can be recorded in Figure 5.5 (page 121).

The hand grip test provides a rough estimate of strength.

© Fitness & Wellness, Inc.

KeyTerms

Anabolic steroids Synthetic versions of the male sex hormone testosterone, which promotes muscle development and hypertrophy.

Muscular strength The ability of a muscle to exert maximum force against resistance (for example, 1 repetition maximum [or 1 RM] of the bench press exercise).

Muscular endurance The ability of a muscle to exert submaximal force repeatedly over time.

One repetition maximum (1 RM) The maximum amount of resistance an individual is able to lift in a single effort.

FIGURE 5.2 Procedure for the hand grip strength test.

1. Adjust the width of the dynamometer* so the middle bones (middle phalanges) of your fingers rest on the distant end of the dynamometer grip.

Proper grip size for the hand grip test.

© Fitness & Wellness, Inc.

2. Use your dominant hand for this test. Place your elbow at a 90° angle and about 2" away from the body.

3. Grip as hard as you can for a few seconds. Do not move any other body part as you perform the test (do not flex or extend the elbow, do not move the elbow away or toward the body, and do not lean forward or backward during the test).

4. Record the dynamometer reading in pounds (if reading is in kilograms, multiply by 2.2046).

5. Three trials are allowed for this test. Use the highest reading for your final test score. Record your test results in Figure 5.5, and look up your percentile rank in Table 5.1.

6. Based on your percentile rank, obtain the hand grip strength fitness category according to the following guidelines:

Percentile Rank	Fitness Category
≥90	Excellent
70–80	Good
50–60	Average
30–40	Fair
≤20	Poor

*A Lafayette model 78010 dynamometer is recommended for this test. Lafayette Instruments Co., Sagamore and North 9th Street, Lafayette, IN 47903.

TABLE 5.1 Scoring Table for Hand Grip Strength Test

Percentile Rank	Men	Women
99	153	101
95	145	94
90	141	91
80	139	86
70	132	80
60	124	78
50	122	74
40	114	71
30	110	66
20	100	64
10	91	60
5	76	58

High physical fitness standard
Health fitness standard

Changes in strength may be more difficult to evaluate with this test. Most strength-training programs are dynamic in nature (body segments are moved through a range of motion), whereas this test provides an isometric assessment. Further, grip strength exercises are seldom used in strength training, and increases in strength are specific to the body parts exercised. This test also can be used to supplement the following strength tests.

Muscular Endurance

Three exercises were selected to assess the endurance of the upper body, lower body, and mid-body muscle groups (see Figure 5.3). The advantage of this test is that it does not require strength-training equipment—only a stopwatch, a metronome, a bench or gymnasium bleacher 16¼" high, a cardboard strip 3½" by 30", and a partner. A percentile rank is given for each exercise according to the number of repetitions performed (see Table 5.2). An overall endurance rating can be obtained by totaling the number of points obtained on each exercise. A form to record the results of this test is provided in Figure 5.5 (page 121).

FIGURE **5.3** Procedure for muscular endurance test.

Three exercises are conducted in this test: bench-jumps, modified dips (men) or modified push-ups (women), and bent-leg curl-ups or abdominal crunches. All exercises should be conducted with the aid of a partner. The correct procedure for performing each exercise is as follows:

Bench-jump.

Using a bench or gymnasium bleacher 16¼" high, attempt to jump up and down the bench as many times as possible in 1 minute. If you cannot jump the full minute, you may step up and down. A repetition is counted each time both feet return to the floor.

Bench jump.

Modified dip.
Men only: Using a bench or gymnasium bleacher, place the hands on the bench with the fingers pointing forward. Have a partner hold your feet in front of you. Bend the hips at approximately 90° (you also may use three sturdy chairs, put your hands on two chairs placed by the sides of your body, and place your feet on the third chair in front of you). Lower your body by flexing the elbows until they reach a 90° angle, then return to the starting position. Perform the repetitions to a two-step cadence (down-up) regulated with a

Modified dip.

metronome set at 56 beats per minute. Perform as many continuous repetitions as possible. Do not count any more repetitions if you fail to follow the metronome cadence.

Modified push-up.
Women: Lie down on the floor (face down), bend the knees (feet up in the air), and place the hands on the floor by the shoulders with the fingers pointing forward. The lower body will be supported at the knees (as opposed to the feet) throughout the test. The chest must touch the floor on each repetition. As with the modified-dip exercise, perform the repetitions to a two-step cadence (up-down) regulated with a metronome set at 56 beats per minute. Perform as many continuous repetitions as possible. Do not count any more repetitions if you fail to follow the metronome cadence.

Modified push-up.

Bent-leg curl-up.
Lie down on the floor (face up) and bend both legs at the knees at approximately 100°. The feet should be on the floor, and you must hold them in place yourself throughout the test. Cross the arms in front of the chest, each hand on the opposite shoulder. Now raise the head off the floor, placing the chin against the chest. This is the starting and finishing position for each curl-up. **The back of the head may not come in contact with the floor, the hands cannot be removed from the shoulders, nor may the feet or hips be raised off the floor at any time during the test. The test is terminated if any of these four conditions occur.** When you curl

Bent-leg curl-up.

up, the upper body must come to an upright position before going back down. The repetitions are performed to a two-step cadence (up-down) regulated with the metronome set at 40 beats per minute. For this exercise, you should allow a brief practice period of 5 to 10 seconds to familiarize yourself with the cadence (the *up* movement is initiated with the first beat, then you must wait for the next beat to initiate the *down* movement; one repetition is accomplished every two beats of the metronome). Count as many repetitions as you are able to perform following the proper cadence. The test is also terminated if you fail to maintain the appropriate cadence or if you accomplish 100 repetitions. Have your partner check the angle at the knees throughout the test to make sure to maintain the 100° angle as close as possible.

Abdominal crunch.
This test is recommended only for individuals who are unable to perform the bent-leg curl-up test because of susceptibility to low-back injury. Exercise form must be carefully monitored during the test. Several authors and researchers have indicated that proper form during this test is extremely difficult to control. Subjects often slide their bodies, bend their elbows, or shrug

(continued)

(Figure 5.3 Procedure for muscular endurance test—continued)

their shoulders during the test. Such actions facilitate the performance of the test and misrepresent the actual test results. Biomechanical factors also limit the ability to perform this test. Further, lack of spinal flexibility keeps some individuals from being able to move the full 3½" range of motion. Others are unable to keep their heels on the floor during the test. The validity of this test as an effective measure of abdominal strength or abdominal endurance has also been questioned in recent research.

Tape a 3½" × 30" strip of cardboard onto the floor. Lie down on the floor in a supine position (face up) with the knees bent at approximately 100° and the legs slightly apart. The feet should be on the floor, and you must hold them in place yourself throughout the test. Straighten out your arms and place them on the floor alongside the trunk with the palms down and the fingers fully extended. The fingertips of both hands should barely touch the closest edge of the cardboard (A). Bring the head off the floor until the chin is 1" to 2" away from your chest. Keep the head in this position during the entire test (do not move the head by flexing or extending the neck). You are now ready to begin the test.

Perform the repetitions to a two-step cadence (up-down) regulated with a metronome set at 60 beats per minute. As you curl up, slide the fingers over the cardboard until the fingertips reach the far edge (3½") of the board (B), then return to the starting position.

Allow a brief practice period of 5 to 10 seconds to familiarize yourself with the cadence. Initiate the up movement with the first beat and the down movement with the next beat. Accomplish one repetition every two beats of the metronome. Count as many repetitions as you are able to perform following the proper cadence. You may not count a repetition if the fingertips fail to reach the distant edge of the cardboard.

Terminate the test if you (a) fail to maintain the appropriate cadence, (b) bend the elbows, (c) shrug the shoulders, (d) slide the body, (e) lift heels off the floor, (f) raise the chin off the chest, (g) accomplish 100 repetitions, or (h) no longer can perform the test. Have your partner check the angle at the knees throughout the test to make sure that the 100° angle is maintained as close as possible.

For this test you may also use a Crunch-Ster Curl-Up Tester, available from Novel Products.* An illustration of the test performed with this equipment is provided in C and D.

Abdominal crunch test.

Photos © Fitness & Wellness, Inc.

---

*Novel Products, Inc. Figure Finder Collection. P.O. Box 408, Rockton, IL 61072-0408. 1-800-323-5143, fax 815-624-4866.

Photos © Fitness & Wellness, Inc.

Abdominal crunch test using the Crunch-Ster Curl-Up Tester

According to the results, look up your percentile rank for each exercise in the far left column of Table 5.2 and determine your muscular endurance fitness category according to the following classification:

Average Score	Fitness Category	Points
≥90	Excellent	5
70–80	Good	4
50–60	Average	3
30–40	Fair	2
≤20	Poor	1

Look up the number of points assigned for each fitness category above. Total the number of points and determine your overall strength endurance fitness category according to the following ratings:

Total Points	Strength Endurance Category
≥13	Excellent
10–12	Good
7–9	Average
4–6	Fair
≤3	Poor

TABLE **5.2** Muscular Endurance Scoring Table

Percentile Rank	MEN				WOMEN			
	Bench Jumps	Modified Dips	Bent-Leg Curl-Ups	Abdominal Crunches	Bench Jumps	Modified Push-Ups	Bent-Leg Curl-Ups	Abdominal Crunches
99	66	54	100	100	58	95	100	100
95	63	50	81	100	54	70	100	100
90	62	38	65	100	52	50	97	69
80	58	32	51	66	48	41	77	49
70	57	30	44	45	44	38	57	37
60	56	27	31	38	42	33	45	34
50	54	26	28	33	39	30	37	31
40	51	23	25	29	38	28	28	27
30	48	20	22	26	36	25	22	24
20	47	17	17	22	32	21	17	21
10	40	11	10	18	28	18	9	15
5	34	7	3	16	26	15	4	0

  High physical fitness standard   Health fitness standard

FIGURE **5.4** Procedure for muscular strength and endurance test.

1. Familiarize yourself with the six lifts used for this test: lat pull-down, leg extension, bench press, bent-leg curl-up or abdominal crunch,* leg curl, and arm curl. Graphic illustrations for each lift are given on pages 140, 141, 137, 133, 133, and 135, respectively. For the leg curl exercise, the knees should be flexed to 90°. A description and illustration of the bent-leg curl-up and the abdominal crunch exercises is provided in Figure 5.3.

For the lateral pull-down exercise, use a sitting position and have your partner hold you down by the waist or shoulders. On the leg extension lift, maintain the trunk in an upright position.

2. Determine your body weight in pounds.
3. Determine the amount of resistance to be used on each lift. To obtain this number, multiply your body weight by the percent given in the following table for each lift.

Lift	Percent of Body Weight	
	Men	Women
Lat Pull-Down	.70	.45
Leg Extension	.65	.50
Bench Press	.75	.45
Bent-Leg Curl-Up or Abdominal Crunch*	NA**	NA**
Leg Curl	.32	.25
Arm Curl	.35	.18

* The abdominal crunch exercise should be used only by individuals who suffer or are susceptible to low-back pain.

** NA = not applicable — see Figure 5.3.

4. Perform the maximum continuous number of repetitions possible.

Muscular Strength and Endurance Test

In this test you will lift a submaximal resistance as many times as possible during six different strength-training exercises. The resistance for each lift is determined according to selected percentages of body weight (see Figure 5.4).

With this test, if an individual does only a few repetitions, the test will primarily measure absolute strength. For those who are able to do a lot of repetitions, the test will be an indicator of muscular endurance. If you are not familiar with the different lifts, review the illustrations on pages 137–144.

Strength/endurance ratings for this test can be established only if the same equipment is used at all times. Unfortunately—because the industry has no standard calibration procedure for strength equipment—a certain resistance (for example, 50 pounds) is seldom the same on two different weight machines (for example, Universal Gym versus Nautilus). Consequently, even though you lift a certain resistance on one machine, you may not be able to lift the same amount on a different machine. Thus reliable fitness ratings cannot be established if you switch equipment.

Even though no fitness ratings are given, test results can be used to evaluate changes in fitness. For example, you may be able to do 7 repetitions at first attempt, but if you can perform 14 repetitions after 12 weeks of training, that's your measure of improvement. The results for the muscular strength and endurance test can also be recorded in Figure 5.5.

STRENGTH TRAINING PRESCRIPTION

The capacity of muscle cells to exert force increases and decreases according to the demands placed upon the muscular system. If muscle cells are overloaded beyond their normal use, such as in strength-training programs, the cells increase in size (a condition known as hypertrophy) and strength. If the demands placed on the muscle cells decrease, such as in sedentary living or required rest because of illness or injury, the cells **atrophy** (that is, decrease in size) and lose strength. A good level of muscular strength is important to develop and maintain fitness, health, and total well-being.

Factors that Affect Strength

Several physiological factors combine to create muscle contraction and subsequent strength gains: neural stimulation, type of muscle fiber, the overload principle, and specificity of training. Basic knowledge of these concepts is important to understand the principles involved in strength training.

NEURAL STIMULATION

Within the neuromuscular system, single **motor neurons** branch and attach to multiple muscle fibers. The motor neuron and the fibers it innervates (supplies with nerves) form a **motor unit**. The number of fibers a motor neuron can innervate varies from just a few in muscles that require precise control (eye muscles, for example) to as many as 1,000 or more in large muscles that do not perform refined or precise movements.

Stimulation of a motor neuron causes the muscle fibers to contract maximally or not at all. Variations in the number of fibers innervated and the frequency of their stimulation determine the strength of the muscle contraction. As the number of fibers innervated and frequency of stimulation increases, so does the strength of the muscular contraction.

> **Muscular strength seems to be the most important health-related component of physical fitness in the older adult population.**

TYPES OF MUSCLE FIBER

The human body has two basic types of muscle fibers: (a) slow-twitch, or red, fibers and (b) fast-twitch, or white, fibers. **Slow-twitch fibers** have a greater capacity for aerobic work. **Fast-twitch fibers** have a greater capacity for anaerobic work and produce more overall force. The latter are important for quick and powerful movements commonly used in strength-training activities.

The proportion of slow- and fast-twitch fibers is determined genetically and consequently varies from one person to another. Nevertheless, training increases the functional capacity of both types of fiber and, more specifically, strength training increases their ability to exert force.

During muscular contraction, slow-twitch fibers always are recruited first. As the force and speed of muscle contraction increase, the relative importance of the fast-twitch fibers increases. To activate the fast-twitch fibers, an activity must be intense and powerful.

OVERLOAD PRINCIPLE

Strength gains are achieved in two ways:

1. Through increased ability of individual muscle fibers to generate a stronger contraction.

2. By recruiting a greater proportion of the total available fibers for each contraction.

Key Terms

Atrophy Decrease in the size of a cell.

Motor neurons Nerves connecting the central nervous system to the muscle.

Motor unit The combination of a motor neuron and the muscle fibers that neuron innervates.

Slow-twitch fibers Muscle fibers with greater aerobic potential and slow speed of contraction.

Fast-twitch fibers Muscle fibers with greater anaerobic potential and fast speed of contraction.

FIGURE 5.5 Strength test report.

Name:_____ Date: _____

Course: _____ Section: _____ Gender:_____ Age: _____

I. Hand Grip Strength Test

Instructions are provided in Figure 5.2, page 116. Perform the test according to the instructions and look up your results in Table 5.1, page 116.

Hand used: ☐ Right ☐ Left

Reading: [   ] lbs.

Fitness category (see Figure 5.2, page 116): [   ]

II. Muscular Endurance Test

Conduct and score this test using the guidelines provided in Figure 5.3 and Table 5.2, pages 117–119.
Record your repetitions, fitness category, and points in the spaces provided below.

Exercise	Metronome Cadence	Repetitions	Fitness Category	Points
Bench jumps	none	[ ]	[ ]	[ ]
Modified dips—men only	56 bpm	[ ]	[ ]	[ ]
Modified push-ups—women only	56 bpm	[ ]	[ ]	[ ]
Bent-leg curl-ups	40 bpm	[ ]	[ ]	[ ]
Abdominal crunches	60 bpm	[ ]	[ ]	[ ]

Total Points: [   ]

Overall muscular endurance fitness category (see end of Figure 5.3, page 118): [   ]

(continued)

(Figure 5.5 Strength test report—continued)

III. Muscular Strength and Endurance Test

Perform the Muscular Strength and Endurance Test according to the procedure outlined in Figure 5.4, page 119. Record the results, fitness category, and points in the appropriate blanks provided below.

Body weight: [   ] lbs.

Lift	Body Weight	Percent of (pounds)	Resistance	Repetitions
	Men	Women		
Lat pull-down	.70	.45	[ ]	[ ]
Leg extension	.65	.50	[ ]	[ ]
Bench press	.75	.45	[ ]	[ ]
Bent-leg curl-up or abdominal crunch	NA*	NA*		[ ]
Leg curl	.32	.25	[ ]	[ ]
Arm curl	.35	.18	[ ]	[ ]

*Not applicable—no resistance required. Use test described in Figure 5.3, pages 117–118.

IV. Muscular Strength and Endurance Goals

Indicate the muscular strength/endurance classification that you would like to achieve by the end of the term:

[   ]

conclusion Briefly state your feelings about your current strength level and indicate how you are planning to achieve your strength objective.

_____

_____

_____

_____

_____

_____

_____

_____

_____

_____

These two factors combine in the **overload principle**. The demands placed on the muscle must be increased systematically and progressively over time, and the resistance must be of a magnitude significant enough to cause physiological adaptation. In simpler terms, just like all other organs and systems of the human body, to increase in physical capacity, muscles have to be taxed repeatedly beyond their accustomed loads. Because of this principle, strength training is also called "progressive resistance training."

SPECIFICITY OF TRAINING

The principle of **specificity of training** states that, for a muscle to increase in strength or endurance, the training program must be specifically tailored to obtain the desired effects (also see the section titled "Resistance" on page 126). In other words, you don't do bench presses to improve your hurdles.

PRINCIPLES OF STRENGTH TRAINING

Because muscular strength and endurance are important in developing and maintaining overall fitness and well-being, the principles necessary to develop a strength-training program have to be understood, just as in the prescription for cardio-respiratory exercise. These principles are mode of training, resistance, sets, and frequency of training.

Mode of Training

Two types of training methods are used to improve strength: isometric (static) and dynamic (previously called "isotonic"). In isometric training, muscle contractions produce little or no movement, such as pushing or pulling against an immovable object. In dynamic training, the muscle contractions produce movement, such as extending the knees with resistance on the ankles (leg extension, Exercise 24). The specificity of training principle applies here, too. To increase isometric versus dynamic strength, an individual must use static instead of dynamic training to achieve the desired results.

Isometric Training

Even though **isometric training** does not require much equipment, its popularity of several years ago has waned. Because strength gains with isometric training are specific to the angle of muscle contraction, this type of training is beneficial in a sport such as gymnastics, which requires regular static contractions during routines.

In isometric training, muscle contraction produces little or no movement.

Dynamic Training

Dynamic training is the most popular mode for strength training. The primary advantage is that strength is gained through the full range of motion. Most daily activities are dynamic in nature. We are constantly lifting, pushing, and pulling objects, and strength is needed through a complete range of motion. Another advantage is that improvements are measured easily by the amount lifted.

Dynamic training consists of two action phases when an exercise is performed: **concentric** or **positive resistance** and **eccentric** or **negative resistance**. In the concentric phase, the muscle

Key Terms

Overload principle Training concept that the demands placed on a system (cardiorespiratory or muscular) must be increased systematically and progressively over time to cause physiological adaptation (development or improvement).

Specificity of training Principle that training must be done with the specific muscle the person is attempting to improve.

Isometric training Strength-training method referring to a muscle contraction that produces little or no movement, such as pushing or pulling against an immovable object.

Dynamic training Strength-training method referring to a muscle contraction with movement.

Concentric Shortening of a muscle during muscle contraction.

Positive resistance The lifting, pushing, or concentric phase of a repetition during the performance of a strength-training exercise.

Eccentric Lengthening of a muscle during muscle contraction.

Negative resistance The lowering or eccentric phase of a repetition during the performance of a strength-training exercise.

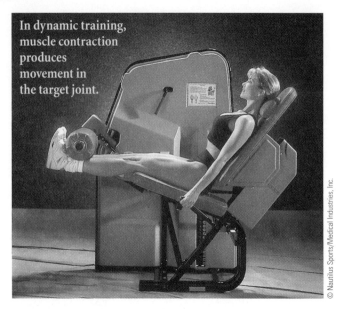

In dynamic training, muscle contraction produces movement in the target joint.

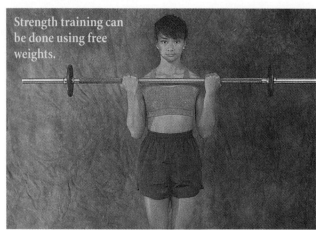

Strength training can be done using free weights.

shortens as it contracts to overcome the resistance; in the eccentric phase, it lengthens to overcome the resistance. For example, during a bench press exercise, when the person lifts the resistance from the chest to full-arm extension, the triceps muscle on the back of the upper arm shortens to extend the elbow. During the eccentric phase, the same triceps muscle must lengthen to lower the weight during elbow flexion, but it lengthens slowly to avoid dropping the resistance. Both motions work the same muscle against the same resistance.

Eccentric muscle contractions allow us to lower weights in a smooth, gradual, and controlled manner. Without eccentric contractions, weights would be dropped on the way down. Because the same muscles work when you lift and lower a resistance, always be sure to execute both actions in a controlled manner. Failure to do so diminishes the benefits of the training program and increases the risk for injuries.

Dynamic training programs can be conducted without hand-held weights, with exercise bands, **free weights**, **fixed-resistance** machines, variable-resistance machines, or isokinetic equipment. When you perform dynamic exercises without hand-held weights (for example, pull-ups and push-ups), with free weights, or with fixed-resistance machines, you move a constant resistance through a joint's full **range of motion**. In this situation, the greatest resistance that can be lifted equals the maximum weight that can be moved at the weakest angle of the joint. This is because of changes in muscle length and angle of pull as the joint moves through its range of motion.

As strength training became more popular, new strength-training machines were developed. This technology brought about **isokinetic training** and **variable-resistance** training programs, which require special machines that provide differing amounts of resistance, with the intent of overloading the muscle group maximally through the entire range of motion. A distinction of isokinetic training is that the speed of the muscle contraction is kept constant because the machine provides resistance to match the user's force through the range of motion. The mode of training an individual selects depends mainly on the type of equipment available and the specific objective the training program is attempting to accomplish.

The benefits of isokinetic and variable-resistance training are similar to the other dynamic training methods. Theoretically, strength gains should be better because maximum resistance is applied at all angles. Research, however, has not shown this type of training to be more effective than other modes of dynamic training. A possible advantage, though, is that specific speeds used in various sport skills can be duplicated more closely with isokinetic strength training, which may enhance performance (based on the principle of specificity of training). A disadvantage is that the equipment is not readily available to many people.

FREE WEIGHTS VERSUS MACHINES IN DYNAMIC TRAINING

Plate-loaded barbells (free weights) were the most popular weight-training equipment available during the first half of the twentieth century. Strength-training machines were developed in the middle of the century, but did not become popular until the 1970s. With subsequent technological improvements on these machines, a stirring debate surfaced over which of the two training modalities was better.

Free weights require that the individual balance the resistance through the entire lifting motion. Thus, a logical assumption could be made that free weights are a better training modality because additional stabilizing muscles are needed to balance the resistance as it is moved through the muscle's range of motion.

In isokinetic training, the speed of muscle contraction is constant.

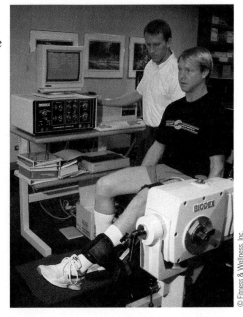

© Fitness & Wellness, Inc.

Research studies, however, have not shown any differences in strength development between the free-weight or training-machine modalities.[5] Although there are pros and cons to each modality, muscles do not know whether the source of a resistance is a barbell, a dumbbell, a Universal Gym machine, a Nautilus machine, or a simple cinder block. What determines the degree of a person's strength development is the quality of the program and the individual's effort during the training program itself—not the type of equipment used.

Advantages of Free Weights Following are the advantages of using free weights instead of machines in a strength-training program.

1. Cost: Free weights are much less expensive than most exercise machines. On a limited budget, free weights are a better option.

2. Variety: A bar and a few plates can be used to perform many exercises to strengthen most muscles in the body.

3. Portability: Free weights are portable and can be easily moved from one area or station to another.

4. Balance: Free weights require that a person balance the weight through the entire range of motion. This feature requires the involvement of additional (stabilizing) muscles to keep the weight moving properly.

5. One size fits all: Free weights can be used by people of almost all ages. A drawback of machines is that individuals who are at the extremes in terms of height or limb length often do not fit into the machines. In particular, small women and adolescents are at a disadvantage.

Advantages of Machines Strength training machines have the following advantages over free weights.

1. Safety: Machines are safer because spotters are rarely needed to monitor exercises.

2. Selection: A few exercises—such as hip flexion, hip abduction, leg curls (Exercise 18), lat pulldown (Exercise 21), and neck exercises—can be performed only with machines.

3. Variable resistance: Most machines provide variable resistance. Free weights provide only fixed resistance.

4. Isolation: Individual muscles are better isolated with machines because stabilizing muscles are not used to balance the weight during the exercise.

5. Time: Exercising with machines requires less time because the resistance is quickly set using a selector pin instead of having to manually change dumbbells or weight plates on both sides of a barbell.

6. Flexibility: Most machines can provide resistance over a greater range of movement during the exercise, thus contributing to greater flexibility in the joints. For example, a barbell pullover exercise provides resistance over a range of 100 degrees, whereas a weight machine may allow for as much as 260 degrees.

7. Rehabilitation: Machines are more useful during injury rehabilitation. A knee injury, for instance, is practically impossible to rehab using free weights, whereas small loads can be easily selected through a limited range of motion with a weight machine.

8. Skill acquisition: Learning a new exercise movement—and performing it correctly—is faster because the machine controls the direction of the movement.

KeyTerms

Free weights Barbells and dumbbells.

Fixed resistance Type of exercise in which a constant resistance is moved through a joint's full range of motion.

Range of motion Entire arc of movement of a given joint.

Isokinetic training Strength-training method in which the speed of the muscle contraction is kept constant because the equipment (machine) provides an accommodating resistance to match the user's force (maximal) through the range of motion.

Variable resistance Training using special machines equipped with mechanical devices that provide differing amounts of resistance through the range of motion.

Resistance

Resistance in strength training is the equivalent of intensity in cardiorespiratory exercise prescription. It is the amount of resistance, load, or weight lifted—which depends on whether the individual is trying to develop muscular strength or muscular endurance.

To stimulate strength development, a resistance of approximately 80 percent of the maximum capacity (1 RM) is recommended.[6] For example, a person who can press 150 pounds should work with at least 120 pounds (150 × .80). Using less than 80 percent will help increase muscular endurance rather than strength.

Because of the time factor involved in constantly determining the 1 RM on each lift to ensure that the person is indeed working above 80 percent, a rule of thumb accepted by many authors and coaches is that individuals should be able to perform more than 3 but no more than 12 repetitions (3 to 12 RM) for adequate strength gains. For example, if a person is training with a resistance of 120 pounds and cannot lift it more than 12 times, the training stimulus (weight) is adequate for development of strength.

Once the person can lift the resistance more than 12 times, the resistance should be increased by 5 to 10 pounds and the person again should build up to 12 repetitions. This is referred to as "**progressive resistance training**."

Research on strength indicates that the closer a person trains to the 1 RM, the greater the strength gains. A disadvantage of working constantly at or near the 1 RM is that it increases the risk for injury.

Highly trained athletes seeking maximum strength development often use 1 to 6 repetitions maximum. Working around 10 repetitions maximum seems to produce the best results in terms of muscular hypertrophy. If training is conducted with more than 12 repetitions, primarily muscular endurance will be developed.

Body builders tend to work with moderate resistance levels (60 to 85 percent of the 1 RM) and perform 8 to 20 repetitions to near-fatigue. A foremost objective of body building is to increase muscle size. Moderate resistance promotes blood flow to the muscles, "pumping up the muscles" (also known as "the pump") and making them look much larger than they do in a rested state.

From a health-fitness point of view, 8 to 12 repetitions maximum are recommended for adequate development. We live in a dynamic world in which muscular strength and endurance are both required to lead an enjoyable life. Therefore, working near a 10-repetition threshold seems to improve overall performance most effectively.

Sets

In strength training, a **set** is the number of repetitions performed for a given exercise. For example, a person lifting 120 pounds eight times has performed one set of eight repetitions (1 × 8 × 120).

When you work with 8 to 12 repetitions maximum, three sets per exercise are recommended. Because of the characteristics of muscle fiber, the number of sets that can be done is limited. As the number of sets increases, so does the amount of muscle fatigue and subsequent recovery time. Therefore, strength gains may be lessened by performing too many sets.

A recommended program for beginners in their first year of training is one or two light warm-up sets using about 50 percent of the 1 RM (no warm-up sets are necessary for subsequent exercises that will use the same muscle group) followed by three heavy sets, up to the maximum number of repetitions selected. Because of the lower resistances used in body building, four to eight sets can be done for each heavy exercise.

To avoid muscle soreness and stiffness, new participants ought to build up gradually to the three sets of maximal repetitions. This can be done by performing only one set of each exercise with a lighter resistance on the first day, two sets of each exercise on the second day (one light and the second with the regular, heavy resistance), and three sets on the third day (one light and two heavy). After that, a person should be able to do all three heavy sets.

The time necessary to recover between sets depends mainly on the resistance used during each set. In strength training, the energy to lift heavy weights is derived primarily from the ATP-CP or phosphagen system (see Chapter 8, "Energy [ATP] Production"). Ten seconds of maximal exercise nearly depletes the CP stores in the exercised muscle(s). These stores are replenished in about 3 minutes of recovery.

Based on this principle, a rest period of about 3 minutes between sets is necessary for people who are trying to maximize their strength gains. Individuals training for health-fitness purposes might allow 2 minutes of rest between sets. Body builders should rest no more than 1 minute to maximize the pumping effect. The exercise program will be more time-effective by alternating two or three exercises that require different muscle groups (called "**circuit training**"). In this way, an individual will not have to wait 2 to 3 minutes before proceeding to a new set on a different exercise. For example, the bench press, leg extension, and abdominal curl-up exercises may be combined so the person can go almost directly from one set to the next.

Frequency of Training

Strength training should be done either through a total body workout two to three times a week, or more frequently if using a split-body routine (upper body one day, lower body the next). After a maximum strength workout, the muscles should be rested for about 2 to 3 days to allow adequate recovery. If not completely recovered in 2 to 3 days, the person most likely is overtraining and therefore not reaping the full benefits of the program. In that case, the person should do fewer sets of exercises than in the previous workout. A summary of strength-training guidelines for health-fitness purposes is provided in Figure 5.6.

To achieve significant strength gains, a minimum of 8 weeks of consecutive training is necessary. After achieving a recommended strength level, from a health-fitness standpoint, one training session per week will be sufficient to maintain the new strength level. Highly trained athletes will need to train two times per week to maintain their strength level.

Frequency of strength training for body builders varies from person to person. Because they use moderate resistance, daily or even two-a-day workouts are common. The frequency depends on the amount of resistance, number of sets performed per session, and the person's ability to recover from the previous exercise bout (see Table 5.3). The latter often is dictated by level of conditioning.

TABLE 5.3 Guidelines for Various Strength Training Programs

Strength-Training Program	Resistance	Sets	Rest Between Sets*	Frequency (workouts per week)**
Health fitness	8–12 reps max	3	2 min	2–3
Maximal strength	1–6 reps max	3–6	3 min	2–3
Muscular endurance	10–30 reps	3–6	2 min	3–6
Body building	8–20 reps near max	3–8	0–1 min	4–12

*Recovery between sets can be decreased by alternating exercises that use different muscle groups.

**Weekly training sessions can be increased by using a split-body routine.

Plyometrics

Strength, speed, and explosiveness are all crucial for success in athletics. All three of these factors are enhanced with a progressive-resistance training program, but greater increases in speed and explosiveness are thought possible with **plyometric exercise**. The objective is to generate the greatest amount of force in the shortest time. A sound strength base is necessary before attempting plyometric exercises.

Plyometric training is popular in sports that require powerful movements, such as basketball, volleyball, sprinting, jumping, and gymnastics. A typical plyometric exercise involves jumping off and back onto a box, attempting to rebound as quickly as possible on each jump. Box heights are increased progressively from about 12 to 22 inches.

The bounding action attempts to take advantage of the stretch-recoil and stretch reflex characteristics

FIGURE 5.6 Strength-training guidelines.

Mode:	8 to 10 dynamic strength-training exercises involving the body's major muscle groups
Resistance:	Enough resistance to perform 8 to 12 repetitions to near-fatigue (10 to 15 repetitions for older and more frail individuals)
Sets:	A minimum of 1 set
Frequency:	At least two times per week

Based on the recommended quantity and quality of exercise for developing and maintaining cardiorespiratory and muscular fitness, and flexibility in healthy adults by the American College of Sports Medicine, *Medical Science Sports Exercise* 30 (1998): 975–991.

KeyTerms

Resistance Amount of weight that is lifted.

Progressive resistance training A gradual increase of resistance over a period of time.

Set A fixed number of repetitions. One set of bench presses might be 10 repetitions.

Circuit training Alternating exercises by performing them in a sequence of three to six or more.

Plyometric exercise Explosive jump training, incorporating speed and strength training to enhance explosiveness.

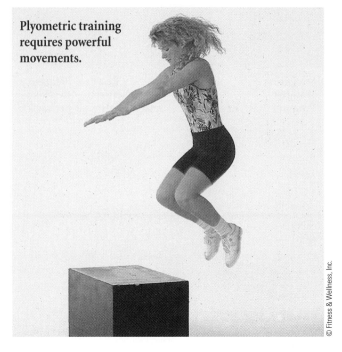

Plyometric training requires powerful movements.

© Fitness & Wellness, Inc.

of muscle. The rapid stretch applied to the muscle at contact with the ground is thought to augment muscle contraction, leading to more explosiveness. Plyometrics can be used, too, for strengthening upper body muscles. An example is push-ups with a forceful enough extension of the arms to drive the hands (and body) completely off the floor during each repetition.

A drawback of plyometric training is its higher risk for injuries compared with conventional modes of progressive resistance training. For instance, the potential for injury escalates as the box height or the number of repetitions increases.

STRENGTH-TRAINING EXERCISES

The two strength-training programs introduced on pages 132–144 provide a complete body workout. The major muscles of the human body referred to in the exercises are pointed out in Figure 5.7.

Only a minimum of equipment is required for the first program, Strength-Training Exercises without Weights (Exercises 1 through 12). This program can be conducted within your own home. Your body weight is used as the primary resistance for most exercises. A few exercises call for a friend's help or some basic implements from around your house to provide greater resistance.

Strength-Training Exercises with Weights (Exercises 13 through 32) require machines such as those shown in the accompanying photographs. These exercises can be conducted on either fixed-resistance

or variable-resistance equipment. Many of these exercises can also be performed with free weights. The first twelve exercises (13 to 24) are recommended to get a complete workout. You can do these exercises as circuit training. If time is a factor, as a minimum, perform the first eight (13 through 20) exercises. Exercises 25 to 32 are supplemental or can be used to replace some of the basic twelve (for instance, substitute Exercise 25 or 26 for 13; 27 for 14; 28 for 17; 29 for 18; 30 for 21; 31 or 32 for 23).

Exercise Guidelines

As you prepare to design your strength-training program, keep the following guidelines in mind:

1. Select exercises that will involve all major muscle groups: chest, shoulders, back, legs, arms, hip, and trunk.

2. Never lift weights alone. Always have someone work out with you in case you need a spotter or help with an injury. When using free weights, one to two spotters are recommended for certain exercises (bench press, squats, overhead press).

3. Warm up properly prior to lifting weights by performing a light- to moderate-intensity aerobic activity (5 to 7 minutes) and some gentle stretches for a few minutes.

4. Exercise larger muscle groups (such as those in the chest, back, and legs) before exercising smaller muscle groups (arms, abdominals, ankles, neck). For example, the bench press exercise works the chest, shoulders, and back of the upper arms (triceps), whereas the triceps extension works the back of the upper arms only.

5. Exercise opposing muscle groups for a balanced workout. When you work the chest (bench press), also work the back (rowing torso). If you work the biceps (arm curl), also work the triceps (triceps extension).

6. Perform all exercises in a controlled manner. Avoid fast and jerky movements and do not throw the entire body into the lifting motion. Failure to do so increases the risk of injury and decreases the effectiveness of the exercise. Do not arch the back when lifting a weight.

7. Perform each exercise through the entire possible range of motion.

8. Breathe naturally. Inhale during the eccentric phase (bringing the weight down) and exhale during the concentric phase (lifting or pushing the weight up). Practice proper breathing with lighter weights when you are learning a new exercise.

FIGURE 5.7 Major muscles in the human body.

Temporalis
(closes jaw)

Masseter
(flexes jaw)

Sterno-cleido-mastoid
(rotates head)

Intercostals
(breathing)

Pectoralis minor
(abducts ribs)

Biceps brachii
(flexes elbow)

Serratus
(adducts shoulder)

Rectus abdominus

Deep flexors
(flexes fingers)

Internal oblique
(flattens abdomen)

Tendons
from forearm
flexors to fingers

Sartorius
(rotates thigh)

Rectus femoris
(extends knee)

Gastrocnemius
(points toe, flexes knee)

Soleus
(points toe)

Tendons of toes

Frontalis
(raises eyebrow)

Orbicularis oculi (closes eye)

Orbicularis oris (purses lips)

Throat muscles
(aids swallowing)

Pectoralis major
(adducts arm)

Deltoid
(abducts arm)

Brachialis
(flexes arm)

External oblique
(flattens abdomen)

Superficial flexors
(flexes fingers)

Vastus lateralis
(extends knee)

Vastus medialis
(extends knee)

Tibialis anterior
(raises feet)

Splenius capitus

Sternomastoid

Trapezius

Deltoid

Triceps

Latissimus dorsi

Serratus posterior
inferior

Extensors
of forearm

Gluteus
maximus

Tendons
from
forearm,
extensors
to fingers

Biceps femoris

Semitendonosus

Gastrocnemius

Tendon of Achilles

9. Avoid holding your breath while straining to lift a weight. Holding your breath greatly increases the pressure inside the chest and abdominal cavity, making it practically impossible for the blood in the veins to return to the heart. Although rare, a sudden high intrathoracic pressure may lead to dizziness, a blackout, a stroke, a heart attack, or a hernia.

10. Based on the program selected, allow adequate recovery time between sets of exercises (see Table 5.3).

11. Discontinue training if you experience unusual discomfort or pain. High tension loads used in strength training can exacerbate potential injuries. Discomfort and pain are signals to stop and determine what's wrong. Be sure to properly evaluate your condition before you continue training.

12. Stretch out for a few minutes at the end of each strength-training workout to help muscles return to their normal resting length and to minimize muscle soreness and risk of injury.

SETTING UP YOUR OWN STRENGTH-TRAINING PROGRAM

The same pre-exercise guidelines outlined for cardiorespiratory endurance training apply to strength training (see Figure 1.22, page 27). If you have any concerns about your present health status or ability to safely participate in strength training, consult a physician before you start. Strength training is not advised for people with advanced heart disease.

Before you proceed to write your strength-training program, you should determine your stage of change for this fitness component in Figure 5.8 (page 145). Next, if you are prepared to do so and depending on the facilities available, you can choose one of the training programs outlined in this chapter. Using Figure 5.8 you can also develop your own strength-training program. You may then use the form provided in Figure 5.9 (pages 147–148) to keep a record of your training sessions.

The resistance and the number of repetitions you use with your program should be based on whether you want to increase muscular strength or muscular endurance:

- **For strength gains,** do up to 12 repetitions maximum, and, for muscular endurance, more than 12. For most people, three training sessions per week on nonconsecutive days is an ideal arrangement for proper development.

- **For both strength and endurance gains,** three sets of about 12 repetitions maximum for each exercise are recommended. In doing this, you will obtain good strength gains and yet be close to the endurance threshold.

- If you are training for reasons other than health fitness, review Table 5.3 for a summary of the guidelines.

Perhaps the only exercise that calls for more than 12 repetitions is the abdominal group of exercises. The abdominal muscles are considered primarily antigravity or postural muscles. Hence, a little more endurance may be required. When doing abdominal work, most people perform about 20 repetitions.

If time is a concern in completing a strength training exercise program, the American College of Sports Medicine[7] recommends as a minimum (a) one set of 8 to 12 repetitions performed to near-fatigue, and (b) 8 to 10 exercises involving the major muscle groups of the body, conducted twice a week. The recommendation is based on research showing that this training generates 70 to 80 percent of the improvements reported in other programs using three sets of about 10 RM.

WEB INTERACTIVE

American Council on Exercise: Strength and Resistance Training
This site features tips on strength training, crunches, plyometrics, and an article on how women build muscle.
http://www.acefitness.org/fitfacts/fitfacts_list.cfm#7

Weight Training and Weight-lifting Safety
Information from the *American Family Physician* journal.
http://www.familydoctor.org/handouts/198.html

Weight Training FAQ
This site contains answers to frequently asked questions regarding weight training.
http://www.touchofwellness.com

INTERACTIVE SITES

Strength Training Muscle Map & Explanation
This site provides an anatomical map of the body's muscles. Click on a muscle for exercises designed to strengthen that particular muscle, complete with a video and safety information.
http://www.global-fitness.com/strength/s_map.html

The Virtual Gym
Get the most out of exercise equipment found at the gym, with less risk of injury. You can select a specific muscle and learn what piece of gym equipment to use to improve strength and endurance of that muscle.
http://www.fitnesslink.com/virtualgym

n*tes

1. W. Campbell, M. Crim, V. Young, and W. J. Evans, "Increased Energy Requirements and Changes in Body Composition with Resistance Training in Older Adults," *Journal of Clinical Nutrition* 60 (1994): 167–175.

2. W. J. Evans, "Exercise, Nutrition and Aging," *Journal of Nutrition* 122 (1992): 796–801.

3. See note 1.

4. P. E. Allsen, *Strength Training* (Dubuque, IA: Kendall/Hunt, 1996).

5. S. P. Messier and M. Dill, "Alterations in Strength and Maximal Oxygen Uptake Consequent to Nautilus Circuit Weight Training," *Research Quarterly for Exercise and Sport* 56 (1985): 345–351.

   T. V. Pipes, "Variable Resistance Versus Constant Resistance Strength Training in Adult Males," *European Journal of Applied Physiology* 39 (1978): 27–35.

6. W. W. K. Hoeger, D. R. Hopkins, S. L. Barette, and D. F. Hale, "Relationship Between Repetitions and Selected Percentages of One Repetition Maximum: A Comparison Between Untrained and Trained Males and Females," *Journal of Applied Sport Science Research* 4, no. 2 (1990): 47–51.

7. "The Recommended Quantity and Quality of Exercise for Developing and Maintaining Cardiorespiratory and Muscular Fitness and Flexibility in Healthy Adults," *Medicine and Science in Sports and Exercise* 30 (1998): 975–991.

Suggested Readings

- Allsen, P. E. Strength Training. Dubuque, IA: Kendall/Hunt, 1996.

- Brzycki, M. "Free Weights and Machines." *Fitness Management* 15 (1999): 36–37, 40.

- Foss, M. L., and S. J. Keteyian. *Fox's Physiological Basis for Exercise and Sport*. Boston: WCB McGraw-Hill, 1998.

- Hesson, J. L. *Weight Training for Life*. Belmont, CA: Wadsworth/Thomson Learning, 2003.

- Heyward, V. H. *Advanced Fitness Assessment & Exercise Prescription*. Champaign, IL: Human Kinetic Press, 1998.

- Hoeger, W. W. K., and S. A. Hoeger. *Principles and Labs for Fitness and Wellness*. Belmont, CA: Wadsworth/ Thomson Learning, 2002.

- Mannie, K. "Barbells Versus Machines: Balancing a Weighty Issue." *Coach and Athletic Director* 67 (1998): 6–7.

- McArdle, W. D., F. I. Katch, and V. L. Katch. *Essentials of Exercise Physiology*. Philadelphia: Lippincott Williams & Wilkins, 2000.

- Munnings, F. "Strength Training: Not Only for the Young." *Physician and Sportsmedicine* 21 (1993): 133–140.

- Wescott, W. L., and T. R. Baechle. *Strength Training for Seniors*. Champaign, IL: Human Kinetic Press, 1999.

- Wilmore, J. H., and D. L. Costill. *Physiology of Sport and Exercise*. Champaign, IL: Human Kinetic Press, 1999.

Strength-Training Exercises without Weights

1 Step-Up

ACTION Step up and down using a box or chair approximately 12 to 15 inches high (a). Conduct one set using the same leg each time you go up, and then conduct a second set using the other leg. You also could alternate legs on each step-up cycle. You may increase the resistance by holding an object in your arms (b). Hold the object close to the body to avoid increased strain in the lower back.

MUSCLES DEVELOPED Gluteal muscles, quadriceps, gastrocnemius, and soleus

Back   Front   Back

A   B

Photos © Fitness & Wellness, Inc.

2 Rowing Torso

ACTION Raise your arms laterally (abduction) to a horizontal position and bend your elbows to 90°. Have a partner apply enough pressure on your elbows to gradually force your arms forward (horizontal flexion) while you try to resist the pressure. Next, reverse the action, horizontally forcing the arms backward as your partner applies sufficient forward pressure to create resistance.

© Fitness & Wellness, Inc.

Back

MUSCLES DEVELOPED Posterior deltoid, rhomboids, and trapezius

3 Push-Up

ACTION Maintaining your body as straight as possible (a), flex the elbows, lowering the body until you almost touch the floor (b), then raise yourself back up to the starting position. If you are unable to perform the push-up as indicated, decrease the resistance by supporting the lower body with the knees rather than the feet (c) or using an incline plane and supporting your hands at a higher point than the floor (d). If you wish to increase the resistance, have someone else add resistance to your shoulders as you are coming back up (e).

MUSCLES DEVELOPED Triceps, deltoid, pectoralis major, abdominals, and erector spinae

Back   Front   Front

Back

A   B   C

D   E

Photos © Fitness & Wellness, Inc.

4 Abdominal Crunch and Bent-Leg Curl-Up

ACTION Start with your head and shoulders off the floor, arms crossed on your chest, and knees slightly bent (a). The greater the flexion of the knee, the more difficult the curl-up. Now curl up to about 30° (abdominal crunch—illustration b) or curl up all the way (abdominal curl-up—illustration c), then return to the starting position without letting the head or shoulders touch the floor or allowing the hips to come off the floor. If you allow the hips to raise off the floor and the head and shoulders to touch the floor, you most likely will "swing up" on the next crunch or curl-up, which minimizes the work of the abdominal muscles. If you cannot curl up with the arms on the chest, place the hands by the side of the hips or even help yourself up by holding on to your thighs (illustrations d and e). Do not perform the sit-up exercise with your legs completely extended, because this will strain the lower back. For additional resistance during the abdominal crunch, have a partner add slight resistance to your shoulders as you "crunch up."

MUSCLES DEVELOPED Abdominal muscles and hip flexors

NOTE: *The abdominal curl-up exercise should be used only by individuals of at least average fitness without a history of lower back problems. New participants and those with a history of lower back problems should use the abdominal crunch exercise in its place.*

Front

Photos © Fitness & Wellness, Inc.

5 Leg Curl

Action   Lie on the floor face down. Cross the right ankle over the left heel (a). Apply resistance with your right foot while you bring the left foot up to 90° at the knee joint (b). Apply enough resistance so the left foot can only be brought up slowly. Repeat the exercise, crossing the left ankle over the right heel.

MUSCLES DEVELOPED Hamstrings (and quadriceps)

Front   Back

Photos © Fitness & Wellness, Inc.

EXERCISES

6 Modified Dip

ACTION Place your hands on two opposite chairs; feet on a third chair with knees slightly bent (make sure that the chairs are well stabilized). Dip down at least to a 90° angle at the elbow joint, then return to the initial position. To increase the resistance, have someone else hold you down by the shoulders on the way up (see illustration c). You may also perform this exercise using a gymnasium bleacher or box and with the help of a partner, as illustrated in photo d.

Front   Back

MUSCLES DEVELOPED Triceps, deltoid, and pectoralis major

Photos © Fitness & Wellness, Inc.

7 Pull-Up

ACTION Suspend yourself from a bar with a pronated (thumbs-in) grip (a). Pull your body up until your chin is above the bar (b), then lower the body slowly to the starting position. If you are unable to perform the pull-up as described, either have a partner hold your feet to push off and facilitate the movement upward (illustrations c and d) or use a lower bar and support your feet on the floor (e).

MUSCLES DEVELOPED Biceps, brachioradialis, brachialis, trapezius, and latissimus dorsi

Front   Back

Photos © Fitness & Wellness, Inc.

8 Arm Curl

ACTION Using a palms-up grip, start with the arm completely extended and, with the aid of a sandbag or bucket filled (as needed) with sand or rocks (a), curl up as far as possible, (b) then return to the initial position. Repeat the exercise with the other arm.

MUSCLES DEVELOPED Biceps, brachioradialis, and brachialis

Front

Photos © Fitness & Wellness, Inc.

9 Heel Raise

ACTION From a standing position with feet flat on the floor (a), raise and lower your body weight by moving at the ankle joint only (b). For added resistance, have someone else hold your shoulders down as you perform the exercise.

MUSCLES DEVELOPED Gastrocnemius and soleus

Back

Photos © Fitness & Wellness, Inc.

10 Leg Abduction and Adduction

ACTION Both participants sit on the floor. The person on the left places the feet on the inside of the other person's feet. Simultaneously, the person on the left presses the legs laterally (to the outside—abduction), while the person on the right presses the legs medially (adduction). Hold the contraction for 5 to 10 seconds. Repeat the exercise at all three angles, and then reverse the pressing sequence. The person on the left places the feet on the outside and presses inward, while the person on the right presses outward.

MUSCLES DEVELOPED Hip abductors (rectus femoris, sartori, gluteus medius and minimus) and adductors (pectineus, gracilis, adductor magnus, adductor longus, and adductor brevis)

© Fitness & Wellness, Inc.

EXERCISES

11 Reverse Crunch

ACTION Lie on your back with arms crossed on your chest and knees and hips flexed at 90° (a). Now attempt to raise the pelvis off the floor by lifting vertically from the knees and lower legs (b). This is a challenging exercise that may be difficult for beginners to perform.

MUSCLES DEVELOPED Abdominals

Front

A

B

Photos © Fitness & Wellness, Inc.

12 Pelvic Tilt

ACTION Lie flat on the floor with the knees bent at about a 90° angle (a). Tilt the pelvis by tightening the abdominal muscles, flattening your back against the floor, and raising the lower gluteal area ever so slightly off the floor (b). Hold the final position for several seconds. The exercise can also be performed against a wall (c).

AREAS STRETCHED Low back muscles and ligaments

AREAS STRENGTHENED Abdominal and gluteal muscles

Front   Back

A

B

C

Photos © Fitness & Wellness, Inc.

EXERCISES

Strength-Training with Weights

13 Bench Press

MACHINE Lie down on the bench with the head by the weight stack, the bench press bar above the chest, and the knees bent so the feet rest on the far end of the bench (a). Grasp the bar handles and press upward until the arms are completely extended (b), then return to the original position. Do not arch the back during this exercise.

Front   Back

MUSCLES DEVELOPED Pectoralis major, triceps, and deltoid

Photos © Nautilus Sports/Medical Industries, Inc.

FREE WEIGHTS Lie on the bench with arms extended and have one or two spotters help you place the barbell directly over your shoulders (a). Lower the weight to your chest (b) and then push it back up until you achieve full extension of the arms. Do not arch the back during this exercise.

Eric Risberg

14 Leg Press

ACTION From a sitting position with the knees flexed at about 90° and both feet on the footrest (a), extend the legs fully (b), then return slowly to the starting position.

MUSCLES DEVELOPED Quadriceps and gluteal muscles

Front   Back

Photos © Universal Gym Equipment, Inc.

15 Abdominal Crunch

ACTION Sit in an upright position. Grasp the handles over your shoulders and crunch forward. Return slowly to the original position.

MUSCLES DEVELOPED Abdominals

Front

Photos © Nautilus Sports/Medical Industries, Inc.

EXERCISES

16 Rowing Torso

ACTION Sit in the machine with your arms in front of you, elbows bent and resting against the padded bars (a). Press back as far as possible, drawing the shoulder blades together (b). Return to the original position.

Back

MUSCLES DEVELOPED Posterior deltoid, rhomboids, and trapezius

Photos © Nautilus Sports/Medical Industries, Inc.

Bent-Over Lateral Raise

ACTION Bend over with your back straight and knees bent at about 5 to 10° (a). Hold one dumbbell in each hand. Raise the dumbbells laterally to about shoulder level (b) and then slowly return them to the starting position.

Eric Risberg

17 Arm Curl

MACHINE Using a supinated or palms-up grip, start with the arms almost completely extended (a). Curl up as far as possible (b), then return to the starting position.

Front

FREE WEIGHTS Standing upright, hold a barbell in front of you at about shoulder width with arms extended and the hands in a thumbs-out position (supinated grip) (a). Raise the barbell to your shoulders (b) and slowly return it to the starting position.

Photos © Universal Gym Equipment, Inc.

MUSCLES DEVELOPED Biceps, brachioradialis, and brachialis

Eric Risberg

E X E R C I S E S

18 | Leg Curl

ACTION Lie with the face down on the bench, legs straight, and place the back of the feet under the padded bar (a). Curl up to at least 90° (b), and return to the original position.

MUSCLES DEVELOPED Hamstrings

Back

A   B

Photos © Universal Gym Equipment, Inc.

19 | Seated Back

ACTION Sit in the machine with your trunk flexed and the upper back against the shoulder pad. Place the feet under the padded bar and hold on with your hands to the bars on the sides (a). Start the exercise by pressing backward, simultaneously extending the trunk and hip joints (b). Slowly return to the original position.

MUSCLES DEVELOPED Erector spinae and gluteus maximus

Back   Back

A   B

Photos © Universal Gym Equipment, Inc.

20 | Heel Raise

MACHINE Start with your feet either flat on the floor or the front of the feet on an elevated block (a), then raise and lower yourself by moving at the ankle joint only (b). If additional resistance is needed, you can use a squat strength-training machine.

Back

MUSCLES DEVELOPED
Gastrocnemius, soleus

FREE WEIGHTS In a standing position, place a barbell across the shoulders and upper back. Grip the bar away from the shoulders as far out as needed (a). Place the ball of your feet over a weight plate or a small board so that your heels are lower than the front of your feet. Raise your heels off the floor as far as possible (b) and then slowly return them to the starting position.

A   B

Photos © Universal Gym Equipment, Inc.

A   B

Eric Risberg

EXERCISES

21 Lat Pull-Down

ACTION Starting from a sitting position, hold the exercise bar with a wide grip (a). Pull the bar down in front of you until it reaches the base of the neck (b), then return to the starting position. If heavy resistance is used, stabilization of the body may be required either by using equipment as shown or by having someone else hold you down by the waist or shoulders.

MUSCLES DEVELOPED Latissimus dorsi, pectoralis major, and biceps

Back   Front

A

B

Photos © Fitness & Wellness, Inc.

22 Rotary Torso

MACHINE Sit upright in the machine and place the elbows behind the padded bars. Rotate the torso as far as possible to one side and then return slowly to the starting position. Repeat the exercise to the opposite side.

Front

FREE WEIGHTS Stand with your feet slightly apart. Place a barbell across your shoulders and upper back, holding on to the sides of the barbell. Now gently, and in a controlled manner, twist your torso to one side as far as possible and then do so in the opposite direction.

Photos © Nautilus Sports/Medical Industries, Inc.

© Fitness & Wellness, Inc.

MUSCLES DEVELOPED Internal and external obliques (abdominal muscles)

23 Triceps Extension

MACHINE Sit in an upright position, arms up, elbows bent, and place the little finger side of the hands and wrists against the pads, palms of the hands facing each other (a). Fully extend one arm at a time (b), and then return to the original position. Repeat with the other arm.

MUSCLES DEVELOPED Triceps

Back

A   B

Photos © Nautilus Sports/Medical Industries, Inc.

FREE WEIGHTS In a standing position, hold a barbell with both hands overhead and with the arms in full extension (a). Slowly lower the barbell behind your head (b) and then return it to the starting position.

A   B

Eric Risberg

24 Leg Extension

ACTION Sit in an upright position with the feet under the padded bar and grasp the handles at the sides (a). Extend the legs until they are completely straight (b), then return to the starting position.

MUSCLES DEVELOPED
Quadriceps

Front

A

B

Photos © Universal Gym Equipment, Inc.

25 Shoulder Press

MACHINE Sit in an upright position and grasp the bar wider than shoulder width (a). Press the bar all the way up until the arms are fully extended (b), then return to the initial position.

A

B

Photos © Universal Gym Equipment, Inc.

MUSCLES DEVELOPED
Triceps, deltoid, and pectoralis major

Back   Front

FREE WEIGHTS Place a barbell on your shoulders in front of the body (a) and press the weight overhead until complete extension of the arms is achieved (b). Then return the weight to the original position. Be sure not to arch the back or lean back during this exercise.

A

B

Eric Risberg

EXERCISES

26 Chest Press

ACTION Start with the arms up to the side, hands resting against the handle bars, and elbows bent at 90° (a). Press the movement arms forward as far as possible, leading with the elbows (b). Slowly return to the starting position.

Front

MUSCLES DEVELOPED
Pectoralis major and deltoid

Photos © Nautilus Sports/Medical Industries, Inc.

Bent-Arm Flyes

ACTION Lie down on your back on a bench and hold a dumbbell in each hand directly overhead (a). Keeping your elbows slightly bent, lower the weights laterally to a horizontal position (b) and then bring them back up to the starting position.

Eric Risberg

27 Squat

MACHINE Place the shoulders under the padded bars by bending the knees to about 120°. Completely extend the legs, then return to the original position.

Back   Front   Back   Back

MUSCLES DEVELOPED Quadriceps, gluteus maximus, erector spinae, gastrocnemius, soleus

Photos © Universal Gym Equipment, Inc.

FREE WEIGHTS From a standing position, and with a spotter to each side, support a barbell over your shoulders and upper back (a). Keeping your head up and back straight, bend at the knees and the hips until you achieve an approximate 120° angle at the knees (b). Then return to the starting position. *Do not perform this exercise alone.* If no spotters are available, use a squat rack to ensure that you will not get trapped under a heavy weight.

Eric Risberg

28 Upright Rowing

MACHINE Start with the arms extended and grip the handles with the palms down (a). Pull all the way up to the chin (b), then return to the starting position.

Photos © Universal Gym Equipment, Inc.

MUSCLES DEVELOPED Biceps, brachioradialis, brachialis, deltoid, and trapezius

Front   Front   Back

FREE WEIGHTS Hold a barbell in front of you, with the arms fully extended and hands in a thumbs-in grip (pronated) less than shoulder-width apart (a). Pull the barbell up until it reaches shoulder level (b) and then slowly return it to the starting position.

Eric Risberg

29 Seated Leg Curl

ACTION Sit in the unit and place the strap over the upper thighs. With legs extended, place the back of the feet over the padded rollers (a). Flex the knees until you reach a 90° to 100° angle (b). Slowly return to the starting position.

MUSCLES DEVELOPED
Hamstrings

Back

Photos © Nautilus Sports/Medical Industries, Inc.

EXERCISES

30 Bent-Arm Pullover

MACHINE Sit back into the chair and grasp the bar behind your head (a). Pull the bar over your head all the way down to your abdomen (b) and slowly return to the original position.

MUSCLES DEVELOPED Latissimus dorsi, pectoral muscles, deltoid, and serratus anterior

Back   Front

FREE WEIGHTS Lie on your back on an exercise bench with the head over the edge of the bench. Hold a barbell over your chest with the hands less than shoulder-width apart (a). Keeping the elbows shoulder-width apart, lower the weight over your head until your shoulders are completely extended (b). Slowly return the weight to the starting position.

Photos © Universal Gym Equipment, Inc.

Photos © Universal Gym Equipment, Inc.

Eric Risberg

31 Triceps Extension

ACTION Using a palms-down grip, grasp the bar slightly closer than shoulder width and start with the elbows almost completely bent (a). Extend the arms fully (b), then return to starting position.

MUSCLES DEVELOPED Triceps

Back

32 Dip

ACTION Start with the elbows flexed (a), then extend the arms fully and return slowly to the initial position.

MUSCLES DEVELOPED Triceps, deltoid, and pectoralis major

Back   Front

Photos © Universal Gym Equipment, Inc.

Photos © Universal Gym Equipment, Inc.

FIGURE 5.8 Strength-training program.

Name: _____ Date: _____

Course: _____ Section: _____ Gender: _____ Age: _____

I. Stage of Change for Muscular Strength or Endurance

Using Figure 2.4 (page 45) and Table 2.3 (page 43), identify your current stage of change for participation in a muscular strength or muscular endurance program:

[   ]

II. Instructions

Select one of the two strength-training exercise programs. Perform all of the recommended exercises and, with the exception of the abdominal curl-up exercises, determine the resistance required to do approximately 10 repetitions maximum. For "Strength-Training Exercises without Weights," simply indicate the total number of repetitions performed. For the abdominal crunches or curl-up exercises, perform or build up to about 20 repetitions.

1. Strength-Training Exercises without Weights

Exercise	Repetitions
Rowing torso	
Push-up	
Bent-leg curl-up or abdominal crunch	
Leg curl	
Modified dip	
Pull-up or arm curl	
Heel raise	
Leg abduction and adduction	
Reverse crunch	
Pelvic tilt	

(continued)

(Figure 5.8 Strength-training program—continued)

2. Strength-Training Exercises with Weights

Exercise	Repetitions	Resistance
Bench press, shoulder press, or chest press (select and circle one)		
Leg press or squat (select one)		
Abdominal curl-up or abdominal crunch		N/A
Rowing torso		
Arm curl or upright rowing (select one)		
Leg curl or seated leg curl (select one)		
Seated back		
Heel raise		
Lat pull-down or bent-arm pullover (select one)		
Rotary torso		
Triceps extension or dip (select one)		
Leg extension		

III. Your Personalized Strength-Training Program

Once you have performed activity 1 or 2 above (or both), and depending on your personal goal (strength versus endurance), design your strength-training program using a minimum of eight exercises. Indicate the number of sets, repetitions, and approximate resistance that you will use. Also state the days of the week, time, and facility that will be used for this program.

Strength-training days: M ☐ T ☐ W ☐ Th ☐ F ☐ Sa ☐ Su ☐

Time of day: ☐ Facility: ☐

Exercise	Sets / Reps / Resistance		Exercise	Sets / Reps / Resistance
1.		9.		
2.		10.		
3.		11.		
4.		12.		
5.		13.		
6.		14.		
7.		15.		
8.		16.		

FIGURE 5.9 Strength training record form.

Name: _____   Course: _____   Section: _____

Exercise	St/Reps/Res*	St/Reps/Res*	St/Reps/Res*	St/Reps/Res*	St/Reps/Res*	St/Reps/Res*	St/Reps/Res*	St/Reps/Res*	St/Reps/Res*	St/Reps/Res*
Date										

*St/Reps/Res = Sets, Repetitions, and Resistance (e.g., 1/6/125 = 1 set of 6 repetitions with 125 pounds)

FIGURE 5.9 Strength training record form.

Name: _____ Course: _____ Section: _____

Date								
Exercise	St/Reps/Res*	St/Reps/Res*	St/Reps/Res*	St/Reps/Res*	St/Reps/Res*	St/Reps/Res*	St/Reps/Res*	St/Reps/Res*

*St/Reps/Res = Sets, Repetitions, and Resistance (e.g., 1/6/125 = 1 set of 6 repetitions with 125 pounds)

Muscular Flexibility Assessment and Prescription

Understand the importance of muscular flexibility to adequate fitness and preventive health care.

Identify the factors that affect muscular flexibility.

Become familiar with a battery of tests to assess overall body flexibility (modified sit-and-reach test, total body rotation test, shoulder rotation test).

Learn to interpret flexibility test results according to health-fitness and physical-fitness standards.

Define ballistic stretching, slow-sustained stretching, and proprioceptive neuromuscular facilitation stretching.

Understand the factors that contribute to the development of muscular flexibility.

Be introduced to a program for the prevention and rehabilitation of low back pain.

ealth-care professionals and practitioners generally have underestimated and over-looked the contribution of good muscular **flexibility** to overall fitness and preventive health care. Flexibility is defined as the ability of a joint to move freely through its full range of motion. Most people who exercise don't take the time to stretch. And a large number of those who do stretch don't stretch properly.

Sports medicine specialists believe that many muscular/skeletal problems and injuries are related to a lack of flexibility. In daily life, we often have to make rapid or strenuous movements we are not accustomed to making. A tight muscle that is abruptly forced beyond its normal range of motion often injures adjacent tendons, ligaments, or the muscle itself.

A decline in flexibility can cause poor posture and subsequent aches and pains that lead to limited and painful joint movement. Inordinate tightness is uncomfortable and debilitating. Approximately 80 percent of all low back problems in the United States stem from improper alignment of the vertebral column and pelvic girdle, a direct result of inflexible and weak muscles. This backache syndrome costs U.S. industry billions of dollars each year in lost productivity, health services, and worker compensation.[1]

Improving and maintaining a good range of motion in the joints enhances the quality of life. Good flexibility promotes healthy muscles and joints. Improving elasticity of muscles and connective tissue around joints enhances freedom of movement and the individual's ability to participate in all types of activities.

Taking part in a regular stretching program also increases resistance to muscle injury and soreness, prevents low back and other spinal column problems, improves and maintains good postural alignment, promotes proper and graceful body movement, improves personal appearance and self-image, and helps to develop and maintain motor skills throughout life. In addition, flexibility exercises have been prescribed successfully to treat **dysmenorrhea**[2] (painful menstruation) and general neuromuscular tension (stress). Regular **stretching** helps decrease the aches and pains caused by psychological stress and contributes to a decrease in anxiety, blood pressure, and breathing rate.[3]

Further, stretching exercises, in conjunction with calisthenics, are helpful in warm-up routines to prepare the human body for more vigorous aerobic or strength-training exercises, as well as in cool-down routines following exercise to help the person return to a normal resting state. Fatigued muscles tend to contract to a shorter-than-average resting length, and stretching exercises help fatigued muscles reestablish their normal resting length.

Similar to muscular strength, good range of motion is critical in older life. Because of decreased flexibility, older adults lose mobility and are unable to perform simple daily tasks such as bending forward or turning. Many older adults do not turn their head or rotate their trunk to look over their shoulder, but rather step around 90° to 180° to see behind them.

Physical activity and exercise can also be hampered severely by lack of good range of motion. Because of the pain during activity, older people who have tight hip flexors (muscles) cannot jog or walk very far. A vicious circle ensues, because the condition usually worsens with further inactivity. A simple stretching program can alleviate or prevent this problem and help people return to an exercise program.

Lack of physical activity and excessive sitting lead to chronic back pain.

© Fitness & Wellness, Inc.

FACTORS AFFECTING FLEXIBILITY

Total range of motion around a joint is highly specific and varies from one joint to another (hip, trunk, shoulder), as well as from one individual to the next. Muscular flexibility relates primarily to genetic factors and to physical activity. Beyond that, factors such as joint structure, ligaments, tendons, muscles, skin, previous injury, adipose tissue (fat), body temperature, age, and gender influence range of motion about a joint. Because of the specificity of flexibility, indicating an "ideal" level of flexibility is difficult. Nevertheless, flexibility is important to health and independent living.

The range of motion about a given joint depends mostly on the structure of that joint. Greater range of

motion, however, can be attained through plastic and elastic elongation. **Plastic elongation** is the permanent lengthening of soft tissue. Even though joint capsules, ligaments, and tendons are basically non-elastic, they can undergo plastic elongation. This permanent lengthening, accompanied by increases in range of motion, is best attained through slow-sustained stretching exercises.

> **Plastic elongation is permanent lengthening of soft tissue. Elastic elongation is the temporary lengthening of soft tissue.**

Elastic elongation is the temporary lengthening of soft tissue. Muscle tissue has elastic properties and responds to stretching exercises by undergoing elastic or temporary lengthening. This elastic elongation increases the extensibility of the muscles.

Changes in muscle temperature can increase or decrease flexibility by as much as 20 percent. Properly warmed-up individuals have better flexibility than non-warmed–up people. Cool temperatures have the opposite effect, impeding range of motion. Because of the effects of temperature on muscular flexibility, many people prefer to do their stretching exercises after the aerobic phase of their workout. Aerobic activities raise body temperature, facilitating plastic elongation.

Another factor that influences flexibility is the amount of adipose (fat) tissue in and around joints and muscle tissue. Excess adipose tissue will increase resistance to movement, and the added bulk also hampers joint mobility because of the contact between body surfaces.

On the average, women have more flexibility than men do, and they seem to retain this advantage throughout life. Aging does decrease the extensibility of soft tissue, though, resulting in less flexibility in both sexes.

The two most significant contributors to lower flexibility levels are sedentary living and lack of exercise. With less physical activity, muscles lose their elasticity, and tendons and ligaments tighten and shorten. Inactivity also tends to be accompanied by an increase in adipose tissue, which further decreases joint range of motion. Finally, injury to muscle tissue and tight skin from excessive scar tissue have negative effects on joint range of motion.

ASSESSMENT OF FLEXIBILITY

Most of the flexibility tests developed over the years are specific to certain sports and are not practical for the general population. Their application in health and fitness programs is limited. For example, the front-to-rear splits test and the bridge-up test have applications in sports such as gymnastics and several track-and-field events, but they do not represent actions most people encounter in daily life.

Because of the lack of practical flexibility tests, most health and fitness centers rely strictly on the sit-and-reach test as an indicator of overall flexibility. This test measures flexibility of the hamstring muscles (back of the thigh) and, to a lesser extent, the lower back muscles.

Flexibility is joint-specific. This means that a lot of flexibility in one joint does not necessarily indicate that other joints are just as flexible. Therefore, the total body rotation test and the shoulder rotation test—indicators of everyday movements such as reaching, bending, and turning—are included to determine your flexibility profile.

The sit-and-reach test has been modified from the traditional test so that arm and leg lengths are taken into consideration to determine the score (see Figure 6.1). In the original sit-and-reach test, the 15-inch mark of the yardstick used to measure flexibility was always set at the edge of the box where the feet are placed. This does not take into consideration an individual with long arms and/or short legs or one with short arms and/or long legs.[4] All other factors being equal, an individual with longer arms or shorter legs, or both, receives a better rating because of the structural advantage.

The procedures and norms for the flexibility tests are described in Figures 6.1 through 6.3 and Tables 6.1 through 6.3. The flexibility test results in these three tables are provided both in inches and centimeters (cm). Be sure to use the proper column to read your percentile score based on your test results. For the flexibility profile, you should take all three tests.

Key Terms

Flexibility The ability of a joint to move freely through its full range of motion.

Dysmenorrhea Painful menstruation.

Stretching Moving the joints beyond the accustomed range of motion.

Plastic elongation Permanent lengthening of soft tissue.

Elastic elongation Temporary lengthening of soft tissue.

FIGURE 6.1 Procedure for modified sit-and-reach test.

To perform this test, you will need the Acuflex I* Sit-and-Reach Flexibility Tester, or you may simply place a yardstick on top of a box approximately 12" (30 cm) high.

1. Warm up properly before the first trial.
2. Remove your shoes for the test. Sit on the floor with the hips, back, and head against a wall, the legs fully extended, and the bottom of the feet against the Acuflex I or sit-and-reach box.
3. Place the hands one on top of the other, and reach forward as far as possible without letting the head and back come off the wall (the shoulders may be rounded as much as possible, but neither the head nor the back should come off the wall at this time). The technician then can slide the reach indicator on the Acuflex I (or yardstick) along the top of the box until the end of the indicator touches the participant's fingers. The indicator then must be held firmly in place throughout the rest of the test.
4. Now your head and back can come off the wall. Gradually reach forward three times, the third time stretching forward as far as possible on the indicator (or yardstick) and holding the final position at least 2 seconds. Be sure that during the test you keep the backs of the knees flat against the floor.
5. Record the final number of inches reached to the nearest one-half inch or centimeter.

You are allowed two trials, and an average of the two scores is used as the final test score. The respective percentile ranks and fitness categories for this test are given in Tables 6.1 and 6.4.

Starting position for the modified sit-and-reach test.

Modified sit-and-reach test.

* The Acuflex I Flexibility Tester for the modified sit-and-reach test can be obtained from Figure Finder Collection, Novel Products, P. O. Box 408, Rockton, IL 61072-0480. Phone: 800-323-5143, fax 815-624-4866.

TABLE 6.1 Percentile Ranks for Modified Sit-and-Reach Test

	MEN								WOMEN							
	Age Category									Age Category						
Percentile Rank	≤18		19–35		36–49		≥50		Percentile Rank	≤18		19–35		36–49		≥50	
	in.	cm	in.	cm	in.	cm	in.	cm		in.	cm	in.	cm	in.	cm	in.	cm
99	20.8	52.8	20.1	51.1	18.9	48.0	16.2	41.1	99	22.6	57.4	21.0	53.3	19.8	50.3	17.2	43.7
95	19.6	49.8	18.9	48.0	18.2	46.2	15.8	40.1	95	19.5	49.5	19.3	49.0	19.2	48.8	15.7	39.9
90	18.2	46.2	17.2	43.7	16.1	40.9	15.0	38.1	90	18.7	47.5	17.9	45.5	17.4	44.2	15.0	38.1
80	17.8	45.2	17.0	43.2	14.6	37.1	13.3	33.8	80	17.8	45.2	16.7	42.4	16.2	41.1	14.2	36.1
70	16.0	40.6	15.8	40.1	13.9	35.3	12.3	31.2	70	16.5	41.9	16.2	41.1	15.2	38.6	13.6	34.5
60	15.2	38.6	15.0	38.1	13.4	34.0	11.5	29.2	60	16.0	40.6	15.8	40.1	14.5	36.8	12.3	31.2
50	14.5	36.8	14.4	36.6	12.6	32.0	10.2	25.9	50	15.2	38.6	14.8	37.6	13.5	34.3	11.1	28.2
40	14.0	35.6	13.5	34.3	11.6	29.5	9.7	24.6	40	14.5	36.8	14.5	36.8	12.8	32.5	10.1	25.7
30	13.4	34.0	13.0	33.0	10.8	27.4	9.3	23.6	30	13.7	34.8	13.7	34.8	12.2	31.0	9.2	23.4
20	11.8	30.0	11.6	29.5	9.9	25.1	8.8	22.4	20	12.6	32.0	12.6	32.0	11.0	27.9	8.3	21.1
10	9.5	24.1	9.2	23.4	8.3	21.1	7.8	19.8	10	11.4	29.0	10.1	25.7	9.7	24.6	7.5	19.0
05	8.4	21.3	7.9	20.1	7.0	17.8	7.2	18.3	05	9.4	23.9	8.1	20.6	8.5	21.6	3.7	9.4
01	7.2	18.3	7.0	17.8	5.1	13.0	4.0	10.2	01	6.5	16.5	2.6	6.6	2.0	5.1	1.5	3.8

High physical fitness standard   Health fitness standard

FIGURE **6.2**   Procedure for the total body rotation test.

An Acuflex II* Total Body Rotation Flexibility Tester or a measuring scale with a sliding panel is needed to administer this test. The Acuflex II or scale is placed on the wall at shoulder height and should be adjustable to accommodate individual differences in height. If you need to build your own scale, use two measuring tapes and glue them above and below the sliding panel centered at the 15" (38 cm) mark. Each tape should be at least 30" (76 cm) long. If no sliding panel is available, simply tape the measuring tapes onto a wall. A line also must be drawn on the floor and centered with the 15" (38 cm) mark.

1. Warm up properly before beginning this test.

2. Stand sideways, an arm's length away from the wall, with the feet straight ahead, slightly separated, and the toes right up to the line drawn on the floor. Hold out the arm opposite to the wall horizontally from the body, making a fist with the hand. The Acuflex II, measuring scale, or tapes should be shoulder height at this time.

3. Rotate the trunk, the extended arm going backward (always maintaining a horizontal plane) and making contact with the panel, gradually sliding it forward as far as possible. If no panel is available, slide the fist alongside the tapes as far as possible. Hold the final position at least 2 seconds. Position the hand with the little finger side forward during the entire sliding movement. **Proper hand position is crucial. Many people attempt to open the hand, or push with extended fingers, or slide the panel with the knuckles—none** of which is acceptable. During the test the knees can be slightly bent, **but the feet cannot be moved, always pointing straight forward.** The body must be kept as straight (vertical) as possible.

4. Conduct the test on either the right or the left side of the body. Perform two trials on the selected side. Record the farthest point reached, measured to the nearest half inch or centimeter and held for at least 2 seconds. Use the average of the two trials as the final test score. Use Tables 6.2 and 6.4, determine the percentile rank and flexibility fitness classification for this test.

---

*The Acuflex II Flexibility Tester for the total body rotation test can be obtained from Figure Finder Collection, Novel Products, P.O. Box 408, Rockton, IL 61072-0408. Phone: 800-323-5143, fax 815-624-4866.

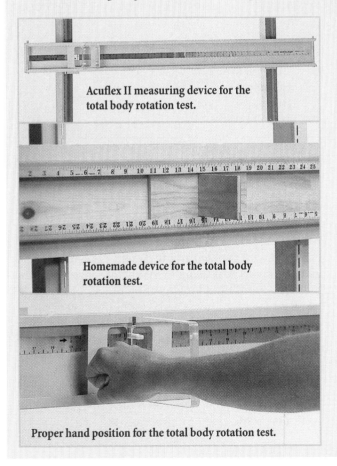

Acuflex II measuring device for the total body rotation test.

Homemade device for the total body rotation test.

Proper hand position for the total body rotation test.

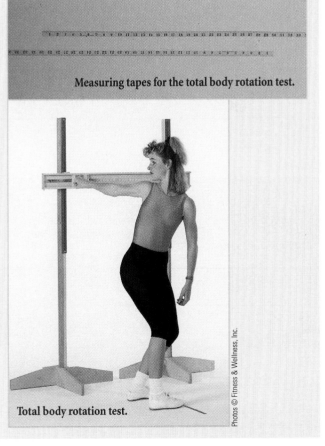

Measuring tapes for the total body rotation test.

Total body rotation test.

Photos © Fitness & Wellness, Inc.

TABLE 6.2 Percentile Ranks for Total Body Rotation Test

MEN

Percentile Rank	Left Rotation								Right Rotation							
	≤18		19–35		36–49		≥50		≤18		19–35		36–49		≥50	
	in.	cm	in.	cm	in.	cm	in.	cm	in.	cm	in.	cm	in.	cm	in.	cm
99	29.1	73.9	28.0	71.1	26.6	67.6	21.0	53.3	28.2	71.6	27.8	70.6	25.2	64.0	22.2	56.4
95	26.6	67.6	24.8	63.0	24.5	62.2	20.0	50.8	25.5	64.8	25.6	65.0	23.8	60.5	20.7	52.6
90	25.0	63.5	23.6	59.9	23.0	58.4	17.7	45.0	24.3	61.7	24.1	61.2	22.5	57.1	19.3	49.0
80	22.0	55.9	22.0	55.9	21.2	53.8	15.5	39.4	22.7	57.7	22.3	56.6	21.0	53.3	16.3	41.4
70	20.9	53.1	20.3	51.6	20.4	51.8	14.7	37.3	21.3	54.1	20.7	52.6	18.7	47.5	15.7	39.9
60	19.9	50.5	19.3	49.0	18.7	47.5	13.9	35.3	19.8	50.3	19.0	48.3	17.3	43.9	14.7	37.3
50	18.6	47.2	18.0	45.7	16.7	42.4	12.7	32.3	19.0	48.3	17.2	43.7	16.3	41.4	12.3	31.2
40	17.0	43.2	16.8	42.7	15.3	38.9	11.7	29.7	17.3	43.9	16.3	41.4	14.7	37.3	11.5	29.2
30	14.9	37.8	15.0	38.1	14.8	37.6	10.3	26.2	15.1	38.4	15.0	38.1	13.3	33.8	10.7	27.2
20	13.8	35.1	13.3	33.8	13.7	34.8	9.5	24.1	12.9	32.8	13.3	33.8	11.2	28.4	8.7	22.1
10	10.8	27.4	10.5	26.7	10.8	27.4	4.3	10.9	10.8	27.4	11.3	28.7	8.0	20.3	2.7	6.9
05	8.5	21.6	8.9	22.6	8.8	22.4	0.3	0.8	8.1	20.6	8.3	21.1	5.5	14.0	0.3	0.8
01	3.4	8.6	1.7	4.3	5.1	13.0	0.0	0.0	6.6	16.8	2.9	7.4	2.0	5.1	0.0	0.0

WOMEN

Percentile Rank	Left Rotation								Right Rotation							
	≤18		19–35		36–49		≥50		≤18		19–35		36–49		≥50	
	in.	cm	in.	cm	in.	cm	in.	cm	in.	cm	in.	cm	in.	cm	in.	cm
99	29.3	74.4	28.6	72.6	27.1	68.8	23.0	58.4	29.6	75.2	29.4	74.7	27.1	68.8	21.7	55.1
95	26.8	68.1	24.8	63.0	25.3	64.3	21.4	54.4	27.6	70.1	25.3	64.3	25.9	65.8	19.7	50.0
90	25.5	64.8	23.0	58.4	23.4	59.4	20.5	52.1	25.8	65.5	23.0	58.4	21.3	54.1	19.0	48.3
80	23.8	60.5	21.5	54.6	20.2	51.3	19.1	48.5	23.7	60.2	20.8	52.8	19.6	49.8	17.9	45.5
70	21.8	55.4	20.5	52.1	18.6	47.2	17.3	43.9	22.0	55.9	19.3	49.0	17.3	43.9	16.8	42.7
60	20.5	52.1	19.3	49.0	17.7	45.0	16.0	40.6	20.8	52.8	18.0	45.7	16.5	41.9	15.6	39.6
50	19.5	49.5	18.0	45.7	16.4	41.7	14.8	37.6	19.5	49.5	17.3	43.9	14.6	37.1	14.0	35.6
40	18.5	47.0	17.2	43.7	14.8	37.6	13.7	34.8	18.3	46.5	16.0	40.6	13.1	33.3	12.8	32.5
30	17.1	43.4	15.7	39.9	13.6	34.5	10.0	25.4	16.3	41.4	15.2	38.6	11.7	29.7	8.5	21.6
20	16.0	40.6	15.2	38.6	11.6	29.5	6.3	16.0	14.5	36.8	14.0	35.6	9.8	24.9	3.9	9.9
10	12.8	32.5	13.6	34.5	8.5	21.6	3.0	7.6	12.4	31.5	11.1	28.2	6.1	15.5	2.2	5.6
05	11.1	28.2	7.3	18.5	6.8	17.3	0.7	1.8	10.2	25.9	8.8	22.4	4.0	10.2	1.1	2.8
01	8.9	22.6	5.3	13.5	4.3	10.9	0.0	0.0	8.9	22.6	3.2	8.1	2.8	7.1	0.0	0.0

☐ High physical fitness standard   ☐ Health fitness standard

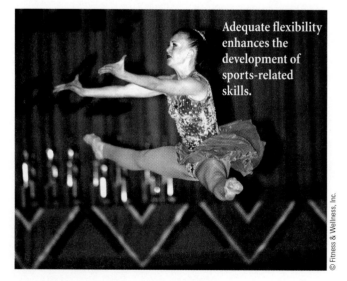

Adequate flexibility enhances the development of sports-related skills.

© Fitness & Wellness, Inc.

Interpreting Flexibility Test Results

After obtaining your scores and fitness ratings for each test, you can determine the fitness category for each flexibility test using the guidelines given in Table 6.4. You also should look up the number of points assigned for each fitness category in this table. The overall flexibility fitness classification is obtained by totaling the number of points from all three tests and using the ratings given in Table 6.5

You can use Figure 6.8 on page 165 to record your flexibility fitness results. You also should record your overall flexibility results in the fitness and wellness profile given in Appendix A.

FIGURE 6.3 Procedure for shoulder rotation test.

This test can be done using the Acuflex III* Flexibility Tester, which consists of a shoulder caliper and a measuring device for shoulder rotation. If unavailable, you can construct your own device quite easily. The caliper can be built with three regular yardsticks. Glue two of the yardsticks at one end at a 90° angle and use the third one as the sliding end of the caliper. Construct the rotation device by placing a 60" (150 cm) measuring tape on an aluminum or wood stick, starting at about 6" (15 cm) from the end of the stick.

1. Warm up before the test.

2. Using the shoulder caliper, measure the biacromial width to the nearest fourth inch or half centimeter (use the top scale on the Acuflex III). Measure biacromial width between the lateral edges of the acromion processes of the shoulders.

3. Place the Acuflex III or homemade device behind the back and **use a reverse grip (thumbs out)** to hold on to the device. Place the right hand next to the zero point of the scale or tape (lower scale on the Acuflex III) and hold it firmly in place throughout the test. Place the left hand on the other end of the measuring device, as wide as needed.

4. Standing straight up and extending both arms to full length, with elbows locked, slowly bring the measuring device over the head until it reaches forehead level. For subsequent trials, depending on the resistance encountered when rotating the shoulders, move the left grip in ½" to 1" (1 to 2 cm) at a time and repeat the task until you no longer can rotate the shoulders without undue strain or start bending the elbows to do so. Always keep the righthand grip against the zero point of the scale. Measure the last successful trial to the nearest half inch or centimeter. Take this measurement at the inner edge of the left hand on the side of the little finger.

5. Determine the final score for this test by subtracting the biacromial width from the best score (shortest distance) between both hands on the rotation test. For example, if the best score is 35" and the biacromial width is 15", the final score is 20" (35 − 15 = 20). Using Tables 6.3 and 6.4, determine the percentile rank and flexibility fitness classification for this test.

* The Acuflex III Flexibility Tester for the shoulder rotation test can be obtained from Figure Finder Collection, Novel Products, Inc., P. O. Box 408, Rockton, IL 61072-0408. Phone: (800) 323-5143, fax 815-624-4866.

Measuring biacromial width.

Starting position for the shoulder rotation test (note the reverse grip—thumbs out—used for this test).

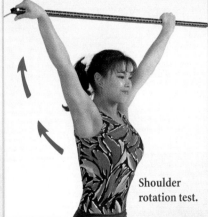

Shoulder rotation test.

Photos © Fitness & Wellness, Inc.

TABLE 6.3 Percentile Ranks for Shoulder Rotation Test

Percentile Rank	≤18 in.	cm	19–35 in.	cm	36–49 in.	cm	≥50 in.	cm
				Age Category				
MEN								
99	2.2	5.6	−1.0	−2.5	18.1	46.0	21.5	54.6
95	15.2	38.6	10.4	26.4	20.4	51.8	27.0	68.6
90	18.5	47.0	15.5	39.4	20.8	52.8	27.9	70.9
80	20.7	52.6	18.4	46.7	23.3	59.2	28.5	72.4
70	23.0	58.4	20.5	52.1	24.7	62.7	29.4	74.7
60	24.2	61.5	22.9	58.2	26.6	67.6	29.9	75.9
50	25.4	64.5	24.4	62.0	28.0	71.1	30.5	77.5
40	26.3	66.8	25.7	65.3	30.0	76.2	31.0	78.7
30	28.2	71.6	27.3	69.3	31.9	81.0	31.7	80.5
20	30.0	76.2	30.1	76.5	33.3	84.6	33.1	84.1
10	33.5	85.1	31.8	80.8	36.1	91.7	37.2	94.5
05	34.7	88.1	33.5	85.1	37.8	96.0	38.7	98.3
01	40.8	103.6	42.6	108.2	43.0	109.2	44.1	112.0
WOMEN								
99	2.6	6.6	−2.4	−6.1	11.5	29.2	13.1	33.3
95	8.0	20.3	6.2	15.7	15.4	39.1	16.5	41.9
90	10.7	27.2	9.7	24.6	16.8	42.7	20.9	53.1
80	14.5	36.8	14.5	36.8	19.2	48.8	22.5	57.1
70	16.1	40.9	17.2	43.7	21.5	54.6	24.3	61.7
60	19.2	48.8	18.7	47.5	23.1	58.7	25.1	63.8
50	21.0	53.3	20.0	50.8	23.5	59.7	26.2	66.5
40	22.2	56.4	21.4	54.4	24.4	62.0	28.1	71.4
30	23.2	58.9	24.0	61.0	25.9	65.8	29.9	75.9
20	25.0	63.5	25.9	65.8	29.8	75.7	31.5	80.0
10	27.2	69.1	29.1	73.9	31.1	79.0	33.1	84.1
05	28.0	71.1	31.3	79.5	33.4	84.8	34.1	86.6
01	32.5	82.5	37.1	94.2	34.9	88.6	35.4	89.9

High physical fitness standard

Health fitness standard

TABLE 6.4 Flexibility Fitness Categories According to Percentile Ranks

Percentile Rank	Fitness Category	Points
≥90	Excellent	5
70–80	Good	4
50–60	Average	3
30–40	Fair	2
≤20	Poor	1

TABLE 6.5 Overall Flexibility Fitness Category

Total Points	Flexibility Category
≥13	Excellent
10–12	Good
7–9	Average
4–6	Fair
≤3	Poor

PRINCIPLES OF MUSCULAR FLEXIBILITY PRESCRIPTION

Even though heredity, or genetics, plays a crucial role in body flexibility, the range of joint mobility can be increased and maintained through a regular flexibility exercise program. Because range of motion is highly specific to each body part (ankle, trunk, shoulder), a comprehensive stretching program should include all body parts and follow the basic guidelines for flexibility development.

The overload and specificity of training principles (discussed in conjunction with strength development in Chapter 5) apply as well to the development of muscular flexibility. To increase the total range of motion of a joint, the specific muscles surrounding that joint have to be stretched progressively beyond their accustomed length. The principles of mode, intensity, repetitions, and frequency of exercise also can be applied to flexibility programs.

Mode of Training

Three modes of stretching exercises can increase flexibility:

1. Ballistic stretching.
2. Slow-sustained stretching.
3. Proprioceptive neuromuscular facilitation (PNF) stretching.

Although research has indicated that all three types of stretching are effective in improving flexibility, each technique has certain advantages.

BALLISTIC STRETCHING

Ballistic (or dynamic) **stretching** exercises are done with jerky, rapid, and bouncy movements that provide the necessary force to lengthen the muscles. This type of stretching helps to develop flexibility, but the ballistic actions may cause muscle soreness and injury from small tears to the soft tissue.

Precautions must be taken not to overstretch ligaments, because they undergo plastic or permanent elongation. If the stretching force cannot be controlled, as in fast, jerky movements, ligaments easily can be overstretched. This, in turn, leads to excessively loose joints, increasing the risk for injuries, including joint dislocation and **subluxation**. Slow, gentle, and **controlled-ballistic stretching** (instead of jerky, rapid, and bouncy movements), however, is quite effective in developing flexibility and can be performed safely by most individuals.

SLOW-SUSTAINED STRETCHING

With the **slow-sustained stretching** technique, muscles are lengthened gradually through a joint's complete range of motion, and the final position is held for a few seconds. A slow-sustained stretch causes the muscles to relax and thereby achieve greater length. This type of stretch causes little pain and has a low risk for injury. Slow-sustained stretching exercises are the most frequently used and recommended in flexibility-development programs.

PROPRIOCEPTIVE NEUROMUSCULAR FACILITATION (PNF)

Proprioceptive neuromuscular facilitation (PNF) stretching has become more popular in the last few years. This technique, based on a "contract-and-relax" method, requires the assistance of another person. The procedure is as follows:

1. The person assisting with the exercise provides initial force by pushing slowly in the direction of the desired stretch. This first stretch does not cover the entire range of motion.

2. The person being stretched then applies force in the opposite direction of the stretch, against the assistant, who tries to hold the initial degree of stretch as close as possible. This results in an isometric contraction at the angle of the stretch.

3. After 4 or 5 seconds of isometric contraction, the muscle being stretched is relaxed completely. The assistant then increases the degree of stretch slowly to a greater angle.

4. The isometric contraction is repeated for another 4 or 5 seconds, following which the muscle is relaxed again. The assistant then can increase the degree of stretch, slowly, one more time. Steps 1 through 4 are repeated two to five times, until the exerciser feels mild discomfort. On the last trial, the final stretched position should be held for several seconds.

Theoretically, with the PNF technique, the isometric contraction helps relax the muscle being

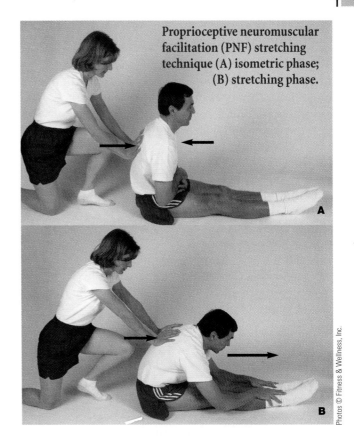

Proprioceptive neuromuscular facilitation (PNF) stretching technique (A) isometric phase; (B) stretching phase.

Photos © Fitness & Wellness, Inc.

stretched, which results in greater muscle length. Some fitness leaders believe PNF is more effective than slow-sustained stretching. Another benefit of PNF is an increase in strength of the muscle(s) being stretched. Research has shown approximately 17 and 35 percent increases in absolute strength and muscular endurance, respectively, in the hamstring muscle group after 12 weeks of PNF stretching.[5] The results were consistent in both men and women. These increases are attributed to the isometric contractions performed during PNF. The disadvantages of PNF are (1) more pain, (2) need for a second person to assist, and (3) need for more time to conduct each session.

KeyTerms

Ballistic stretching Exercises done with jerky, rapid, bouncy movements.

Subluxation Partial dislocation of a joint.

Controlled ballistic stretching Exercises done with slow, short, and sustained movements.

Slow-sustained stretching Exercises in which the muscles are lengthened gradually through a joint's complete range of motion.

Proprioceptive neuromuscular facilitation (PNF) Stretching technique in which muscles are stretched out sequentially with intermittent isometric contractions.

Intensity

The **intensity**, or degree of stretch, when doing flexibility exercises should be only to a point of mild discomfort. Pain does not have to be part of the stretching routine. Excessive pain is an indication that the load is too high and may cause injury.

All stretching should be done to slightly below the pain threshold. As participants reach this point, they should try to relax the muscle being stretched as much as possible. After completing the stretch, the body part is brought back gradually to the starting point.

> **Pain does not have to be part of the stretching routine. Excessive pain is an indication that the load is too high and may cause injury.**

Repetitions

The time required for an exercise session for flexibility development is based on the number of repetitions and the length of time each **repetition** (final stretched position) is held. The general recommendation is that each exercise be done four or five times, holding the final position each time for about 10 to 30 seconds.

As flexibility increases, a person can gradually increase the time each repetition is held, to a maximum of 1 minute. Individuals who are susceptible to flexibility injuries, however, should limit each stretch to 20 seconds.

Frequency

Flexibility exercises should be conducted five to six times a week in the early stages of the program. After a minimum of 6 to 8 weeks of almost daily stretching, flexibility levels can be maintained with only two or three sessions per week, doing about three repetitions of 10 to 15 seconds each. Figure 6.4 summarizes the flexibility development guidelines.

WHEN TO STRETCH?

Many people do not differentiate a warm-up from stretching. Warming up means starting a workout slowly with walking, cycling, or slow jogging, followed by gentle stretching (not through the entire range of motion). Stretching implies movement of joints through their full range of motion and holding the

---

FIGURE 6.4 Guidelines for development of flexibility.

Mode:	Static or dynamic (slow ballistic or proprioceptive neuromuscular facilitation) stretching to include every major joint of the body
Intensity:	Stretch to the point of mild discomfort
Repetitions:	Repeat each exercise at least 4 times and hold the final stretched position for 10 to 30 seconds
Frequency:	2–3 days per week

Based on the recommended quantity and quality of exercise for developing and maintaining cardiorespiratory and muscular fitness and flexibility in healthy adults by the American College of Sports Medicine, *Medical Science Sports Exercise*, 30 (1998): 975–991.

---

final degree of stretch according to recommended guidelines.

Gentle stretching is recommended in conjunction with warm-up routines. Two to three minutes are recommended before steady activities (walking, jogging, cycling) and up to ten minutes before stop-and-go activities (racquet sports, basketball, soccer) and athletic participation in general (football, gymnastics). Activities that require abrupt changes in direction are more likely to cause muscle strains if performed without proper warm-up that includes mild stretching.

A good time to do flexibility exercises is after aerobic workouts. Surveys have shown that individuals who stretch intensely before workouts without an adequate warm-up actually have a higher rate of injuries than those who do not stretch at all. Higher body temperature in itself helps to increase the joint range of motion. Muscles also are fatigued following exercise. A fatigued muscle tends to shorten, which can lead to soreness and spasms. Stretching exercises help fatigued muscles reestablish their normal resting length and prevent unnecessary pain.

FLEXIBILITY EXERCISES

To improve body flexibility, each major muscle group should be subjected to at least one stretching exercise. A complete set of exercises for developing muscular flexibility is presented on pages 167–170.

You may not be able to hold a final stretched position with some of these exercises (such as lateral head tilts and arm circles), but you still should perform the exercise through the joint's full range of motion. Depending on the number and length of repetitions, a complete workout will last between 15 and 30 minutes.

Contraindicated Exercises

Most strength and flexibility exercises are relatively safe to perform, but even safe exercises can be hazardous if performed incorrectly. Some exercises may be safe to perform occasionally but, when executed repeatedly, may cause trauma and injury. Preexisting muscle or joint conditions (old sprains or injuries) can further increase the risk of harm when performing certain exercises. As you develop your exercise program, you are encouraged to follow the exercise descriptions and guidelines given in this book.

A few exercises, however, are not recommended because of the potential high risk for injury. These exercises are sometimes performed in videotaped workouts and some fitness classes. **Contraindicated exercises** may cause harm because of the excessive strain placed on muscles and joints; in particular the spine, lower back, knees, neck, or shoulders.

Illustrations of contraindicated exercises are presented in Figure 6.5. Safe alternate exercises are listed below each contraindicated exercise and are illustrated in the strength (pages 137–148) and flexibility (pages 167–170) exercises sections. In isolated instances, a qualified physical therapist may select one or a few of the contraindicated exercises to treat a certain injury or disability in a carefully supervised setting. Unless you are specifically instructed to use one of these exercises, it is best that you select safe exercises from this book.

KeyTerms

Intensity In flexibility exercises, the degree of stretch.

Repetitions Number of times a given resistance is performed.

Contraindicated exercises Exercises that are not recommended because they may cause injury.

FIGURE 6.5 Contraindicated exercises.

Swan Stretch
Excessive strain on the spine; may harm intervertebral disks.
Alternative: Flexibility Exercise 20, page 170

Cradle
Excessive strain on the spine, knees, and shoulders.
Alternatives: Flexibility Exercises 20, 8, and 6, pages 170, 168, and 167

Windmill
Excessive strain on the spine and knees.
Alternatives: Flexibility Exercises 12 and 21, pages 168 and 170

Straight-Leg Sit-Ups **Alternating Bent-Leg Sit-Ups**
These exercises strain the lower back.
Alternatives: Strength Exercises 4 and 15, pages 138 and 141

Photos © Fitness & Wellness, Inc.

(continued)

(Figure 6.5 Contraindicated exercises—continued)

Hurdler Stretch
Excessive strain on the bent knee.
Alternatives: Flexibility Exercises 8 and 12, page 168

The Hero
Excessive strain on the knees.
Alternatives: Flexibility Exercises 8 and 14, pages 168 and 169

Sit-Ups with Hands Behind the Head
Excessive strain on the neck.
Alternatives: Strength Exercises 4 and 15, pages 138 and 141

Double-Leg Lift **Upright Double-Leg Lifts**
All three of these exercises cause excessive strain on the spine and may harm disks.   **V-Sits**
Alternatives: Strength Exercises 4 and 15, pages 138 and 141

Head Rolls
May injure neck disks.
Alternative: Flexibility Exercise 1, page 167

Donkey Kicks
Excessive strain on the back, shoulders, and neck.
Alternatives: Flexibility Exercises 20, 14, and 1, pages 170, 169, and 167

Yoga Plow
Excessive strain on the spine, neck, and shoulders.
Alternatives: Flexibility Exercises 12, 15, 16, 17, and 19, pages 168, 169, and 170

Standing Toe Touch
Excessive strain on the knee and lower back.
Alternative: Flexibility Exercise 12, page 168

Knee to Chest (with hands over the shin)
Excessive strain on the knee.
Alternative: Flexibility Exercises 15 and 16, page 169

Full Squat
Excessive strain on the knees.
Alternatives: Flexibility Exercise 8, Strength Exercises 1, 14, 24, pages 167, 169, and 170

PREVENTING AND REHABILITATING LOW BACK PAIN

Few people make it through life without having low back pain at some point. An estimated 75 million Americans have chronic low back pain each year. Back pain is considered chronic if it persists longer than three months. About 80 percent of the time, backache syndrome is preventable and is caused by (a) physical inactivity, (b) poor postural habits and body mechanics, or (c) excessive body weight.

People tend to think of back pain as a skeleton problem. In fact, the spine's curvature, alignment, and movement are controlled by surrounding muscles. Lack of physical activity is the most common reason for chronic low back pain. In particular, a major contributor to back pain is excessive sitting, which causes back muscles to shorten, stiffen, and become weaker.

Deterioration or weakening of the abdominal and gluteal muscles, along with tightening of the lower back (erector spinae) muscles, brings about an unnatural forward tilt of the pelvis (Figure 6.6). This tilt puts extra pressure on the spinal vertebrae, causing pain in the lower back. Accumulation of fat around the midsection of the body contributes to the forward tilt of the pelvis, which further aggravates the condition.

Low back pain frequently is associated with faulty posture and improper body mechanics (body positions in all of life's daily activities, including sleeping, sitting, standing, walking, driving, working, and exercising). Incorrect posture and poor mechanics, as explained in Figure 6.7, increase strain not only on the lower back, but on many other bones, joints, muscles, and ligaments as well.

Back pain can be reduced greatly by including some specific stretching and strengthening exercises in the regular fitness program. In most cases back pain is present only with movement and physical activity.

If the pain is severe and persists even at rest, the first step is to consult a physician, who can rule out any disk damage and may prescribe proper bed rest using several pillows under the knees for leg support (see Figure 6.7). This position helps release muscle spasms by stretching the muscles involved. In addition, a physician may prescribe a muscle relaxant or anti-inflammatory medication (or both) and some type of physical therapy.

In most cases of low back pain, even with severe pain, people feel better within days or weeks without

> Faulty posture and weak and inelastic muscles are the leading causes of chronic low back problems in the United States.

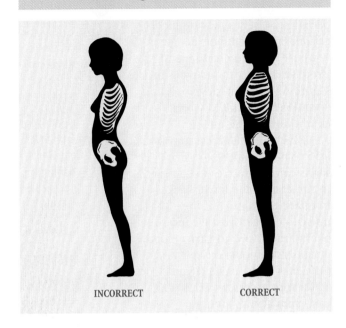

FIGURE 6.6 Incorrect and correct pelvic alignment.

INCORRECT   CORRECT

treatment from health care professionals.[6] To relieve symptoms, you may use over-the-counter pain relievers and hot or cold packs. You should also stay active to avoid further weakening of the back muscles. Low-impact activities like walking, swimming, water aerobics, and cycling are recommended. Once you are pain-free in the resting state, you need to start correcting the muscular imbalance by stretching the tight muscles and strengthening the weak ones. Stretching exercises always are performed first.

If there is no indication of disease or injury (such as leg numbness or pain), a herniated disk, or fractures, spinal manipulation by a chiropractor or other health care professional can provide pain relief. Spinal manipulation as a treatment modality for low back pain has been endorsed by the federal Agency for Health Care Policy and Research. The guidelines suggest that spinal manipulation may help to alleviate discomfort and pain during the first few weeks of an acute low back pain episode. Generally, benefits are seen within ten treatments. People who have had chronic pain for over 6 months should avoid spinal manipulation until they have been thoroughly examined by a physician.

Several exercises for preventing and rehabilitating the backache syndrome are given on pages 169–170. These exercises can be done twice or more daily when a person has back pain. Under normal circumstances, doing these exercises three to four times a week is enough to prevent the syndrome. Data has shown that the recurrence of back pain is higher in people who rely solely on medication, compared with people who use both medication and exercise therapy to recover.[7] In Figure 6.9 you can develop your own flexibility and low back conditioning programs.

Psychological stress may also lead to back pain.[8] Excessive stress causes muscles to contract. In the case of the lower back, frequent tightening of the muscles can throw the back out of alignment and constrict blood vessels that supply oxygen and nutrients to the back. If you suffer from excessive stress and back pain at the same time, proper stress management (see Chapter 12) should be a part of your comprehensive back-care program.

WEB INTERACTIVE

Stretching and Flexibility: Everything You Never Wanted to Know
This very comprehensive and academic site describes the physiology of muscles, types of flexibility, types of stretching, factors limiting flexibility, how to stretch, and specific exercises. Recommendations for further research.

http://www.enteract.com/~bradapp/docs/rec/stretching

The Basics of Stretching
By Dr. C. Everett Koop, Former U.S. Surgeon General. This site describes the fundamentals of what stretching means, what it can achieve, the advantages, the disadvantages, exercise tips and a glossary description of a few common stretching terms to get started.

http://www.drkoop.com/wellness/fitness/facts/stretching.asp

Stretching Exercises
This site features a series of stretches for the calves, gluteus, hamstrings, hips, and quadriceps. It also describes in detail the position of the body, duration and intensity needed to obtain a good stretch.

http://www.kirtland.cc.mi.us/~balbackl/stretch/htm

INTERACTIVE SITES:

The YMCA Site and Reach Test
Step-by-step instructions tell you how to measure your flexibility. Enter your score in inches and then click to compare your scores with standards for your age and gender.

http://www.shapeup.org/fitness/assess/fset2.htm

Ten Basic Stretches
This site features ten exercises to improve flexibility, complete with photographs.

http://www.drkoop.com/wellness/fitness/exercise/stretch.asp

n*tes

1. S. A. Plowman, "Physical Fitness and Healthy Low Back Function," *President's Council on Physical Fitness and Sports: Physical Activity and Fitness Research Digest*, Series 1, no 3, (1993): 3.
2. American College of Obstetricians and Gynecologists, *Guidelines for Exercise During Pregnancy*, 1994.
3. "Stretch Yourself Younger," *Consumer Reports on Health* 11 (August 1999): 6–7.
4. W. W. K. Hoeger and D. R. Hopkins, "A Comparison Between the Sit and Reach and the Modified Sit and Reach in the Measurement of Flexibility in Women," *Research Quarterly for Exercise and Sport* 63 (1992): 191–195.

W. W. K. Hoeger, D. R. Hopkins, S. Button, and T. A. Palmer, "Comparing the Sit and Reach with the Modified Sit and Reach in Measuring Flexibility in Adolescents," *Pediatric Exercise Science* 2 (1990): 156–162.

D. R. Hopkins and W. W. K. Hoeger, "A Comparison of the Sit and Reach and the Modified Sit and Reach in the Measurement of Flexibility for Males," *Journal of Applied Sports Science Research* 6 (1992): 7–10.

5. J. Kokkonen and S. Lauritzen, "Isotonic Strength and Endurance Gains Through PNF Stretching," *Medicine and Science in Sports and Exercise* 27 (1995): S22, 127.
6. R. Deyo, "Chiropractic Care for Back Pain: The Physician's Perspective," *HealthNews* 4 (September 10, 1998).
7. J. A. Hides, G. A. Jull, and C. A. Richardson, "Long-term Effects of Specific Stabilizing Exercises for First-episode Low Back Pain," *Spine* 26 (2001): E243–248.
8. A. Brownstein, "Chronic Back Pain Can Be Beaten," *Bottom Line Health* 13 (October 1999): 3–4.

 Suggested Readings

■ Alter, M. J. *The Science of Stretching*. Champaign, IL: Human Kinetic Press, 1996.
■ Alter, M. J. *Sports Stretch*. Champaign, IL: Human Kinetic Press, 1997.
■ Anderson, B. *Stretching*. Bolinas, CA: Shelter Publications, 1999.
■ Heyward, V. H. *Advanced Fitness Assessment and Exercise Prescription*. Champaign, IL: Human Kinetic Press, 1998.
■ Hoeger, W. W. K., and D. R. Hopkins. "Assessing Muscular Flexibility." *Fitness Management* 6, no. 2 (1990): 34–36, 42.
■ Kurz, T. *Stretching Scientifically: A Guide to Flexibility Training*. Island Pond, VT: Stadion Publishers, 1994.
■ McAtee, R. E. *Facilitated Stretching*. Champaign, IL: Human Kinetic Press, 1993.

FIGURE 6.7   Your back and how to care for it.

Your back and how to care for it

Whatever the cause of low back pain, part of its treatment is the correction of faulty posture. But good posture is not simply a matter of "standing tall." It refers to correct use of the body at all times. In fact, for the body to function in the best of health it must be so used that no strain is put upon the muscles, joints, bones, and ligaments. To prevent low back pain, avoiding strain must become a way of life, practiced while lying, sitting, standing, walking, working, and exercising. When body position is correct, internal organs have enough room to function normally and blood circulates more freely.

With the help of this guide, you can begin to correct the positions and movements which bring on or aggravate backache. Particular attention should be paid to the positions recommended for resting, since it is possible to strain the muscles of the back and neck even while lying in bed. By learning to live with good posture, under all circumstances, you will gradually develop the proper carriage and stronger muscles needed to protect and support your hard-working back.

HOW TO STAY ON YOUR FEET WITHOUT TIRING YOUR BACK

To prevent strain and pain in everyday activities, it is restful to change from one task to another before fatigue sets in. You can lie down between chores; others should check body position frequently, drawing in the abdomen, flattening the back, bending the knees slightly.

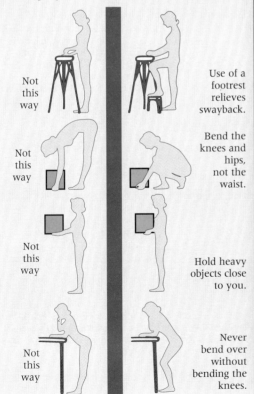

Not this way

Not this way

Not this way

Not this way

Use of a footrest relieves swayback.

Bend the knees and hips, not the waist.

Hold heavy objects close to you.

Never bend over without bending the knees.

CHECK YOUR CARRIAGE HERE

In correct, fully erect posture, a line dropped from the ear will go through the tip of the shoulder, middle of hip, back of kneecap, and front of anklebone.

Incorrect
Lower back is arched or hollow.

Incorrect
Upper back is stooped, lower back is arched, abdomen sags.

Incorrect
Note how, in strained position pelvis tilts forward, chin is out, and ribs are down, crowding internal organs.

Correct
In correct position, chin is in, head up back flattened, pelvis held straight.

To find the correct standing position: Stand one foot away from wall. Now sit against wall, bending knees slightly. Tighten abdominal and buttock muscles. This will tilt the pelvis back and flatten the lower spine. Holding this position, inch up the wall to standing position, by straightening the legs. Now walk around the room, maintaining the same posture. Place back against wall again to see if you have held it.

HOW TO SIT CORRECTLY

A back's best friend is a straight, hard chair. If you can't get the chair you prefer, learn to sit properly on whatever chair you get. *To correct sitting position from forward slump:* Throw head well back, then bend it forward to pull in the chin. This will straighten the back. Now tighten abdominal muscles to raise the chest. Check position frequently.

Relieve strain by sitting well forward, flatten back by tightening abdominal muscles, and cross knees.

Use of footrest relieves swayback. Aim is to have knees higher than hips.

Correct way to sit while driving, close to pedals. Use seat belt or hard backrest, available commercially.

TV slump leads to "dowager's hump," strains neck and shoulders.

If chair is too high, swayback is increased.

Keep neck and back in as straight a line as possible with the spine. Bend forward from hips.

Driver's seat too far from pedals emphasizes curve in lower back.

Strained reading position. Forward thrusting strains muscles of neck and head.

(continued)

(Figure 6.7 Your back and how to care for it—continued)

HOW TO PUT YOUR BACK TO BED

For proper bed posture, a firm mattress is essential. Bed-boards, sold commercially or devised at home, may be used with soft mattresses. Bedboards, preferably, should be made of 3/4-inch plywood. Faulty sleeping positions intensify swayback and result not only in backache but in numbness, tingling, and pain in arms and legs.

Incorrect:
Lying flat on back makes swayback worse.

Use of high pillow strains neck, arms, shoulders.

Sleeping face down exaggerates swayback, strains neck and shoulders.

Bending one hip and knee does not relieve swayback.

Correct:
Lying on side with knees bent effectively flattens the back. Flat pillow may be used to support neck, especially when shoulders are broad.

Sleeping on back is restful and correct when knees are properly supported.

Raise the foot of the mattress 8 inches to discourage sleeping on the abdomen.

Proper arrangement of pillows for resting or reading in bed.

A straight-back chair used behind a pillow makes a serviceable backrest.

WHEN DOING NOTHING, DO IT RIGHT

Rest is the first rule for the tired, painful back. The following positions relieve pain by taking all pressure and weight off the back and legs.

Note pillows under knees to relieve strain on spine.

For complete relief and relaxing effect, these positions should be maintained from 5 to 25 minutes.

EXERCISE — WITHOUT GETTING OUT OF BED

Exercises to be performed while lying in bed are aimed not so much at strengthening muscles as at teaching correct positioning. But muscles used correctly become stronger and in time are able to support the body with the least amount of effort.

Do all exercises in this position. Legs should not be straightened.

Bring knee up to chest. Lower slowly but do not straighten leg. Relax. Repeat with each leg 10 times.

Bring both knees slowly up to chest. Tighten muscles of abdomen, press back flat against bed. Hold knees to chest 20 seconds, then lower slowly. Relax. Repeat 5 times. This exercise gently stretches the shortened muscles of the lower back, while strengthening abdominal muscles. Clasp knees, bring them up to chest, at the same time coming to a sitting position. Rock back and forth.

EXERCISE — WITHOUT ATTRACTING ATTENTION

Use these inconspicuous exercises whenever you have a spare moment during the day, both to relax tension and improve the tone of important muscle groups.
1. Rotate shoulders, forward and backward.
2. Turn head slowly side to side.
3. Watch an imaginary plane take off, just below the right shoulder. Stretch neck, follow it slowly as it moves up, around and down, disappearing below the other shoulder. Repeat, starting on left side.
4. Slowly, slowly, touch left ear to left shoulder, right ear to right shoulder. Raise both shoulders to touch ears, drop them as far down as possible.
5. At any pause in the day—waiting for an elevator to arrive, for a specific traffic light to chang—pull in abdominal muscles, tighten, hold it for the count of eight without breathing. Relax slowly. Increase the count gradually after the first week, practice breathing normally with the abdomen flat and contracted. Do this sitting, standing, and walking.

RULES TO LIVE BY—FROM NOW ON

1. Never bend from the waist only; bend the hips and knees.
2. Never lift a heavy object higher than your waist.
3. Always turn and face the object you wish to lift.
4. Avoid carrying unbalanced loads; hold heavy objects close to your body.
5. Never carry anything heavier than you can manage with ease.
6. Never lift or move heavy furniture. Wait for someone to do it who knows the principles of leverage.
7. Avoid sudden movements, sudden "overloading" of muscles. Learn to move deliberately, swinging the legs from the hips.
8. Learn to keep the head in line with the spine, when standing, sitting, lying in bed.
9. Put soft chairs and deep couches on your "don't sit" list. During prolonged sitting, cross your legs to rest your back.
10. Your doctor is the only one who can determine when low back pain is due to faulty posture. He is the best judge of when you may do general exercises for physical fitness. When you do, omit any exercise which arches or overstrains the lower back: backward bends, or forward bends, touching the toes with the knees straight.
11. Wear shoes with moderate heels, all about the same height. Avoid changing from high to low heels.
12. Put a footrail under the desk, and a footrest under the crib.
13. Diaper the baby sitting next to him or her on the bed.
14. Beg or buy a rocking chair. Rocking rests the back by changing the muscle groups used.
15. Train yourself vigorously to use your abdominal muscles to flatten your lower abdomen. In time, this muscle contraction will become habitual, making you the envied possessor of a youthful body-profile!
16. Don't strain to open windows or doors.
17. For good posture, concentrate on strengthening "nature's corset"— the abdominal and buttock muscles. The pelvic roll exercise is especially recommended to correct the postural relation between the pelvis and the spine.

FIGURE 6.8 Muscular flexibility report.

Name: _____ Date: _____

Course: _____ Section: _____ Gender: _____ Age: _____

Test	Score	Fitness Category	Points
Modified Sit-and-Reach			
Total Body Rotation ☐ Right ☐ Left			
Shoulder Rotation			

Total Points: _____

Overall Flexibility Category: _____

FIGURE 6.9 Flexibility fitness program and back conditioning program.

I. Stage of Change for Flexibility Training

Using Figure 2.4 (page 45) and Table 2.3 (page 43), identify your current stage of change for participation in a muscular stretching program: _____

II. Instruction

Perform all of the recommended flexibility exercises given on pages 167–170. Use a combination of slow-sustained and proprioceptive neuromuscular facilitation stretching techniques. Indicate the technique(s) used for each exercise and, where applicable, the number of repetitions performed and the length of time that the final degree of stretch was held.

Stretching Exercises

Exercise	Stretching Technique	Repetitions	Length of Final Stretch
Lateral head tilt			NA*
Arm circles			NA
Side stretch			
Body rotation			
Chest stretch			
Shoulder hyperextension stretch			
Shoulder rotation stretch			NA
Quad stretch			
Heel cord stretch			
Adductor stretch			
Sitting adductor stretch			
Sit-and-reach stretch			
Triceps stretch			

*Not Applicable

(continued)

(Figure 6.9 Flexibility fitness program and back conditioning program—continued)

Stretching Schedule (Indicate days, time, and place where you will stretch):

Flexibility-training days: M ☐ T ☐ W ☐ Th ☐ F ☐ Sa ☐ Su ☐ Time of day: ☐ Place: ☐

Low Back Conditioning Program

Perform all of the recommended exercises for the prevention and rehabilitation of low back pain given on pages 169–170. Indicate the number of repetitions performed for each exercise.

Exercise	Repetitions
Hip flexors stretch	☐
Single-knee-to-chest stretch	☐
Double-knee-to-chest stretch	☐
Upper and lower back stretch	☐
Sit-and-reach stretch	☐
Gluteal stretch	☐
Back extension stretch	☐
Trunk rotation and lower back stretch	☐
Pelvic tilt	☐
Cat stretch	☐
Abdominal crunch or abdominal curl-up	☐

Proper Body Mechanics

Perform the following tasks using the proper body mechanics given in Figure 6.7 (pages 163–164). Check off each item as you perform the task:

☐ Standing (carriage) position   ☐ Resting position for tired and painful back

☐ Sitting position   ☐ Lifting an object

☐ Bed posture

conclusion

"Rules To Live By—From Now On"

Read the 18 "Rules To Live By—From Now On" given in Figure 6.7 (page164) and indicate below those rules that you need to work on to improve posture and body mechanics and prevent low back pain.

_____

_____

_____

_____

_____

_____

_____

Flexibility Stretches

1 Neck Stretches

ACTION Slowly and gently tilt the head laterally (A). You may increase the degree of stretch by gently pulling with one hand (B). You may also turn the head about 30° to one side and stretch the neck by raising your head toward the ceiling (see photo C—do not extend your head backward, look straight forward). Now gradually bring the head forward until you feel adequate stretch in the muscles on the back of the neck (D). Perform the exercises on both the right and left sides. Repeat each exercise several times and hold the final stretched position for a few seconds.

AREAS STRETCHED Neck flexors and extensors; ligaments of the cervical spine

2 Arm Circles

ACTION Gently circle the arms all the way around. Conduct the exercise in both directions.

AREAS STRETCHED Shoulder muscles and ligaments

3 Side Stretch

ACTION Stand straight up, feet separated to shoulder width, and place the hands on the waist. Now move the upper body to one side and hold the final stretch for a few seconds. Repeat on the other side.

AREAS STRETCHED Muscles and ligaments in the pelvic region

4 Body Rotation

ACTION Place the arms slightly away from the body and rotate the trunk as far as possible, holding the final position for several seconds. Conduct the exercise for both the right and left sides of the body. You also can perform this exercise by standing about 2 feet away from the wall (back toward the wall) and then rotating the trunk, placing the hands against the wall.

AREAS STRETCHED Hip, abdominal, chest, back, neck, and shoulder muscles; hip and spinal ligaments

5 Chest Stretch

ACTION Place your hands on the shoulders of your partner, who will in turn push you down by your shoulders. Hold the final position for a few seconds.

AREAS STRETCHED Chest (pectoral) muscles; shoulder ligaments

6 Shoulder Hyperextension Stretch

ACTION Have a partner grasp your arms from behind by the wrists and slowly push them upward. Hold the final position for a few seconds.

AREAS STRETCHED Deltoid and pectoral muscles; ligaments of the shoulder joint

EXERCISES

7 Shoulder Rotation Stretch

ACTION With the aid of surgical tubing or an aluminum or wood stick, place the tubing or stick behind the back and grasp the two ends using a reverse (thumbs-out) grip. Slowly bring the tubing or stick over your head, keeping the elbows straight. Repeat several times (bring the hands closer together for additional stretch).

AREAS STRETCHED Deltoid, latissimus dorsi, and pectoral muscles; shoulder ligaments

© Fitness & Wellness, Inc.

8 Quad Stretch

ACTION Lie on the side and move one foot back by flexing the knee. Grasp the front of the ankle and pull the ankle toward the gluteal region. Hold for several seconds. Repeat with the other leg.

AREAS STRETCHED Quadriceps muscle; knee and ankle ligaments

© Fitness & Wellness, Inc.

9 Heel Cord Stretch

ACTION Stand against the wall or at the edge of a step and stretch the heel downward, alternating legs. Hold the stretched position for a few seconds.

AREAS STRETCHED Heel cord (Achilles tendon); gastrocnemius and soleus muscles

© Fitness & Wellness, Inc.

10 Adductor Stretch

ACTION Stand with the feet about twice shoulder width and place the hands slightly above the knee. Flex one knee and slowly go down, holding the final position for a few seconds. Repeat with the other leg.

AREAS STRETCHED Hip adductor muscles

© Fitness & Wellness, Inc.

11 Adductor Stretch

ACTION Sit on the floor and bring the feet in close to you, allowing the soles of the feet to touch each other. Now place the forearms (or elbows) on the inner part of the thigh and push the legs downward, holding the final stretch for several seconds.

AREAS STRETCHED Hip adductor muscles

© Fitness & Wellness, Inc.

12 Sit-and-Reach Stretch

ACTION Sit on the floor with legs together and gradually reach forward as far as possible. Hold the final position for a few seconds. This exercise also may be performed with the legs separated, reaching to each side as well as to the middle.

AREAS STRETCHED Hamstrings and lower back muscles; lumbar spine ligaments

© Fitness & Wellness, Inc.

EXERCISES

13 Triceps Stretch

ACTION Place the right hand behind the neck. Grasp the right arm above the elbow with the left hand. Gently pull the elbow backward. Repeat the exercise with the opposite arm.

AREAS STRETCHED Back of upper arm (triceps muscle); shoulder joint

NOTE: Exercises 14 through 21, and 23, are also flexibility exercises and can be added to your stretching program.

Exercises for the Prevention and Rehabilitation of Low Back Pain

14 Hip Flexors Stretch

ACTION Kneel down on an exercise mat, a soft surface, or place a towel under your knees. Raise the left knee off the floor and place the left foot about three feet in front of you. Place the left hand over the left knee and the right hand over the back of the right hip. Keeping the lower back flat, slowly move forward and downward as you apply gentle pressure over the right hip. Repeat the exercise with the opposite leg forward.

AREAS STRETCHED Flexor muscles in front of the hip joint

15 Single-Knee-to-Chest Stretch

ACTION Lie down flat on the floor. Bend one leg at approximately 100° and gradually pull the opposite leg toward the chest. Hold the final stretch for a few seconds. Switch legs and repeat the exercise.

AREAS STRETCHED Lower back and hamstring muscles; lumbar spine ligaments

16 Double-Knee-to-Chest Stretch

ACTION Lie flat on the floor and then curl up slowly into a fetal position. Hold for a few seconds.

AREAS STRETCHED Upper and lower back and hamstring muscles; spinal ligaments

17 Upper and Lower Back Stretch

ACTION Sit on the floor and bring the feet in close to you, allowing the soles of the feet to touch each other. Holding on to your feet, bring your head and upper chest gently toward your feet.

AREAS STRETCHED Upper and lower back muscles and ligaments

18 Sit-and-Reach Stretch

(see Exercise 12 on page 168)

E X E R C I S E S

19 Gluteal Stretch

ACTION Sitting on the floor, bend the right leg and place the right ankle slightly above the left knee. Grasp the left thigh with both hands and gently pull the leg toward the chest. Repeat the exercise with the opposite leg.

AREAS STRETCHED
Buttock area
(gluteal muscles)

20 Back Extension Stretch

ACTION Lie face down on the floor with the elbows by the chest, forearms on the floor, and the hands beneath the chin. Gently raise the trunk by extending the elbows until you reach an approximate 90° angle at the elbow joint. Be sure the forearms remain in contact with the floor at all times. DO NOT extend the back beyond this point. Hyperextension of the lower back may lead to or aggravate an existing back problem. Hold the stretched position for about 10 seconds.

AREAS STRETCHED Abdominal region

ADDITIONAL BENEFITS Restore lower back curvature

21 Trunk Rotation and Lower Back Stretch

ACTION Sit on the floor and bend the right leg, placing the right foot on the outside of the left knee. Place the left elbow on the right knee and push against it. At the same time, try to rotate the trunk to the right (clockwise). Hold the final position for a few seconds. Repeat the exercise with the other side.

AREAS STRETCHED Lateral side of the hip and thigh; trunk and lower back

22 Pelvic Tilt

(see Exercise 12 in Chapter 5, page 140)

NOTE:

This is perhaps the most important exercise for the care of the lower back. It should be included as a part of the daily exercise routine and should be performed several times throughout the day when pain in the lower back is present as a result of muscle imbalance.

23 Cat Stretch

ACTION Kneel on the floor and place the hands in front of you (on the floor) about shoulder width apart. Relax the trunk and lower back (a). Now arch the spine and pull in the abdomen as far as you can and hold this position for a few seconds (b). Repeat the exercise 4–5 times.

AREAS STRETCHED Low back muscles and ligaments

AREAS STRENGTHENED Abdominal and gluteal muscles

24 Abdominal Crunch or Abdominal Curl-Up

(see Exercise 4 in Chapter 5, page 138)

It is important that you do not stabilize your feet when performing either of these exercises, because doing so decreases the work of the abdominal muscles. Also, remember not to "swing up" but, rather, to curl up as you perform these exercises.

Body Composition Assessment

Objectives

Define body composition and understand its relationship to recommended body weight assessment.

Identify the difference between essential and storage fat.

Explain various techniques used to assess body composition.

Be able to assess body composition using the skinfold thickness technique.

Be able to assess body composition using the girth measurements technique.

Understand the importance of waist-to-hip ratio and body mass index.

Be able to determine recommended weight according to recommended percent body fat values.

What does body composition mean? To understand **body composition,** we must recognize that the human body consists of fat and nonfat components. The fat component is usually called "fat mass" or "**percent body fat**." The nonfat component is termed "**lean body mass.**"

For many years people relied on height/weight charts to determine their recommended body weight. We know, however, that these tables can be highly inaccurate and they fail to identify critical fat values associated with higher risk for disease. The proper way to determine recommended weight is to determine body composition—that is, to find out what percent of total body weight is fat and what amount is lean tissue.

Once the fat percentage is known, **recommended body weight** can be calculated from recommended body fat. Recommended body weight, also called "healthy weight," implies the absence of any medical condition that would improve with weight loss and a fat distribution pattern that is not associated with higher risk for illness.

Although various techniques for determining percent body fat were developed several years ago, many people are still unaware of these procedures and continue to depend on height/weight charts to find their recommended body weight. The standard height/weight tables, first published in 1912, were based on average weights (including shoes and clothing) for men and women who obtained life insurance policies between 1888 and 1905. The recommended body weight on these tables is obtained according to gender, height, and frame size. Because no scientific guidelines are given to determine frame size, most people choose their frame size based on the column in which the weight comes closest to their own!

To determine whether people are truly **overweight** or falsely at recommended body weight, body composition must be established. **Obesity** is related to an excess of body fat. If body weight is the only criterion, an individual can easily be overweight according to height/weight charts, yet not have too much body fat. Football players, body builders, weight lifters, and other athletes with large muscle size are typical examples. Some of these athletes who appear to be 20 or 30 pounds overweight really have little body fat.

> To determine whether people are truly overweight or falsely at recommended body weight, body composition must be established.

The inaccuracy of height/weight charts was illustrated clearly when a young man who weighed about 225 pounds applied to join a city police force but was turned down without having been granted an interview. The reason? He was "too fat," according to the height/weight charts. When this young man's body composition later was assessed at a preventive medicine clinic, he was shocked to find out that only 5 percent of his total body weight was in the form of fat—considerably lower than the recommended standard. In the words of the technical director of the clinic, "The only way this fellow could come down to the chart's target weight would have been through surgical removal of a large amount of his muscle tissue."

At the other end of the spectrum, some people who weigh very little and may be viewed as skinny or underweight actually can be classified as overweight because of their high body fat content. People who weigh as little as 100 pounds but are more than 30 percent fat (about one-third of their total body weight) are not uncommon. These cases are found more readily in the sedentary population and among people who are always dieting. Physical inactivity and a constant negative caloric balance both lead to a loss in lean body mass (see Chapter 9). From these examples, body weight alone clearly does not always tell the true story.

ESSENTIAL AND STORAGE FAT

Total fat in the human body is classified into two types: essential fat and storage fat. **Essential fat** is needed for normal physiological function. Without it, human health deteriorates. This type of fat is found in tissues such as muscles, nerve cells, bone marrow, intestines, heart, liver, and lungs. This essential fat constitutes about 3 percent of the total weight in men and 12 percent in women (see Figure 7.1). The percentage is higher in women because it includes sex-specific fat, such as that found in the breast tissue, the uterus, and other sex-related fat deposits.

> In terms of body composition, the lowest limit for normal physiological function is 3 percent body fat for men and 12 percent for women.

Storage fat is the fat stored in adipose tissue, mostly beneath the skin (subcutaneous fat) and around major organs in the body. This fat serves three basic functions:

1. As an insulator to retain body heat.

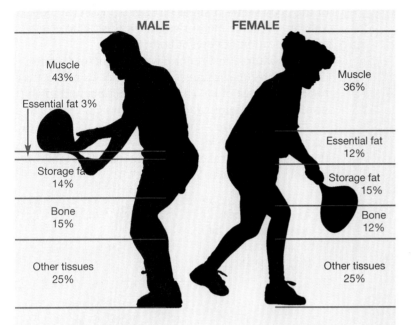

FIGURE **7.1** Typical body composition of an adult man and woman.

MALE

Muscle 43%

Essential fat 3%

Storage fat 14%

Bone 15%

Other tissues 25%

FEMALE

Muscle 36%

Essential fat 12%

Storage fat 15%

Bone 12%

Other tissues 25%

2. As energy substrate for metabolism.
3. As padding against physical trauma to the body.

The amount of storage fat does not differ between men and women except that men tend to store fat around the waist and women more so around the hips and thighs.

TECHNIQUES FOR ASSESSING BODY COMPOSITION

Body composition can be assessed through several procedures. The most common techniques are (a) hydrostatic or underwater weighing, (b) skinfold thickness, (c) girth measurements, (d) bioelectrical impedance, and (e) air displacement. Because these procedures yield estimates of body fat, each technique may yield slightly different values. Therefore, when assessing body composition before and after any exercise or nutrition program, the same technique should be used for pre- and post-program comparisons.

More sophisticated techniques to assess body composition are presently available, but the equipment is costly and not readily accessible to the general population. These procedures are used primarily in research and medical facilities. In addition to lean tissue and body fat, some of these newer methods also provide information on total body water and bone mass. Among these techniques are magnetic resonance imaging (MRI), dual energy X-ray absorptiometry (DEXA), computed tomography (CT), and total body electrical conductivity (TOBEC). In terms of predicting percent body fat, they do not appear to be more accurate than hydrostatic weighing.

Hydrostatic Weighing

Hydrostatic weighing has been used for decades as the standard of body composition in exercise laboratories. Almost all other techniques to determine body composition are validated against hydrostatic weighing. It is the most accurate technique if it is done properly and if the individual is able to perform the test adequately. The procedure requires a considerable amount of time, skill, space, and equipment and must be administered by a well-trained technician.

Because each individual assessment can take as long as 30 minutes, hydrostatic weighing is not

KeyTerms

Body composition The fat and nonfat components of the human body; important in assessing recommended body weight.

Percent body fat Proportional amount of fat in the body based on the person's total weight; includes both essential and storage fat.

Lean body mass Body weight without body fat.

Recommended body weight Body weight at which there seems to be no harm to human health; healthy weight.

Overweight An excess amount of weight against a given standard, such as height or recommended percent body fat.

Obesity An excessive accumulation of body fat, usually at least 30 percent above recommended body weight.

Essential fat Minimal amount of body fat needed for normal physiological functions; constitutes about 3 percent of total weight in men and 12 percent in women.

Storage fat Body fat in excess of essential fat; stored in adipose tissue.

Hydrostatic weighing Underwater technique to assess body composition; considered the most accurate of the body composition assessment techniques.

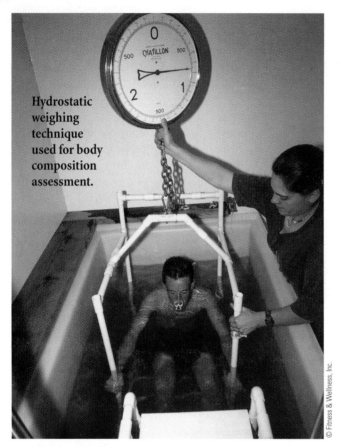

Hydrostatic weighing technique used for body composition assessment.

© Fitness & Wellness, Inc.

Skinfold Thickness

Assessing body composition using **skinfold thickness** is based on the principle that approximately half of the body's fatty tissue is directly beneath the skin. Valid and reliable measurements of this tissue give a good indication of percent body fat.

The skinfold test is done with the aid of pressure calipers. Several sites must be measured to reflect the total percentage of fat: triceps, suprailium, and thigh skinfolds for women; and chest, abdomen, and thigh for men (see Figure 7.2). All measurements should be taken on the right side of the body. A sum of these three sites is then taken and the percent body fat can be looked up in Table 7.1, 7.2, or 7.3.

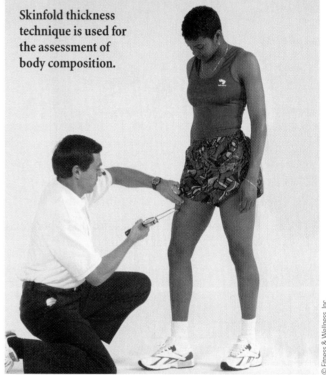

Skinfold thickness technique is used for the assessment of body composition.

© Fitness & Wellness, Inc.

feasible when testing a lot of people. Furthermore, the person's residual lung volume (amount of air left in the lungs following complete forceful exhalation) should be measured before testing. If residual volume cannot be measured, as is the case in many laboratories and health/fitness centers, it must be estimated using the predicting equations, which may decrease the accuracy of hydrostatic weighing. Also, the psychological variables in being weighed while submerged underwater makes hydrostatic weighing difficult to administer to **aquaphobic** people.

For each underwater weighing trial, the person has to: (a) force out all of the air in the lungs, (b) lean forward and completely submerge underwater in a sitting position for about 5 to 10 seconds (long enough to take a reading on the scale), and (c) remain as calm as possible (chair movement makes reading the scale difficult). This procedure has to be repeated 8 to 10 times.

Because of the cost, time, and complexity of hydrostatic weighing, most health and fitness programs prefer **anthropometric measurement techniques**, which correlate quite well with hydrostatic weighing. These techniques, primarily skinfold thickness and girth measurements, allow a quick, simple, and inexpensive estimate of body composition.

Various types of skinfold calipers can be used to assess skinfold thickness.

© Fitness & Wellness, Inc.

FIGURE **7.2** Procedure and anatomical landmarks for skinfold measurements.

Skinfold Measurement

1. Select the proper anatomical sites. For men, use chest, abdomen, and thigh skinfolds. For women, use triceps, suprailium, and thigh skinfolds. Take all measurements on the right side of the body with the person standing.

2. Measure each site by grasping a double thickness of skin firmly with the thumb and forefinger, pulling the fold slightly away from the muscular tissue. Hold caliper perpendicular to the fold and take the measurement 1/2" below the finger hold. Measure each site three times and read the values to the nearest .1 to .5 mm. Record the average of the two closest readings as the final value for that site. Take the readings without delay to avoid excessive compression of the skinfold. Release and refold the skinfold between readings.

3. When doing pre- and post-assessments, conduct the measurement at the same time of day. The best time is early in the morning to avoid water hydration changes resulting from activity or exercise.

4. Obtain percent fat by adding the skinfold measurements from all three sites and looking up the respective values in Tables 7.1, 7.2, or 7.3.

For example, if the skinfold measurements for an 18-year-old female are (a) triceps = 16, (b) suprailium = 4, and (c) thigh = 30 (total = 50), the percent body fat is 20.6%.

Chest (diagonal fold halfway between shoulder crease and nipple)

Abdomen (vertical fold taken about 1" to the right of umbilicus)

Triceps (vertical fold on back of upper arm, halfway between shoulder and elbow)

Suprailium (diagonal fold above crest of ilium, on the side of the hip)

Thigh (vertical fold on front of thigh, midway between knee and hip)

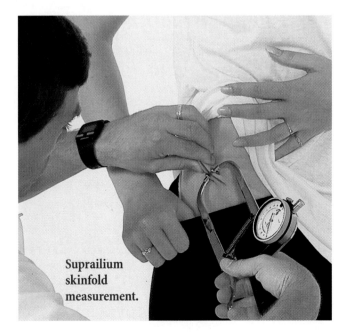

Suprailium skinfold measurement.

Even with the skinfold technique, training is necessary to obtain accurate measurements. Also, different technicians may produce slightly different measurements from the same person. Therefore, the same technician should take pre- and post-program measurements.

Measurements should be done at the same time of the day, preferably in the morning, because changes in water hydration from activity and exercise can affect skinfold girth. If skinfold calipers are available to you, you may assess your percent body fat with the help of your instructor or an experienced technician. You can record your results in Figure 7.6 at the end of this chapter.

KeyTerms

Aquaphobic Having a fear of water.

Anthropometric measurement techniques Measurement of body girths at different sites.

Skinfold thickness Technique to assess body composition by measuring a double thickness of skin at specific body sites.

TABLE 7.1 Percent Fat Estimates for Women Calculated from Triceps, Suprailium, and Thigh Skinfold Measurements

	Age at Last Birthday								
Sum of 3 Skinfolds	22 or Under	23 to 27	28 to 32	33 to 37	38 to 42	43 to 47	48 to 52	53 to 57	58 and Over
23– 25	9.7	9.9	10.2	10.4	10.7	10.9	11.2	11.4	11.7
26– 28	11.0	11.2	11.5	11.7	12.0	12.3	12.5	12.7	13.0
29– 31	12.3	12.5	12.8	13.0	13.3	13.5	13.8	14.0	14.3
32– 34	13.6	13.8	14.0	14.3	14.5	14.8	15.0	15.3	15.5
35– 37	14.8	15.0	15.3	15.5	15.8	16.0	16.3	16.5	16.8
38– 40	16.0	16.3	16.5	16.7	17.0	17.2	17.5	17.7	18.0
41– 43	17.2	17.4	17.7	17.9	18.2	18.4	18.7	18.9	19.2
44– 46	18.3	18.6	18.8	19.1	19.3	19.6	19.8	20.1	20.3
47– 49	19.5	19.7	20.0	20.2	20.5	20.7	21.0	21.2	21.5
50– 52	20.6	20.8	21.1	21.3	21.6	21.8	22.1	22.3	22.6
53– 55	21.7	21.9	22.1	22.4	22.6	22.9	23.1	23.4	23.6
56– 58	22.7	23.0	23.2	23.4	23.7	23.9	24.2	24.4	24.7
59– 61	23.7	24.0	24.2	24.5	24.7	25.0	25.2	25.5	25.7
62– 64	24.7	25.0	25.2	25.5	25.7	26.0	26.2	26.4	26.7
65– 67	25.7	25.9	26.2	26.4	26.7	26.9	27.2	27.4	27.7
68– 70	26.6	26.9	27.1	27.4	27.6	27.9	28.1	28.4	28.6
71– 73	27.5	27.8	28.0	28.3	28.5	28.8	29.0	29.3	29.5
74– 76	28.4	28.7	28.9	29.2	29.4	29.7	29.9	30.2	30.4
77– 79	29.3	29.5	29.8	30.0	30.3	30.5	30.8	31.0	31.3
80– 82	30.1	30.4	30.6	30.9	31.1	31.4	31.6	31.9	32.1
83– 85	30.9	31.2	31.4	31.7	31.9	32.2	32.4	32.7	32.9
86– 88	31.7	32.0	32.2	32.5	32.7	32.9	33.2	33.4	33.7
89– 91	32.5	32.7	33.0	33.2	33.5	33.7	33.9	34.2	34.4
92– 94	33.2	33.4	33.7	33.9	34.2	34.4	34.7	34.9	35.2
95– 97	33.9	34.1	34.4	34.6	34.9	35.1	35.4	35.6	35.9
98–100	34.6	34.8	35.1	35.3	35.5	35.8	36.0	36.3	36.5
101–103	35.2	35.4	35.7	35.9	36.2	36.4	36.7	36.9	37.2
104–106	35.8	36.1	36.3	36.6	36.8	37.1	37.3	37.5	37.8
107–109	36.4	36.7	36.9	37.1	37.4	37.6	37.9	38.1	38.4
110–112	37.0	37.2	37.5	37.7	38.0	38.2	38.5	38.7	38.9
113–115	37.5	37.8	38.0	38.2	38.5	38.7	39.0	39.2	39.5
116–118	38.0	38.3	38.5	38.8	39.0	39.3	39.5	39.7	40.0
119–121	38.5	38.7	39.0	39.2	39.5	39.7	40.0	40.2	40.5
122–124	39.0	39.2	39.4	39.7	39.9	40.2	40.4	40.7	40.9
125–127	39.4	39.6	39.9	40.1	40.4	40.6	40.9	41.1	41.4
128–130	39.8	40.0	40.3	40.5	40.8	41.0	41.3	41.5	41.8

Body density is calculated based on the generalized equation for predicting body density of women developed by A. S. Jackson, M. L. Pollock, and A. Ward and published in *Medicine and Science in Sports and Exercise* 12 (1980): 175–182. Percent body fat is determined from the calculated body density using the Siri formula.

TABLE 7.2 Percent Fat Estimates for Men Under 40 Calculated from Chest, Abdomen, and Thigh Skinfold Measurements

	Age at Last Birthday							
Sum of 3 Skinfolds	19 or Under	20 to 22	23 to 25	26 to 28	29 to 31	32 to 34	35 to 37	38 to 40
8– 10	.9	1.3	1.6	2.0	2.3	2.7	3.0	3.3
11– 13	1.9	2.3	2.6	3.0	3.3	3.7	4.0	4.3
14– 16	2.9	3.3	3.6	3.9	4.3	4.6	5.0	5.3
17– 19	3.9	4.2	4.6	4.9	5.3	5.6	6.0	6.3
20– 22	4.8	5.2	5.5	5.9	6.2	6.6	6.9	7.3
23– 25	5.8	6.2	6.5	6.8	7.2	7.5	7.9	8.2
26– 28	6.8	7.1	7.5	7.8	8.1	8.5	8.8	9.2
29– 31	7.7	8.0	8.4	8.7	9.1	9.4	9.8	10.1
32– 34	8.6	9.0	9.3	9.7	10.0	10.4	10.7	11.1
35– 37	9.5	9.9	10.2	10.6	10.9	11.3	11.6	12.0
38– 40	10.5	10.8	11.2	11.5	11.8	12.2	12.5	12.9
41– 43	11.4	11.7	12.1	12.4	12.7	13.1	13.4	13.8
44– 46	12.2	12.6	12.9	13.3	13.6	14.0	14.3	14.7
47– 49	13.1	13.5	13.8	14.2	14.5	14.9	15.2	15.5
50– 52	14.0	14.3	14.7	15.0	15.4	15.7	16.1	16.4
53– 55	14.8	15.2	15.5	15.9	16.2	16.6	16.9	17.3
56– 58	15.7	16.0	16.4	16.7	17.1	17.4	17.8	18.1
59– 61	16.5	16.9	17.2	17.6	17.9	18.3	18.6	19.0
62– 64	17.4	17.7	18.1	18.4	18.8	19.1	19.4	19.8
65– 67	18.2	18.5	18.9	19.2	19.6	19.9	20.3	20.6
68– 70	19.0	19.3	19.7	20.0	20.4	20.7	21.1	21.4
71– 73	19.8	20.1	20.5	20.8	21.2	21.5	21.9	22.2
74– 76	20.6	20.9	21.3	21.6	22.0	22.2	22.7	23.0
77– 79	21.4	21.7	22.1	22.4	22.8	23.1	23.4	23.8
80– 82	22.1	22.5	22.8	23.2	23.5	23.9	24.2	24.6
83– 85	22.9	23.2	23.6	23.9	24.3	24.6	25.0	25.3
86– 88	23.6	24.0	24.3	24.7	25.0	25.4	25.7	26.1
89– 91	24.4	24.7	25.1	25.4	25.8	26.1	26.5	26.8
92– 94	25.1	25.5	25.8	26.2	26.5	26.9	27.2	27.5
95– 97	25.8	26.2	26.5	26.9	27.2	27.6	27.9	28.3
98–100	26.6	26.9	27.3	27.6	27.9	28.3	28.6	29.0
101–103	27.3	27.6	28.0	28.3	28.6	29.0	29.3	29.7
104–106	27.9	28.3	28.6	29.0	29.3	29.7	30.0	30.4
107–109	28.6	29.0	29.3	29.7	30.0	30.4	30.7	31.1
110–112	29.3	29.6	30.0	30.3	30.7	31.0	31.4	31.7
113–115	30.0	30.3	30.7	31.0	31.3	31.7	32.0	32.4
116–118	30.6	31.0	31.3	31.6	32.0	32.3	32.7	33.0
119–121	31.3	31.6	32.0	32.3	32.6	33.0	33.3	33.7
122–124	31.9	32.2	32.6	32.9	33.3	33.6	34.0	34.3
125–127	32.5	32.9	33.2	33.5	33.9	34.2	34.6	34.9
128–130	33.1	33.5	33.8	34.2	34.5	34.9	35.2	35.5

Body density is calculated based on the generalized equation for predicting body density of men developed by A. S. Jackson and M. L. Pollock and published in the *British Journal of Nutrition* 40 (1978): 497–504. Percent body fat is determined from the calculated body density using the Siri formula.

TABLE **7.3** Percent Fat Estimates for Men Over 40 Calculated from Chest, Abdomen, and Thigh Skinfold Measurements

	Age at Last Birthday							
Sum of 3 Skinfolds	41 to 43	44 to 46	47 to 49	50 to 52	53 to 55	56 to 58	59 to 61	62 and Over
8– 10	3.7	4.0	4.4	4.7	5.1	5.4	5.8	6.1
11– 13	4.7	5.0	5.4	5.7	6.1	6.4	6.8	7.1
14– 16	5.7	6.0	6.4	6.7	7.1	7.4	7.8	8.1
17– 19	6.7	7.0	7.4	7.7	8.1	8.4	8.7	9.1
20– 22	7.6	8.0	8.3	8.7	9.0	9.4	9.7	10.1
23– 25	8.6	8.9	9.3	9.6	10.0	10.3	10.7	11.0
26– 28	9.5	9.9	10.2	10.6	10.9	11.3	11.6	12.0
29– 31	10.5	10.8	11.2	11.5	11.9	12.2	12.6	12.9
32– 34	11.4	11.8	12.1	12.4	12.8	13.1	13.5	13.8
35– 37	12.3	12.7	13.0	13.4	13.7	14.1	14.4	14.8
38– 40	13.2	13.6	13.9	14.3	14.6	15.0	15.3	15.7
41– 43	14.1	14.5	14.8	15.2	15.5	15.9	16.2	16.6
44– 46	15.0	15.4	15.7	16.1	16.4	16.8	17.1	17.5
47– 49	15.9	16.2	16.6	16.9	17.3	17.6	18.0	18.3
50– 52	16.8	17.1	17.5	17.8	18.2	18.5	18.8	19.2
53– 55	17.6	18.0	18.3	18.7	19.0	19.4	19.7	20.1
56– 58	18.5	18.8	19.2	19.5	19.9	20.2	20.6	20.9
59– 61	19.3	19.7	20.0	20.4	20.7	21.0	21.4	21.7
62– 64	20.1	20.5	20.8	21.2	21.5	21.9	22.2	22.6
65– 67	21.0	21.3	21.7	22.0	22.4	22.7	23.0	23.4
68– 70	21.8	22.1	22.5	22.8	23.2	23.5	23.9	24.2
71– 73	22.6	22.9	23.3	23.6	24.0	24.3	24.7	25.0
74– 76	23.4	23.7	24.1	24.4	24.8	25.1	25.4	25.8
77– 79	24.1	24.5	24.8	25.2	25.5	25.9	26.2	26.6
80– 82	24.9	25.3	25.6	26.0	26.3	26.6	27.0	27.3
83– 85	25.7	26.0	26.4	26.7	27.1	27.4	27.8	28.1
86– 88	26.4	26.8	27.1	27.5	27.8	28.2	28.5	28.9
89– 91	27.2	27.5	27.9	28.2	28.6	28.9	29.2	29.6
92– 94	27.9	28.2	28.6	28.9	29.3	29.6	30.0	30.3
95– 97	28.6	29.0	29.3	29.7	30.0	30.4	30.7	31.1
98–100	29.3	29.7	30.0	30.4	30.7	31.1	31.4	31.8
101–103	30.0	30.4	30.7	31.1	31.4	31.8	32.1	32.5
104–106	30.7	31.1	31.4	31.8	32.1	32.5	32.8	33.2
107–109	31.4	31.8	32.1	32.4	32.8	33.1	33.5	33.8
110–112	32.1	32.4	32.8	33.1	33.5	33.8	34.2	34.5
113–115	32.7	33.1	33.4	33.8	34.1	34.5	34.8	35.2
116–118	33.4	33.7	34.1	34.4	34.8	35.1	35.5	35.8
119–121	34.0	34.4	34.7	35.1	35.4	35.8	36.1	36.5
122–124	34.7	35.0	35.4	35.7	36.1	36.4	36.7	37.1
125–127	35.3	35.6	36.0	36.3	36.7	37.0	37.4	37.7
128–130	35.9	36.2	36.6	36.9	37.3	37.6	38.0	38.5

Body density is calculated based on the generalized equation for predicting body density of men developed by A. S. Jackson and M. L. Pollock and published in the *British Journal of Nutrition* 40 (1978): 497–504. Percent body fat is determined from the calculated body density using the Siri formula.

Girth Measurements

A simpler method to determine body fat is by measuring circumferences (**girth measurements**) at various body sites. This technique requires only a standard measuring tape. Good accuracy can be achieved with little practice. The limitation is that it may not be valid for athletic individuals (men or women) who participate actively in strenuous physical activity or for people who can be classified visually as thin or obese.

The required procedure for girth measurements is given in Figure 7.3, and the estimated percent body fat based on these measurements can be found in Table 7.4 (for women) and Table 7.5 (for men). Measurements for women include the upper arm, hip, and wrist; for men, the waist and wrist.

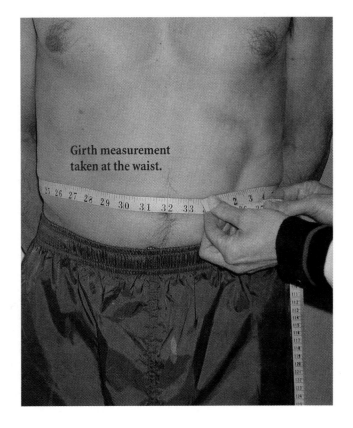

Girth measurement taken at the waist.

KeyTerms

Girth measurements Technique to assess body composition by measuring circumferences at specific body sites.

FIGURE 7.3 Procedure for body fat assessment according to girth measurements.

Girth Measurements for Women*

1. Using a regular tape measure, determine the following girth measurements in centimeters (cm):

   Upper Arm: take the measure halfway between the shoulder and the elbow.

   Hip: measure at the point of largest circumference.

   Wrist: take the girth in front of the bones where the wrist bends.

2. Obtain the person's age.

3. Using Table 7.4, find the girth measurement for each site and age in the lefthand columns. Look up the constant values in the righthand columns. These values will allow you to derive body density (BD) by substituting the constants in the following formula:

   $BD = A - B - C + D$

4. Using the derived body density, calculate percent body fat (%F) according to the following equation:

   $\%F = (495 \div BD) - 450**$

   Example: Jane is 20 years old, and the following girth measurements were taken: biceps = 27 cm, hip = 99.5 cm, wrist = 15.4 cm.

Data	Constant
Upper Arm = 27 cm	A = 1.0813
Age = 20	B = .0102
Hip = 99.5 cm	C = .1206
Wrist = 15.4 cm	D = .0971

$BD = A - B - C + D$
$BD = 1.0813 - .0102 - .1206 + .0971 = 1.0476$

$\%F = (495 \div BD) - 450$
$\%F = (495 \div 1.0476) - 450 = 22.5\%$

Girth Measurements for Men***

1. Using a regular tape measure, determine the following girth measurements in inches (the men's measurements are taken in inches as contrasted with centimeters for women):

   Waist: measure at the umbilicus (belly button).

   Wrist: measure in front of the bones where the wrist bends.

2. Subtract the wrist from the waist measurement.

3. Obtain the person's weight in pounds.

4. Look up the percent body fat (%F) in Table 7.5 by using the difference obtained in Step 2 above and the person's body weight.

   Example: John weighs 160 pounds, and his waist and wrist girth measurements are 36.5 and 7.5 inches, respectively.

   Waist girth = 36.5 inches
   Wrist girth = 7.5 inches
   Difference = 29.0 inches
   Body weight = 160.0 lbs.
   %F = 22

---

* Reproduced by permission from R. B. Lambson, *Generalized Body Density Prediction Equations for Women Using Simple Anthropometric Measurements*, unpublished doctoral dissertation, Brigham Young University, Provo, UT, August 1987.

** From W. E. Siri, *Body Composition From Fluid Spaces and Density* (Berkeley: University of California, Donner Laboratory of Medical Physics, 1956).

*** Table 7.5 reproduced by permission from A. G. Fisher, and P. E. Allsen, *Jogging* (Dubuque, IA: Wm. C. Brown, 1987). This table was developed according to the generalized body composition equation for men using simple measurement techniques by K. W. Penrouse, A. G. Nelson, and A. G. Fisher, *Medicine and Science in Sports and Exercise* 17(2):189, 1985. © American College of Sports Medicine 1985.

TABLE **7.4** Conversion Constants from Girth Measurements (Centimeters) to Calculate Body Density for Women

Upper Arm (cm)	Constant A	Age	Constant B	Hip (cm)	Constant C	Hip (cm)	Constant C	Wrist (cm)	Constant D
20.5	1.0966	17	.0086	79	.0957	114.5	.1388	13.0	.0819
21.0	1.0954	18	.0091	79.5	.0963	115	.1394	13.2	.0832
21.5	1.0942	19	.0096	80	.0970	115.5	.1400	13.4	.0845
22.0	1.0930	20	.0102	80.5	.0976	116	.1406	13.6	.0857
22.5	1.0919	21	.0107	81	.0982	116.5	.1412	13.8	.0870
23.0	1.0907	22	.0112	81.5	.0988	117	.1418	14.0	.0882
23.5	1.0895	23	.0117	82	.0994	117.5	.1424	14.2	.0895
24.0	1.0883	24	.0122	82.5	.1000	118	.1430	14.4	.0908
24.5	1.0871	25	.0127	83	.1006	118.5	.1436	14.6	.0920
25.0	1.0860	26	.0132	83.5	.1012	119	.1442	14.8	.0933
25.5	1.0848	27	.0137	84	.1018	119.5	.1448	15.0	.0946
26.0	1.0836	28	.0142	84.5	.1024	120	.1454	15.2	.0958
26.5	1.0824	29	.0147	85	.1030	120.5	.1460	15.4	.0971
27.0	1.0813	30	.0152	85.5	.1036	121	.1466	15.6	.0983
27.5	1.0801	31	.0157	86	.1042	121.5	.1472	15.8	.0996
28.0	1.0789	32	.0162	86.5	.1048	122	.1479	16.0	.1009
28.5	1.0777	33	.0168	87	.1054	122.5	.1485	16.2	.1021
29.0	1.0775	34	.0173	87.5	.1060	123	.1491	16.4	.1034
29.5	1.0754	35	.0178	88	.1066	123.5	.1497	16.6	.1046
30.0	1.0742	36	.0183	88.5	.1072	124	.1503	16.8	.1059
30.5	1.0730	37	.0188	89	.1079	124.5	.1509	17.0	.1072
31.0	1.0718	38	.0193	89.5	.1085	125	.1515	17.2	.1084
31.5	1.0707	39	.0198	90	.1091	125.5	.1521	17.4	.1097
32.0	1.0695	40	.0203	90.5	.1097	126	.1527	17.6	.1109
32.5	1.0683	41	.0208	91	.1103	126.5	.1533	17.8	.1122
33.0	1.0671	42	.0213	91.5	.1109	127	.1539	18.0	.1135
33.5	1.0666	43	.0218	92	.1115	127.5	.1545	18.2	.1147
34.0	1.0648	44	.0223	92.5	.1121	128	.1551	18.4	.1160
34.5	1.0636	45	.0228	93	.1127	128.5	.1558	18.6	.1172
35.0	1.0624	46	.0234	93.5	.1133	129	.1563		
35.5	1.0612	47	.0239	94	.1139	129.5	.1569		
36.0	1.0601	48	.0244	94.5	.1145	130	.1575		
36.5	1.0589	49	.0249	95	.1151	130.5	.1581		
37.0	1.0577	50	.0254	95.5	.1157	131	.1587		
37.5	1.0565	51	.0259	96	.1163	131.5	.1593		
38.0	1.0554	52	.0264	96.5	.1169	132	.1600		
38.5	1.0542	53	.0269	97	.1176	132.5	.1606		
39.0	1.0530	54	.0274	97.5	.1182	133	.1612		
39.5	1.0518	55	.0279	98	.1188	133.5	.1618		
40.0	1.0506	56	.0284	98.5	.1194	134	.1624		
40.5	1.0495	57	.0289	99	.1200	134.5	.1630		
41.0	1.0483	58	.0294	99.5	.1206	135	.1636		
41.5	1.0471	59	.0300	100	.1212	135.5	.1642		

(continued)

Upper Arm (cm)	Constant A	Age	Constant B	Hip (cm)	Constant C	Hip (cm)	Constant C	Wrist (cm)	Constant D
42.0	1.0459	60	.0305	100.5	.1218	136	.1648		
42.5	1.0448	61	.0310	101	.1224	136.5	.1654		
43.0	1.0434	62	.0315	101.5	.1230	137	.1660		
43.5	1.0424	63	.0320	102	.1236	137.5	.1666		
44.0	1.0412	64	.0325	102.5	.1242	138	.1672		
		65	.0330	103	.1248	138.5	.1678		
		66	.0335	103.5	.1254	139	.1685		
		67	.0340	104	.1260	139.5	.1691		
		68	.0345	104.5	.1266	140	.1697		
		69	.0350	105	.1272	140.5	.1703		
		70	.0355	105.5	.1278	141	.1709		
		71	.0360	106	.1285	141.5	.1715		
		72	.0366	106.5	.1291	142	.1721		
		73	.0371	107	.1297	142.5	.1728		
		74	.0376	107.5	.1303	143	.1733		
		75	.0381	108	.1309	143.5	.1739		
				108.5	.1315	144	.1745		
				109	.1321	144.5	.1751		
				109.5	.1327	145	.1757		
				110	.1333	145.5	.1763		
				110.5	.1339	146	.1769		
				111	.1345	146.5	.1775		
				111.5	.1351	147	.1781		
				112	.1357	147.5	.1787		
				112.5	.1363	148	.1794		
				113	.1369	148.5	.1800		
				113.5	.1375	149	.1806		
				114	.1382	149.5	.1812		
						150	.1818		

TABLE 7.5 Estimated Percent Body Fat for Men Obtained from Waist Minus Wrist Girth Measurements and Body Weight

Waist Minus Wrist Girth Measurement (Inches)

Body Weight (pounds)	22	22.5	23	23.5	24	24.5	25	25.5	26	26.5	27	27.5	28	28.5	29	29.5	30	30.5	31	31.5	32	32.5	33	33.5	34	34.5	35	35.5	36	36.5	37	37.5	38	38.5	39	39.5	40	40.5	41	41.5	42	42.5	43	43.5	44	44.5	45	45.5	46	46.5	47	47.5	48	48.5	49	49.5	50
120	4	6	8	10	12	14	16	18	20	21	23	25	27	29	31	33	35	37	39	41	43	45	47	49																																
125	4	6	7	9	11	13	15	17	19	20	22	24	26	28	30	32	33	35	37	39	41	43	45	47	49	51	53	55	58																											
130	3	5	7	9	11	12	14	16	18	20	21	23	25	27	28	30	32	33	35	37	39	41	43	44	46	48	50	52	55	57	58																								
135	3	5	7	8	10	12	14	16	18	19	21	23	24	26	28	29	31	33	34	36	38	39	41	43	44	46	48	50	53	55	56																								
140	3	5	6	8	10	11	13	15	16	18	20	22	24	26	27	29	31	32	34	36	38	39	41	43	44	46	48	50	52	54	56																								
145	3	4	6	7	9	11	12	14	16	17	19	21	23	24	26	28	29	31	33	34	36	38	39	41	43	44	46	47	49	52	54	55																							
150	2	4	6	7	9	10	12	13	15	17	19	20	22	23	25	26	28	29	31	32	34	35	36	38	40	41	43	44	46	47	49	50	52	53	55																				
155	2	4	5	7	8	10	11	13	15	16	18	19	21	22	24	25	27	28	30	31	32	34	35	37	38	40	41	43	44	46	47	49	50	52	53	55																			
160	2	4	5	6	8	9	11	12	14	15	17	19	20	22	23	25	26	28	29	31	32	34	35	37	38	40	41	43	44	46	47	48	50	51	53	54																			
165	2	3	5	6	8	9	10	12	13	15	16	18	19	21	22	24	25	27	28	30	31	33	34	35	37	38	40	41	43	44	45	47	48	50	51	52	54																		
170	2	3	4	6	7	9	10	11	13	14	16	17	19	20	22	23	25	26	27	29	30	32	33	35	36	37	39	40	41	43	44	45	47	48	50	51	52	54																	
175	2	3	4	6	7	8	10	11	12	14	15	17	18	19	21	22	24	25	27	28	29	31	32	33	35	36	38	39	40	41	43	44	45	47	48	50	52	53																	
180	3	4	5	7	8	9	11	12	13	15	16	17	19	20	22	23	24	26	27	28	30	31	32	34	35	36	38	39	40	41	43	44	45	47	48	49	50	52	53																
185	3	4	5	6	8	9	10	12	13	14	16	17	18	20	21	23	24	25	27	28	29	30	32	33	34	36	37	38	39	41	42	43	44	46	47	48	49	50	51	53														
190	3	4	5	6	7	9	10	11	13	14	15	17	18	19	21	22	23	24	26	27	28	29	31	32	33	34	36	37	38	39	41	42	43	44	45	46	48	49	50	51	52													
195	2	3	5	6	7	8	10	11	12	14	15	16	17	19	20	21	22	24	25	26	28	29	30	31	32	34	35	36	37	38	40	41	42	43	44	45	47	48	49	50	51	52												
200	2	3	4	6	7	8	9	11	12	13	14	16	17	18	19	21	22	23	24	26	27	28	29	31	32	33	34	35	37	38	39	40	41	43	44	45	46	47	48	50	51	52												
205	2	3	4	5	6	8	9	10	11	13	14	15	16	18	19	20	21	23	24	25	26	28	29	30	31	32	34	35	36	37	38	40	41	42	43	44	46	47	48	49	50	51	52											
210	2	3	4	5	7	8	9	10	11	13	14	15	16	18	19	20	21	22	24	25	26	27	28	30	31	32	33	34	36	37	38	39	40	42	43	44	45	46	47	48	49	50	51	52										
215	2	3	4	5	6	8	9	10	11	12	13	15	16	17	18	19	21	22	23	24	25	27	28	29	30	31	32	34	35	36	37	38	39	41	42	43	44	45	46	47	48	49	50	51	53									
220	2	3	4	5	6	7	9	10	11	12	13	14	16	17	18	19	20	22	23	24	25	26	27	29	30	31	32	33	34	36	37	38	39	40	41	42	43	44	45	46	47	48	49	50	51	52								
225	2	3	4	5	6	7	8	9	11	12	13	14	15	16	18	19	20	21	22	23	24	26	27	28	29	30	31	32	33	35	36	37	38	39	40	41	42	43	44	45	46	47	48	49	50	51								
230	2	3	4	5	6	7	8	9	10	11	13	14	15	16	17	18	19	20	22	23	24	25	26	27	28	30	31	32	33	34	35	36	37	38	39	41	42	43	44	45	46	47	48	49	50	51								
235	2	3	4	5	6	7	8	9	10	11	12	13	14	15	17	18	19	20	21	22	23	24	25	26	28	29	30	31	32	33	34	35	36	37	38	40	41	42	43	44	45	46	47	48	49	50	51						
240	2	3	4	5	6	7	8	9	10	11	12	13	14	15	16	17	18	20	21	22	23	24	25	26	27	28	29	30	31	32	33	35	36	37	38	39	40	41	42	43	44	45	46	47	48	49	50	51					
245	2	3	4	4	5	6	7	8	9	10	11	12	13	14	15	16	18	19	20	21	22	23	24	25	26	27	28	29	30	31	32	33	34	35	36	37	38	39	40	41	42	43	44	45	46	47	48	49	50				
250	2	3	3	4	5	6	7	8	9	10	11	12	13	14	15	16	17	18	19	20	21	22	23	24	25	26	27	28	29	30	31	32	33	34	35	36	37	38	39	40	41	42	43	44	45	46	47	48	49	50			
255	2	3	3	4	5	6	7	8	9	10	11	12	13	14	15	16	17	18	19	20	21	22	23	24	25	26	26	27	28	29	30	31	32	33	34	35	36	37	38	39	40	41	42	43	44	45	46	47	48	49	50		
260	2	3	3	4	5	5	6	7	8	9	10	11	12	13	14	15	16	17	18	19	20	21	22	23	24	25	26	26	27	28	29	30	31	32	33	34	35	36	37	38	39	40	41	42	43	44	45	46	47	48	49		
265	2	3	3	4	5	5	6	7	8	9	10	11	12	13	14	15	16	17	18	19	20	21	22	23	23	24	25	26	27	28	29	30	31	32	33	34	35	36	37	38	39	40	41	42	43	44	45	46	47	48	49		
270	2	2	3	4	5	5	6	7	7	8	9	10	11	12	13	14	15	16	17	18	19	20	21	22	23	24	25	26	27	28	29	30	31	31	32	33	34	35	36	37	38	39	40	41	42	43	44	45	46	47	48		
275	2	2	3	4	4	5	6	7	7	8	9	10	11	12	13	14	15	16	17	18	19	20	21	22	23	23	24	25	26	27	28	29	30	31	32	33	34	35	36	37	38	39	40	41	42	43	44	45	46	47	48		
280	2	2	3	4	4	5	6	6	7	8	9	10	11	12	13	14	15	16	16	17	18	19	20	21	22	23	24	25	26	27	28	29	30	31	32	33	34	35	36	37	38	39	40	41	42	43	43	44	45	46	47		
285	2	2	3	3	4	5	6	6	7	8	9	10	10	11	12	13	14	15	16	17	18	19	20	21	22	23	24	25	26	27	28	29	30	31	32	33	34	35	36	37	38	38	39	40	41	42	43	44	45	46		
290	2	2	3	3	4	5	5	6	7	8	8	9	10	11	12	13	14	15	16	17	18	19	20	21	22	23	23	24	25	26	27	28	29	30	31	32	33	34	35	36	36	37	38	39	40	41	42	43	43	44	45		
295	2	2	3	3	4	5	5	6	7	7	8	9	10	11	12	13	14	15	15	16	17	18	19	20	21	22	23	24	25	26	27	28	29	30	31	32	33	34	35	36	36	37	38	39	40	41	42	43	43	44		
300	2	2	3	4	5	5	6	7	8	9	9	10	11	12	13	14	15	16	17	18	19	20	21	22	23	24	25	26	26	27	28	29	30	31	32	33	34	35	36	37	38	39	40	41	42	43	43						

Bioelectrical Impedance

The **bioelectrical impedance** technique is simple to administer, but it does require costly equipment. In this technique the individual is hooked up to a machine and a weak (totally painless) electrical current is run through the body to analyze body composition (body fat, lean body mass, and body water). The technique is based on the principle that lean tissue is a better conductor of electrical tissue than fat tissue is. The easier the conductance, the leaner the individual.

The accuracy of current equations used to estimate percent body fat with this technique is still questionable. More research is required before the equations approach the accuracy of hydrostatic weighing, skinfolds, or girth measurements.

An advantage of bioelectrical impedance is that the results are highly reproducible. Unlike other techniques, in which experienced technicians are necessary to obtain valid results, almost anyone can administer bioelectrical impedance. And, although the test results may not be completely accurate, this instrument is valuable in assessing changes in body composition over time.

If this instrument or some other type of equipment for assessing body composition is available to you, you can use it to determine your percent body fat. You may want to compare the results with other techniques. Following all manufacturer's instructions will ensure the best possible result.

Air Displacement

Air displacement is a new technique that holds considerable promise. With this technique, an individual sits inside a small chamber, commercially known as the **Bod Pod**. Computerized pressure sensors determine the amount of air displaced by the person inside the chamber. Body volume is calculated by subtracting the air volume with the person inside the chamber from the volume of the empty chamber. The amount of air in the person's lungs is also taken into consideration when determining the actual body volume. Body density and percent body fat are then calculated from the obtained body volume.

Initial research has shown that this technique compares very favorably with hydrostatic weighing and it is less cumbersome to administer. The procedure takes only about 5 minutes. Additional research is needed, however, to determine its accuracy among different age groups, ethnic backgrounds, and athletic populations. Administering this assessment is a relatively easy procedure but, because of its high cost, the Bod Pod is not readily available in fitness centers and exercise laboratories.

Waist-to-Hip Ratio

Scientific evidence suggests that the way people store fat affects the risk for disease. Some individuals tend to store fat in the abdominal area (called the "apple shape"). Others store it mainly around the hips and thighs (gluteal femoral fat or "pear shape").

Obese individuals with a lot of abdominal fat clearly are at higher risk for coronary heart disease, congestive heart failure, hypertension, Type II diabetes (also called "adult-onset" or "non-insulin–dependent" diabetes), and strokes than are obese people with similar amounts of total body fat stored primarily in the hips and thighs. Evidence also indicates that, among individuals with a lot of abdominal fat, those whose fat deposits are around internal organs (visceral fat) have an even greater risk for disease than those whose abdominal fat is mainly beneath the skin (subcutaneous fat).[1]

Because of the higher risk for disease in individuals who tend to store a lot of fat in the abdominal area, as contrasted with the hips and thighs, a **waist-to-hip ratio** test was designed to estimate the risk. The waist measurement is taken at the point of smallest circumference, and the hip measurement is taken at the point of greatest circumference.

The waist-to-hip ratio differentiates the "apples" from the "pears." Most men are apples, and most women are pears. The panel recommends that men need to lose weight if the waist-to-hip ratio is 1.0 or higher. Women need to lose weight if the ratio is .85 or higher (see Table 7.6). More conservative estimates indicate that the risk starts to increase when the ratio exceeds .95 and .80 for men and women, respectively. For example, the waist-to-hip ratio for a man with a 40-inch waist and a 38-inch hip would be 1.05 (40 ÷ 38). This ratio may indicate higher risk for disease.

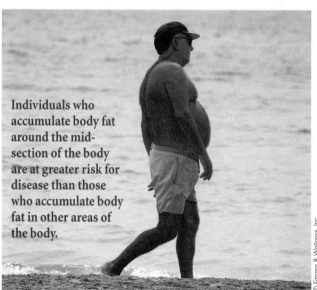

Individuals who accumulate body fat around the midsection of the body are at greater risk for disease than those who accumulate body fat in other areas of the body.

Body Mass Index

Another technique scientists use to determine thinness and excessive fatness is the **body mass index (BMI)**. This index incorporates height and weight to estimate critical fat values at which the risk for disease increases.

BMI is calculated by (a) dividing the weight in kilograms by the square of the height in meters or (b) multiplying body weight in pounds by 705 and dividing this figure by the square of the height in inches. For example, the BMI for an individual who weighs 172 pounds (78 kg) and is 67 inches (1.7 mts) tall would be 27: $[78 \div (1.7)^2]$ or $[172 \times 705 \div (67)^2]$. You can also look up your BMI in Table 7.7 according to your height and weight.

Key Terms

Bioelectrical impedance Technique to assess body composition by running a weak electrical current through the body.

Air displacement Technique to assess body composition by calculating the body volume from the air displaced by an individual sitting inside a small chamber.

Bod Pod Commercial name of the equipment used for the assessment of body composition through the air displacement technique.

Waist-to-hip ratio A measurement to assess potential risk for disease based on distribution of body fat.

Body mass index (BMI) A technique to determine thinness and excessive fatness that incorporates height and weight to estimate critical fat values at which the risk for disease increases.

TABLE 7.6 Disease Risk According to Waist-to-Hip Ratio

Waist-to-Hip Ratio		
Men	Women	Disease Risk
≤0.95	≤0.80	Very low
0.96–0.99	0.81–0.84	Low
≥1.00	≥0.85	High

TABLE 7.7 Body Mass Index

Determine your BMI by looking up the number where your weight and height intersect on the table. According to your results, look up your disease risk in Table 7.8

Height / Weight	110	115	120	125	130	135	140	145	150	155	160	165	170	175	180	185	190	195	200	205	210	215	220	225	230	235	240	245	250
5'0"	21	22	23	24	25	26	27	28	29	30	31	32	33	34	35	36	37	38	39	40	41	42	43	44	45	46	47	48	49
5'1"	21	22	23	24	25	26	26	27	28	29	30	31	32	33	34	35	36	37	38	39	40	41	42	43	43	44	45	46	47
5'2"	20	21	22	23	24	25	26	27	27	28	29	30	31	32	33	34	35	36	37	37	38	39	40	41	42	43	44	45	46
5'3"	19	20	21	22	23	24	25	26	27	27	28	29	30	31	32	33	34	35	35	36	37	38	39	40	41	42	43	43	44
5'4"	19	20	21	21	22	23	24	25	26	27	27	28	29	30	31	32	33	33	34	35	36	37	38	39	39	40	41	42	43
5'5"	18	19	20	21	22	22	23	24	25	26	27	27	28	29	30	31	32	32	33	34	35	36	37	37	38	39	40	41	42
5'6"	18	19	19	20	21	22	23	23	24	25	26	27	27	28	29	30	31	31	32	33	34	35	36	36	37	38	39	40	40
5'7"	17	18	19	20	20	21	22	23	23	24	25	26	27	27	28	29	30	31	31	32	33	34	34	35	36	37	38	38	39
5'8"	17	17	18	19	20	21	21	22	23	24	24	25	26	27	27	28	29	30	30	31	32	33	33	34	35	36	36	37	38
5'9"	16	17	18	18	19	20	21	21	22	23	24	24	25	26	27	27	28	29	30	30	31	32	32	33	34	35	35	36	37
5'10"	16	17	17	18	19	19	20	21	22	22	23	24	24	25	26	27	27	28	29	29	30	31	32	32	33	34	34	35	36
5'11"	15	16	17	17	18	19	20	20	21	22	22	23	24	24	25	26	26	27	28	29	29	30	31	31	32	33	33	34	35
6'0"	15	16	16	17	18	18	19	20	20	21	22	22	23	24	24	25	26	26	27	28	28	29	30	31	31	32	33	33	34
6'1"	15	15	16	16	17	18	18	19	20	20	21	22	22	23	24	24	25	26	26	27	28	28	29	30	30	31	32	32	33
6'2"	14	15	15	16	17	17	18	19	19	20	21	21	22	22	23	24	24	25	26	26	27	28	28	29	30	30	31	31	32
6'3"	14	14	15	16	16	17	17	18	19	19	20	21	21	22	22	23	24	24	25	26	26	27	27	28	29	29	30	31	31
6'4"	13	14	15	15	16	16	17	18	18	19	19	20	21	21	22	23	23	24	24	25	26	26	27	27	28	29	29	30	30

According to BMI, the lowest risk for chronic disease is in the 22 to 25 range[2] (see Table 7.8). Individuals are classified as overweight between 25 and 30. BMIs above 30 are defined as obese and below 20 as **underweight**. As compared with individuals with a BMI below 25, mortality rates are up to 25 percent higher for people with a BMI between 25 and 30, and 50 to 100 percent higher for those with a BMI above 30.[3] Approximately 20 percent of U. S. adults have a body BMI of 30 or more.

BMI is a useful tool to screen the general population, but its weaknesses, similar to height/weight charts, is that it fails to differentiate fat from lean body mass or to identify where most of the fat is located (waist-to-hip ratio). Using BMI, athletes with a large amount of muscle mass (such as body builders and football players) can easily fall in the moderate- or even high-risk categories. Therefore, body composition and waist-to-hip ratios are better procedures to determine health risk and recommended body weight.

DETERMINING RECOMMENDED BODY WEIGHT

After finding your percent body fat, you can determine your current body composition classification by consulting Table 7.9. In this table you will find the health fitness and the high physical fitness percent fat standards.

For example, the recommended health fitness fat percentage for a 20-year-old female is 28 percent or less. The health fitness standard is established at the point at which there seems to be no harm to health in terms of percent body fat. A high physical fitness range for this same woman would be between 18 percent and 23 percent.

The high physical fitness standard does not mean you cannot be somewhat below this number. Many highly trained male athletes are as low as 3 percent, and some female distance runners have been measured at 6 percent body fat (which may not be healthy).

Although people generally agree that the mortality rate is higher for obese people, some evidence indicates that the same is true for underweight people.

TABLE 7.8 Disease Risk According to Body Mass Index (BMI)

BMI	Disease Risk	Classification
<20.00	Moderate to Very high	Underweight
20.00 to 21.99	Low	Acceptable
22.00 to 24.99	Very low	Acceptable
25.00 to 26.99	Low	Overweight
27.00 to 29.99	Moderate	Overweight
30.00 to 39.99	High	Obese
≥40.00	Very high	Obese

TABLE 7.9 Body Composition Classification According to Percent Body Fat

MEN

Age	Underweight	Excellent	Good	Moderate	Overweight	Significantly Overweight
≤19	<3	12.0	12.1–17.0	17.1–22.0	22.1–27.0	≥27.1
20–29	<3	13.0	13.1–18.0	18.1–23.0	23.1–28.0	≥28.1
30–39	<3	14.0	14.1–19.0	19.1–24.0	24.1–29.0	≥29.1
40–49	<3	15.0	15.1–20.0	20.1–25.0	25.1–30.0	≥30.1
≥50	<3	16.0	16.1–21.0	21.1–26.0	26.1–31.0	≥31.i

WOMEN

Age	Underweight	Excellent	Good	Moderate	Overweight	Significantly Overweight
≤19	<12	17.0	17.1–22.0	22.1–27.0	27.1–32.0	≥32.1
20–29	<12	18.0	18.1–23.0	23.1–28.0	28.1–33.0	≥33.1
30–39	<12	19.0	19.1–24.0	24.1–29.0	29.1–34.0	≥34.1
40–49	<12	20.0	20.1–25.0	25.1–30.0	30.1–35.0	≥35.1
≥50	<12	21.0	21.1–26.0	26.1–31.0	31.1–36.0	≥36.1

High physical fitness standard   Health fitness standard

"Underweight" and "thin" do not necessarily mean the same thing. The body fat of a healthy thin person is around the high physical fitness standard, whereas an underweight person has extremely low body fat, even to the point of compromising the essential fat.

The 3 percent essential fat for men and 12 percent for women seem to be the lower limits for people to maintain good health. Below these percentages, normal physiological functions can be seriously impaired. Some experts point out that a little storage fat (over the essential fat) is better than none at all. As a result, the health and high fitness standards for percent fat in Table 7.9 are set higher than the minimum essential fat requirements, at a point beneficial to optimal health and well-being. Finally, because lean tissue decreases with age, one extra percentage point is allowed for every additional decade of life.

Your recommended body weight is computed based on the selected health or high fitness fat percentage for your age and gender. Your decision to select a "desired" fat percentage should be based on your current percent body fat and your personal health/fitness objectives. Following is the procedure to compute your own recommended body weight:

1. Determine the pounds of body weight in fat (FW). Multiply your body weight (BW) by the current percent fat (%F) expressed in decimal form (FW = BW × %F).

2. Determine lean body mass (LBM) by subtracting the weight in fat from the total body weight (LBM = BW − FW). (Anything that is not fat must be part of the lean component.)

3. Select a desired body fat percentage (DFP) based on the health or high fitness standards given in Table 7.9.

4. Compute recommended body weight (RBW) according to the formula: RBW = LBM ÷ (1.0 − DFP).

As an example of these computations, a 19-year-old female who weighs 160 pounds and is 30 percent fat would like to know what her recommended body weight would be at 22 percent:

Gender: female
Age: 19
BW: 160 lbs
%F: 30% (.30 in decimal form)

1. FW = BW × %F
   FW = 160 × .30 = 48 lbs
2. LBM = BW − FW
   LBM = 160 − 48 = 112 lbs
3. DFP: 22% (.22 in decimal form)
4. RBW = LBM ÷ (1.0 − DFP)

RBW = 112 ÷ (1.0 − .22)
RBW = 112 ÷ .78 = 143.6 lbs

Figure 7.6 at the end of this chapter provide the opportunity for you to record your own body composition, recommended body weight, and disease risk according to waist-to-hip ratio and BMI. A second column is provided in each of these figures for a follow-up assessment at a future date. In Figure 7.6 you also have the opportunity to express your feelings about and personal goals for body composition.

Other than hydrostatic weighing, skinfold thickness seems to be the most practical and valid technique to estimate body fat. If skinfold calipers are available, use this technique to assess your percent body fat. If calipers are not available, estimate your percent fat according to the girth measurements technique or another technique available to you. (You may wish to use several techniques and compare the results.)

IMPORTANCE OF REGULAR BODY COMPOSITION ASSESSMENT

Children in the United States do not start with a weight problem. Although a small group struggles with weight throughout life, most are not overweight when they reach age 20.

Current trends indicate that starting at age 25, the average man and woman in the United States gain 1 pound of weight per year. Thus, by age 65, the average American will have gained 40 pounds of weight. Because of the typical reduction in physical activity in our society, however, each year the average person also loses a half a pound of lean tissue. Therefore, over this span of 40 years there has been an actual fat gain of 60 pounds accompanied by a 20-pound loss of lean body mass[4] (see Figure 7.4). These changes cannot be detected unless body composition is assessed periodically.

If you are on a diet/exercise program, you should repeat your percent body fat assessment and recommended weight computations about once a month. This is important because lean body mass is affected by weight reduction programs and amount of physical activity. As lean body mass changes, so will your recommended body weight. To make valid comparisons, the same technique should be used for pre- and post-program assessments.

Key Terms

Underweight Extremely low body weight.

Changes in body composition resulting from a weight control/exercise program were illustrated in a coed aerobics (aerobic dance) course taught during a 6-week summer term. Students participated in aerobics routines four times a week, 60 minutes each time. On the first and last days of class, several physiological parameters, including body composition, were assessed. Students also were given information on diet and nutrition, and they basically followed their own dietary program.

> **Starting at age 25, the average adult in the United States gains 1.5 pounds of body fat per year.**

At the end of the 6 weeks, the average weight loss for the entire class was 3 pounds (see Figure 7.5). But, because body composition was assessed, class members were surprised to find that the average fat loss was actually 6 pounds, accompanied by a 3-pound increase in lean body mass.

When you diet, body composition should be re-assessed periodically because of the effects of negative caloric balance on lean body mass. As discussed in Chapter 9, dieting does decrease lean body mass. The loss of lean body mass can be offset or eliminated by combining a sensible diet with physical exercise.

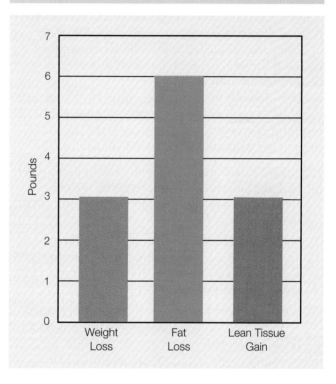

FIGURE 7.5 Effects of a 6-week aerobics exercise program on body composition.

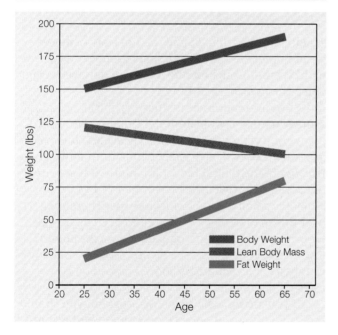

FIGURE 7.4 Typical body composition changes for adults in the United States.

WEB INTERACTIVE

Body Mass Index

This comprehensive site from *Shape Up, America!* describes body mass measurements and includes a Body Mass Index chart.

http://www.shapeup.org/bmi/index.html

Body Composition Tests from the American Heart Association

This site describes the importance of waist-to-hip ratio and body mass index as body composition measurements. The site contains tables for adult measurements for each.

http://www.justmove.org/myfitness/lowarticles/
lowframes.cfm?Target=bodycomp.html

Skinfold caliper measurements

This site describes how and where to take these measurements and explains the equations used to determine body fat.

http://www.solid.net/lowcarb/lylemcd/skinfold.htm

INTERACTIVE SITES

Count Your Calories Because Your Calories Count

This interactive site, sponsored by Wake Forest University Baptist Medical Center, features a four-step assessment of your diet, including "How's Your Diet?," "Fit or Not Quiz," "Calorie Calculator," and "Drive-Thru Diet." There is also an "Eating Disorders Quiz."

http://www.bgsm.edu/nutrition/in.html

Measuring Your Percentage of Body Fat

This site features a wellness link, nutrition information, and a virtual gym. It also enables you to determine your exercise efficiency by calculating your body mass index and your target heart rate.

http://www.fitnesslink.com/exercise/bodyfat.shtml

Calculate Your BMI

using your height and weight. BMI stands for Body Mass Index, a ratio between weight and height, and is a better predictor of disease risk than body weight alone. This site also features tools to calculate your ideal weight and your target heart rate.

http://www.drkoop.com/dyncon/article.asp?atE&id=1402

n*tes

1. C. Bouchard, G. A. Bray, and V. S. Hubbard, "Basic and Clinical Aspects of Regional Fat Distribution," *American Journal of Clinical Nutrition* 52 (1990): 946–950.

2. E. E. Calle, M. J. Thun, J. M. Petrelli, C. Rodriguez, and C. W. Heath, "Body-Mass Index and Mortality in a Prospective Cohort of U.S. Adults," *The New England Journal of Medicine* 341 (1999): 1097–1105.

3. K. M. Flegal, M. D. Carrol, R. J. Kuczmarski, and C. L. Johnson, "Overweight and Obesity in the United States: Prevalence and Trends, 1960–1994," *International Journal of Obesity and Related Metabolic Disorders* 22 (1998): 39–47.

4. J. H. Wilmore, "Exercise and Weight Control: Myths, Misconceptions, and Quackery" (lecture given at annual meeting of American College of Sports Medicine, Indianapolis, June 1994).

Suggested Readings

■ Bouchard, C., and F. E. Johnson, Editors. *Fat Distribution During Growth and Later Health Outcomes.* New York: Alan R. Liss, 1988.

■ Bouchard, C., G. A. Bray, and V. S. Hubbard. "Basic and Clinical Aspects of Regional Fat Distribution." *American Journal of Clinical Nutrition* 52 (1990): 946–950.

■ Bray, G. A. "Pathophysiology of Obesity." *American Journal of Clinical Nutrition* 55 (1992): 488S–494S.

■ Davies, P. S. W., T. J. Cole, and C. Davies. *Body Composition Techniques in Health and Disease.* Cambridge, England: Cambridge University Press, 1995.

■ Heyward, V. H., and L. M. Stolarczyk. *Applied Body Composition Assessment.* Champaign, IL: Human Kinetics, 1996.

■ Hoeger, W. W. K., and S. A. Hoeger. *Principles and Labs for Fitness and Wellness.* Belmont, CA: Wadsworth/ Thompson Learning, 2002.

■ Jackson, A. S., and M. L. Pollock. "Generalized Equations for Predicting Body Density of Men." *British Journal of Nutrition* 40 (1978): 497–504.

■ Jackson, A. S., M. L. Pollock, and A. Ward. "Generalized Equations for Predicting Body Density of Women." *Medicine and Science in Sports and Exercise* 3 (1980): 175–182.

■ Lambson, R. B. "Generalized Body Density Prediction Equations for Women Using Simple Anthropometric Measurements." (Unpublished doctoral dissertation, Brigham Young University, Provo, UT, August 1987).

■ Lohman, T. G. *Advances in Body Composition Assessment*. Champaign, IL: Human Kinetics, 1992.

■ Penrouse, K. W., A. G. Nelson, and A. G. Fisher. "Generalized Body Composition Equation for Men Using Simple Measurement Techniques." *Medicine and Science in Sports and Exercise* 17, no. 2 (1985): 189.

■ Roche, A. F., S. B. Heymsfield, and T. G. Lohman. *Human Body Composition*. Champaign, IL: Human Kinetics, 1996.

■ Siri, W. E. "Body Composition from Fluid Spaces and Density." Berkeley, CA: Donner Laboratory of Medical Physics, University of California, 1956.

■ Stensland, S. H., and S. Margolis. "Simplifying the Calculation of Body Mass Index for Quick Reference." *Journal of the American Dietetic Association* 90 (1990): 856.

FIGURE 7.6 Percent body fat and recommended body weight assessment (use second column for a retest or post-test).

Name: _____ Date: _____

Course: _____ Section: _____ Gender: _____ Age: _____

I. Percent Body Fat According to Skinfold Thickness

Men

Chest (mm): [   ]

Abdomen (mm): [   ]

Thigh (mm): [   ]

Total (mm): [   ]

% Fat: [   ]

Women

Triceps (mm): [   ]

Suprailium (mm): [   ]

Thigh (mm): [   ]

Total (mm): [   ]

% Fat: [   ]

Follow-up

% Fat [   ] %

II. Percent Fat According to Girth Measurements

Men

Waist (inches): [   ]

Wrist (inches): [   ]

Difference: [   ]

Body Weight: [   ]

% Fat: [   ]

Women

Upper Arm (cm): [   ]   Constant A = [   ]

Age: [   ]   Constant B = [   ]

Hip (cm): [   ]   Constant C = [   ]

Wrist (cm): [   ]   Constant D = [   ]

BD* = A − B − C + D

BD = [   ] − [   ] − [   ] + [   ] = [   ]

% Fat = (495 ÷ BD) − 450 = (495 ÷ [   ]) − 450 = [   ]

*Body density

Follow-up

% Fat [   ] %

III. Disease Risk According to Waist-to-Hip Ratio and Body Mass Index

Waist-to-Hip Ratio

Waist (inches): [   ]

Hip (inches): [   ]

Ratio (waist − hip): [   ]

Disease Risk: [   ]

Follow-up

[   ]

[   ]

[   ]

[   ]

Recommended Standards

Waist-to-Hip Ratio		
Men	**Women**	**Disease Risk**
≤ 0.95	≤ 0.80	Very low
0.96–0.99	0.81–0.84	Low
≥ 1.00	≥ 0.85	High

(continued)

Body Mass Index

Weight: [ ] lbs   [ ] kg

Height: [ ] inches   [ ] meters

BMI = Weight (lbs) × 705 ÷ Height (in) ÷ Height (in)

BMI = [ ] (lbs) × 705 ÷ [ ] (in) ÷ [ ] (in)

BMI = Weight (kg) ÷ Height (m) ÷ Height (m)

BMI = [ ] (kg) ÷ [ ] (m) ÷ [ ] (m)

Disease Risk: [ ]

Follow-up BMI = [ ]   Disease Risk: [ ]

Recommended Standards

BMI	Disease Risk	Classification
<20.00	Moderate to Very high	Underweight
20.00 to 21.99	Low	Acceptable
22.00 to 24.99	Very low	
25.00 to 26.99	Low	Overweight
27.00 to 29.99	Moderate	
30.00 to 39.99	High	Obese
≥40.00	Very high	

IV. Recommended Body Weight Determination

A. Body weight (BW): [ ]

B. Current %F*: [ ] %

C. Fat weight (FW) = BW × %F

   FW = [ ] × [ ] = [ ]

D. Lean body mass (LBM) = BW − FW = [ ] − [ ] = [ ]

E. Age: [ ]

F. Desired fat percent (DFP − see Table 7.9, page 184): [ ] %

G. Recommended body weight (RBW) = LBM ÷ (1.0 − DFP*)

   RBW = [ ] ÷ (1.0 − [ ]) = [ ]

*Express percentages in decimal form (for example, 25% = .25)

Follow Up

A. BW: [ ]

B. %F: [ ] %

C. FW: [ ]

D. LBM: [ ]

E. Age: [ ]

F. DFP: [ ] %

G. RBW: [ ]

V. Body Composition Results and Goals

Briefly indicate if you are satisfied with your current body weight and body composition results. If not, state your goals in terms of percent body fat and lean body mass and how you plan to achieve these goals by the end of the term.

_____

_____

_____

_____

_____

_____

_____

_____

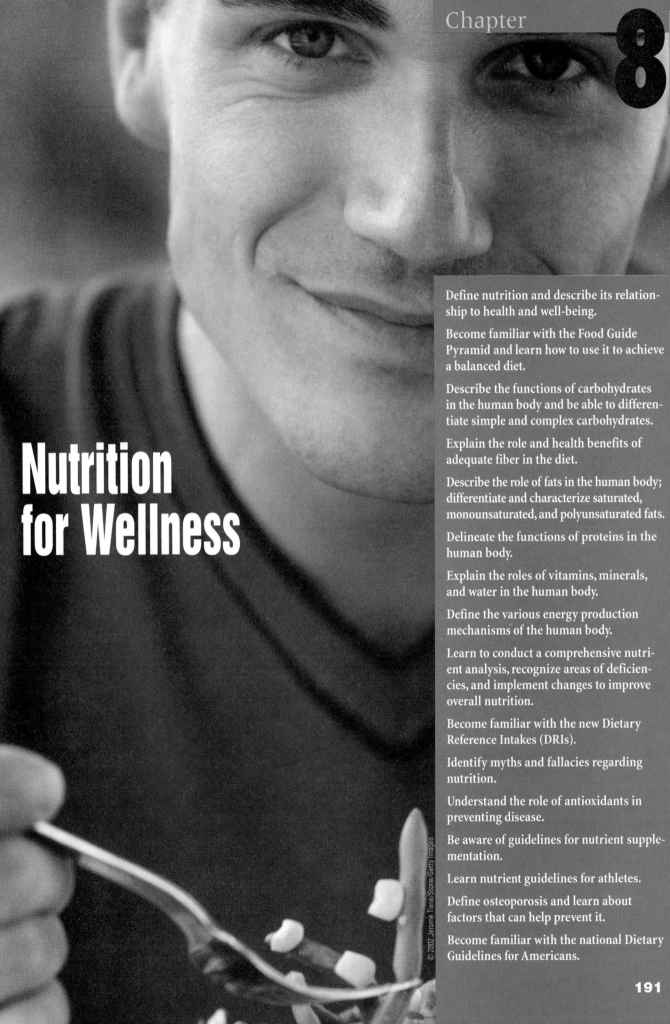

Nutrition for Wellness

© 2002 Jerome Tisne/Stone/Getty Images.

Define nutrition and describe its relationship to health and well-being.

Become familiar with the Food Guide Pyramid and learn how to use it to achieve a balanced diet.

Describe the functions of carbohydrates in the human body and be able to differentiate simple and complex carbohydrates.

Explain the role and health benefits of adequate fiber in the diet.

Describe the role of fats in the human body; differentiate and characterize saturated, monounsaturated, and polyunsaturated fats.

Delineate the functions of proteins in the human body.

Explain the roles of vitamins, minerals, and water in the human body.

Define the various energy production mechanisms of the human body.

Learn to conduct a comprehensive nutrient analysis, recognize areas of deficiencies, and implement changes to improve overall nutrition.

Become familiar with the new Dietary Reference Intakes (DRIs).

Identify myths and fallacies regarding nutrition.

Understand the role of antioxidants in preventing disease.

Be aware of guidelines for nutrient supplementation.

Learn nutrient guidelines for athletes.

Define osteoporosis and learn about factors that can help prevent it.

Become familiar with the national Dietary Guidelines for Americans.

Scientific evidence has long linked good **nutrition** to overall health and well-being. Proper nutrition means that a person's diet supplies all the essential nutrients needed to carry out normal tissue growth, repair, and maintenance. The diet also should provide enough **substrates** to produce the energy necessary for work, physical activity, and relaxation. These nutrients should be obtained from a wide variety of sources. Figure 8.1 shows the Food Guide Pyramid with the recommended number of servings from each food group for proper nutrition.

Too much or too little of any nutrient can precipitate serious health problems. The typical U.S. diet is too high in calories, sugar, fat, saturated fat, and sodium, and not high enough in fiber—factors that undermine good health. Food availability is not the problem. The problem is overconsumption.

According to the 1988 report on nutrition and health issued by the U.S. Surgeon General—the first ever of its kind—diseases of dietary excess and imbalance are among the leading causes of death in the United States.[1] Similar trends are observed in developed countries throughout the world. In the report, based on more than 2,000 scientific studies, the Surgeon General said that dietary changes can bring better health to all Americans. Other surveys reveal that, on a given day, nearly half of the people in the United States eat no fruit and almost a fourth eat no vegetables.

Diet and nutrition often play a crucial role in the development and progression of chronic diseases. A diet high in saturated fat and cholesterol increases the risk for atherosclerosis and coronary heart disease. In sodium-sensitive individuals, high salt intake has been linked to high blood pressure. Some researchers believe that 30 to 50 percent of all cancers are diet-related. Obesity, diabetes, and osteoporosis also have been associated with faulty nutrition.

> The typical U.S. diet is too high in calories, sugar, fat, saturated fat, and sodium. Food availability is not a problem. The problem is overconsumption.

To lower the risk for chronic disease, an effective wellness program must incorporate the dietary recommendations for Americans, as follows:

- Let the Food Guide Pyramid guide your food choices.
- Eat a variety of foods daily, especially grains, fruits, and vegetables. Many of these foods are high in nutrients, starch, and fiber.
- Avoid too much fat, saturated fat, and cholesterol.
- Avoid too much sugar and sodium.
- Maintain adequate calcium intake.
- Keep food safe to eat—which means that the food poses little risk of food-borne illness.
- Maintain recommended body weight.
- Drink alcoholic beverages in moderation, if at all.

These guidelines will be discussed throughout this chapter and in later chapters of this book.

NUTRIENTS

The essential **nutrients** the human body requires are carbohydrates, fat, protein, vitamins, minerals, and water. The first three are called "fuel nutrients" because they are the only substances the body uses to supply the energy (commonly measured in calories) needed for work and normal body functions. The three others—vitamins, minerals, and water—are regulatory nutrients. They have no caloric value, but still are necessary for a person to function normally and maintain good health. Many nutritionists add a seventh nutrient to this list: fiber. This nutrient has received a great deal of attention recently. Recommended amounts appear to provide protection against several diseases, including cardiovascular disease and some cancers.

Carbohydrates, fats, proteins, and water are termed "macronutrients" because we need them in proportionately large amounts daily. Vitamins and minerals are required in only small amounts—grams, milligrams, and micrograms instead of, say, ounces—and nutritionists therefore refer to them as "micronutrients."

Depending on the amount of nutrients and calories they contain, foods can be classified by their **nutrient density**. Foods that contain few or a moderate number of calories but are packed with nutrients are said to have high nutrient density. Foods that have a lot of calories but few nutrients

KeyTerms

Nutrition Science that studies the relationship of foods to optimal health and performance.

Substrate Substance acted upon by an enzyme (examples: carbohydrates and fats).

Nutrients Substances found in food that provide energy, regulate metabolism, and help with growth and repair of body tissues.

Nutrient density A measure of the amount of nutrients and calories in various foods.

FIGURE 8.1 Food guide pyramid.

Fats, Oils, and Sweets
USE SPARINGLY

KEY
● Fat (naturally occurring and added)
▼ Sugars (added)

These symbols show fats, oils, and added sugars in foods.

Milk, Yogurt, and Cheese Group
2–3 SERVINGS

Meat, Poultry, Fish, Dry Beans, Eggs, and Nuts Group
2–3 SERVINGS

Vegetable Group
3–5 SERVINGS

Fruit Group
2–4 SERVINGS

Bread, Cereal, Rice, and Pasta Group
6–11 SERVINGS

What counts as one serving?

Breads, Cereals, Rice, and Pasta
1 slice of bread
1/2 cup of cooked rice or pasta
1/2 cup of cooked cereal
1 ounce of ready-to-eat cereal

Vegetables
1/2 cup of chopped raw or cooked vegetables
1 cup of leafy raw vegetables

Fruits
1 piece of fruit or melon wedge
3/4 cup of juice
1/2 cup of canned fruit
1/4 cup of dried fruit

Milk, Yogurt, and Cheese
1 cup of milk or yogurt
1½ to 2 ounces of cheese

Meat, Poultry, Fish, Dry Beans, Eggs, and Nuts
2½ to 3 ounces of cooked lean meat, poultry, or fish
Count 1/2 cup of cooked beans, or 1 egg, or 2 tablespoons of peanut butter as 1 ounce of lean meat (about 1/3 serving)

Fats, Oils, and Sweets
LIMIT CALORIES FROM THIS GROUP especially if you need to lose weight

The amount you eat may be more than one serving. For example, a dinner portion of spaghetti would count as two or three servings of pasta.

How many servings do you need each day?

	Women & some older adults	Children, teen girls, active women, most men	Teen boys & active men
Calorie level*	about 1,600	about 2,200	about 2,800
Bread group	6	9	11
Vegetable group	3	4	5
Fruit group	2	3	4
Milk group	2–3**	2–3**	2–3**
Meat group	2, for a total of 5 ounces	2, for a total of 6 ounces	3, for a total of 7 ounces

* These are the calorie levels if you choose low-fat, lean foods from the 5 major food groups and use foods from the fats, oils, and sweets group sparingly.

** Women who are pregnant or breastfeeding, teenagers, and young adults to age 24 need 3 servings.

A Closer Look at Fat and Added Sugars

The small tip of the pyramid shows fats, oils, and sweets. These are foods such as salad dressings, cream, butter, margarine, sugars, soft drinks, candies, and sweet

desserts. Alcoholic beverages are also part of this group. These foods provide calories but few vitamins and minerals. Most people should go easy on foods from this group.

Some fat or sugar symbols are shown in the other food groups. That's to remind you that some foods in these groups can also be high in fat and added sugars, such as cheese or ice cream from the milk group, or french fries from the vegetable group. When choosing foods for a healthful diet, consider the fat and added sugars in your choices from all the food groups, not just fats, oils, and sweets from the pyramid tip.

SOURCE: Developed by the U.S. Department of Agriculture to promote a healthy diet for people in the United States.

are of low nutrient density and are commonly called "junk food."

A **calorie** is the unit of measure indicating the energy value of food to the person who consumes it. It is also used to express the amount of energy a person expends in physical activity. Technically, a kilocalorie (kcal), or large calorie, is the amount of heat necessary to raise the temperature of 1 kilogram of water 1 degree Centigrade. For simplicity, people call it a calorie rather than a kcal. For example, if the caloric value of a food is 100 calories (that is, 100 kcal), the energy in this food would raise the temperature of 100 kilograms of water 1 degree Centigrade. Similarly, walking 1 mile would burn about 100 calories (again, 100 kcal).

Carbohydrates

Carbohydrates constitute the major source of calories the body uses to provide energy for work, maintain cells, and generate heat. They also help regulate fat and metabolize protein. Each gram of carbohydrates provides the human body with 4 calories. The major sources of carbohydrates are breads, cereals, fruits, vegetables, and milk and other dairy products. Carbohydrates are classified into simple carbohydrates and complex carbohydrates (Figure 8.2).

SIMPLE CARBOHYDRATES

Often called "sugars," **simple carbohydrates** have little nutritive value. Examples are candy, soda, and cakes. Simple carbohydrates are divided into monosaccharides and disaccharides. These carbohydrates—whose names end with "-ose"—often take the place of more nutritive foods in the diet.

Monosaccharides The simplest sugars are **monosaccharides**. The three most common monosaccharides are glucose, fructose, and galactose:

1. Glucose is a natural sugar found in food; it also is produced in the body from other simple and complex carbohydrates. It is used as a source of energy, or it may be stored in the muscles and liver in the form of glycogen (a long chain of glucose molecules hooked together). Excess glucose in the blood is converted to fat and stored in **adipose tissue**.

2. Fructose, or fruit sugar, occurs naturally in fruits and honey and is converted to glucose in the body.

3. Galactose is produced from milk sugar in the mammary glands of lactating animals and is converted to glucose in the body.

Disaccharides The three major **disaccharides** are

1. Sucrose or table sugar (glucose + fructose).
2. Lactose (glucose + galactose).
3. Maltose (glucose + glucose).

These disaccharides are broken down in the body and the resulting simple sugars (monosaccharides) are used as indicated above.

COMPLEX CARBOHYDRATES

Complex carbohydrates are also called "polysaccharides." Anywhere from about ten to thousands of monosaccharide molecules can unite to form a single polysaccharide. Examples of complex carbohydrates are starches, dextrins, and glycogen.

1. Starch, the storage form of glucose in plants, is needed to promote their earliest growth. Starch is commonly found in grains, seeds, corn, nuts, roots, potatoes, and legumes. In a healthful diet, grains, the richest source of starch, should supply most of the energy. Once eaten, starch is converted to glucose for the body's own energy use.

2. Dextrins are formed from the breakdown of large starch molecules exposed to dry heat, such as in baking bread or producing cold cereals. These complex carbohydrates of plant origin provide many valuable nutrients and can be an excellent source of fiber.

3. Glycogen is the animal polysaccharide synthesized from glucose and is found only in tiny amounts in meats—in essence, we manufacture it; we don't consume it. **Glycogen** constitutes the body's

FIGURE 8.2 Major types of carbohydrates.

Simple Carbohydrates (simple sugars)	Monosaccharides	Glucose Fructose Galactose
	Disaccharides	Sucrose (glucose + fructose) Lactose (glucose + galactose) Maltose (glucose + glucose)
Complex Carbohydrates	Polysaccharides	Starches Glycogen Dextrins
	Fiber	Cellulose Hemicellulose Pectins Gums Mucilages

reservoir of glucose. Thousands of glucose molecules are linked to be stored as glycogen in liver and muscle. When a surge of energy is needed, enzymes in the muscle and the liver break down glycogen and thus make glucose readily available for energy transformation. (This process is discussed under "Nutrition for Athletes," page 226.)

FIBER

Fiber is a form of complex carbohydrate. A high-fiber diet gives a person a feeling of fullness without adding too many calories to the diet. **Dietary fiber** is present mainly in plant leaves, skins, roots, and seeds. Processing and refining foods removes almost all of the natural fiber. In our diet, the main sources of fiber are whole-grain cereals and breads, fruits, vegetables, and legumes.

Fiber is important in the diet because it decreases the risk for cardiovascular disease and cancer. Increased fiber intake also may lower the risk of coronary heart disease, because saturated fats often take the place of fiber in the diet, increasing the absorption and formation of cholesterol. Other health disorders that have been tied to low intake of fiber are constipation, diverticulitis, hemorrhoids, gallbladder disease, and obesity.

The recommended amount of fiber intake is about 25 to 30 grams per day. Most people in the United States eat only 10 to 12 grams of fiber per day, putting them at increased risk for disease. A person can increase fiber intake by eating more fruits, vegetables, legumes, grains, and cereals. A 6-year follow-up study provided further evidence linking increased fiber intake (to 30 grams per day) to a significant reduction in heart attacks, cancer of the colon, breast cancer, diabetes, and diverticulitis.[2] Table 8.1 provides the fiber content of selected foods.

Fibers are typically classified according to their solubility in water. Soluble fiber dissolves in water

TABLE 8.1 Dietary Fiber Content of Selected Foods

Food (gm)	Serving Size	Dietary Fiber
Almonds, shelled	¼ cup	3.9
Apple	1 medium	3.7
Banana	1 small	1.2
Beans (red, kidney)	½ cup	8.2
Blackberries	½ cup	4.9
Beets, red, canned (cooked)	½ cup	1.4
Brazil nuts	1 oz	2.5
Broccoli (cooked)	½ cup	3.3
Brown rice (cooked)	½ cup	1.7
Carrots (cooked)	½ cup	3.3
Cauliflower (cooked)	½ cup	5.0
Cereal		
All Bran	1 oz	8.5
Cheerios	1 oz	1.1
Cornflakes	1 oz	0.5
Fruit and Fibre	1 oz	4.0
Fruit Wheats	1 oz	2.0
Just Right	1 oz	2.0
Wheaties	1 oz	2.0
Corn (cooked)	½ cup	2.2
Eggplant (cooked)	½ cup	3.0
Lettuce (chopped)	½ cup	0.5
Orange	1 medium	4.3
Parsnips (cooked)	½ cup	2.1
Pear	1 medium	4.5
Peas (cooked)	½ cup	4.4
Popcorn (plain)	1 cup	1.2
Potato (baked)	1 medium	4.9
Strawberries	½ cup	1.6
Summer squash (cooked)	½ cup	1.6
Watermelon	1 cup	0.1

Calorie The amount of heat necessary to raise the temperature of 1 gram of water 1 degree Centigrade; used to measure the energy value of food and cost (energy expenditure) of physical activity.

Carbohydrates A classification of dietary nutrient containing carbon, hydrogen, and oxygen; the major source of energy for the human body.

Simple carbohydrates Formed by simple or double sugar units with little nutritive value; divided into monosaccharides and disaccharides.

Monosaccharides The simplest carbohydrates (sugars), formed by five- or six-carbon skeletons. The three most common monosaccharides are glucose, fructose, and galactose.

Adipose tissue Fat cells in the body.

Disaccharides Simple carbohydrates formed by two monosaccharide units linked together, one of which is glucose. The major disaccharides are sucrose, lactose, and maltose.

Complex carbohydrates Carbohydrates formed by three or more simple sugar molecules linked together; also referred to as "polysaccharides."

Glycogen Form in which glucose is stored in the body.

Dietary fiber A complex carbohydrate in plant foods that is not digested but is essential to the digestion process.

and forms a gel-like substance that encloses food particles. This property allows soluble fiber to bind and excrete fats from the body. This type of fiber has been shown to lower blood cholesterol and blood sugar levels. Soluble fibers are found primarily in oats, fruits, barley, and legumes.

Insoluble fiber is not easily dissolved in water, and the body cannot digest it. This type of fiber is important because it binds water, causing a softer and bulkier stool that increases **peristalsis**—involuntary muscle contractions of intestinal walls that force the stool through the intestines and enable quicker excretion of food residues. Speeding up passage of food residues through the intestines seems to lower the risk for colon cancer, mainly because it reduces the amount of time that cancer-causing agents are in contact with the intestinal wall. Insoluble fiber is also thought to bind with carcinogens (cancer-producing substances), and more water in the stool may dilute the cancer-causing agents, lessening their potency. Sources of insoluble fiber include wheat, cereals, vegetables, and skins of fruits.

> The recommended amount of fiber intake is about 25 to 30 grams per day. Most people in the United States eat only 10 to 12 grams of fiber per day.

The most common types of fiber are

1. Cellulose, water-soluble fiber found in plant cell walls.
2. Hemicellulose, water-soluble fiber found in cereal fibers.
3. Pectins, water-insoluble fiber found in vegetables and fruits.
4. Gums and mucilages, water-insoluble fiber also found in small amounts in foods of plant origin.

Surprisingly, too much fiber can be detrimental to health. It can produce loss of calcium, phosphorus, and iron, not to mention gastrointestinal discomfort. If you increase the fiber in your diet, do so gradually over several weeks to avoid gastrointestinal disturbances. While increasing fiber intake, be sure to drink more water to avoid constipation and even dehydration.

Fats

The human body uses **fats** as a source of energy. Fat is the most concentrated energy source. Each gram of fat supplies 9 calories to the body (in contrast to 4 for carbohydrates). Fats are a part of the human cell structure. Deposits of fat cells are used as stored energy and as an insulator to preserve body heat. They absorb shock, supply essential fatty acids, and carry the fat-soluble vitamins A, D, E, and K. Fats can be classified into three main groups: simple, compound, and derived (Figure 8.3). The most familiar sources of fat are whole milk and other dairy products, meats, and meat alternatives such as eggs and nuts.

SIMPLE FATS

A simple fat consists of a glyceride molecule linked to one, two, or three units of fatty acids. According to the number of fatty acids attached, simple fats are divided into monoglycerides (one fatty acid), diglycerides (two fatty acids), and triglycerides (three fatty acids). More than 90 percent of the weight of fat in foods and more than 95 percent of the stored fat in the human body are in the form of triglycerides.

The length of the carbon atom chain and the amount of hydrogen saturation (that is, the number of hydrogen molecules attached to the carbon chain) in fatty acids vary. Based on the extent of saturation, fatty acids are said to be "saturated" or "unsaturated." Unsaturated fatty acids are classified further into monounsaturated and polyunsaturated. Saturated fatty acids are mainly of animal origin; unsaturated fats are found mostly in plant products.

Saturated Fats In saturated fatty acids (often called "saturated fats"), the carbon atoms are fully saturated with hydrogen atoms; only single bonds link the carbon atoms on the chain (see Figure 8.4). Foods high in saturated fatty acids are meats, animal fat, lard, whole milk, cream, butter, cheese, ice cream, hydrogenated oils (hydrogenation makes oils saturated), coconut oil, and palm oils. Saturated fats typically do not melt at room temperature. Coconut and palm oils are exceptions. In general, saturated fats raise the blood cholesterol level.

> Saturated fats raise blood cholesterol and increases the risk for coronary heart disease.

Unsaturated Fats In unsaturated fatty acids (often called "unsaturated fats"), double bonds form between unsaturated carbons. In monounsaturated fatty acids (MUFA), only one double bond is found along the chain. Examples of monounsaturated fatty acids are olive, canola, rapeseed, peanut, and sesame oils. Polyunsaturated fatty acids (PUFA) contain two or more double bonds between unsaturated carbon atoms along the chain. Corn, cottonseed, safflower, walnut, sunflower, and soybean oils are high in polyunsatu-

FIGURE **8.3** Major types of fats (lipids).

Simple Fats	Monoglyceride (glyceride + one fatty acid*)
	Diglycerides (glyceride + two fatty acids)
	Triglycerides (glyceride + three fatty acids)
Compound Fats	Phospholipids
	Glucolipids
	Lipoproteins
Derived Fats	Sterols (cholesterol)

*Fatty acids can be saturated or unsaturated.

FIGURE **8.4** Chemical structure of saturated and unsaturated fats.

Saturated Fatty Acid

```
     H    H    H    H    H   OH
     |    |    |    |    |    |
G* - C -  C -  C -  C -  C -  C = O
     |    |    |    |    |
     H    H    H    H    H
```

Monounsaturated Fatty Acid

```
     H    H    H    H    H   OH
     |    |    |    |    |    |
G* - C -  C -  C =  C -  C -  C = O
     |    |              |
     H    H              H
                ↑
            Double Bond
```

Polyunsaturated Fatty Acid

```
     H    H    H    H    H    H    H    H   OH
     |    |    |    |    |    |    |    |    |
G* - C -  C -  C -  C =  C -  C =  C -  C -  C = O
     |    |    |         |              |
     H    H    H         H              H
                     ↑           ↑
                 Double Bonds
```

*Glyceride component

Earlier studies had suggested that polyunsaturated fats also seemed to cause reduction of "good" (HDL) cholesterol (a high HDL-cholesterol level is desirable because it helps to decrease the risk of diseases of the cardiovascular system). Additional research, however, does not support the lowering effect on HDL-cholesterol.[3] At typical levels found in the diet, both polyunsaturated and monounsaturated fats now seem to have similar effects on blood cholesterol.

Other Fatty Acids Hydrogen is often added to monounsaturated and polyunsaturated fats to increase shelf life and to solidify them so they are more spreadable. During this process, called "partial hydrogenation," the position of hydrogen atoms may be changed along the carbon chain, transforming the fat into a **transfatty acid**.

Margarine and spreads, crackers, cookies, and french fries often contain transfatty acids. Health-conscious people minimize the intake of these types of fats, because studies suggest that diets high in transfatty acids elevate LDL cholesterol and lower HDL cholesterol to the same extent as saturated fats.[4] Paying attention to food labels is important, because the words "partially hydrogenated" and "transfatty acids" indicate that the product carries a health risk just as high as that of saturated fat.

One type of polyunsaturated fatty acids that gained attention in recent years is **omega-3 fatty acids**, which seem to decrease cancer risk and lower triglycerides (which are a risk factor for coronary heart disease). Fish—especially fresh or frozen mackerel, herring, tuna, salmon, and lake trout—and flaxseed contain omega-3 fatty acids. Canned fish is not recommended for this purpose, because the canning process destroys most of the omega-3 oil. These fatty acids are also found, but to a lesser extent, in canola oil, walnuts, soybeans, and wheat germ.

rated fatty acids. Unsaturated fats usually are liquid at room temperature. Shorter fatty acid chains also tend to be liquid at room temperature.

Polyunsaturated and monounsaturated fats tend to lower blood cholesterol. When unsaturated fats replace saturated fats in the diet, the former tend to stimulate the liver to clear cholesterol from the blood.

KeyTerms

Peristalsis Involuntary muscle contractions of intestinal walls that facilitate excretion of wastes.

Fats Nutrients containing carbon, hydrogen, some oxygen, and sometimes other chemical elements.

Transfatty acid Solidified fat formed by adding hydrogen to monounsaturated and polyunsaturated fats to increase shelf life.

Omega-3 fatty acids Polyunsaturated fatty acids found primarily in cold-water seafood, flaxseed, and flaxseed oil; thought to lower blood cholesterol and triglycerides.

One of the simplest ways to increase omega-3 is by consuming flaxseed oil. One half of a daily tablespoon is recommended. The strong taste of flaxseed oil, however, makes this oil difficult to consume by itself. Various brands are commercially available and some are better tasting than others. Using flaxseed oil in a Caesar or other salad dressing mix is an excellent way to make it palatable. Flaxseed oil must be kept refrigerated and it should not be used for cooking.

Another essential fatty acid is **omega-6**. Our diets are typically high in omega-6-rich oils, found in corn, sunflower, and most oils in processed foods. For a healthful diet, a balance of about the same amount of omega-3 and omega-6 should be achieved. We usually consume 10 to 20 times more omega-6 than omega-3. Omega-6 fatty acids amplify inflammatory processes; without a balance, uncontrolled inflammatory reactions can damage organs in the body.

Some data suggest that fish oil, obtained eating one or two servings of fish weekly, lessens the risk for coronary heart disease. However, people who have diabetes or a history of hemorrhaging or strokes, who are on aspirin or blood-thinning therapy, and who are presurgical patients should not consume fish oil except under a physician's instruction.

COMPOUND FATS

Compound fats are a combination of simple fats and other chemicals. Examples are

1. Phospholipids—similar to triglycerides, except that choline (or another compound) and phosphoric acid take the place of one of the fatty acid units.
2. Glucolipids—a combination of carbohydrates, fatty acids, and nitrogen.
3. Lipoproteins—water-soluble aggregates of protein and triglycerides, phospholipids, or cholesterol.

Lipoproteins (a combination of lipids and proteins) are especially important because they transport fats in the blood. The major forms of lipoproteins are high-density (HDL), low-density (LDL), and very-low-density (VLDL) lipoproteins. Lipoproteins play a large role in developing or in preventing heart disease. High HDL levels have been associated with lower risk for coronary heart disease, whereas high LDL levels have been linked to increased risk for this disease. HDL is more than 50 percent protein and contains little cholesterol; LDL is approximately 25 percent protein and nearly 50 percent cholesterol. VLDL contains about 50 percent triglycerides, only about 10 percent protein, and 20 percent cholesterol.

DERIVED FATS

Derived fats combine simple and compound fats. **Sterols** are an example. Although sterols contain no fatty acids, they are considered lipids because they do not dissolve in water. The most often mentioned sterol is cholesterol, which is found in many foods or can be manufactured in the body—primarily from saturated fats.

Proteins

Proteins are the main substances the body uses to build and repair tissues such as muscles, blood, internal organs, skin, hair, nails, and bones. They form a part of hormone, antibody, and **enzyme** molecules. Enzymes play a key role in all of the body's processes. Because all enzymes are formed by proteins, this nutrient is necessary for normal functioning. Proteins also help maintain the normal balance of body fluids.

Proteins can be used as a source of energy, too, but only if sufficient carbohydrates are not available. Each gram of protein yields 4 calories of energy (the same as carbohydrates). The main sources of protein are meats and alternatives, milk, and other dairy products. Excess proteins may be converted to glucose or fat or even excreted in the urine.

The human body uses 20 **amino acids** to form different types of protein. Amino acids contain nitrogen, carbon, hydrogen, and oxygen. Of the 20 amino acids, 9 are called "essential amino acids" because the body cannot produce them. The other 11, termed "nonessential amino acids," can be manufactured in the body if food proteins in the diet provide enough nitrogen (see Table 8.2). For the body to function normally, all amino acids shown in the table must be present in the diet.

Proteins that contain all the essential amino acids, known as "complete" or "higher-quality" protein, are usually of animal origin. If one or more of the essential amino acids is missing, the proteins are termed "incomplete" or "lower-quality" protein. Individuals have to take in enough protein to ensure nitrogen for adequate production of amino acids and also to get enough high-quality protein to obtain the essential amino acids.

Protein deficiency is not a problem in the typical U.S. diet. Two glasses of skim milk combined with about 4 ounces of poultry or fish meet the daily protein requirement. Too much animal protein, on the other hand, can cause serious health problems. Some people eat twice as much protein as they need. Protein

Protein foods from animal sources often are high in fat, saturated fat, and cholesterol, which can lead to cardiovascular disease and cancer.

TABLE **8.2** Amino Acids

Essential Amino Acids*	Nonessential Amino Acids
Histidine	Alanine
Isoleucine	Arginine
Leucine	Asparagine
Lysine	Aspartic acid
Methionine	Cysteine
Phenylalanine	Glutamic acid
Threonine	Glutamine
Tryptophan	Glycine
Valine	Proline
	Serine
	Tyrosine

*Must be provided in the diet, because the body cannot manufacture them.

foods from animal sources are often high in fat, saturated fat, and cholesterol, which can lead to cardiovascular disease and cancer. Too much animal protein also decreases blood enzymes that prevent precancerous cells from developing into tumors.

As mentioned earlier, a well-balanced diet contains a variety of foods from all five basic food groups, including wise selection of foods from animal sources (see also "Balancing the Diet," page 202). Based on current nutrition data, meat (poultry and fish included) should be replaced by grains, legumes, vegetables, and fruits as main courses. Meats should be used more for flavoring than for volume. Daily consumption of beef, poultry, or fish should be limited to 3 ounces (about the size of a deck of cards) to 6 ounces.

Vitamins

Vitamins are necessary for normal bodily metabolism, growth, and development. Vitamins are classified into two types based on their solubility: fat-soluble (A, D, E, and K) and water-soluble (B complex and C). The body does not manufacture most vitamins, so they can be obtained only through a well-balanced diet. To decrease loss of vitamins during cooking, natural foods should be microwaved or steamed rather than boiled in water that is thrown out later.

A few exceptions, such as vitamin A, D, and K, are formed in the body. Vitamin A is produced from beta-carotene, found mainly in yellow foods such as carrots, pumpkin, and sweet potatoes. Vitamin D is created when ultraviolet light from the sun transforms 7-dehydrocholesterol, a compound in human skin. Vitamin K is created in the body by intestinal bacteria. The major functions of vitamins are outlined in Table 8.3.

Vitamins C, E, and beta-carotene also function as antioxidants, which are thought to play a key role in preventing chronic diseases. The specific function of these antioxidant nutrients and of the mineral selenium (also an antioxidant) are discussed under "Antioxidants" (page 220) and "Folate," (page 223).

Minerals

Approximately 25 **minerals** have important roles in body functioning. Minerals are contained in all cells, especially those in hard parts of the body (bones, nails, teeth). Minerals are crucial to maintaining water balance and the acid-base balance. They are essential components of respiratory pigments, enzymes, and enzyme systems, and they regulate muscular and nervous tissue impulses, blood clotting, and normal heart rhythm.

The three minerals mentioned most often are calcium, iron, and sodium. Calcium deficiency may result in osteoporosis, and low iron intake can induce iron-deficiency anemia (both are discussed under "Special Nutrient Needs of Women," page 229). High sodium intake may contribute to high blood pressure. The specific functions of some of the most important minerals are given in Table 8.4

Key Terms

Omega-6 fatty acids Polyunsaturated fatty acids found primarily in corn and sunflower oils and most oils in processed foods.

Lipoproteins Lipids covered by proteins, they transport fats in the blood; types are LDL, HDL, and VLDL.

Sterols Derived fats, of which cholesterol is the best-known example.

Proteins Complex organic compounds containing nitrogen and formed by combinations of amino acids; the main substances used in the body to build and repair tissues.

Enzymes Catalysts that facilitate chemical reactions in the body.

Amino acids Chemical compounds that contain nitrogen, carbon, hydrogen, and oxygen; the basic building blocks the body uses to build different types of protein.

Vitamins Organic nutrients essential for normal metabolism, growth, and development of the body.

Minerals Inorganic elements found in the body and in food; essential for normal body functions.

TABLE 8.3 Major Functions of Vitamins

Nutrient	Good Sources	Major Functions	Deficiency Symptoms
Vitamin A	Milk, cheese, eggs, liver, yellow and dark green fruits and vegetables	Required for healthy bones, teeth, skin, gums, and hair; maintenance of inner mucous membranes, thus increasing resistance to infection; adequate vision in dim light.	Night blindness; decreased growth; decreased resistance to infection; rough, dry skin
Vitamin D	Fortified milk, cod liver oil, salmon, tuna, egg yolk	Necessary for bones and teeth; needed for calcium and phosphorus absorption.	Rickets (bone softening), fractures, muscle spasms
Vitamin E	Vegetable oils, yellow and green leafy vegetables, margarine, wheat germ, whole grain breads and cereals	Related to oxidation and normal muscle and red blood cell chemistry.	Leg cramps, red blood cell breakdown
Vitamin K	Green leafy vegetables, cauliflower, cabbage, eggs, peas, potatoes	Essential for normal blood clotting.	Hemorrhaging
Vitamin B_1 (Thiamin)	Whole grain or enriched bread, lean meats and poultry, fish, liver, pork, poultry, organ meats, legumes, nuts, dried yeast	Assists in proper use of carbohydrates; normal functioning of nervous system; maintenance of good appetite.	Loss of appetite, nausea, confusion, cardiac abnormalities, muscle spasms
Vitamin B_2 (Riboflavin)	Eggs, milk, leafy green vegetables, whole grains, lean meats, dried beans and peas	Contributes to energy release from carbohydrates, fats, and proteins; needed for normal growth and development, good vision, and healthy skin.	Cracking of the corners of the mouth, inflammation of the skin, impaired vision
Vitamin B_6 (Pyridoxine)	Vegetables, meats, whole grain cereals, soybeans, peanuts, potatoes	Necessary for protein and fatty acid metabolism and for normal red blood cell formation.	Depression, irritability, muscle spasms, nausea
Vitamin B_{12}	Meat, poultry, fish, liver, organ meats, eggs, shellfish, milk, cheese	Required for normal growth, red blood cell formation, nervous system and digestive tract functioning.	Impaired balance, weakness, drop in red blood cell count
Niacin	Liver and organ meats, meat, fish, poultry, whole grains, enriched breads, nuts, green leafy vegetables, dried beans and peas	Contributes to energy release from carbohydrates, fats, and proteins; normal growth and development; and formation of hormones and nerve-regulating substances.	Confusion, depression, weakness, weight loss
Biotin	Liver, kidney, eggs, yeast, legumes, milk, nuts, dark green vegetables	Essential for carbohydrate metabolism and fatty acid synthesis.	Inflamed skin, muscle pain, depression, weight loss
Folic Acid	Leafy green vegetables, organ meats, whole grains and cereals, dried beans	Needed for cell growth and reproduction and for red blood cell formation.	Decreased resistance to infection
Pantothenic Acid	All natural foods, especially liver, kidney, eggs, nuts, yeast, milk, dried peas and beans, green leafy vegetables	Related to carbohydrate and fat metabolism.	Depression, low blood sugar, leg cramps, nausea, headaches
Vitamin C (Ascorbic acid)	Fruits, vegetables	Helps protect against infection; required for formation of collagenous tissue, normal blood vessels, teeth, and bones.	Slow-healing wounds, loose teeth, hemorrhaging, rough scaly skin, irritability

TABLE **8.4**	Major Functions of Minerals		
Nutrient	Good Sources	Major Functions	Deficiency Symptoms
Calcium	Milk, yogurt, cheese, green leafy vegetables, dried beans, sardines, salmon	Required for strong teeth and bone formation; maintenance of good muscle tone, heartbeat, and nerve function.	Bone pain and fractures, periodontal disease, muscle cramps
Copper	Seafood, meats, beans, nuts, whole grains	Helps with iron absorption and hemoglobin formation; required to synthesize the enzyme cytochrome oxidase.	Anemia (although deficiency is rare in humans)
Iron	Organ meats, lean meats, seafoods, eggs, dried peas and beans, nuts, whole and enriched grains, green leafy vegetables	Major component of hemoglobin; aids in energy utilization.	Nutritional anemia, overall weakness
Phosphorus	Meats, fish, milk, eggs, dried beans and peas, whole grains, processed foods	Required for bone and teeth formation; energy release regulation.	Bone pain and fracture, weight loss, weakness
Zinc	Milk, meat, seafood, whole grains, nuts, eggs, dried beans	Essential component of hormones, insulin, and enzymes; used in normal growth and development.	Loss of appetite, slow-healing wounds, skin problems
Magnesium	Green leafy vegetables, whole grains, nuts, soybeans, seafood, legumes	Needed for bone growth and maintenance; carbohydrate and protein utilization; nerve function; temperature regulation.	Irregular heartbeat, weakness, muscle spasms, sleeplessness
Sodium	Table salt, processed foods, meat	Needed for body fluid regulation; transmission of nerve impulses; heart action.	Rarely seen
Potassium	Legumes, whole grains, bananas, orange juice, dried fruits, potatoes	Required for heart action; bone formation and maintenance; regulation of energy release; acid-base regulation.	Irregular heartbeat, nausea, weakness
Selenium	Seafood, meat, whole grains	Component of enzymes; functions in close association with vitamin E.	Muscle pain, possible heart muscle deterioration, possible hair and nail loss

Water

Water is the most important nutrient, involved in almost every vital body process: in digesting and absorbing food, in energy production, in the circulatory process, in body heat regulation, in removing waste products, in building and rebuilding cells, and in transporting other nutrients. Approximately 60 percent of total body weight is water (see Figure 8.5).

Water is contained in almost all foods, but primarily in liquid foods, fruits, and vegetables. Besides the water content obtained from food, every person needs between 8 to 12 glasses of fluids a day. Water loss during the day must be replenished regularly—if you wait for the thirst signal, you may already have lost too much water. At 2 percent body weight loss within one day, you are dehydrated. At 5 percent, you may become dizzy and disoriented, have trouble with cognitive skills and heart function, and even lose consciousness.

ENERGY (ATP) PRODUCTION

The energy derived from food is not used directly by the cells. It is first transformed into **adenosine triphosphate (ATP)**. The subsequent breakdown of this compound provides the energy used by all

KeyTerms

Adenosine triphosphate (ATP) A high-energy chemical compound that the body uses for immediate energy.

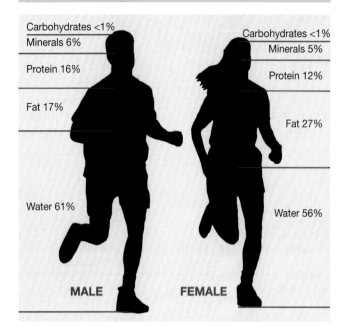

FIGURE 8.5 Approximate proportions of nutrients in the human body.

Carbohydrates <1%
Minerals 6%
Protein 16%
Fat 17%
Water 61%

MALE

Carbohydrates <1%
Minerals 5%
Protein 12%
Fat 27%
Water 56%

FEMALE

FIGURE 8.6 Contributions of different energy formation mechanisms during various forms of physical activity.

Aerobic System
Anaerobic System
ATP-CP System

Duration of Activity

energy-requiring processes of the body (also see Figure 8.6). ATP must be recycled continually to sustain life and work. ATP can be resynthesized in three ways:

1. ATP and ATP-CP system. The body stores small amounts of ATP and creatine phosphate (CP). These stores are used during all-out activities such as sprinting, long jumping, and weight lifting. The amount of stored ATP provides energy for just one or two seconds. During brief all-out efforts, ATP is resynthesized from CP, another high-energy phosphate compound. This is the ATP-CP, or phosphagen, system.

   Depending on the amount of physical training, the concentration of CP stored in cells is sufficient to allow maximum exertion for up to 10 seconds. Once the CP stores are depleted, the person is forced to slow down or rest to allow ATP to form through anaerobic and aerobic pathways.

2. Anaerobic or lactic acid system. During maximal intensity exercise that is sustained between 10 and 180 seconds, ATP is replenished from the breakdown of glucose through a series of chemical reactions that do not require oxygen (hence "anaerobic"). In the process, though, **lactic acid** is produced. As lactic acid accumulates, it leads to muscular fatigue.

   Because of the accumulation of lactic acid with high-intensity exercise, the formation of ATP during anaerobic activities is limited to about 3

minutes. A recovery period is then necessary to allow for the elimination of lactic acid. Formation of ATP through the anaerobic system requires glucose (carbohydrates).

3. Aerobic system. The production of energy during slow-sustained exercise is derived primarily through aerobic metabolism. Glucose (carbohydrates), fatty acids (fat), and oxygen (hence "aerobic") are required to form ATP using this process and, under steady-state exercise conditions, lactic acid accumulation is minimal.

   Because oxygen is required, a person's capacity to utilize oxygen is crucial for successful athletic performance in aerobic events. The higher one's maximal oxygen uptake (VO_{2max}), the greater one's capacity to generate ATP through the aerobic system—and the better the athletic performance in long distance events.

BALANCING THE DIET

One of the fundamental ways to enjoy good health and live life to its fullest is through a well-balanced diet. As illustrated in Table 8.5, the generally recommended guideline states that daily caloric intake should be distributed so that 50 to 60 percent of the total calories come from carbohydrates (mostly complex carbohydrates and less than 10 percent from sugar), about 30 percent of the total calories from fat (as long as saturated fat constitutes less than 7 percent,

TABLE **8.5** The American Diet: Current and Recommended Carbohydrates, Fat, and Protein Intake (expressed as a percentage of total calories)

Current	Recommended
Carbohydrates 50%	Carbohydrates 50–60%
Simple 26%	Simple <10%
Complex 24%	Complex 40–50%
Fat 34%	Fat 30%
Monounsaturated 11%	Monounsaturated Up to 20%
Polyunsaturated 10%	Polyunsaturated Up to 10%
Saturated 13%	Saturated Less than 7%
Protein 15%	Protein 15%

* Adapted from the 2001 National Cholesterol Education Program (NCEP) guidelines.

polyunsaturated up to 10 percent, and monounsaturated fat up to 20 percent of total calories) and approximately 15 percent of the total calories from protein.[5] The diet also must include all of the essential vitamins, minerals, and water. Rating a particular diet accurately is difficult without a complete nutrient analysis.

Most health organizations have endorsed the 30 percent–fat guideline during the last two decades. More recently, however, nutritionists and preventive medicine specialists are beginning to suggest a daily fat intake lower than the currently recommended 30 percent of total calories. Most scientific studies have shown that a 30 percent–fat diet provides little or no improvement in lowering cholesterol levels.[6] The role of high fat intake in increasing cancer risk is undeniable. An intake of about 20 percent calories from fat is better for overall reduction in risk for cancer.[7] Although the 30 percent guideline is still valid, a gradual change to a lower value might be more beneficial for overall disease prevention.

Diets in most developed countries have changed significantly since the turn of the twentieth century. Today people eat more fat, fewer carbohydrates, and about the same amount of

> **Daily caloric intake should be distributed so 50 to 60 percent of the total calories come from carbohydrates, less than 30 percent of the total calories come from fat, and 15 percent of the total calories come from protein.**

protein, but fewer calories. At the same time, people weigh more than they did in 1900, an indication that they are not as physically active as their grandparents were.

Diets also were much healthier at the turn of the twentieth century. In the United States in 1909, carbohydrates accounted for 57 percent of the total daily caloric intake, 67 percent of which were complex carbohydrates. Today, carbohydrate intake has decreased to 50 percent, and complex carbohydrates account for only 24 percent of this intake. The proportion of fat has risen from 32 percent to 34 percent. Protein intake has increased from about 12 percent to 15 percent of the total caloric intake.

Nutrition Standards

Nutritionists use a variety of nutrient standards. The most widely known nutrient standard is the RDA, or Recommended Dietary Allowances. However, this is not the only standard. Others include the Dietary Reference Intakes and the Daily Values on food labels. Each standard has a different purpose and utilization in dietary planning and assessment.

DIETARY REFERENCE INTAKES

To help people meet dietary guidelines, the National Academy of Sciences has developed a new set of dietary nutrient intakes for healthy people in the United States and Canada, the **Dietary Reference Intakes (DRIs)**. The DRIs are based on a review of the most current research on nutrient needs of healthy people. The DRI reports are written by the Food and Nutrition Board of the Institute of Medicine in cooperation with scientists from Canada. The DRIs are being released in phases: The first, released in 1997, contained revised recommendations for five nutrients important for bone health. The next set, released in 1998, contained recommendations for eight B-vitamins and choline. In June 2000, recommendations for vitamin C, vitamin E, and selenium were issued.

The general term "DRIs" includes four types of reference values for planning and assessing diets and

Key Terms

Lactic acid End product of anaerobic glycolysis (metabolism).

Dietary Reference Intakes (DRIs) A general term that describes four types of nutrient standards that establish adequate amounts and maximum safe nutrient intakes in the diet. These standards are Estimated Average Requirements (EAR), Recommended Dietary Allowances (RDA), Adequate Intakes (AI), and Tolerable Upper Intake Levels (UL).

for establishing adequate amounts and maximum safe nutrient intakes in the diet. The type of reference value used for a given nutrient and a specific age/gender group is determined according to available scientific information and the intended use of the dietary standard. The reference values are as follows:

The **Estimated Average Requirement (EAR)** is the amount of a nutrient that is estimated to meet the nutrient requirement of half the healthy people in specific age and gender groups. At this nutrient intake level, the upper 50 percent of the people do not have their nutritional requirements met. If, for example, we look at 300 healthy women of age 26, the EAR would meet the nutritional requirement for only one half of these women.

The **Recommended Dietary Allowance (RDA)** is the daily amount of a nutrient considered adequate to meet the known nutrient needs of practically all healthy people in the United States. Because the committee must decide what level of intake to recommend for everybody, the RDA is set well above the EAR and covers about 98 percent of the population. Stated another way, the RDA recommendation for any nutrient is well above almost everyone's actual requirement. The RDA could be considered a goal for adequate intake. The process for determining the RDA depends on being able to set an EAR. RDAs are statistically determined from the EAR values. If an EAR cannot be set, no RDA can be established.

When data is insufficient or inadequate to set an EAR, an **Adequate Intake (AI)** value is determined instead of the RDA. The AI value is derived from approximations of observed nutrient intakes by a group or groups of healthy people. The AI value for children and adults is expected to meet or exceed the nutritional requirements of a corresponding healthy population. Nutrients for which DRIs have been set are presented in Table 8.6.

The **Upper Intake Level (UL)**, which eventually will be available for all nutrients, establishes the highest level of nutrient intake that appears safe for most healthy people, beyond which exists an increased risk of adverse effects. As intakes increase above the UL, so does the risk of adverse effects. In general terms, the optimum nutrient range for healthy eating is between the RDA and the UL. The established ULs are presented in Table 8.7.

DAILY VALUES

In 1993, the Food and Drug Administration (FDA) revised food labeling regulations and introduced the **Daily Values (DVs)**, which are reference values for nutrients and food components (such as carbohydrate, fiber, and fat) that do not have established RDAs but do have important relationships with health. These values represent dietary intakes to achieve based on a consensus of recommended national standards.

The DVs for use on food labels include fat, saturated fat, and carbohydrate (as a percent of total calories); cholesterol, sodium, and potassium (in milligrams); and fiber and protein (in grams). The DVs for total fat, saturated fat, and carbohydrate are expressed as percentages for a 2,000-calorie diet and may therefore require adjustments depending on an individual's total daily caloric needs. For example, on a 2,000-calorie diet, carbohydrate intake should be about 60 percent of total daily calories (300 grams), and fat intake should be limited to less than 30 percent (65 grams) (see Figure 8.7). The vitamin, mineral, and protein DVs were adapted from the RDAs but are not the most current recommendations. The DVs are also not as specific for age and gender groups as are the DRIs. Both the DRIs and the DVs apply only to healthy adults. They are not intended for people who are ill and may require additional nutrients.

Nutrient Analysis

The first step in evaluating your diet is to conduct a nutrient analysis. This can be quite educational, because most people do not realize how harmful and nonnutritious many common foods are. The analysis covers calories, carbohydrates, fats, cholesterol, and sodium, as well as eight crucial nutrients: protein, calcium, iron, vitamin A, thiamin, riboflavin, niacin, and vitamin C. If the diet has enough of these eight nutrients, the foods consumed in natural form to provide these nutrients typically contain all the other nutrients the human body needs.

To do your own nutrient analysis, keep a 3-day record of everything you eat on the form in Figure 8.8 (make additional copies of this form as needed). At the end of each day, look up the nutrient content for those foods in the list of Nutritive Values of Selected Foods (located in Appendix B). Record this information on the form in Figure 8.8. If you do not find a food in Appendix B, the information may be on the food container itself.

When you have recorded the nutritive values for each day, add up each column and write the totals at the bottom of the chart. After the third day, fill in your totals on Figure 8.9 and compute an average for the 3 days. To rate your diet, compare your figures with those in the Recommended Dietary Allowances (RDA) provided in the bottom half of Figure 8.9 or in Table 8.6. The results give a good indication of areas of strength and deficiency in your current diet.

If you are using the software available with this book to conduct a nutrient analysis, type in the food name and the number of servings based on the

TABLE 8.6 Dietary Reference Intakes (DRIs): Recommended Intakes for Individuals

Recommended Dietary Allowances (RDA) — Adequate Intakes (AI)

	Calcium (mg)	Vitamin D (mcg)	Thiamin (mg)	Riboflavin (mg)	Niacin (mg NE)	Vitamin B$_6$ (mg)	Folate (mcg DFE)	Vitamin B$_{12}$ (mcg)	Phosphorus (mg)	Magnesium (mg)	Fluoride (mg)	Vitamin A (mcg)	Vitamin C (mg)	Vitamin E (mg)	Selenium (mcg)	Iron (mg)	Pantothenic acid (mg)	Biotin (mg)	Choline (mg)
Males																			
14–18	1,300	5	1.2	1.3	16	1.3	400	2.4	1,250	410	3	900	75	15	55	11	5.0	25	550
19–30	1,000	5	1.2	1.3	16	1.3	400	2.4	700	400	4	900	90	15	55	8	5.0	30	550
31–50	1,000	5	1.2	1.3	16	1.3	400	2.4	700	420	4	900	90	15	55	8	5.0	30	550
51–70	1,200	10	1.2	1.3	16	1.7	400	2.4	700	420	4	900	90	15	55	8	5.0	30	550
>70	1,200	15	1.2	1.3	16	1.7	400	2.4	700	420	4	900	90	15	55	8	5.0	30	550
Females																			
14–18	1,300	5	1.0	1.0	14	1.2	400	2.4	1,250	360	3	700	65	15	55	15	5.0	25	400
19–30	1,000	5	1.1	1.1	14	1.3	400	2.4	700	310	3	700	75	15	55	18	5.0	30	425
31–50	1,000	5	1.1	1.1	14	1.3	400	2.4	700	320	3	700	75	15	55	18	5.0	30	425
51–70	1,200	10	1.1	1.1	14	1.5	400	2.4	700	320	3	700	75	15	55	8	5.0	30	425
>70	1,200	15	1.1	1.1	14	1.5	400	2.4	700	320	3	700	75	15	55	8	5.0	30	425
Pregnant	*	*	1.4	1.4	18	1.9	600	2.6	*	+40	3	750	85	15	60	27	6.0	30	450
Lactating	*	*	1.5	1.6	17	2.0	500	2.8	*	*	3	1,300	120	19	70	10	7.0	35	550

*Values for these nutrients do not change with pregnancy or lactation. Use the value listed for women of comparable age.

SOURCE: Adapted with permission from *Recommended Dietary Allowances*, 10th Edition, and the first two of the *Dietary Reference Intakes* series, National Academy Press. Copyright 1989, 1997, 1998, 1999, 2000, and 2001, respectively, by the National Academy of Sciences. Courtesy of the National Academy Press, Washington, DC.

TABLE 8.7 Tolerable Upper Intake Levels (UL) of Selected Nutrients for Adults (19–70 years)

Nutrient	UL per Day
Calcium	2.5 gr
Phosphorus	4.0 gr*
Magnesium	350 mg
Vitamin D	50 mcg
Fluoride	10 mg
Niacin	35 mg
Vitamin B$_6$	100 mg
Folate	1000 mcg
Choline	3.5 gr
Vitamin C	2000 mg
Vitamin E	1000 mg
Selenium	400 mcg

*3.5 gr per day for pregnant women 19 years of age and older.

standard amounts given in the list of selected foods in Appendix B (see form provided in Figure 8.10 or follow the instructions given in the software program).

Estimated Average Requirements (EAR) The amount of a nutrient that meets the dietary needs in half the people.

Recommended Dietary Allowances (RDA) The daily amount of a nutrient (statistically determined from the EARs) considered adequate to meet the known nutrient needs of almost 98 percent of all healthy people in the United States.

Adequate Intakes (AI) The recommended amount of a nutrient intake when sufficient evidence is not available to calculate the EAR and subsequent RDA.

Upper Intake Level (UL) The highest level of nutrient intake that appears safe for most healthy people, beyond which exists an increased risk of adverse effects.

Daily Values (DVs) Reference values for nutrients and food components used in food labels.

FIGURE 8.7 Food label with U.S. Recommended Daily Values.

1 Better by Design
How to recognize the new food labels

The new food labels feature a revamped nutrition panel titled "Nutrition Facts," with nutrient listings that reflect current health concerns. Now you'll be able to find information on fat, fiber and other food components fundamental to lowering your risk of cancer and other chronic diseases. Listings for nutrients like thiamin and riboflavin will no longer be required, because Americans generally eat enough of them these days.

2 Size Up the Situation
All serving sizes are created equal

Now you can compare similar products and know that their serving sizes are basically identical. So when you realize how much fat is packed into that carton of double-dutch-chocolate-caramel-chew ice cream you're eyeing, you might opt for lowfat frozen yogurt instead. Serving sizes will also be standardized, so manufacturers can't make nutrition claims for unrealistically small portions. That means a chocolate cake, for example, must be divided into 8 servings sized to satisfy the average person — not 16 servings sized to satisfy the average munchkin.

3 Look Before You Leap
Use the Daily Values

You will find the Daily Values on the bottom half of the "Nutrition Facts" panel. Some represent maximum levels of nutrients that should be consumed each day for a healthful diet (as with fat) while others refer to minimum levels that can be exceeded (as with carbohydrates). They are based on both a 2,000 and 2,500 calorie diet. Your own needs may be more or less, but these figures give you a point from which to compare. For example, the sample label indicates that someone with a 2,000 calorie diet should eat no more than 65 grams of fat per day. This is based on a diet getting 30% of calories as fat. If you normally eat less calories, or want to eat less than 30% of calories as fat, your daily fat consumption will be lower.

4 Rate It Right
Scan the % Daily Values

The % Daily Values make judging the nutritional quality of a food a snap. For instance, you can look at the % Daily Value column and find that a food has 25% of the Daily Value for fiber. This means the product will give you a substantial portion of the recommended amount of fiber for the day. You can also use this column to compare nutrients in similar products. The % Daily Values are based on a 2,000 calorie diet.

5 Trust Adjectives
Descriptors have legal definitions

Terms like "low," "high" and "free" have long been used on food labels. What these words actually mean, however, could vary. Thanks to the new labeling laws, such descriptions must now meet legal definitions. For example, you may be shopping for foods high in vitamin A, which has been linked to lower risk of certain cancers. Under the new label laws, a food described as "high" in a particular nutrient must contain 20% or more of the Daily Value for that nutrient. So if the bottle of juice you're thinking of buying says "high in vitamin A,'" you can now feel confident that it really is a good source of the vitamin.

6 Read Health Claims with Confidence
The nutrient link to disease prevention

You can also expect to see food packages with health claims linking certain nutrients to reduced risk of cancer and other diseases. The federal government has approved three health claims dealing with cancer prevention: a low fat diet may reduce your risk for cancer; high fiber foods may reduce your risk for cancer; and fruits and vegetables may reduce your risk for cancer. A food may not make such a health claim for one nutrient if it contains other nutrients that undermine its health benefits. A high fiber, but high fat, jelly doughnut cannot carry a health claim!

Nutrition Facts
Serving Size ½ cup (91g)
Servings Per Container 5

Amount Per Serving

Calories 58   Calories from Fat 0

% **Daily Value***

Total Fat 0g	**0%**
Saturated Fat 0g	**0%**
Cholesterol 0mg	**0%**
Sodium 45mg	**2%**
Total Carbohydrate 12g	**4%**
Dietary Fiber 3g	**12%**
Sugars 3g	
Protein 3g	

Vitamin A	92%	Vitamin C	16%
Calcium	2%	Iron	5%

* Percent Daily Values are based on a 2,000 calorie diet. Your daily values may be higher or lower depending on your calorie needs:

	Calories	2,000	2,500
Total Fat	Less than	65g	80g
Sat Fat	Less than	20g	25g
Cholesterol	Less than	300mg	300mg
Sodium	Less than	2,400mg	2,400mg
Total Carbohydrate		300g	375g
Fiber		25g	30g

Calories per gram:
Fat 9 • Carbohydrates 4 • Protein 4

Many factors affect cancer risk. Eating a diet low in fat and high in fiber may lower risk of this disease.

- GOOD SOURCE OF FIBER
- LOWFAT

Reprinted with permission from the American Institute for Cancer Research.

FIGURE 8.8 Daily nutrient intake.

Name: _____ Date: _____ Course: _____ Section: _____ Gender: _____ Age: _____

Foods	Amount	Calories	Protein (gm)	Fat (total gm)	Sat. Fat (gm)	Chol- esterol (mg)	Carbo- hydrates (gm)	Cal- cium (mg)	Iron (mg)	Sodium (mg)	Vit. A (IU)	Vit. B$_1$ (mg)	Vit. B$_2$ (mg)	Niacin (mg)	Vit. C (mg)
Totals															

FIGURE 8.9 Nutrient analysis.

Name: _____ Date: _____ Section: _____ Course: _____ Gender: _____ Age: _____

Day	Calories	Protein (gm)	Fat (gm)	Sat. Fat (gm)	Cholesterol (mg)	Carbo-hydrates (gm)	Calcium (mg)	Iron (mg)	Sodium (mg)	Vit. A (µg RE)	Thiamin Vit. B_1 (mg)	Riboflavin Vit. B_2 (mg)	Niacin (mg)	Vit. C (mg)
One														
Two														
Three														
Totals														
Average[a]														
Percentages[b]														
Recommended Dietary Allowances*														
Men 14–18 yrs.	See below[c]	See below[d]	<30%[e]	<10%[e]	<300[e]	>58%[e]	1,300	12	2,400[e]	1,000	1.2	1.3	16	75
19–30 yrs.			<30%[e]	<10%[e]	<300[e]	>58%[e]	1,000	10	2,400[e]	1,000	1.2	1.3	16	90
31–50 yrs.			<30%[e]	<10%[e]	<300[e]	>58%[e]	1,000	10	2,400[e]	1,000	1.2	1.3	16	90
51+ yrs.			<30%[e]	<10%[e]	<300[e]	>58%[e]	1,200	10	2,400[e]	1,000	1.2	1.3	16	90
Women 14–18 yrs.			<30%[e]	<10%[e]	<300[e]	>58%[e]	1,300	15	2,400[e]	800	1.0	1.0	14	65
19–30 yrs.			<30%[e]	<10%[e]	<300[e]	>58%[e]	1,000	15	2,400[e]	800	1.1	1.1	14	75
31–50 yrs.			<30%[e]	<10%[e]	<300[e]	>58%[e]	1,000	15	2,400[e]	800	1.1	1.1	14	75
51+ yrs.			<30%[e]	<10%[e]	<300[e]	>58%[e]	1,200	10	2,400[e]	800	1.1	1.1	14	75
Pregnant			<30%[e]	<10%[e]	<300[e]	>58%[e]	1,200	30	2,400[e]	800	1.4	1.4	18	75
Lactating			<30%[e]	<10%[e]	<300[e]	>58%[e]	1,200	15	2,400[e]	1,300	1.5	1.5	17	95

[a]Divide totals by 3 or number of days assessed.
[b]Percentages: Protein and carbohydrates = multiply average by 4, divide by average calories, and multiply by 100.
Fat and saturated fat = multiply average by 9, divide by average calories, and multiply by 100.
[c]Use Table 9.2 (Page 253) for all categories.
[d]Protein intake should be .8 grams per kilogram of body weight. Pregnant women should consume an additional 15 grams of daily protein, and lactating women should have an extra 20 grams.
[e]Based on recommendations by nutrition experts.

SOURCE: Adapted from *Recommended Dietary Allowances,* © 1989 by the National Academy of Sciences (Washington, DC: National Academy Press).

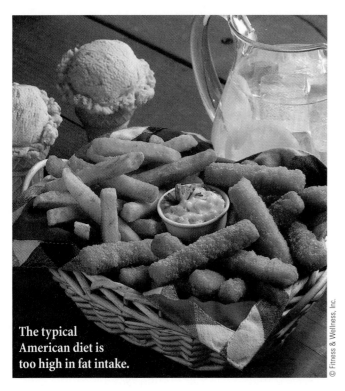

The typical American diet is too high in fat intake.

FIGURE 8.11 Caloric value of food (fuel nutrients).

Some of the most revealing information learned in a nutrient analysis is the source of fat intake in the diet. The average daily fat consumption in the U.S. diet is about 34 percent of the total caloric intake, which increases the risk for chronic diseases such as cardiovascular disease, cancer, diabetes, and obesity. Less than 30 percent of total calories should come from fat.

As illustrated in Figure 8.11, one gram of carbohydrates or of protein supplies the body with 4 calories, and fat provides 9 calories per gram consumed (alcohol yields 7 calories per gram). Therefore, looking at only the total grams consumed for each type of food can be misleading.

For example, a person who eats 160 grams of carbohydrates, 100 grams of fat, and 70 grams of protein has a total intake of 330 grams of food. This indicates that 30 percent of the total grams of food is in the form of fat (100 grams of fat ÷ 330 grams of total food = .30; .30 × 100 = 30 percent). In reality, almost half of that diet is in the form of fat calories.

In the sample diet, 640 calories are derived from carbohydrates (160 grams × 4 calories per gram),

> **The average daily fat consumption in the U.S. diet is too high, which increases the risk for chronic diseases such as cardiovascular disease, cancer, diabetes, and obesity.**

280 calories from protein (70 grams × 4 calories per gram), and 900 calories from fat (100 grams × 9 calories per gram), for a total of 1,820 calories. If 900 calories are derived from fat, almost half of the total caloric intake is in the form of fat (900 ÷ 1,820 (100 = 49.5 percent).

Each gram of fat provides 9 calories. When figuring out the percent fat calories of individual foods, you may find Figure 8.12 a useful guideline. Multiply the grams of fat by 9 and divide by the total calories in that particular food (per serving). Then multiply that number by 100 to get the percentage. For example, the food label in Figure 8.12 lists a total of 120 calories and 5 grams of fat, and the equation

You can restructure your meals so that rice, pasta, beans, breads, and vegetables are in the center of the plate; meats are on the side and added primarily for flavoring; fruits are used for desserts; and low- or nonfat milk products are used.

FIGURE 8.12 Computation of fat content in food.

Nutrition Facts

Serving Size 1 cup (240 ml)
Servings Per Container 4

Amount Per Serving

Calories 120	Calories from Fat 45

	% Daily Value*
Total Fat 5g	**8%**
Saturated Fat 3g	**15%**
Cholesterol 20mg	**7%**
Sodium 120mg	**5%**
Total Carbohydrate 12g	**4%**
Dietary Fiber 0g	**0%**
Sugars 12g	
Protein 8g	

Vitamin A	10%	•	Vitamin C	4%
Calcium	30%	•	Iron	0%

* Percent Daily Values are based on a 2,000 calorie diet. Your daily values may be higher or lower depending on your calorie needs:

	Calories	2,000	2,500
Total Fat	Less than	65g	80g
Sat Fat	Less than	20g	25g
Cholesterol	Less than	300mg	300mg
Sodium	Less than	2,400mg	2,400mg
Total Carbohydrate		300g	375g
Fiber		25g	30g

Calories per gram:
Fat 9 • Carbohydrate 4 • Protein 4

Percent fat calories = (grams of fat × 9)
÷ calories per serving × 100

5 grams of fat × 9 calories per grams of fat =
45 calories from fat

45 calories from fat ÷ 120 calories per serving
× 100 = 38% fat

below shows the fat content to be 38 percent of total calories. This simple guideline can help you decrease the fat in your diet. The fat content of selected foods, given in grams and as a percent of total calories, is presented in Figure 8.13. The percentage of fat is further subdivided into saturated, monounsaturated, polyunsaturated, and other fatty acids.

Beware of products labeled "97 percent fat-free." These products use weight, and not percent of total calories, as a measure of fat. Many of these foods still are in the range of 30 percent fat calories.

ACHIEVING A BALANCED DIET

Anyone who has completed a nutrient analysis and has given careful attention to Tables 8.3 (vitamins) and 8.4 (minerals) will probably realize that a well-balanced diet entails eating a variety of foods and reducing daily intake of fats and sweets. The Food Guide Pyramid in Figure 8.1 (page 193) provides simple and sound instructions for nutrition. The pyramid contains five major food groups, along with fats, oils, and sweets (which are to be used sparingly). The daily recommended number of servings of the five major food groups are as follows:

1. Six to eleven servings of the bread, cereal, rice, and pasta group.

2. Three to five servings of the vegetable group.

3. Two to four servings of the fruit group.

4. Two to three servings of the milk, yogurt, and cheese group.

5. Two to three servings of the meat, poultry, fish, dry beans, eggs, and nuts group.

Grains, vegetables, and fruits provide the nutritional base for a healthy diet. Daily fruits and vegetables should include, as a minimum, one good source of **pro-vitamin** A or carotene (apricots, cantaloupe, broccoli, carrots, pumpkin, dark leafy vegetables) and one good source of vitamin C (citrus fruit, kiwi fruit,

High-fiber foods are essential to a healthy diet.

KeyTerms

Pro-vitamin A compound that can be converted into a vitamin.

FIGURE **8.13** Fat content of selected foods.

FAT CONTENT OF SELECTED FOODS

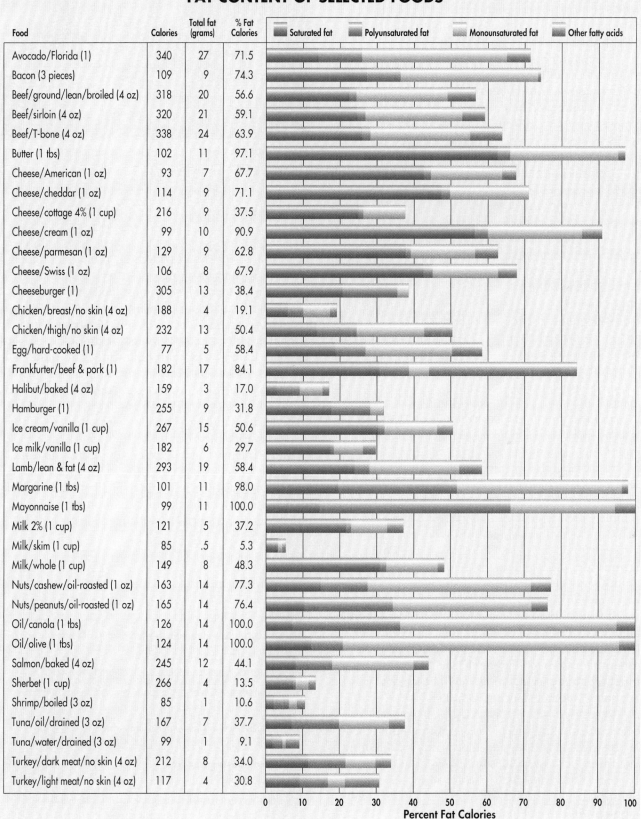

Food	Calories	Total fat (grams)	% Fat Calories
Avocado/Florida (1)	340	27	71.5
Bacon (3 pieces)	109	9	74.3
Beef/ground/lean/broiled (4 oz)	318	20	56.6
Beef/sirloin (4 oz)	320	21	59.1
Beef/T-bone (4 oz)	338	24	63.9
Butter (1 tbs)	102	11	97.1
Cheese/American (1 oz)	93	7	67.7
Cheese/cheddar (1 oz)	114	9	71.1
Cheese/cottage 4% (1 cup)	216	9	37.5
Cheese/cream (1 oz)	99	10	90.9
Cheese/parmesan (1 oz)	129	9	62.8
Cheese/Swiss (1 oz)	106	8	67.9
Cheeseburger (1)	305	13	38.4
Chicken/breast/no skin (4 oz)	188	4	19.1
Chicken/thigh/no skin (4 oz)	232	13	50.4
Egg/hard-cooked (1)	77	5	58.4
Frankfurter/beef & pork (1)	182	17	84.1
Halibut/baked (4 oz)	159	3	17.0
Hamburger (1)	255	9	31.8
Ice cream/vanilla (1 cup)	267	15	50.6
Ice milk/vanilla (1 cup)	182	6	29.7
Lamb/lean & fat (4 oz)	293	19	58.4
Margarine (1 tbs)	101	11	98.0
Mayonnaise (1 tbs)	99	11	100.0
Milk 2% (1 cup)	121	5	37.2
Milk/skim (1 cup)	85	.5	5.3
Milk/whole (1 cup)	149	8	48.3
Nuts/cashew/oil-roasted (1 oz)	163	14	77.3
Nuts/peanuts/oil-roasted (1 oz)	165	14	76.4
Oil/canola (1 tbs)	126	14	100.0
Oil/olive (1 tbs)	124	14	100.0
Salmon/baked (4 oz)	245	12	44.1
Sherbet (1 cup)	266	4	13.5
Shrimp/boiled (3 oz)	85	1	10.6
Tuna/oil/drained (3 oz)	167	7	37.7
Tuna/water/drained (3 oz)	99	1	9.1
Turkey/dark meat/no skin (4 oz)	212	8	34.0
Turkey/light meat/no skin (4 oz)	117	4	30.8

Saturated fat   Polyunsaturated fat   Monounsaturated fat   Other fatty acids

Percent Fat Calories

cantaloupe, strawberries, broccoli, cabbage, cauliflower, green pepper).

In addition to providing nutrients crucial to health, fruits and vegetables are the sole source of **phytochemicals** ("phyto" comes from the Greek word for plant). These compounds, recently discovered by scientists, show promising results in the fight against cancer.

The main function of phytochemicals in plants is to protect them from sunlight. In humans, they seem to have a powerful ability to block the formation of cancerous tumors. Their actions are so diverse that, at almost every stage of cancer, phytochemicals have the ability to block, disrupt, slow down, or even reverse the process. These compounds are not found in pills.

The consistent message is to eat a diet with ample fruits and vegetables. The recommended five to nine servings of fruits and vegetables daily has absolutely no substitute. Science has not yet found a way to allow people to eat a poor diet, pop a few pills, and derive the same benefits.

> Phytochemicals, found in abundance in fruits and vegetables, have a powerful ability to block the formation of cancerous tumors.

Milk, poultry, fish, and meats are to be consumed in moderation. Milk and milk products should be low-fat. The recommendation is to consume 3 ounces of poultry, fish, or meat and not to exceed 6 ounces daily. All visible fat and skin should be trimmed off meats and poultry before cooking.

As an aid in balancing your diet, the form in Figure 8.14 enables you to record your daily food intake. (This record is much easier to keep than the complete dietary analysis in Figures 8.8 and 8.9). Make one copy for each day you wish to record. Whenever you have something to eat, record, in Figure 8.14, the food and the amount eaten. Do this immediately after each meal so you will be able to keep track of your actual food intake more easily.

If you eat twice the amount of a standard serving, double the number of servings. Evaluate your diet by checking whether you ate the minimum required servings for each food group. If you meet the minimum required servings at the end of each day, you are doing well in balancing your diet.

Rearrange your meals on the plate so rice, pasta, beans, breads, and vegetables are in the center, meats are on the side and are added primarily for flavoring. Use fruits for dessert. Substitute low-fat or nonfat milk and milk products. These are all strategies to help you enjoy a healthy diet, prevent disease, and improve your overall quality of life.

© Fitness & Wellness, Inc.

Most fruits and vegetables contain large amounts of cancer-preventing phytochemicals.

Vegetarianism

Over 12 million people in the United States follow vegetarian diets. **Vegetarians** rely primarily on foods from the bread, cereal, rice, pasta, and fruit and vegetable groups and avoid most foods from animal sources in the dairy and protein groups. The five basic types of vegetarians are as follows: **Vegans** eat no animal products at all. **Ovovegetarians** allow eggs in the diet. **Lactovegetarians** allow foods from the milk group. **Ovolactovegetarians** include egg and milk products in the diet. **Semivegetarians** do not eat red meat, but do include fish and poultry in addition to milk products and eggs in their diets.

Vegetarian diets can be healthful and consistent with the Dietary Guidelines for Americans and can meet the DRIs for nutrients. However, vegetarians who do not select their food combinations properly can develop nutritional deficiencies of protein, vitamins, minerals, and even calories. Even greater attention

Key Terms

Phytochemicals Chemical compounds thought to prevent and fight cancer; found in large quantities in fruits and vegetables.

Vegetarians Individuals whose diet is of vegetable or plant origin.

Vegans Vegetarians who eat no animal products at all.

Ovovegetarians Vegetarians who allow eggs in their diet.

Lactovegetarians Vegetarians who eat foods from the milk group.

Ovolactovegetarians Vegetarians who include eggs and milk products in their diet.

Semivegetarians Vegetarians who include milk products, eggs, and fish and poultry in the diet.

FIGURE **8.14** Healthy diet plan.

Name: _____ Course: _____ Section: _____

I. Record your intake immediately after each meal.

No.	Food*	Amount	Calories	Fat (gm)	Bread, Cereal, Rice, and Pasta	Vegetable	Fruit	Milk, Yogurt, and Cheese	Meat, Poultry, Fish, Dry Beans, Eggs, and Nuts
1									
2									
3									
4									
5									
6									
7									
8									
9									
10									
11									
12									
13									
14									
15									
16									
17									
18									
19									
20									
21									
22									
23									
24									
25									
26									
27									
28									
29									
30									
Totals			**		***				
Recommended Amount*					6–11	3–5	2–4	2–3	2–3
Deficiencies*									

*See "List of Nutritive Value of Selected Foods" in Appendix B.

**Compute using Table 9.2, page 253.

***Multiply the recommended amount of calories by .30 (30%) and divide by 9 to obtain the recommended amount of grams of fat (if on a diet, multiply by .20 or .10—see Table 9.4, page 255).

(continued)

(Figure 8.14 Healthy diet plan—continued)

II. Nutrition Stage of Change

Using Figure 2.4 (page 45) and Table 2.3 (page 43) identify your current stage of change for nutrition (healthy diet):

 conclusion What I Learned and What I Can Do to Improve My Nutrition

Based on the nutrient analysis and your daily diet analysis, explain what these experiences have taught you and list specific changes and strategies that you can use to improve your present nutrition habits. Use an extra blank sheet of paper as needed.

I have learned the following about myself/my current diet: _____

_____

_____

_____

_____

Specific changes I plan to make: _____

_____

_____

_____

_____

Strategies I will use: _____

_____

_____

_____

_____

should be paid when planning vegetarian diets for infants and children. Unless carefully planned, a strict plant-based diet will prevent proper growth and development.

NUTRIENT CONCERNS

Protein deficiency can be a concern in some vegetarian diets. Vegans in particular must be careful to eat foods that provide a balanced distribution of essential amino acids, such as grain products and legumes. Strict vegans also need a supplement of vitamin B_{12}. This vitamin is not found in plant foods; its only source is animal foods. Deficiency of this vitamin can lead to anemia and nerve damage.

The key to a healthful vegetarian diet is to eat foods that possess complementary proteins. Most plant-based products lack one or more essential amino acids in adequate amounts. For example, both grains and legumes are good protein sources, but neither provides all the essential amino acids. Grains and cereals are low in the amino acid lysine, and legumes lack methionine. Foods from these two groups—such as combinations of tortillas and beans, rice and beans, rice and soybeans, or wheat bread and peanuts—will complement each other and provide all required protein nutrients. These complementary proteins may be consumed over the course of one day, but it is best if they are consumed during the same meal.

Other nutrients likely to be deficient in vegetarian diets—and ways to overcome them—are as follows:

- Vitamin D can be obtained from moderate sun exposure or by taking a supplement.

- Riboflavin can be found in green leafy vegetables, whole grains, and legumes.

- Calcium can be obtained from fortified soybean milk or fortified orange juice, calcium-rich tofu, and selected cereals. A calcium supplement is also an option.

- Iron can be found in whole grains, dried fruits and nuts, and legumes. To enhance iron absorption, a good source of vitamin C should be consumed with these foods (calcium and iron are the most difficult nutrients to consume in sufficient amounts in a strict vegan diet).

- Zinc can be obtained from whole grains, wheat germ, beans, nuts, and seeds.

Most vegetarians today consume dairy products and eggs. A modified version of the Food Guide Pyramid has been prepared for the ovolactovegetarian. All food groups and number of servings remain the same, except that the meat, poultry, fish, dry beans, eggs, and nuts group has been replaced with an eggs,

legumes, nuts, and seeds group, and two to four servings are recommended from this group (instead of two to three). Those who are interested in vegetarian diets are encouraged to consult additional resources, because special vegetarian diet planning cannot be covered adequately in a few paragraphs.

NUTS

Consumption of nuts and soy foods, commonly used in vegetarian diets, has received considerable attention in recent years. A few years ago, most people regarded nuts as especially high in fat and calories. Although they are 70 to 90 percent fat, most of it is unsaturated fat. And research indicates that people who eat nuts several times a week have a lower incidence of heart disease. Eating two to three ounces (about one-half cup) of almonds, walnuts, or macadamia nuts a day may decrease high blood cholesterol by about 10 percent. Nuts can even enhance the cholesterol-lowering effects of the Mediterranean diet (discussed in the next section).

Heart-health benefits are attributed not only to the unsaturated fats, but to other nutrients found in nuts, such as vitamin E and folic acid. Nuts are also packed with additional B vitamins, calcium, copper, potassium, magnesium, fiber, and phytochemicals. Many of these nutrients are cancer- and cardio-protective, help lower homocysteine levels, and act as antioxidants (discussed in "Antioxidants" (page 220) and "Folate," on page 223).

Nuts do have a drawback: They are still high in calories. A handful of nuts provides as many calories as a piece of cake, so avoid using nuts as a snack. Excessive weight gain is a risk factor for cardiovascular disease. Therefore, nuts are recommended for use in place of high-protein foods such as meats, bacon, eggs, or as part of a meal in fruit or vegetable salads, homemade bread, pancakes, casseroles, yogurt, and oatmeal. Peanut butter is also healthier than cheese or some cold cuts in sandwiches.

SOY PRODUCTS

The increased popularity of soy foods is attributed primarily to Asian research that points to less heart disease, lower cholesterol levels, and fewer hormone-related cancers in people who regularly consume soy foods. The benefits of soy lie in its high protein content and plant chemicals, known as isoflavones, that act as antioxidants and may protect against estrogen-related cancers (breast, ovarian, and endometrial). The compound genistein, one of many

Soy foods may protect against estrogen-related cancers.

phytochemicals in soy, helps to reduce breast cancer risk, and soy consumption has also been linked to a lower risk for prostate cancer.

Additionally, soy proteins can lower blood cholesterol to a greater extent than would be expected just from its low-fat and high-fiber content. The evidence of heart-protecting benefits from soy foods is so strong that the FDA now allows the following claim on food labels: "25 grams of soy proteins a day, as part of a diet low in saturated fat and cholesterol, may reduce the risk of heart disease." One to two cups of soy milk, one-half cup of tofu, one-and-one-half tablespoons of soy protein isolate, or one-fourth cup of soy flour provide about 10 grams of soy protein. Additional information on the health benefits of soy foods is given in Chapters 10 and 11.

Mediterranean Diet

Much attention has been given recently to the **Mediterranean diet**, because people in that region have notably lower rates of diet-linked diseases and a longer life expectancy. The diet focuses on olive oil, red wine, grains, legumes, vegetables, and fruits, with limited amounts of meat, fish, milk, and cheese. Although it is a semivegetarian diet, up to 40 percent of the total daily caloric intake may come from fat—mostly monounsaturated fat from olive oil. Moderate

intake of red wine is included with meals. The dietary plan also encourages regular physical activity (see Figure 8.15).

Critics of the Mediterranean diet believe that regular wine consumption may lead to alcohol abuse and liver damage. Proponents counter with research that supports a lower risk for heart disease in people who consume one to two alcoholic beverages per day. In terms of heart disease, the Mediterranean diet advocates daily exercise and wine in moderation.

Ethnic Diets

As people migrate, they take their dietary practices with them. Many ethnic diets are healthier than the typical American diet, because they emphasize consumption of complex carbohydrates and limit fat intake. The predominant minority ethnic groups in America are African American, Hispanic American, and Asian American. Unfortunately, ethnic diets quickly become Americanized when they enter the United States. Often, vegetables are cut back and meats and salt are added to these diets to please the American consumer. Ethnic dishes, nonetheless, can be prepared at home. They are easy to make and much healthier if the typical (original) variety of vegetables, corn, rice, spices, and condiments are used. Ethnic dietary plans also encourage daily physical

FIGURE 8.15 Mediterranean diet pyramid.

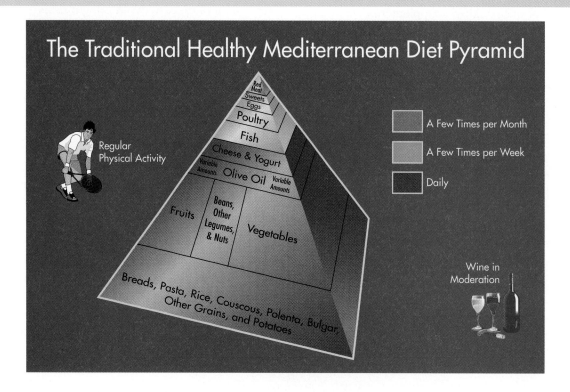

activity and suggest no more than two alcoholic drinks per day.

The African-American diet (soul food) is based on the regional cuisine of the American South. Soul food includes yams, black-eyed peas, okra, and peanuts. The latter were then combined with American foods like corn products and pork. Today, most people view soul food as meat, fried chicken, sweet potatoes, and chitterling.

Hispanic dishes arrived with the conquistadores and evolved through combinations with other ethnic diets and local foods available in Latin America. For example, the Cuban cuisine combined Spanish, Chinese, and native foods; Puerto Rican cuisine developed from Spanish, African, and native products; Mexican diets evolved from Spanish and native food. Corn, beans, squash, chili peppers, avocados, papayas, and fish were primarily used in all these diets. Rice and citrus foods were later added by the colonists. Today a wide variety of foods are used, including red meat; but the staple of the diets still include rice, corn, and beans.

Diets rich in vegetables and using minimal amounts of meat and fat are characteristic in Asian-American diets. The Okinawan diet in Japan, where some of the healthiest and oldest people in the world live, is high in fresh (versus pickled) vegetables, high in fiber, and low in fat and salt. The Chinese cuisine uses more than 200 vegetables, and fat-free sauces and seasoning are used to enhance flavor. The Chinese diet varies somewhat within regions of China. The lowest in fat is that of southern China, with fish, seafood, and stir-fried vegetables used in most meals. Chinese food in American restaurants, however, contains a much higher percentage of fat and protein than the traditional Chinese cuisine.

Table 8.8 provides a list foods to choose from when dining at selected ethnic restaurants.

All healthy diets have similar characteristics. They are high in fruits, vegetables, and grains and low in fat and saturated fat. Low-fat or fat-free dairy products are also used, and portion control is emphasized. The latter is essential in a healthy diet plan, because many people now think that if a food item is labeled "low-fat" or "fat-free," it can be

> **Healthy diets are high in fruits, vegetables, and grains and low in fat and saturated fat.**

Key Terms

Mediterranean diet Typical diet of people around the Mediterranean region that focuses on olive oil, red wine, grains, legumes, vegetables, and fruits, with limited amounts of meat, fish, milk, and cheese.

TABLE 8.8 Ethnic Eating Guide

	Choose Often	Choose Less Often

Chinese	Beef with broccoli
	Chinese greens
	Steamed rice, brown
	  or white
	Steamed beef with
	  pea pods
	Stir-fry dishes
	Teriyaki beef or chicken
	Wonton soup
		Crispy duck
		Egg rolls
		Fried rice
		Kung pao chicken
		  (fried)
		Peking duck
		Pork spareribs

Japanese	Chiri nabe (fish stew)
	Grilled scallops
	Sushi, Sashimi (raw fish)
	Teriyaki
	Yakitori (grilled chicken)
		Tempura (fried
		  chicken, shrimp,
		  or vegetables)
		Tonkatsu
		  (fried pork)

Italian	Cioppino (seafood stew)
	Minestrone
	  (vegetarian soup)
	Pasta with marinara
	  sauce
	Pasta primavera
	  (pasta with vegetables)
	Steamed clams
		Antipasto
		Cannelloni, ravioli
		Fettuccini alfredo
		Garlic bread
		White clam sauce

Mexican	Beans and rice
	Black bean/vegetable
	  soup
	Burritos, bean
	Chili
	Enchiladas, bean
	Fajitas
	Gazpacho
	Taco salad
	Tamales
	Tortillas, steamed
		Chili rellenos
		Chimichangas
		Enchiladas,
		  beef or cheese
		Flautas
		Guacamole
		Nachos
		Quesadillas
		Tostadas
		Sour cream
		  (as topping)

Middle Eastern	Tandoori chicken Curry (yogurt-based) Rice pilaf Lentil soup	Falafel Shish kebab
French	Poached salmon Spinach salad Consommé Salad nicoise	Beef Wellington Escargot French onion soup Sauces in general

Soul Food	Baked chicken
	Baked fish
	Roasted pork
	  (not smothered
	  or "etouffe")
	Sauteed okra
	Baked sweet potato
		Fried chicken
		Fried fish
		Smothered pork
		  tenderloin
		Okra in gumbo
		Sweet potato
		  casserole or pie

Greek	Gyros Pita Lentil soup	Baklava Moussaka

SOURCE: Adapted from P. A. Floyd, S. E. Mimms, and C. Yelding-Howard. *Personal Health: Perspectives & Lifestyles* (Belmont, CA: Wadsworth/Thompson Learning, 1998).

consumed in large quantities. Low-fat or fat-free does not imply calorie-free. Many people who consume low-fat diets increase the amount of food that they eat, which in the long term leads to obesity and its associated health problems.

NUTRIENT SUPPLEMENTATION

Approximately half of all adults in the United States take daily nutrient **supplements**. Nutrient requirements for the body normally can be met by consuming as few as 1,200 calories per day, as long as the diet contains the recommended servings from the five food groups.

Many people consider it necessary to take vitamin supplements. It's true that our bodies cannot retain water-soluble vitamins as long as fat-soluble vitamins. The body excretes excessive intakes readily. Small amounts, however, can be retained for weeks or months in various organs and tissues of the body. Fat-soluble vitamins, on the other hand, are stored in fatty tissue. Therefore, daily intake of these vitamins is not as crucial. Too much vitamin A and vitamin D actually can be detrimental to health.

People should not take **megadoses** of vitamins and minerals. For some nutrients, a dose of five times the RDA taken over several months may create problems. For others, it may not pose any threat to human health. Vitamin and mineral doses should not exceed the ULs. For those nutrients that do not have an established UL, no dosage higher than three times the RDA should be taken.

Iron deficiency (determined through blood testing) is more common in women. Iron supplementation is frequently recommended for women who have heavy menstrual flow. Some pregnant and lactating women also may require supplements. According to 1990 guidelines by the National Academy of Sciences, the average pregnant woman who eats an adequate amount of a variety of foods should take a low dose of iron supplement daily. Women who are pregnant with more than one baby may need additional supplements. Folate supplements also are encouraged prior to and during pregnancy to prevent certain birth defects (see following discussion in "Antioxidants" and "Folate"). In the above instances, supplements should be taken under a physician's supervision.

Other people who may benefit from supplementation are people with nutrient deficiencies (including low calcium intake), alcoholics and street-drug users who do not have a balanced diet, smokers, vegans (strict vegetarians), individuals on extremely low-calorie diets (less than 1,200 calories per day), older adults who don't eat balanced meals regularly, newborn infants (who are usually given a single dose of vitamin K to prevent abnormal bleeding), and people with disease-related disorders or who are taking medications that interfere with proper nutrient absorption. Although some supplements are encouraged (see discussion that follows), most supplements do not seem to provide additional benefits for healthy people who eat a balanced diet. They do not help people run faster, jump higher, relieve stress, improve sexual prowess, cure a common cold, or boost energy levels.

Antioxidants

Much research currently is being done to study the effectiveness of **antioxidants** in thwarting several chronic diseases. Although there are probably over 4,000 antioxidants in foods, the four more studied antioxidants are Vitamins C, E, beta-carotene (a precursor to vitamin A), and the mineral selenium (see Table 8.9).

TABLE 8.9 Antioxidant Nutrients, Sources, and Functions

Nutrient	Good Sources	Antioxidant Effect
Vitamin C	Citrus fruit, kiwi fruit, cantaloupe, strawberries, broccoli, green or red peppers, cauliflower, cabbage	Appears to inactivate oxygen free radicals.
Vitamin E	Vegetable oils, yellow and green leafy vegetables, margarine, wheat germ, oatmeal, almonds, whole-grain breads, cereals	Protects lipids from oxidation.
Beta-carotene	Carrots, squash, pumpkin, sweet potatoes, broccoli, green leafy vegetables	Soaks up oxygen free radicals.
Selenium	Seafood, Brazil nuts, meat, whole grains	Helps prevent damage to cell structures.

Oxygen is used during metabolism to change carbohydrates and fats into energy. During this process, oxygen is transformed into stable forms of water and carbon dioxide. A small amount of oxygen, however, ends up in an unstable form, referred to as **oxygen free radicals**.

A free radical molecule has a normal proton nucleus with a single unpaired electron. Having only one electron makes the free radical extremely reactive, and it looks constantly to pair its electron with one from another molecule. When a free radical steals a second electron from another molecule, that other molecule in turn becomes a free radical. This chain reaction goes on until two free radicals meet to form a stable molecule.

> Antioxidants, found in abundance in fruits and vegetables, thwart chronic diseases.

Free radicals attack and damage proteins and lipids, in particular cell membranes and DNA. This damage is thought to contribute to the development of conditions such as cardiovascular disease, cancer, emphysema, cataracts, Parkinson's disease, and premature aging. Solar radiation, cigarette smoke, air pollution, radiation, some drugs, injury or infection, chemicals (such as pesticides), and other environmental factors also seem to encourage the formation of free radicals. Antioxidants are thought to offer protection by absorbing free radicals before they can cause damage and also by interrupting the sequence of reactions once damage has begun, thwarting certain chronic diseases (see Figure 8.16).

The body's own defense systems typically neutralize free radicals so that they don't cause any damage. However, when free radicals are produced faster than the body can neutralize them, they can damage the cells.

Antioxidants are found abundantly in food, especially in fruits and vegetables. Unfortunately, only 9 percent of Americans eat the minimum five daily servings of fruits and vegetables (five to nine is the recommendation).[8]

Many of the benefits of antioxidants are obtained from food sources themselves, and controversy exists as to the benefits of antioxidants taken in supplement form. Many researchers in this area believe that taking antioxidant supplements prevents free-radical damage. In a departure from past recommendations, the editorial board of the *University of California at Berkeley Wellness Letter* issued the first antioxidant nutrient supplement recommendations in 1994. In 2001, these guidelines were updated and the board now recommends the following:[9]

- Consume between 250 and 500 mg of vitamin C.
- Take 200 to 400 **IU (international units)** of vitamin E (look for natural vitamin E, because synthetic forms are not well used by the body).

KeyTerms

Supplements Tablets, pills, capsules, liquids, or powders that contain vitamins, minerals, amino acids, herbs, or fiber that are taken to increase the intake of these nutrients.

Megadoses For most vitamins, 10 times the RDA or more; for vitamins A and D, 5 and 2 times the RDA, respectively.

Antioxidants Compounds such as vitamins C and E, beta-carotene, and selenium that prevent oxygen from combining with other substances in the body to form harmful compounds.

Oxygen free radicals Substances formed during metabolism that attack and damage proteins and lipids, in particular the cell membrane and DNA, leading to diseases such as heart disease, cancer, and emphysema.

International unit (IU) Measure of nutrients in foods.

FIGURE 8.16 Antioxidant protection: blocking and absorbing oxygen free radicals to prevent chronic diseases.

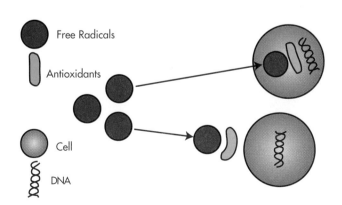

Free Radicals

Antioxidants

Cell

DNA

If supplements are taken, it is recommended that they be taken with meals and split in two to three doses per day.[10] Based on the above recommendations, however, people who consume five or more daily servings of fresh fruits and vegetables can get their daily vitamin C requirements through the diet alone. To obtain the recommended guideline for vitamin E through diet alone, however, is practically impossible. Vitamin E, also called tocopherol, is found primarily in oil-rich seeds and vegetable oils. As shown in Table 8.10, vitamin E is not easily found in large quantities in foods typically consumed in the diet. Thus, a daily vitamin E supplement is encouraged.

Antioxidant nutrients often work in conjunction with other nutrients in food that may further enhance their beneficial actions. Because vitamin E is fat-soluble, it should be taken with a meal that has some fat in it. Vitamin C is water-soluble, and the body eliminates it in about 12 hours. For best results, consume vitamin C–rich foods twice a day or divide your vitamin C supplement in half and take it twice a day.

Some evidence has linked high intake of vitamin E to reduced risk of heart disease, but may not offer additional protection to people who already have the disease.[11] Healthy people who take vitamin E do have fewer heart problems, and the vitamin appears to slow down the progression of plaque (atherosclerosis) in the arteries.[12]

High intake of a vitamin C supplement is no longer recommended. Studies have shown that vitamin C offers benefits against heart disease, cancer, cataracts, and several other health disorders. Thus, a

TABLE 8.10 Antioxidant Content of Selected Foods

Beta-Carotene	IU
Apricot (1 medium)	675
Broccoli (½ cup, frozen)	1,740
Broccoli (½ cup, raw)	680
Cantaloupe (1 cup)	5,160
Carrot (1 medium, raw)	20,255
Green peas (½ cup, frozen)	535
Mango (1 medium)	8,060
Mustard greens (½ cup, frozen)	3,350
Papaya (1 medium)	6,120
Spinach (½ cup, frozen)	7,395
Sweet potato (1 medium, baked)	24,875
Tomato (1 medium)	1,395
Turnip greens (½ cup, boiled)	3,960

Vitamin C	mg
Acerola (1 cup, raw)	1,640
Acerola juice (8 oz)	3,864
Cantaloupe (½ melon, medium)	90
Cranberry juice (8 oz)	90
Grapefruit (½, medium, white)	52
Grapefruit juice (8 oz)	92
Guava (1 medium)	165
Kiwi (1 medium)	75
Lemon juice (8 oz)	110
Orange (1 medium)	66
Orange juice (8 oz)	120
Papaya (1 medium)	85
Pepper (½ cup, red, chopped, raw)	95
Strawberries (1 cup, raw)	88

Vitamin E	IU	mg*
Almond oil (1 tbsp)		5.3
Almonds (1 oz)	10.1	
Canola oil (1 tbsp)		9.0
Cottonseed oil (1 tbsp)		5.2
Hazelnuts (1 oz)	4.4	
Kale (1 cup)	15.0	
Margarine (1 tbsp)		2.0
Peanuts (1 oz)	3.0	
Shrimp (3 oz, boiled)	3.1	
Sunflower seeds (1 oz, dry)	14.2	
Sunflower seed oil (1 tbsp)		6.9
Sweet potato (1 medium, baked)	7.2	
Wheat germ oil (1 tbsp)		20.0

Selenium	mcg
Brazil nuts (1)	100
Bread, whole wheat enriched (1 slice)	15
Beef (3 oz)	33
Cereals (3½ oz)	20
Chicken breast, roasted, no skin (3 oz)	24
Cod, baked (3 oz)	57
Egg, hard boiled (1 large)	15
Fruits (3½ oz)	1
Noodles, enriched, boiled (1 cup)	50
Oatmeal, cooked (1 cup)	23
Red snapper (3 oz)	150
Rice, long grain, cooked (1 cup)	20
Salmon, baked (3 oz)	35
Spaghetti w/meat sauce (1 cup)	36
Tuna, canned, water, drained (3 oz)	68
Turkey breast, roasted, no skin (3 oz)	28
Walnuts, black, chopped (¼ cup)	5
Vegetables (3½ oz)	1

*Vitamin E values for oils are commonly expressed in milligrams (mg). One mg is almost equal to 1 IU (international unit).

diet that supplies 250 to 500 mg of daily vitamin C is recommended.[13] More than 500 daily mg is unnecessary, given that research at the National Institutes of Health showed that the body absorbs very little vitamin C beyond the first 200 mg per serving or dose.[14]

Beta-carotene supplementation was encouraged in the early 1990s. It is better, however, to obtain the daily recommended dose of beta-carotene (20,000 IU) from food sources rather than supplements.[15]

Two separate clinical trials found that beta-carotene supplements offered no protection against heart disease and cancer. One of these studies actually found a higher rate of lung cancer and higher mortality rate in smokers who took beta-carotene supplements. For former smokers and nonsmokers, these supplements do not cause any harm, but neither do they offer additional health benefits. Therefore, it is recommended that you "skip the pill and eat the carrot." One medium raw carrot contains about 20,000 IU of beta-carotene.

Adequate intake of the mineral selenium is encouraged. Research indicates that individuals who take 200 micrograms (mcg) of selenium daily decreased their risk of prostate cancer by 63 percent, colorectal cancer by 58 percent, and lung cancer by 46 percent.[16] Data also points to decreased risk of breast, liver, and digestive tract cancers. According to Dr. Edward Giovannucci of the Harvard Medical School, the evidence for the benefits of selenium in reducing prostate cancer risk is so strong that public health officials should recommend that people increase selenium intake now.[17]

Other evidence suggests that taking 100 mcg of selenium supplements daily will increase energy levels, decrease anxiety, and improve immune function.[18] Because selenium may interfere with the body's absorption of vitamin C, the two nutrients should be taken at separate times.[19] Vitamin E supplements, on the other hand, increase the effectiveness of selenium in the body.

> There is perhaps no more extensive body of evidence for the cancer-preventing potential of a normal dietary component than there is for selenium.
>
> —Dr. Gerald Combs, Jr., Cornell University

One Brazil nut (unshelled) that you crack yourself provides about 100 mcg of selenium. Shelled nuts found in supermarkets average only about 20 mcg each. Based on the current body of research, a dose of 100 to 200 mcg per day seems to provide the necessary amount of antioxidant for this nutrient. There is no reason to take more than 200 mcg daily—in fact,

the UL for selenium has been set at 400 mcg. Too much selenium can damage cells rather than protect them. If you choose to take supplements, take an organic form of selenium from yeast and not selenium selenite. The selenium content of various foods is provided in Table 8.10.

Although much interest has been generated by the previously mentioned supplements, multivitamins are still the preferred supplement of the American people. A low-dose multivitamin complex that provides 100 percent of the DV can help fill in certain dietary deficiencies. Some evidence suggest that regular intake decreases the risk for heart disease and stroke. Multivitamins, however, are no magic pills either. They can help, but they don't provide a license to eat carelessly. Multivitamins don't provide energy, fiber, phytochemicals, or the recommended daily dose of vitamin C (250 to 500 mg) and vitamin E (200 to 400 IU).

Folate

Although it is not an antioxidant, 400 mcg of **folate** (a B vitamin) also is recommended for all premenopausal women.[20] Folate helps prevent certain birth defects and seems to offer protection against colon and cervical cancers. Women who might become pregnant should plan on taking a folate supplement, because studies have shown that folate intake (400 mcg per day) during early pregnancy can prevent serious birth defects.

Increasing evidence also indicates that taking 400 mcg of folate along with vitamins B_6 and B_{12} prevents heart attacks by reducing homocysteine levels in the blood (see Chapter 10). High concentrations of homocysteine accelerate the process of plaque formation (atherosclerosis) in the arteries.[21] Five servings of fruits and vegetables per day usually meet the needs for these nutrients. Currently, almost 9 of 10 adults in the United States do not obtain the recommended 400 mcg of folate per day. Because of the critical role of folate in preventing heart disease, some experts recommend a daily vitamin B complex that includes 400 mcg of folate.[22]

SIDE EFFECTS

Toxic effects from antioxidant supplements are rare when they are taken in the recommended amounts. The daily UL for adults 19 to 70 years of age for vitamin C has been set at 2,000 mg, for vitamin E at 1,000 mg, and for selenium at 400 mcg. Although no

Folate One of the B vitamins.

UL has been given, up to 50,000 IU of beta-carotene seem safe. If any of the following side effects arise, you should stop supplementation and check with your physician:

- Vitamin E: gastrointestinal disturbances, increase in blood lipids (determined through blood tests)
- Vitamin C: nausea, diarrhea, abdominal cramps, kidney stones, liver problems
- Beta-carotene: (although not harmful) yellow pigmentation of the skin
- Selenium: nausea, vomiting, diarrhea, irritability, fatigue, flu-like symptoms, lesions of the skin and nervous tissue, loss of hair and nails, respiratory failure, liver damage

Substantial supplementation of vitamin E is not recommended for individuals on **anticoagulant** therapy. Vitamin E is an anticoagulant in itself. Therefore, if you are on such therapy, check with your physician. Pregnant women need a physician's approval prior to beta-carotene supplementation. It also may be unsafe if taken with alcohol or by people who drink more than 4 ounces of pure alcohol per day (the equivalent of 8 beers).

Benefits of Foods

Even though you may consider taking some supplements, fruits and vegetables are the richest sources of antioxidants and phytochemicals. Researchers at the U.S. Department of Agriculture compared the antioxidant effects of vitamins C and E with those of various common fruits and vegetables.[23] The results indicated that three-fourths cup of cooked kale (which contains only 11 IU of vitamin E and 76 mg of vitamin C) neutralized as many free radicals as approximately 800 IU of vitamin E or 600 mg of vitamin C. Other excellent sources of antioxidants found by these researchers include blueberries, strawberries, spinach, Brussels sprouts, plums, broccoli, beets, oranges, and grapes. A list of top antioxidant foods is presented in Table 8.11.

Many people who regularly eat foods high in fat content or too many sweets think they need supplementation to balance their diet. This is another fallacy about nutrition. The problem here is not necessarily a lack of vitamins and minerals, but a diet too high in calories, fat, and sodium. Vitamin, mineral, and fiber supplements do not supply all of the nutrients and other beneficial substances present in food and needed for good health. Supplements will provide added health benefits, but by no means do they replace a well-balanced diet.

TABLE 8.11 Top Antioxidant Foods (expressed in ORAC* units per serving)

Fruits	ORAC Units	Vegetables	ORAC Units
Blueberries, ½ cup	1,750	Kale, 1 cup	1,190
Blackberries, ½ cup	1,470	Beets, 1 cup	570
Prunes, 3	1,460	Red bell peppers, ½ cup	530
Plums, 2	1,250	Brussel sprouts, ½ cup	430
Strawberries, ½ cup	1,170	Corn, ½ cup	420
Raisins, ¼ cup	1,030	Spinach, 1 cup	380
Raspberries, ½ cup	760	Onions, ½ cup	360
Orange, ½ cup	680	Broccoli, ½ cup	320
Red grapes, ½ cup	590	Eggplant, ½ cup	160
Cherries, ½ cup	520	Alfalfa sprouts, ½ cup	150

SOURCE: Adapted from USDA, Agricultural Research Service, *Food & Nutrition Research Briefs*, April 1999 (downloaded from www.ars.usda.gov/is/np/fnrb).

*ORAC = oxygen radical absorbance capacity

Wholesome foods contain vitamins, minerals, carbohydrates, fiber, proteins, fats, phytochemicals, and other substances not yet discovered. Researchers do not know if the protective effects are caused by the antioxidants alone, in combination with other nutrients (such as phytochemicals), or by some other nutrients in food that have not been investigated yet. Many nutrients work in **synergy**, enhancing chemical processes in the body. Supplementation will not offset poor eating habits. Pills are no substitute for common sense.

If you think your diet is not balanced, you first need to conduct a nutrient analysis (see Figures 8.8, 8.9, and 8.10) to determine which nutrients you lack in sufficient amounts. Eat more of them, as well as foods that are high in antioxidants and phytochemicals. Following a nutrient assessment, a **registered dietician** can help you decide what supplement(s) might be necessary. If you take supplements in pill form, look for products that meet the USP (U.S. Pharmacopoeia) disintegration standards on the bottle. The USP symbol suggests that the supplement should completely dissolve in 45 minutes or less. Supplements that do not dissolve, of course, cannot get into the bloodstream.

Functional Foods

Functional foods are any food or food ingredient that offers specific health benefits beyond those supplied by the traditional nutrients it contains. Many functional foods come in their natural form. A tomato for example, is a functional food because it contains the phytochemical lycopene, thought to reduce prostate cancer risk. Other examples of functional foods are kale, broccoli, blueberries, red grapes, and green tea.

The term "functional food," however, has been used primarily as a marketing tool by the food industry to attract the consumer. Unlike fortified foods, which have been modified to help prevent nutrient deficiencies, functional foods are being created by the food industry by adding ingredients aimed at treating or preventing symptoms or disease. With such "functional foods," the added ingredient(s) is often not typically found in the particular food item in its natural form, but it is added to allow manufacturers to make appealing health claims.

In most cases only one extra ingredient is added (a vitamin, mineral, phytochemical, or herb). An example is calcium added to orange juice to make the claim that this particular brand offers protection against osteoporosis. Thus, food manufacturers now offer cholesterol-lowering margarines (enhanced with plant stanol), cancer-protective (lycopene-fortified) ketchup, memory-boosting (ginkgo-added) candy, calcium-fortified chips, and kava-kava–containing corn chips (to enhance relaxation).

The use of some functional foods, however, may undermine good nutrition. Margarines may contain saturated fats or partially hydrogenated oils. Regular ketchup consumption on top of large orders of fries adds many calories and fat to the diet. Sweets are also high in calories and sugar. Chips are high in calories, salt, and fat. In all of these cases, the consumer would be better off taking the specific ingredient in a supplement form rather than consuming the "functional food" with its extra calories, sugar, salt, and/or fat.

Functional foods can provide added benefits if used in conjunction with a healthful diet. You may use nutrient-dense functional foods in your overall wellness plan as an adjunct to health-promoting strategies and treatments.[24]

Genetically Modified Foods

A genetically modified organism (GMO) is one whose DNA (or basic genetic material) is manipulated to obtain certain results. This is done by inserting genes with desirable traits from one plant, animal, or microorganism into another one to either introduce new traits or enhance existing ones.

Health claims approved by the FDA that link foods and disease prevention

- Calcium-rich foods and reduced risk of osteoporosis
- Low-sodium foods and reduced risk of high blood pressure
- Low-fat diet and reduced risk of cancer
- A diet low in saturated fat and cholesterol and reduced risk of heart disease
- High-fiber foods and reduced risk of cancer
- Soluble fiber in fruits, vegetables, and grains and reduced risk of heart disease
- Soluble fiber in oats and psyllium seed husk and reduced risk of heart disease
- Fruit- and vegetable-rich diet and reduced risk of cancer
- Folate-rich foods and reduced risk of neural tube defects
- Less sugar and reduced risk of dental caries

Crops are genetically modified to make them resist disease and extreme environmental conditions (such as heat and frost) better, require less fertilizers and pesticides, last longer, and improve their nutrient content and taste. Such crops could help save billions of dollars in more productive crops and help feed the hungry in developing countries around the world.

Concerns over the safety of genetically modified (GM) foods have created heated public debates in Europe and to a lesser extent in the United States, although the issue is now receiving more attention. The concern is that genetic modifications create "transgenic" organisms that have not previously existed and that have potentially unpredictable effects on the environment and on humans. Concerns exist that GM foods may cause illness or allergies in humans and that cross-pollination may destroy other plants or create "superweeds" with herbicide-resistant genes.

Genetically modified crops were first introduced in the United States in 1996. This technology is moving forward so rapidly that the USDA has already approved more than 50 GM crops. In 1999, about 25

KeyTerms

Anticoagulant Any substance that inhibits blood clotting.

Synergy A reaction in which the result is greater than the sum of its two parts.

Registered dietician (RD) A person with a college degree in dietetics who meets all certification and continuing education requirements of the American Dietetic Association or Dietitians of Canada.

percent of the U.S. cropland produced GM foods. About 60 percent of our soybeans and 35 percent of corn came from GM crops.

Total avoidance of GM foods is difficult, because over 60 percent of processed foods on the market today contain GM organisms.[25] For people who do not wish to consume GM foods, organic foods are an option because organic trade organizations do not certify foods with genetic modifications. Produce bought at the local farmers' market may also be an option, because small farmers are less likely to use this new technology.

At this point, no evidence indicates that GM foods are harmful—but no compelling evidence guarantees that they are safe, either. Many questions remain and much research is required in this field. As a consumer, you need to continue educating yourself as more evidence becomes available in the next few years.

NUTRITION FOR ATHLETES

The two main fuels that supply energy for physical activity are glucose (sugar) and fat (fatty acids). The body uses amino acids, derived from proteins, as an energy substrate when glucose is low, such as during fasting, prolonged aerobic exercise, or a low-carbohydrate diet.

Glucose is derived from foods high in carbohydrates such as breads, cereals, grains, pasta, beans, fruits, vegetables, and sweets in general. Glucose is stored as glycogen in muscles and the liver. Fatty acids (discussed on page 197) are the product of the breakdown of fats. Unlike glucose, an almost unlimited supply of fatty acids, stored as fat in the body, can be used during exercise.

During resting conditions, fat supplies about two-thirds of the energy to sustain the body's vital processes. During exercise, the body uses both glucose (glycogen) and fat in combination to supply the energy demands. The proportion of fat to glucose changes with the intensity of exercise. When a person is exercising below 60 percent of his or her maximal work capacity (VO_{2max}), fat is used as the primary energy substrate. As the intensity of exercise increases, so does the percentage of glucose utilization—up to 100 percent during maximal work that can only be sustained for 2 to 3 minutes.

In general, athletes do not require special supplementation or any other special type of diet. Unless the diet is deficient in basic nutrients, no special, secret, or magic diet will help people perform better or develop faster as a result of what they eat. As long as the diet is balanced—that is, based on a large variety of nutrients from all basic food groups—athletes do not

TABLE 8.12 Recommended Daily Protein Intake	
Activity level	Intake in grams per kg (2.2 lb) of body weight
Sedentary	0.8
Lightly active	0.9
Moderately active	1.1
Very Active	1.3
Extremely active	1.5

require additional supplements (other than the antioxidant recommendations made under "Antioxidants" and "Folate" in this chapter). Even in strength training and body building, protein in excess of 20 percent of total daily caloric intake is not necessary. The recommended daily protein intake ranges from 0.8 grams per kilogram of body weight for sedentary people to 1.5 grams per kilogram for extremely active individuals (see Table 8.12).

The main difference between a sensible diet for a sedentary person and one for a highly active individual is the total number of calories required daily and the amount of carbohydrate intake needed during prolonged physical activity. People in training consume more calories because of their greater energy expenditure—which is required as a result of intense physical training.

Carbohydrate Loading

On a regular diet, the body is able to store between 1,500 and 2,000 calories in the form of glycogen. About 75 percent of this glycogen is stored in muscle tissue. This amount, however, can be increased greatly through **carbohydrate loading**.

A regular diet should be altered during several days of heavy aerobic training or when a person is going to participate in a long-distance event of more than 90 minutes (for example, marathon, triathlon, or road cycling). For events shorter than 90 minutes, carbohydrate loading does not seem to enhance performance.

During prolonged exercise, glycogen is broken down into glucose, which then is readily available to the muscles for energy production. In comparison to fat, glucose frequently is referred to as the "high-octane fuel," because it provides about 6 percent more energy per unit of oxygen consumed.

Heavy training over several consecutive days leads to depletion of glycogen faster than it can be replaced through the diet. Glycogen depletion with heavy training is common in athletes. Signs of depletion include chronic fatigue, difficulty in maintaining accustomed exercise intensity, and lower performance.

On consecutive days of exhaustive physical training (this means several hours daily), a carbohydrate-rich diet—70 percent of total daily caloric intake or 8 grams of carbohydrate per kilogram (2.2 pounds) of body weight—is recommended. This diet often restores glycogen levels in 24 hours. Along with the high-carbohydrate diet, a day of rest often is needed to allow the muscles to recover from glycogen depletion following days of intense training. For people who exercise less than an hour a day, a 60 percent carbohydrate diet or 6 grams of carbohydrate per 1 kilogram of body weight is enough to replenish glycogen stores.

Following an exhaustive workout, eating a combination of carbohydrates and protein (such as a tuna sandwich) within 30 minutes of exercise seems to speed up glycogen storage even more. Protein intake increases insulin activity, thereby enhancing glycogen replenishment. A 70 percent carbohydrate intake then should be maintained throughout the rest of the day.

> **Carbohydrate loading is necessary only for endurance events that last longer than 90 minutes.**

By following a special diet and exercise regimen 5 days before a long-distance event, highly (aerobically) trained individuals are capable of storing two to three times the amount of glycogen found in the average person. Athletic performance may be enhanced for long-distance events of more than 90 minutes by eating a regular balanced diet (50 to 60 percent carbohydrates) along with intensive physical training the fifth and fourth days before the event, followed by a diet high in carbohydrates (about 70 percent) and a gradual decrease in training intensity over the last 3 days before the event.

The amount of glycogen stored as a result of a carbohydrate-rich diet does not seem to be affected by the proportion of complex and simple carbohydrates. Intake of simple carbohydrates (sugars) can be raised while on a 70 percent carbohydrate diet, as long as 48 percent of the total calories is derived from complex carbohydrates. The latter provide more nutrients and fiber, making them a better choice for a healthier diet.

On the day of the long-distance event, carbohydrates are still the recommended choice of substrate. As a rule of thumb, athletes should consume 1 gram of carbohydrate for each kilogram (2.2 pounds) of body weight 1 hour prior to exercise (that is, if you weigh 160 pounds, you should consume 160 ÷ 2.2 = 72 grams). The amount of carbohydrate can be

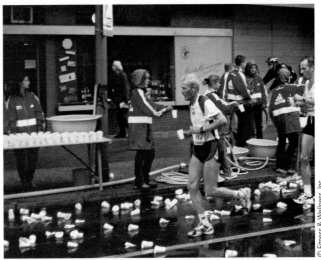

Fluid and carbohydrate replenishment during exercise are essential when participating in long-distance aerobic endurance events, such as a marathon or a triathlon.

increased to 2, 3, or 4 grams per kilogram of weight 2, 3, or 4 hours, respectively, before exercise.

During the long-distance event, researchers recommend that 30 to 60 grams of carbohydrates (120 to 240 calories) be consumed every hour. This is best accomplished by drinking 8 ounces of a 6 to 8 percent-carbohydrate sports drink every 15 minutes. This also lessens the chance of dehydration during exercise, which hinders performance and endangers health. The percentage of the carbohydrate drink is determined by dividing the amount of carbohydrate (in grams) by the amount of fluid (in ml), and multiplying by 100. For example, 18 grams of carbohydrate in 240 ml (8 oz) of fluid yields a drink at 7.5 percent (18 ÷ 240 × 100).

Creatine Supplementation

Creatine is an organic compound obtained in the diet primarily from meat and fish. In the human body, creatine combines with inorganic phosphate and forms the high-energy compound **creatine phosphate (CP)**. CP is then used to resynthesize ATP

Key Terms

Carbohydrate loading Increasing intake of carbohydrates during heavy aerobic training or prior to aerobic endurance events that last longer than 90 minutes.

Creatine An organic compound derived from meat, fish, and amino acids that combines with inorganic phosphate to form creatine phosphate.

Creatine phosphate (CP) A high-energy compound that is used by the cells to resynthesize ATP during all-out activities of very short duration.

during short bursts of all-out physical activity. Individuals on a normal mixed diet consume an average of 1 gram of creatine per day. Each day, 1 additional gram is synthesized from various amino acids. One pound of meat or fish provides approximately 2 grams of creatine.

Creatine supplementation has become popular in recent years among individuals who want to increase muscle mass and improve athletic performance. Creatine monohydrate—a white, tasteless powder that is mixed with fluids prior to ingestion—is the form most popular among people who use the supplement. Supplementation can result in an approximate 20 percent increase in the amount of creatine that is stored in muscles. Most of this creatine binds to phosphate to form CP, and 30 to 40 percent remains as free creatine in the muscle. Increased creatine storage is believed to enable individuals to train more intensely—thus building more muscle mass and enhancing performance in all-out activities of very short duration.

There are two phases to creatine supplementation: the loading phase and the maintenance phase. During the loading phase, the person consumes between 20 and 25 grams (one teaspoonful is about 5 grams) of creatine per day for 5 to 6 days, divided into 4 or 5 dosages of 5 grams each throughout the day (this amount represents the equivalent of consuming 10 or more pounds of meat per day). Research also suggests that the amount of creatine stored in muscle is enhanced by taking creatine in combination with a high-carbohydrate food. Once the loading phase is complete, 2 grams per day appear to be sufficient to maintain the increased muscle stores.

To date, no serious side effects have been documented in people who take up to 25 grams of creatine per day for 5 days. Stomach distress and cramping has been reported only in rare instances. The 2 grams taken per day during the maintenance phase is only slightly above the average intake in our daily diet. Long-term effects of creatine supplementation on health, however, have not been established.

A frequently documented result following 5 to 6 days of creatine loading is an increase of 2 to 3 pounds in body weight. This increase appears to be related to increased water retention necessary to maintain the additional creatine stored in muscles. Some data, however, suggests that the increase in stored water and CP stimulates protein synthesis, thus leading to an increase in lean body mass.

The benefits of elevated creatine stores may be limited to high-intensity/short-duration activities like sprinting, strength training (weight lifting), and sprint cycling. Supplementation is most beneficial during exercise training itself, rather than as an aid to enhance athletic performance a few days before competition.

Enhanced creatine stores do not benefit athletes competing in aerobic endurance events, because CP is not used in energy production for long-distance events. In fact, the additional weight can be detrimental in long-distance running and swimming events, because the athlete must expend more energy to carry the extra weight during competition.

Amino Acid Supplements

A myth regarding athletic performance is that protein (amino acid) supplements will increase muscle mass. The claims and safety of these products have not been proven scientifically. The RDA for protein is .8 grams per kilogram of body weight.

Most athletes, including weight lifters and body builders, increase their caloric intake automatically during intense training. As caloric intake increases, so does the intake of protein, often approaching 2 or more grams per kilogram of body weight. This amount is more than enough to build and repair muscle tissue. Typically, athletes in strength training consume between 3 and 4 grams per kilogram of body weight. In response, supplement manufacturers have created expensive "free-amino acid supplements."

People who buy costly free-amino acid supplements are led to believe that they contribute to the development of muscle mass. However, the human body cannot distinguish between amino acids obtained from food or through supplements. Excess protein is either used for energy or turned into fat. With amino acid supplements, each capsule provides up to 500 milligrams of amino acids and no additional nutrients. In contrast, 3 ounces of meat or fish provide more than 20,000 milligrams of amino acids, along with other essential nutrients such as iron, niacin, and thiamin. The benefits of natural foods to health and budget are clear.

Proponents of free-amino acid supplements further claim that only a small amount of amino acids in food is absorbed and that free-amino acids are absorbed more readily than protein food. Neither claim is correct. The human body absorbs and utilizes between 85 and 99 percent of all protein from food intake. The body handles whole, natural proteins better than single amino acids predigested in the laboratory setting.

Amino acid supplementation can even be dangerous: Supplementation of a group of chemically similar amino acids often prevents the absorption of other amino acids, potentially causing critical imbalances and toxicities. Long-term risks associated with amino acid supplementation have not been determined.

The advertised rate of absorption provides no additional benefit, because building muscle takes hours, not minutes. Muscle overload through heavy training, not supplementation, builds muscle. Expensive protein supplements benefit only those who sell them.

SPECIAL NUTRIENT NEEDS OF WOMEN

Three considerations specific to women are bone health, hormone replacement therapy beginning at menopause, and iron supplementation to offset the iron lost through menstruation.

Bone Health and Osteoporosis

In **osteoporosis**, bones—primarily of the hip, wrist, and spine—become so weak and brittle that they fracture readily. The process begins slowly in the third and fourth decades of life. Women are especially susceptible after menopause because of the accompanying loss of **estrogen**, which increases the rate at which bone mass is broken down.

Approximately 22 million U.S. women have osteoporosis, and 16 million don't know that they have this disease. About 1.5 million fractures are attributed to this condition each year. Of women who have hip fractures, half die within 6 months and the other half do not return to independent living. Based on current trends, a 50-year-old woman in the United States has at least a 50 percent probability of a future fracture because of osteoporosis. The chances of a postmenopausal woman of developing osteoporosis are much greater than her chances of developing breast cancer or suffering a heart attack or stroke. According to Dr. Barbara Drinkwater, a leading researcher in this area, "Shocking as these figures are, they cannot adequately convey the pain and deterioration in the quality of life of women who suffer the crippling effects of osteoporotic fractures."[26]

Although osteoporosis is viewed primarily as a women's disease, more than 30 percent of all men will be affected by age 75. About 100,000 of the yearly 300,000 hip fractures in the United States occur in men.

Although the genetic component is strong, osteoporosis is preventable. Maximizing bone density at a young age and subsequently decreasing the rate of bone loss later in life are critical to preventing osteoporosis. Normal hormone levels (estrogen for women, testosterone at a later age for men), adequate calcium intake, and physical activity cannot be overemphasized.

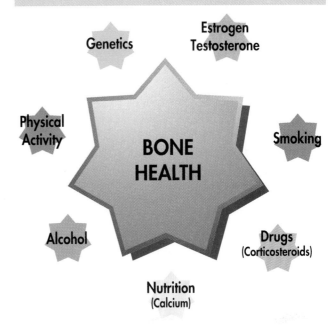

FIGURE 8.17 Factors that affect bone health (osteoporosis).

All three factors are crucial to prevent osteoporosis. The absence of any one of these three factors leads to bone loss for which the other two factors never completely compensate. Smoking, excessive use of alcohol, and corticosteroid drugs also accelerate the rate of bone loss in both women and men. Figure 8.17 depicts these variables.

Estrogen is the most important factor in preventing osteoporosis in women.

Bone health begins at a young age. Some experts have called osteoporosis a "pediatric disease." Bone density can be promoted early in life by making sure the diet has sufficient calcium and participating in weight-bearing activities. Although the RDA for calcium is between 1,000 and 1,300 mg per day, leading researchers in this area recommend even higher intakes (see Table 8.13). Although these recommended daily intakes can be met easily through diet alone, some experts recommend calcium supplements even for children before puberty.

Key Terms

Osteoporosis Softening, deterioration, or loss of bone mass.

Estrogen Female sex hormone; essential for bone formation and conservation of bone density.

TABLE 8.13 Recommended Daily Calcium Intake

Age	Amount (gr)
1–5	800
6–10	800–1,200
11–24	1,200–1,500
25–50 Women	1,000
25–64 Men	1,000
PMW* on HRT**	1,000
PMW not on HRT	1,500
> 65	1,200–1,500

*PMW = Post-menopausal women
**HRT = Hormone replacement therapy

TABLE 8.14 Low-Fat Calcium-Rich Foods

Food	Amount	Calcium (mg)	Calories
Beans, red kidney, cooked	1 cup	70	218
Beet, greens, cooked	½ cup	82	19
Bok choy (Chinese cabbage)	1 cup	158	20
Broccoli, cooked, drained	1 cup	72	44
Burrito, bean (no cheese)	1	57	225
Cottage cheese, 2% low-fat	½ cup	78	103
Ice milk (vanilla)	½ cup	102	100
Instant breakfast, nonfat milk	1 cup	407	216
Kale, cooked, drained	1 cup	94	36
Milk, nonfat, powdered	1 tbs	52	15
Milk, skim	1 cup	296	88
Oatmeal, instant, fortified, plain	½ cup	109	70
Okra, cooked, drained	½ cup	74	23
Orange juice, fortified	1 cup	300	110
Soy milk, fortified, fat free	1 cup	400	110
Spinach, raw	1 cup	56	12
Turnip greens, cooked	1 cup	197	29
Tofu (some types)	½ cup	138	76
Yogurt, fruit	1 cup	372	250
Yogurt, low-fat, plain	1 cup	448	155

To obtain your daily calcium requirement, get as much calcium as possible from calcium-rich foods, including calcium-fortified foods. If you don't get enough (most people don't), take calcium supplements. Supplemental calcium can be obtained in the form of calcium citrate and calcium carbonate. Calcium citrate seems to be equally well absorbed with or without food, whereas calcium carbonate is not well absorbed without food. Thus if your supplement contains calcium carbonate, always take the supplement with meals. Do not take more than 500 mg at a time, because larger amounts are not well absorbed.

Avoid taking calcium supplements with an iron-rich meal or in conjunction with an iron-containing multivitamin. Unfortunately, calcium interferes with iron absorption, thus it is best to separate the intake of these two minerals. The benefit of taking your calcium supplement without food (calcium citrate) is that, in a young menstruating woman who needs iron, calcium won't interfere with the absorption of iron.

Table 8.14 provides a list of selected foods and their calcium content. Along with adequate calcium intake, 400 to 800 IU of vitamin D daily are recommended for optimal calcium absorption. People over 50 may require 800 to 1000 IU. About 40 percent of these adults are deficient in vitamin D.

Excessive protein intake may also affect the body's absorption of calcium. The more protein eaten, the higher the calcium content in the urine (that is, the more calcium excreted). This might be the reason why countries with a high protein intake, including the United States, also have the highest rates of osteoporosis. Aim to achieve the RDA for protein, nonetheless, because people who consume too little protein (less than 35 grams per day), lose more bone mass than those who eat too much (more than 100 grams per day). The RDA for protein is about 50 grams per day for women and 63 for men.

Soft drinks, coffee, and alcoholic beverages can also contribute to a loss in bone density if consumed in large quantities. The damage may not be caused directly by these food items, but rather because they take the place of dairy products in the diet.

Exercise seems to play a key role in preventing osteoporosis by decreasing the rate of bone loss following menopause. Active people are able to maintain bone density much more effectively than their inactive counterparts. A combination of weight-bearing exercises, such as walking or jogging and weight training, is especially helpful. The benefits of exercise go beyond maintaining bone density. Exercise strengthens muscles, ligaments, and tendons—all of which provide support to the bones (skeleton). Exercise also improves balance and coordination, which can help prevent falls and injuries.

Current studies indicate that people who are active have denser bone mineral than inactive people do. Similar to other benefits of participating in exercise, there is no such thing as "bone in the bank." To have good bone health, people need to participate in a regular lifetime exercise program.

Prevailing research also tells us that estrogen is the most important factor in preventing bone loss. Lumbar bone density in women who have always had regular menstrual cycles exceeds that of women with a history of **oligomenorrhea** and **amenorrhea** interspersed with regular cycles. Furthermore, the lumbar density of these two groups of women is higher than that of women who have never had regular menstrual cycles.

As a baseline, women should get a bone density test at menopause to establish bone health at that point in life or to confirm a diagnosis of osteoporosis. The test can also be used to monitor changes in bone mass over time and to predict the risk of future fractures. Bone density tests require small amounts of radiation to determine bone mass of the spine, hip, wrist, heel, or fingers. The amount of radiation is so low that technicians administering the test can sit right next to the person receiving it. The procedure often takes less than 10 minutes.

Following menopause, every woman should consider some type of therapy to prevent bone loss. The various therapy modalities available should be discussed with a physician. Although regular weight-bearing exercise and plenty of calcium in the diet can slow bone loss, osteoporosis can be stopped only through traditional hormone replacement therapy (HRT), such as estrogen and calcitonin, or other more recent nonhormonal modalities.[27]

ESTROGEN REPLACEMENT THERAPY

Estrogen replacement therapy (ERT) is the most common treatment to prevent bone loss following menopause. ERT also may produce a slight increase in bone mass density. Women on ERT do not lose bone mineral density at the rate of women who are not using this therapy. Neither exercise nor calcium supplementation will offset the damaging effects of lower estrogen levels.

For instance, athletes with amenorrhea (who have lower estrogen levels) have lower bone mineral density than even nonathletes with normal estrogen levels. One study showed that amenorrheic athletes at age 25 have the bones of a 52-year-old woman.[28] Other research showed four amenorrheic athletes with a bone density equivalent to that of 70- to 80-year-old women.[29] Over the last few years, it has become clear that sedentary women with normal estrogen levels have better bone mineral density than active amenorrheic athletes. Many experts believe the best predictor of bone mineral content is the history of menstrual regularity.

Many women stop taking estrogen within a year because of unpleasant side effects that include headaches, breast tenderness, bleeding, and fluid retention. To obtain the benefits of ERT on bone mass retention, however, estrogen must be taken over the long term. ERT also reduces the risk of cardiovascular disease. Although the evidence is inconclusive, ERT may increase the risk of breast and endometrial cancer.

A second treatment modality to prevent bone loss is Miacalcin, a synthetic form of the hormone calcitonin. Calcitonin is a thyroid hormone that helps maintain the body's delicate balance of calcium by taking calcium from the blood and depositing it in the bones. Miacalcin is recommended for women who refuse or cannot tolerate ERT. Though it is effective in preventing bone loss, it does not help much in rebuilding bone; therefore, Miacalcin therapy should be started soon after menopause. The drug seems to have no side effects. It is available in injectable and nasal spray forms.

Fosamax (alendronate), a promising non-hormonal drug, has been approved by the FDA for the treatment of osteoporosis.[30] Studies of menopausal women younger than age 60 showed that Fosamax therapy not only prevented bone loss but actually helped increase bone mass by about 6 percent. Fosamax is recommended for women who have osteoporosis already and who cannot or will not take estrogen. Fosamax is used primarily for bone health and does not provide benefits to the cardiovascular system. Although the research is limited, this drug seems to be safe and effective. Like estrogen, it must be taken for the rest of a woman's life.

New treatment modalities being developed to prevent bone loss are the selective estrogen receptor modulators (SERMs). Unlike ERT, these compounds have a positive effect on blood lipids and pose no risk to breast and uterine tissue. SERMs, however, do not help increase bone density. Examples of SERMs currently used to prevent osteoporosis are evista, tamoxifen, and raloxifene.

Adequate Iron Intake

Iron is a key element of **hemoglobin** in blood. The RDA of iron for adult women is between 15 and 18 mg per day (8 to 11 mg for men). According to a survey by the U. S. Department of Agriculture, 19- to

Key Terms

Oligomenorrhea Irregular menstrual cycles.

Amenorrhea Cessation of regular menstrual flow.

Hemoglobin Protein-iron compound in red blood cells that transports oxygen in the blood.

50-year-old women in the United States consumed only 60 percent of the RDA for iron. People who do not have enough iron in the body can develop iron-deficiency anemia, in which the concentration of hemoglobin in the red blood cells is lower than it should be.

Physically active women may also have a greater-than-average need for iron. Heavy training creates a demand for iron that is higher than the recommended intake because small amounts of iron are lost through sweat, urine, and stools. Mechanical trauma, caused by the pounding of the feet on the pavement during extensive jogging, may also lead to destruction of iron-containing red blood cells.

A large percentage of female endurance athletes are reported to have iron deficiency. The blood **ferritin** levels of women who participate in intense physical training should be checked frequently.

The rates of iron absorption and iron loss vary from person to person. In most cases, though, people can get enough iron by eating more iron-rich foods such as beans, peas, green leafy vegetables, enriched grain products, egg yolk, fish, and lean meats. Although organ meats, such as liver, are especially good sources, they also are high in cholesterol. A list of foods high in iron is given in Table 8.15

DIETARY GUIDELINES FOR AMERICANS

In 2000 the Scientific Committee of the U.S. Department of Health and Human Services and the U.S. Department of Agriculture on diet and health issued the fifth edition of the Dietary Guidelines for healthy American adults and children. These guidelines—based on the available scientific research on nutrition, health, and current dietary habits—can potentially reduce the risk of developing certain chronic diseases. The committee issued three goals that include 10 guidelines. These goals, listed here, have been defined as the ABCs for your health and that of your family:[31]

Goal 1: Aim for Fitness

- Aim for a healthy weight.
- Be physically active each day.

Following these two guidelines will help keep you and your family healthy and fit. Healthy eating and regular physical activity enable people of all ages to work productively, enjoy life, and feel their best. They also help children grow, develop, and do well in school.

Balance the food you eat with physical activity to maintain or improve your weight. Excessive body weight increases the risk for heart disease, stroke, diabetes, high blood pressure, and certain cancers. Many people gain weight as adults, and this can be avoided. To maintain body weight, you need to balance food intake with the amount of calories your body uses. Other chapters in this book present extensive information on weight management and exercise programs to help you balance your energy requirements according to your personal needs.

TABLE 8.15 Iron-Rich Foods

Food	Amount	Iron (mg)	Calories	Cholesterol	% Calories From Fat
Beans, red kidney, cooked	1 cup	3.2	218	0	4
Beef, ground lean (21% fat)	3 oz	2.1	237	86	57
Beef, sirloin, lean only	3 oz	2.9	171	76	36
Beef liver, fried	3 oz	5.3	184	409	33
Beet greens, cooked	½ cup	1.4	19	0	—
Broccoli, cooked, drained	1 cup	1.3	44	0	—
Burrito, bean (no cheese)	1	2.3	225	2	28
Egg, hard-cooked	1	.7	77	212	58
Farina (Cream of Wheat), cooked	½ cup	5.2	65	0	—
Instant breakfast, nonfat milk	1 cup	4.8	216	9	4
Peas, frozen, cooked, drained	½ cup	1.3	62	0	—
Shrimp, boiled	3 oz	2.7	87	172	10
Spinach, raw	1 cup	1.5	12	0	—
Vegetables, mixed, cooked	1 cup	1.5	108	0	—

Goal 2: Build a Healthy Base

- Let the Food Pyramid guide your food choices.
- Choose a variety of grains daily, especially whole grains.
- Choose a variety of fruits and vegetables daily.
- Keep food safe to eat.

Following these four guidelines builds a base for healthy eating. Eat a variety of foods. No single food can provide all of the necessary nutrients and other beneficial substances in the amounts the body needs. Consult the Food Guide Pyramid to be sure you get the nutrients your body needs each day.

Make grains, fruits, and vegetables the foundation of your meals. They contain ample vitamins, minerals, complex carbohydrates, and other substances important to good health and have been shown to reduce your risk of certain chronic diseases. Most of your daily calories should come from these food products.

Within each food group, choose a variety of foods. Food items vary, and each item provides different combinations of nutrients and other substances needed for good health. Be flexible and adventurous —try new choices from these three groups in place of some less-nutritious or higher calorie foods you usually eat. Whatever you eat, always take steps to keep your food safe to eat.

Goal 3: Choose Sensibly

- Choose a diet that is low in saturated fat and cholesterol and moderate in total fat.
- Choose beverages and foods to moderate your intake of sugars.
- Choose and prepare foods with less salt.
- If you drink alcoholic beverages, do so in moderation.

These four guidelines help you make sensible choices that promote health and reduce the risk of certain chronic diseases. You can enjoy all foods as part of a healthy diet, as long as you don't overdo it on fat (especially saturated fat), sugars, salt, and alcohol. Read labels to identify foods that are higher in saturated fats, sugars, and salt (sodium).

Choose a diet low in fat, saturated fat, and cholesterol. Reduce fat intake to 30 percent or (preferably) less of total calories. Reduce saturated fatty acid intake to less than 7 percent of total calories and intake of cholesterol to no more than 300 mg daily. Intake of fat and cholesterol can be lowered by substituting fish, poultry without skin, lean meats, and low-fat or nonfat dairy products for fatty meats and whole-milk

Dietary guidelines for Americans

Aim for Fitness ...

- Aim for a healthy weight.
- Be physically active each day.

Build a Healthy Base ...

- Let the Food Pyramid guide your food choices.
- Choose a variety of grains daily, especially whole grains.
- Choose a variety of fruits and vegetables daily.
- Keep food safe to eat.

Choose Sensibly ...

- Choose a diet that is low in saturated fat and cholesterol and moderate in total fat.
- Choose beverages and foods to moderate your intake of sugars.
- Choose and prepare foods with less salt.
- If you drink alcoholic beverages, do so in moderation.

dairy products; by choosing more vegetables, fruits, cereals, and legumes; and by limiting oils, fats, egg yolks, and fried and other fatty foods.

Choose a diet moderate in sugars. Excessive intake of sugar and starch can contribute to weight gain and tooth decay. This guideline advises against frequent and large consumption of food items and snacks high in sugar, which provide unnecessary calories and few nutrients. The more often that high-sugar foods are consumed, and the longer before brushing the teeth following their consumption, the greater the risk for tooth decay.

Choose a diet moderate in salt and sodium. Daily intake of salt (sodium chloride) should be 6 grams or less. Sodium intake can be decreased by limiting the use of salt in cooking and not adding it to food at the table. Salty, highly processed, salt-preserved, and salt-pickled foods (such as bacon, olives, pickles, and lunch meats) should be consumed sparingly.

If you drink alcoholic beverages, do so in moderation. Alcoholic beverages provide calories but few or no nutrients. Moderate drinking has been linked to lower risk for coronary heart disease in some people. Excessive alcohol consumption leads to increased risk for heart disease, stroke, high blood pressure, certain cancers, cirrhosis of the liver, inflammation of the pancreas, brain damage, birth defects, accidents, violence, suicides, and malnutrition. Consumption should be limited to no more than one daily drink

Key Terms

Ferritin Iron stored in the body.

or women and two for men. In general, a 12-ounce bottle of beer, a 4-ounce glass of wine, and a 1.5-ounce shot of 80 proof liquor all contain the same amount of alcohol. Pregnant women should avoid alcoholic beverages altogether.

PROPER NUTRITION: A LIFETIME PRESCRIPTION FOR HEALTHY LIVING

The three factors that do the most for health, longevity, and quality of life are proper nutrition, a sound exercise program, and quitting (or never starting) smoking. Achieving and maintaining a balanced diet is not as difficult as most people would think. If parents did a better job of teaching and reinforcing proper nutrition habits in early youth, the current magnitude of nutrition-related health problems would be much smaller. Although treatment of obesity is important, we should place far greater emphasis on preventing obesity in youth and adults in the first place.

Children tend to eat the way their parents do. If parents adopt a healthy diet, children most likely will follow. The difficult part for most people is retraining themselves to follow a lifetime healthy nutrition plan —a diet that includes lots of grains, legumes, fruits, vegetables, and low-fat dairy products, with moderate use of animal protein, junk food, sodium, and alcohol.

In spite of the ample scientific evidence linking poor dietary habits to early disease and mortality rates, many people remain precontemplators: They are not willing to change their eating patterns. Even when faced with obesity, elevated blood lipids, hypertension, and other nutrition-related conditions, people

do not change. The motivating factor to change one's eating habits seems to be a major health breakdown, such as a heart attack, a stroke, or cancer. By this time the damage has been done already. In many cases it is irreversible and, for some, fatal.

An ounce of prevention is worth a pound of cure. The sooner you implement the dietary guidelines presented in this chapter, the better your chances of preventing chronic diseases and reaching a higher state of wellness.

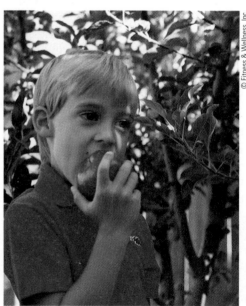

Positive nutrition habits should be taught and reinforced in early youth.

WEB INTERACTIVE

American Dietetic Association
This comprehensive site features daily food tips, frequently asked questions, nutrition resources, and links to other reliable web sites on nutrition.

http://www.eatright.org

Dietary Guidelines from the Food and Nutrition Information Center
This interesting site features not only the 2000 American dietary guidelines, but also has links to historical dietary guidelines (since 1894) and dietary guidelines from 20 countries.

http://www.nal.usda.gov/fnic/dga/index.html

Shape-Up America!'s Eating Smart Menu
This site describes how to establish your dietary goals and plan for success, including tips on how to incorporate physical fitness with your dietary guidelines.

http://www.shapeup.org/publications/eating.smart/textmenu.htm

CyberDiet Succeed at Weight Loss
This site can be accessed at three- or twelve-month intervals and features opportunities to create nutrition profiles, assess body composition, plan diets that meet all varietites of taste, lifestyle, and need.

http://www.cyberdiet.com/reg/index.html

INTERACTIVE SITES:

The Cyberkitchen
This very interactive site, sponsored by Shape Up America, will show you how to balance your dietary intake with your physical activity to maintain healthy weight. You provide personal information regarding your age, gender, height, weight, and activity level; the Cyberkitchen provides you with a healthy diet plan to meet your goals (weight loss or weight gain). It's fun and educational.

http://www.shapeup.org/kitchen/frameset1.htm

The Diet Analysis Web Site
You input the foods you eat and receive a complete nutritional review of your diet based on the Recommended Dietary Allowances for your age and gender.

http://dawp.anet.com/

The Interactive Food Guide Pyramid
Click on the different components of the Food Guide Pyramid to learn how to incorporate the proper nutrients into your daily diet.

http://www.nal.usda.gov:8001/py/pmap.htm

n*tes

1. *Surgeon General's Report on Nutrition and Health: Summary and Recommendations* (DHHS [PHS] Publication no. 88-50211) (Washington, DC: U. S. Government Printing Office, 1988).

2. E. B. Rimm, A. Ascherio, E. Giovannucci, D. Spiegelman, M. J. Stampfer, and W. C. Willett, "Vegetable, Fruit, and Cereal Fiber Intake and Risk of Coronary Heart Disease Among Men," *Journal of the American Medical Association* 275 (1996): 447–451.

3. "The Facts About Fats," *Consumer Reports on Health* (Boulder, CO: The Editors, March, 1997).

4. A. H. Lichtenstein, L. M. Ausman, S. M. Jalbert, and E. J. Schaefer, "Effects of Different Forms of Dietary Hydrogenated Fats on Serum Lipoprotein Cholesterol Levels," *The New England Journal of Medicine* 340 (1999): 1933–1940.

5. National Cholesterol Education Program Expert Panel. "Summary of the Third Report of the National Cholesterol Education Program (NCEP) Expert Panel on Detection, Evaluation, and Treatment of High Blood Cholesterol in Adults (Adult Treatment Panel III)." *Journal of the American Medical Association* 285 (2001): 2486–2497.

6. R. J. Barnard, "Effects of Lifestyle Modification on Serum Lipids," *Archives of Internal Medicine* 151 (1991): 1389–1394.

7. J. H. Weisburger and G. M. Williams, "Causes of Cancer," in *Textbook of Clinical Oncology*, ed. G. P. Murphy, W. Lawrence, Jr., and R.E. Lenhard, Sr. (Atlanta: American Cancer Society, 1995).

8. "Vitamin Report," *University of California at Berkeley Wellness Letter* (Palm Coast, FL: The Editors, October 1994).

9. "Should You Take Vitamin C and E Supplements?" *University of California at Berkeley Wellness Letter* (Palm Coast, FL: The Editors, June 2001).

10. S. Kalish, "The Free Radical Radical: Kenneth Cooper, M.D., on Antioxidants and the Dangers of Hard Running," *Running Times* (March 1995): 16–17.

11. S. Yusunf, et al., "Vitamin E Supplementation and Cardiovascular Events in High-Risk Patients," *The New England Journal of Medicine* 342 (2000): 154–160.

12. "Vitamin E: Have We Jumped the Gun?" *Tufts University Health & Nutrition Letter* (Palm Coast, FL, The Editors, January 2000).

13. "Vitamin C: We Still Take It, and So Should You," *University of California at Berkeley Wellness Letter* (Palm Coast, FL: The Editors, May 2000).

14. "Megadoses of Vitamin C," *Consumer Reports on Health* (Boulder, CO: The Editors, February 2000).

15. "Beta Carotene Pills: Should You Take Them?" *University of California at Berkeley Wellness Letter* 12, no. 7 (1996): 1–2.

16. L. C. Clark, et al., "Effects of Selenium Supplementation for Cancer Prevention in Patients with Carcinoma of the Skin: A Randomized Controlled Trial," *Journal of the American Medical Association* 276 (1996): 1957–1963.

17. "Does This Mineral Prevent Cancer?" *University of California at Berkeley Wellness Letter* 16, no. 9 (2000): 1–2.

18. J. Carper, "Selenium: A Cancer Knockout?" *USA Weekend* (October 2–4, 1996): 8.

19. A. Weil, "Dr. Andrew Weil's Surprising Secrets of Optimum Health," *Bottom Line Health* 18, no. 13 (1997): 9–10.

20. See note 8.

21. C. J. Boushey, S. A. A. Beresford, G. S. Omenn, and A. G. Motulsky, "A Quantitative Assessment of Plasma Homocysteine as a Risk Factor for Vascular Disease," *Journal of the American Medical Association* 274 (1995): 1049–1057.

22. W. Castelli, "Smart Heart Strategies: Best Ways to Beat Heart Disease," *Bottom Line Health* 19, no. 4 (1998): 1–3.

23. "The Antioxidant All-Stars," *University of California at Berkeley Wellness Letter* (March 1997).

24. C. M. Hasler, "How to Use the New 'Functional Foods,' What Works . . . What Doesn't Work," *Bottom Line/Personal Health* (April 2000).

25. "Genetically Modified Foods: What You Should Know," *Self-Healing* (June 2000).

26. Pacific Medical Center, *Nutrition, Exercise, and Bone Health* (Seattle: PMC, 1990).

27. "Preventing Osteoporosis," *Health News* 4, no. 3 (1998): 1–2.

28. B. L. Drinkwater, "Osteoporosis and the Female Masters Athlete," in *Sports Medicine for the Mature Athlete*, ed. J. R. Sutton and R. M. Brock (Carmel, IN: Benchmark Press, 1986), 353–359.

29. K. H. Myburgh, L. K. Bachrach, B. Lewis, K. Kent, and R. Marcus, "Low Bone Mineral Density at Axial and Appendicular Sites in Amenorrheic Athletes," *Medicine and Science in Sports and Exercise* 25, no. 11 (1993): 1197–1202.

30. "Will this Drug Prevent Osteoporosis?" *University of California at Berkeley Wellness Letter* 14, no. 9 (1998): 1–2.

31. U. S. Department of Health and Human Services, Department of Agriculture. *Nutrition and Your Health: Dietary Guidelines for Americans. Home and Garden Bulletin No. 232* (Washington, DC: DHHS, 2000).

- Coleman, E. *Eating for Endurance*. Palo Alto, CA: Bull Publishing, 1997.

- Drinkwater, B. L. "Does Physical Activity Play a Role in Preventing Osteoporosis?" *Research Quarterly for Exercise and Sport* 65 (1994): 197–206.

- Hoeger, W. W. K., and S. A. Hoeger. *Lifetime Physical Fitness and Wellness*. Belmont, CA: Wadsworth/ Thompson Learning, 1999.

- McArdle, W. D., F. I. Katch, and V. L. Katch. *Sports & Exercise Nutrition*. Baltimore: Lippincott Williams & Wilkins, 1999.

- National Academy of Sciences, Institute of Medicine. *Dietary Reference Intakes*. Washington, DC: National Academy Press, 1998.

- National Academy of Sciences, Institute of Medicine. *Eat for Life: The Food and Nutrition Board's Guide to Reducing Your Risk of Chronic Disease*. Edited by C. E. Woteki and P. R. Thomas. Washington, DC: National Academy Press, 1992.

- Volek, J. S. "Creatine Supplementation and Its Possible Role in Improving Physical Performance." *ACSM's Health & Fitness Journal* 1, no. 4, (1997): 23–29.

- Wardlaw, G. M. *Contemporary Nutrition: Issues and Insights*. Boston: McGraw Hill, 2000.

- Whitney, E. N., and S. R. Rolfes. *Understanding Nutrition*. St. Paul: West Publishing, 1996.

- Williams, M. H., R. B. Kreider, and J. D. Branch. *Creatine: The Power Supplement*. Champaign, IL: Human Kinetics, 1999.

- Wynder, E. L., J. H. Weisburger, and S. K. Ng. "Nutrition: The Need to Define 'Optimal' Intake as a Basis for Public Policy Decisions." *American Journal of Public Health* 82 (1992): 346–350.

Weight Management

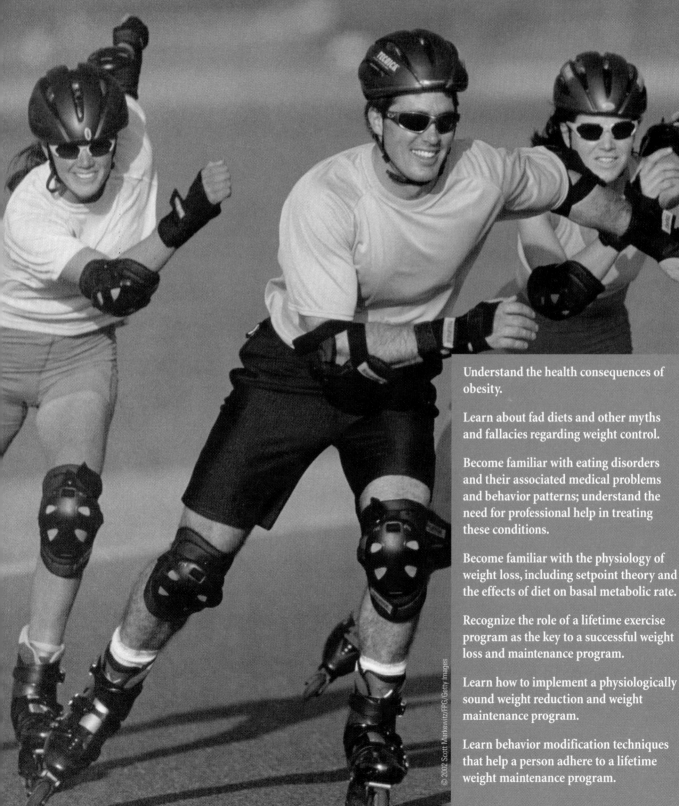

Understand the health consequences of obesity.

Learn about fad diets and other myths and fallacies regarding weight control.

Become familiar with eating disorders and their associated medical problems and behavior patterns; understand the need for professional help in treating these conditions.

Become familiar with the physiology of weight loss, including setpoint theory and the effects of diet on basal metabolic rate.

Recognize the role of a lifetime exercise program as the key to a successful weight loss and maintenance program.

Learn how to implement a physiologically sound weight reduction and weight maintenance program.

Learn behavior modification techniques that help a person adhere to a lifetime weight maintenance program.

wo terms commonly used to describe the condition of weighing more than recommended are "overweight" and "obesity." Overweight is defined as having a body mass index (BMI) greater than 25 and obesity as a BMI of 30 or higher. Obesity levels are the point at which excess body fat can lead to serious health problems. Obesity is a health hazard of epidemic proportions in most developed countries around the world. According to the World Health Organization, an estimated 35 percent of the adult population in industrialized nations is obese.

A 1999 study estimated that, in the United States, 63 percent of men and 55 percent of women are overweight and 21 percent of men and 27 percent of women are obese (see Figure 9.1).[1] An estimated 97 million people are overweight and 30 million are obese.[2] Between 1960 and 1994, the overall (men and women combined) prevalence of adult obesity increased from about 13 percent to 22.5 percent. Most of this increase occurred in the 1990s.[3] In the last decade alone, the average weight of American adults increased by about 15 pounds. The prevalence of obesity is even higher in ethnic groups, especially African Americans and Hispanic Americans.

About 44 percent of all women and 29 percent of all men are on a diet at any given moment.[4] People spend about $40 billion yearly attempting to lose weight. More than $10 billion goes to memberships in weight reduction centers and another $30 billion to diet food sales. Furthermore, according to the National Institutes of Health, the total cost attributable to obesity-related disease is approximately $100 billion per year.

> The lack of physical activity, not the weight problem itself, may cause many of the health risks associated with obesity.

As the second leading cause of preventable death in the United States, overweight and obesity have been associated with several serious health problems and account for 15 to 20 percent of the annual mortality rate. Over 300,000 deaths each year are caused by excessive body weight. Furthermore, obesity is more prevalent than smoking (19%), poverty (14%), and problem drinking (6%) and is associated with at least as much morbidity and poor quality of life as the latter three conditions.[5]

In 1998, the American Heart Association identified obesity as one of the six major risk factors for coronary heart disease. Obesity also is a risk factor for hypertension, congestive heart failure, high blood lipids, atherosclerosis, stroke, thromboembolitic disease,

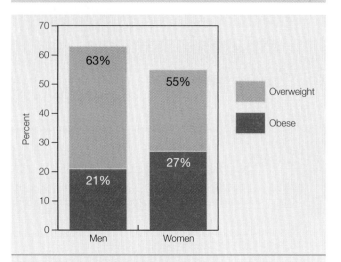

FIGURE 9.1 Percentage of the adult population that is obese (BMI ≥ 30) and overweight (BMI = 25 to 29.9) in the United States.

SOURCE: A. Must et al., "The Disease Burden Associated with Overweight and Obesity," *Journal of the American Medical Association* 282 (1999): 1523–1529.

varicose veins, Type II diabetes, osteoarthritis, gall-bladder disease, sleep apnea, respiratory problems, ruptured intervertebral disks, and for endometrial, breast, prostate, and colon cancers. Furthermore, it is implicated in psychological maladjustment and a higher accidental death rate. Extremely obese people have worse mental health-related quality of life.

OVERWEIGHT VERSUS OBESITY

Overweight and **obesity** are not the same thing. Many overweight people (that is, people who weigh 10 to 20 pounds over the recommended weight) are not obese. Although research findings are inconsistent, the health consequences of a few extra pounds of body fat might be exaggerated and may apply primarily to severely overweight individuals.

Data from the Aerobics Research Institute in Dallas confirm that, as body fat increases, so do blood cholesterol and triglycerides. This study showed that the higher the fitness level, the lower the mortality rate, regardless of body weight.[6] This finding is significant because obese men who were fit had a lower risk of death than unfit men of average weight and as low as fit men of average weight. Thus, at least partially, lack of physical activity and not the weight problem itself may be the cause of premature death in some obese people.

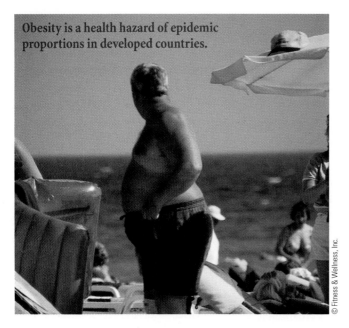

Obesity is a health hazard of epidemic proportions in developed countries.

© Fitness & Wellness, Inc.

Although the premature mortality of obese men in the study who became active decreased regardless of whether they lost weight, few obese men in the study were fit. This pattern holds true in life. Most obese people either don't or can't exercise because of functional limitations when they attempt to participate in traditional fitness activities such as jogging, walking, and cycling. Those who do exercise tend to lose weight.

A few pounds of excess weight may not be harmful to most people, but this is not always the case. People with excessive body fat who have diabetes and other cardiovascular risk factors (elevated blood lipids, high blood pressure, physical inactivity, and poor eating habits) benefit from weight loss. Even a modest reduction of 5 to 10 percent can reduce high blood pressure and total cholesterol levels. People who have a few extra pounds of weight but who otherwise are healthy and physically active, exercise regularly, and eat a healthy diet may not be at greater risk for early death.

Recommended body composition is a primary objective to achieve overall physical fitness and enhanced quality of life. Individuals at recommended body weight are able to participate in a wide variety of moderate-to-vigorous activities without functional limitations. These people have the freedom to enjoy most of life's recreational activities to their fullest potential. Excessive body weight does not afford an individual the fitness level to enjoy vigorous lifetime activities such as basketball, soccer, racquetball, surfing, mountain cycling, or mountain climbing. Maintaining high fitness and recommended body weight gives a person a degree of independence throughout life that most people in developed nations no longer enjoy.

Scientific evidence also recognizes problems with being underweight. Although the social pressure to be thin has declined slightly in recent years, the pressure to attain model-like thinness is still with us and contributes to the gradual increase in the number of people who develop eating disorders (anorexia nervosa and bulimia, discussed later in this chapter).

Extreme weight loss can lead to medical conditions such as heart damage, gastrointestinal problems, shrinkage of internal organs, immune system abnormalities, disorders of the reproductive system, loss of muscle tissue, damage to the nervous system, and even death. About 14 percent of people in the United States are underweight.

TOLERABLE WEIGHT

Many people want to lose weight so they will look better. That's a noteworthy goal. The problem, however, is that they have a distorted image of what they would really look like if they were to reduce to what they think is their ideal weight. Hereditary factors play a big role, and only a small fraction of the population has the genes for a "perfect body."

When people set their own target weight, they should be realistic. Attaining the "Excellent" percent of body fat shown in Table 7.9 (page 184) is extremely difficult for some. It is even more difficult to maintain, unless the person makes a commitment to a vigorous lifetime exercise program and permanent dietary changes. Few people are willing to do that. The "Moderate" percent body fat category may be more realistic for many people.

A question you should ask yourself is: Am I happy with my weight? Part of enjoying a higher quality of life is being happy with yourself. If you are not, you either need to do something about it or learn to live with it.

If your percent of body fat is higher than those in the Moderate category of Table 7.9, you should try to come down and stay in this category, for health reasons. This is the category that seems to pose no detriment to health.

If you are in the Moderate category but would like to reduce your percent of body fat further, you need to ask yourself a second question: How badly do I want it? Do I want it badly enough to implement

KeyTerms

Overweight Excess weight according to a given standard, such as height or recommended percent body fat; less than obese.

Obesity A chronic disease characterized by excessive body fat in relation to lean body mass.

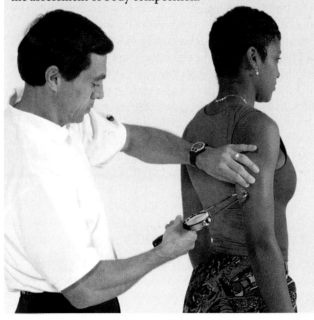

Recommended body weight is best determined through the assessment of body composition.

© Fitness & Wellness, Inc.

lifetime exercise and dietary changes? If you are not willing to change, you should stop worrying about your weight and deem the Moderate category "tolerable" for you.

THE WEIGHT LOSS DILEMMA

Yo-yo dieting carries as great a health risk as being overweight and remaining overweight in the first place. Epidemiological data show that frequent fluctuations in weight (up or down) markedly increase the risk of dying of cardiovascular disease.

Based on the findings that constant losses and regains can be hazardous to health, quick-fix diets should be replaced by a slow but permanent weight loss program (as described under "Losing Weight the Sound and Sensible Way"). Individuals reap the benefits of recommended body weight when they get to that weight and stay there throughout life.

Unfortunately, only about 10 percent of all people who begin a traditional weight-loss program without exercise are able to lose the desired weight. Worse, only 5 in 100 are able to keep the weight off. The body is highly resistant to permanent weight changes through caloric restrictions alone.

Traditional diets have failed because few of them incorporate lifetime changes in food selection and an overall increase in physical activity and exercise as fundamental to successful weight loss and weight maintenance. When the diet stops, weight gain begins.

The $40-billion diet industry tries to capitalize on the idea that weight can be lost quickly without considering the consequences of fast weight loss or the importance of lifetime behavioral changes to ensure proper weight loss and maintenance.

> The body is highly resistant to permanent weight loss through caloric restrictions alone.

In addition, various studies indicate that most people, especially obese people, underestimate their energy intake. Those who try to lose weight but apparently fail to do so are often described as "diet-resistant." One study found that, while on a "diet," a group of obese individuals with a self-reported history of diet resistance underreported their average daily caloric intake by almost 50 percent (1,028 self-reported versus 2,081 actual calories—see Figure 9.2).[7] These individuals also overestimated their amount of daily physical activity by about 25 percent (1,022 self-reported versus 771 actual calories). These differences

FIGURE 9.2 Differences between self-reported and actual daily caloric intake and exercise in obese individuals attempting to lose weight.

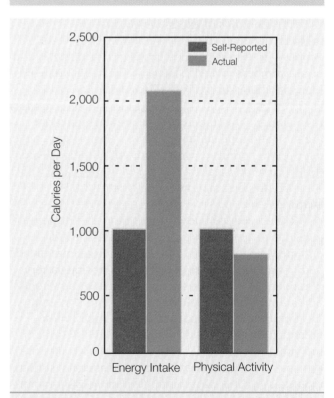

SOURCE: S. W. Lichtman et al., "Discrepancy Between Self-Reported and Actual Caloric Intake and Exercise in Obese Subjects." *New England Journal of Medicine*, 327 (1992): 1893–1898.

represent an additional 1,304 calories of energy per day unaccounted for by the subjects in the study. The findings indicate that failing to lose weight often is related to misreports of actual food intake and level of physical activity.

The Diet Craze

Capitalizing on hopes that the latest diet to hit the market will really work this time, fad diets continue to appeal to people of all shapes and sizes. These diets may work for awhile, but their success is usually short-lived. These diets deceive people and claim that dieters will lose weight by following all instructions. Most fad diets are very low in calories and deprive the body of certain nutrients, generating a metabolic imbalance. Under these conditions, a lot of the weight lost is in the form of water and protein, and not fat.

On a crash diet, close to half the weight loss is in lean (protein) tissue. When the body uses protein instead of a combination of fats and carbohydrates as a source of energy, weight is lost as much as 10 times faster. This is because a gram of protein produces half the amount of energy that fat does. In the case of muscle protein, one-fifth of protein is mixed with four-fifths water. Therefore, each pound of muscle yields only one-tenth the amount of energy of a pound of fat. As a result, most of the weight lost is in the form of water, which on the scale, of course, looks good.

The largest diet craze in the market today are the low-carbohydrate diet plans. Although small variations exist among them, in general, "low-carb" diets limit the intake of carbohydrate-rich foods like bread, potatoes, rice, pasta, cereals, crackers, juices, sodas, sweets (candy, cake, cookies), and even fruits and vegetables. Dieters are allowed to eat all the protein-rich foods they desire, including steak, ham, chicken, fish, bacon, eggs, nuts, cheese, tofu, high-fat salad dressings, butter, and small amounts of a few fruits and vegetables. Examples of these diets are the Atkins Diet, The Zone, Protein Power, the Scarsdale Diet, The Carb Addict's Diet, and Sugar Busters.

During digestion, carbohydrates are converted into glucose, a basic fuel used by every cell in the body. As blood glucose rises, insulin is released from the pancreas. Insulin is a hormone that facilitates the entry of glucose into the cells, thus lowering the glucose level in the bloodstream.

Not all carbohydrates cause a similar rise in blood glucose. The rise in glucose is based on the speed of

> When I get calls about the latest diet fad, I imagine a trick birthday cake candle that keeps lighting up and we have to keep blowing it out.
>
> —Dr. Kelly Brownell
> Yale University

Food Item	Index	Food Item	Index
Glucose	100	Frosted Flakes	55
Carrots	92	Fruit cocktail	55
Honey	87	Sweet corn	55
Baked potatoes	85	Sweet potato	51
Jelly beans	80	Peas	51
White rice	72	White pasta	50
White bread	69	Oatmeal	59
Whole-wheat bread	69	Whole-wheat pasta	42
Pineapple	66	Spaghetti	41
Table sugar	65	Oranges	40
Bananas	62	Apples	39
Boiled potatoes	62	Low-fat yogurt	33
Corn	59	Fructose	20
Muesli	56	Peanuts	13

TABLE 9.1 Glycemic Index of Selected Foods

digestion, which depends on a number of factors, including the size of the food particles. Small-particle carbohydrates break down rapidly and cause a quick, sharp rise in blood glucose. Thus, to gauge a food's effect on blood glucose, carbohydrates are classified by the **glycemic index**.

A high glycemic index signifies a quick rise in blood glucose. At the top of the 100-point scale is glucose itself. This index is not directly related to simple and complex carbohydrates, and the glycemic values are not always what one might expect. Rather, the index is based on the actual laboratory-measured speed of absorption. Processed foods generally have a high glycemic index, whereas high-fiber foods tend to have a lower index (see Table 9.1).

The body functions best when blood sugar remains at a constant level. Although this is best accomplished with low-glycemic index foods, elimination of all high-glycemic index foods from the diet is not necessary (foods with a high glycemic index are useful to replenish depleted glycogen stores following prolonged or exhaustive exercise). Combining high- with

Key Terms

Yo-yo dieting Constantly losing and gaining weight.

Glycemic index An index that is used to rate the plasma glucose response of carbohydrate-containing foods versus the response produced by the same amount of carbohydrate from a standard source, usually glucose or white bread.

low-glycemic index items or with some fat and protein brings the average index down. Regular consumption of high-glycemic foods, nonetheless, can increase the risk of cardiovascular disease, especially in people at risk for diabetes.

Proponents of low-carb diets indicate that if a person eats fewer carbohydrates and more protein, the pancreas will produce less insulin, and as insulin drops, the body will turn to its own fat deposits for energy. There is no scientific proof, however, that high levels of insulin lead to weight gain. None of the authors of these diets have published any studies that validate their claims. Yet, these authors base their diets on the faulty premise that high insulin leads to obesity. In fact, we know the opposite to be true—excessive body fat causes insulin levels to rise, thus increasing the risk for developing diabetes.

The reason for rapid weight loss during low-carb diets is because a low carbohydrate intake forces the liver to produce glucose. The source for most of this glucose is body proteins. As indicated earlier, protein is mostly water, thus weight is lost rapidly. When a person terminates the diet, the body rebuilds some of the protein tissue and some weight is quickly regained.

Low-carb diets are contrary to the nutrition advice of most national leading health organizations (who recommend a diet low in animal fat and saturated fat and high in complex carbohydrates). Without fruits, vegetables, and grains, high-protein diets lack many vitamins, minerals, and fiber—all dietary factors that protect against an array of ailments

> **Promoters of fad diets often claim to be unfairly targeted by the scientific community.**

How to recognize fad diets

Fad diets share common characteristics. These diets typically

- are based on testimonials.
- were developed according to confidential research.
- promote rapid and "painless" weight loss.
- promise miraculous results.
- restrict food selection.
- require the use of selected products.
- do not involve physical activity.
- do not encourage healthy behavioral changes.
- are not supported by the scientific community or national health organizations.

and diseases. The major risk associated with low-carb diets is an increased risk of heart disease because high-protein foods are also high in fat content. A low carbohydrate intake also produces a loss of vitamin B, calcium, and potassium. Potential bone loss can further accentuate the risk for osteoporosis. Weakness, nausea, bad breath, constipation, irritability, lightheadedness, and fatigue are side effects commonly associated with these diets. Long-term adherence to a high-protein diet can also increase the risk of certain types of cancer.

In addition to the low-carb diets, "combo-diets" such as the Schwarzbein and Suzanne Somers diets are also popular of late. The Schwarzbein diet claims that eating proteins and nonstarchy carbohydrates together will keep the food from being stored as fat. The Suzanne Somers diet doesn't allow you to eat proteins within 3 hours of carbohydrates, and if fruits are eaten, the dieter must wait at least 20 minutes before eating other carbohydrate foods. Both of these diets allow consumption of high-protein and high-fat food items, which increases risk for heart disease.

Other diets allow only certain specialized foods. If people would realize that no magic foods will provide all of the necessary nutrients, that a person has to eat a variety of foods to be well-nourished, the diet industry would not be as successful. Most of these diets create a nutritional deficiency, which at times may be fatal.

The reason many of these diets succeed is because a large number of foods are restricted on the diet, thus people tend to eat less food overall. With the extraordinary variety of foods available to us, it is unrealistic to think that people will adhere to these diets for very long. People eventually get tired of eating the

Low-carbohydrate/high-protein diets create nutritional deficiencies and contribute to the development of cardiovascular disease, cancer, and osteoporosis.

© Fitness & Wellness, Inc.

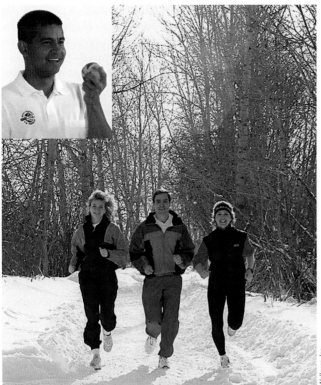

Achieving and maintaining a high physical fitness percent body fat standard requires a lifetime commitment to regular physical activity and proper nutrition.

same thing day in and day out and start eating less, thus leading to weight loss. If they happen to achieve the lower weight but do not make permanent dietary changes, they regain the weight quickly once they go back to their previous eating habits.

A few diets recommend exercise along with caloric restrictions—the best method for weight reduction, of course. People who adhere to these programs will succeed, so the diet has achieved its purpose. Unfortunately, if the people do not change their food selection and activity level permanently, they gain back the weight once they discontinue dieting and exercise.

Also, let's not forget that we eat for reasons other than to lose weight—we eat for pleasure and for health. Healthy eating along with regular physical activity are two of the most essential components of a wellness lifestyle, and they provide the best weight management program available today.

EATING DISORDERS

Anorexia nervosa and bulimia nervosa are physical and emotional conditions thought to stem from some combination of individual, family, and social pressures. These disorders are characterized by an intense fear of becoming fat that does not disappear even when losing extreme amounts of weight. Anorexia nervosa and bulimia nervosa are increasing steadily in most industrialized nations where society encourages low-calorie diets and thinness.

Anorexia Nervosa

Approximately 19 of every 20 individuals with **anorexia nervosa** are young women. An estimated 1 percent of the female population in the United States is anorexic. Anorexic individuals seem to fear weight gain more than death from starvation. Furthermore, they have a distorted image of their body and think of themselves as being fat even when they are emaciated.

Although a genetic predisposition may contribute to the syndrome, the anorexic person often comes from a mother-dominated home, with possible drug addictions in the family. The syndrome may emerge following a stressful life event and uncertainty about one's ability to cope efficiently.

The female role in society is changing rapidly, and women seem to be especially susceptible. Life experiences such as gaining weight, starting the menstrual period, beginning college, losing a boyfriend, having poor self-esteem, being socially rejected, starting a professional career, or becoming a wife or a mother can trigger the syndrome.

Anorexic individuals seem to fear weight gain more than death from starvation.

These individuals typically begin a diet and at first feel in control and happy about the weight loss, even if they are not overweight. To speed the weight loss, they frequently combine extreme dieting with exhaustive exercise and overuse of laxatives and diuretics.

Anorexics commonly develop obsessive and compulsive behaviors and emphatically deny their condition. They are preoccupied with food, meal planning, and grocery shopping, and they have unusual eating habits. As they lose weight and their health begins to deteriorate, anorexics feel weak and tired. They might realize they have a problem, but they will not stop the starvation and will refuse to consider the behavior abnormal.

Key Terms

Anorexia nervosa An eating disorder characterized by self-imposed starvation to lose and maintain very low body weight.

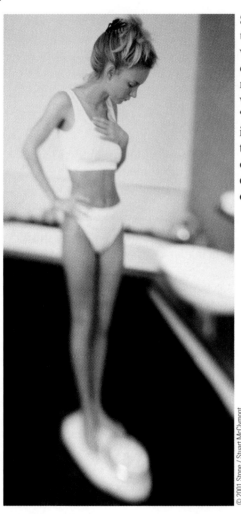

Society's unrealistic view of what constitutes recommended weight and "ideal" body image contributes to the development of eating disorders.

© 2001 Stone / Stuart McClymont

Once anorexics have lost a lot of weight and malnutrition sets in, physical changes become more visible. Typical changes are amenorrhea (stopping menstruation), digestive problems, extreme sensitivity to cold, hair and skin problems, fluid and electrolyte abnormalities (which may lead to an irregular heartbeat and sudden stopping of the heart), injuries to nerves and tendons, abnormalities of immune function, anemia, growth of fine body hair, mental confusion, inability to concentrate, lethargy, depression, dry skin, lower skin and body temperature, and osteoporosis.

Diagnostic criteria for anorexia nervosa are[8]

- Refusal to maintain body weight over a minimal normal weight for age and height (weight loss leading to maintenance of body weight less than 85 percent of that expected or failure to make expected weight gain during periods of growth, leading to body weight less than 85 percent of that expected).

- Intense fear of gaining weight or becoming fat, even though underweight.

- Disturbance in the way in which one perceives one's own body weight, size, or shape; undue influences of body weight or shape on self-evaluation; or denial of the seriousness of the current low body weight.

- In postmenarcheal females, amenorrhea (absence of at least three consecutive menstrual cycles). (A woman is considered to have amenorrhea if her periods occur only following estrogen therapy.)

Many of the changes induced by anorexia nervosa can be reversed. Treatment almost always requires professional help, and the sooner it is started, the better the chances for reversibility and cure. Therapy consists of a combination of medical and psychological techniques to restore proper nutrition, prevent medical complications, and modify the environment or events that triggered the syndrome. Anorexics seldom overcome the problem by themselves. They strongly deny their condition. They are able to hide it and deceive friends and relatives. In their behavior, many of them meet all of the characteristics of anorexia nervosa, but it goes undetected because both thinness and dieting are socially acceptable. Only a well-trained clinician is able to diagnose anorexia nervosa.

Bulimia Nervosa

Bulimia nervosa is more prevalent than anorexia nervosa. For many years it was thought to be a variant of anorexia nervosa, but now it is identified as a separate condition. It afflicts mainly young people. As many as 1 in every 5 women on college campuses may be bulimic, according to some estimates. Bulimia nervosa also is more prevalent than anorexia nervosa in males, although bulimia is still much more prevalent in females.

Bulimics usually are healthy-looking people, well-educated, and near recommended body weight. They seem to enjoy food and often socialize around it. In actuality, they are emotionally insecure, rely on others, and lack self-confidence and self-esteem. Recommended weight and food are abnormally important to them.

The binge-purge cycle usually occurs in stages. As a result of stressful life events or the simple compulsion to eat, bulimics periodically engage in binge eating that may last an hour or longer. With some apprehension, bulimics anticipate and plan the cycle. Next they feel an urgency to begin, followed by large and uncontrollable food consumption during which they may eat several thousand calories (up to 10,000 calories in extreme cases). After a short period of relief and satisfaction, feelings of deep guilt, shame, and intense fear of gaining weight ensue. Purging seems to be an easy answer, because the bingeing cycle can continue without fear of gaining weight.

The diagnostic criteria for bulimia nervosa are[9]

- Recurrent episodes of binge eating. An episode of binge eating is characterized by both of the following:

  1. Eating, in a discrete period of time (for example, within any 2-hour period), an amount of food that is definitely more than most people would eat during a similar period and under similar circumstances.

  2. A sense of lack of control over eating during the episode (a feeling that one cannot stop eating or control what or how much one is eating).

- Recurring inappropriate compensatory behaviors to prevent weight gain, such as self-induced vomiting; misuse of laxatives, diuretics, enemas, or other medications; fasting; or excessive exercise.

- The binge eating and inappropriate compensatory behaviors both occur, on average, at least twice a week for 3 months.

- Self-evaluation is unduly influenced by body shape and weight.

- The binge eating causes marked distress.

> The sooner treatment for eating disorders is initiated, the better the chances for recovery.

The most typical form of purging is self-induced vomiting. Bulimics, too, frequently ingest strong laxatives and emetics. Near-fasting diets and strenuous bouts of exercise are common. Medical problems associated with bulimia nervosa include cardiac arrhythmias, amenorrhea, kidney and bladder damage, ulcers, colitis, tearing of the esophagus or stomach, tooth erosion, gum damage, and general muscular weakness.

Unlike anorexics, bulimics realize their behavior is abnormal and feel great shame about it. Fearing social rejection, they pursue the binge-purge cycle in secrecy and at unusual hours of the day.

Bulimia nervosa can be treated successfully when the person realizes that this destructive behavior is not the solution to life's problems. A change in attitude can prevent permanent damage or death.

Treatment for anorexia nervosa and bulimia nervosa is available on most school campuses through the school's counseling center or the health center. Local hospitals also offer treatment for these conditions. Many communities have support groups, frequently led by professional personnel and usually free of charge.

PHYSIOLOGY OF WEIGHT LOSS

Only a few years ago the principles governing a weight loss and maintenance program seemed to be clear, but now we know the final answers are not in yet. Traditional concepts related to weight control have centered on three assumptions: (a) that balancing food intake against output allows a person to achieve recommended weight, (b) that all fat people just eat too much, and (c) that the human body doesn't care how much (or little) fat it stores. Although these statements contain some truth, they still are open to much debate and research. We now know that the causes of obesity are complex, including a combination of genetics, behavior, and lifestyle factors.

Energy-Balancing Equation

The principle embodied in the **energy-balancing equation** is simple: If daily energy requirements could be determined accurately, caloric intake could be balanced against output. This is not always the case, though, because genetic and lifestyle-related individual differences determine the number of calories required to maintain or lose body weight.

Table 9.2 (page 253) offers some general guidelines for estimating daily caloric intake according to lifestyle patterns. This is only an estimated figure, and (as discussed under "Losing Weight the Sound and Sensible Way") it serves only as a starting point from which individual adjustments have to be made.

One pound of fat represents 3,500 calories. Assuming that a person's basic daily caloric expenditure is 2,500 calories, if this person were to decrease intake by 500 calories per day, it should result in a loss of one pound of fat in 7 days ($500 \times 7 = 3,500$). But research has shown—and many people have experienced—that even when dieters carefully balance caloric input against caloric output, weight loss does not always happen as predicted. Furthermore, two people with similar measured caloric intake and output seldom lose weight at the same rate.

KeyTerms

Bulimia nervosa An eating disorder characterized by a pattern of binge eating and purging in an attempt to lose weight and maintain low body weight.

Energy-balancing equation A principle holding that as long as caloric input equals caloric output, the person will not gain or lose weight. If caloric intake exceeds output, the person gains weight; when output exceeds input, the person loses weight.

The most common explanation of individual differences in weight loss and weight gain has been the variation in human metabolism from one person to another. We are all familiar with people who can eat "all day long" and not gain an ounce of weight, whereas others cannot even "dream about food" without gaining weight. Because experts did not believe that human metabolism alone could account for such extreme differences, they developed several theories that might better explain these individual variations.

Setpoint Theory

Results of several research studies point toward a **weight-regulating mechanism (WRM)** that has a **setpoint** for controlling both appetite and the amount of fat stored. Setpoint is hypothesized to work like a thermostat for body fat, maintaining fairly constant body weight, because it "knows" at all times the exact amount of adipose tissue stored in the fat cells. Some people have high settings; others have low settings.

If body weight decreases (as in dieting), the setpoint senses this change and triggers the WRM to increase the person's appetite or make the body conserve energy to maintain the "set" weight. The opposite also may be true. Some people have a hard time gaining weight. In this case, the WRM decreases appetite or causes the body to waste energy to maintain the lower weight.

SETPOINT AND CALORIC INPUT

Every person has his or her own certain body fat percentage (as established by the setpoint) that the body attempts to maintain. The genetic instinct to survive tells the body that fat storage is vital, and therefore it sets an acceptable fat level. This level may remain somewhat constant or may climb gradually because of poor lifestyle habits.

For instance, under strict calorie reduction, the body may make extreme metabolic adjustments in an effort to maintain its setpoint for fat. The **basal metabolic rate (BMR)**, the lowest level of caloric intake necessary to sustain life, may drop dramatically when operating under a consistent negative caloric balance, and that person's weight loss may plateau for days or even weeks. A low metabolic rate compounds a person's problems in maintaining recommended body weight.

These findings were substantiated by research conducted at Rockefeller University in New York.[10] The authors showed that the body resists maintaining altered weight. Obese and lifetime non-obese individuals were used in the investigation. Following a 10 percent weight loss, in an attempt to regain the lost weight, the body compensated by burning up to 15 percent fewer calories than expected for the new reduced weight (after accounting for the 10 percent loss). The effects were similar in the obese and non-obese participants. These results imply that after a 10 percent weight loss, a person would have to eat even less or exercise more to account for the estimated difference of about 200 to 300 calories.

In this same study, when the participants were allowed to increase their weight to 10 percent above their "normal" body (pre-weight loss) weight, the body burned 10 to 15 percent more calories than expected—the body's attempt to waste energy and maintain the pre-set weight. This is another indication that the body is highly resistant to weight changes unless additional lifestyle changes are incorporated to ensure successful weight management. (These methods will be discussed under "Losing Weight the Sound and Sensible Way".)

Dietary restriction alone will not lower the setpoint, even though the person may lose weight and fat. When the dieter goes back to the normal or even below-normal caloric intake (at which the weight may have been stable for a long time), he or she quickly regains the fat loss as the body strives to regain a comfortable fat store.

Let's use a practical illustration. A person would like to lose some body fat and calculates that his or her current, stable body weight has been reached at an average daily caloric intake of 1,800 calories (no weight gain or loss occurs at this daily intake). In an attempt to lose weight rapidly, this person now goes on a strict low-calorie diet, or even worse, a near-fasting diet. Immediately the body activates its survival mechanism and readjusts its metabolism to a lower caloric balance. After a few weeks of dieting at fewer than 400 to 600 calories per day, the body becomes able to maintain its normal functions at 1,000 calories per day.

Having lost the desired weight, the person terminates the diet, but realizes that the original intake of 1,800 calories per day will have to be lower to maintain the new lower weight. To adjust to the new lower body weight, the person restricts intake to about 1,500 calories per day. The individual is surprised to find that, even at this lower daily intake (300 fewer calories), weight comes back at a rate of 1 pound every 1 to 2 weeks. After the diet is over, this new lowered metabolic rate may take several months to kick back up to its normal level.

From this explanation, individuals clearly should not go on very low-calorie diets. Not only will this slow down resting metabolic rate, but it will also deprive the body of basic daily nutrients required for normal function.

Daily caloric intakes of 1,200 to 1,500 calories provide the necessary nutrients if they are distributed properly over the five basic food groups (meeting the daily required servings from each group). Of course, the individual will have to learn which foods meet the requirements and yet are low in fat and sugar.

Under no circumstances should a person go on a diet that calls for less than 1,200 calories for women or 1,500 calories for men. Weight (fat) is gained over months and years, not overnight. Likewise, weight loss should be gradual, not abrupt.

A second way in which the setpoint may work is by keeping track of the nutrients and calories consumed daily. It is thought that the body, like a cash register, records the daily food intake and that the brain will not feel satisfied until the calories and nutrients have been "registered."

This setpoint for calories and nutrients seems to operate even when people participate in moderately intense exercise. Some evidence suggests that people do not become hungrier with moderate physical activity. Therefore, people can choose to lose weight either by going hungry or by stepping up their daily physical activity. Burning more calories through physical activity helps to lower body fat.

LOWERING THE SETPOINT

The most common question regarding the setpoint is how it can be lowered so the body will feel comfortable at a reduced fat percentage. These factors seem to affect the setpoint directly by lowering the fat thermostat:

1. Aerobic exercise.
2. A diet high in complex carbohydrates.
3. Nicotine.
4. Amphetamines.

The last two are more destructive than the extra fat weight, so they are not reasonable alternatives (as far as the extra strain on the heart is concerned, smoking one pack of cigarettes per day is said to be the equivalent of carrying 50 to 75 pounds of excess body fat).

On the other hand, a diet high in fats and refined carbohydrates, near-fasting diets, and perhaps even artificial sweeteners seem to raise the setpoint. Therefore, the only practical and sensible way to lower the setpoint and lose fat weight is a combination of aerobic exercise and a diet high in complex carbohydrates and low in fat.

Because of the effects of proper food management on the body's setpoint, many nutritionists believe the source of calories should be the main concern in a weight-control program, instead of simply total number of calories consumed. In this regard, most of the successful dieter's effort is spent in redirecting eating habits, increasing the intake of complex carbohydrates and high-fiber foods, and decreasing the consumption of refined carbohydrates (sugars) and fats. In most cases, this change in eating habits will bring about a decrease in total daily caloric intake. Because 1 gram of carbohydrates provides only 4 calories, as opposed to 9 calories per gram of fat, you could eat twice the volume of food (by weight) when substituting carbohydrates for fat.

In 1996 the Food and Drug Administration (FDA) approved a new fat substitute, **olestra**, for use in "savory snacks." According to the *University of California at Berkeley Wellness Letter*, consumers should "just say no" to olestra and not buy products that contain this fat substitute.[11]

Olestra can cause diarrhea and cramping, and it can deplete the body of fat-soluble vitamins, including A, D, E, and K. Vitamin E is a strong antioxidant, and shortages of vitamin K pose a risk for people with bleeding disorders and those on blood-thinning medication. In addition, potential cancer-causing changes in liver cells have been found in animal studies of olestra. Although the fat and caloric content of olestra-containing foods is lower than that of foods cooked with natural fats, consuming snacks using this fat substitute not only can pose a risk to good health but also will reinforce unhealthy eating habits.

A "diet" is no longer viewed as a temporary tool to aid in weight loss but, instead, as a permanent change in eating behaviors to ensure weight management and better health. The role of increased physical activity must also be considered, because successful weight loss, maintenance of healthy weight, and recommended body composition are seldom attained without a moderate reduction in caloric intake combined with a regular exercise program.

Key Terms

Weight-regulating mechanism (WRM) A feature of the hypothalamus of the brain that controls how much the body should weigh.

Setpoint Weight control theory that the body has an established weight and strongly attempts to maintain that weight.

Basal metabolic rate (BMR) The lowest level of oxygen consumption necessary to sustain life.

Olestra Fat substitute made from sugar and fatty acids; provides no calories to the body because it passes through the digestive system without being absorbed.

DIET AND METABOLISM

Fat can be lost by selecting the proper foods, exercising, or restricting calories. When a person tries to lose weight by dietary restrictions alone, lean body mass (muscle protein, along with vital organ protein) always decreases. The amount of lean body mass lost depends entirely on caloric limitation.

When people go on a near-fasting diet, up to half of the weight loss is lean body mass and the other half is actual fat loss (see Figure 9.3).[12] When diet is combined with exercise, close to 100 percent of the weight loss is in the form of fat, and lean tissue actually may increase. Loss of lean body mass is never good, because it weakens the organs and muscles and slows down metabolism. Large losses in lean tissue can cause disturbances in heart function and damage to other organs. Equally important is not to overindulge (binge) following a very low-calorie diet. This may cause changes in metabolic rate and electrolyte balance, which could trigger fatal cardiac arrhythmias.

Contrary to some beliefs, aging is not the main reason for the lower metabolic rate. It is not so much that metabolism slows down as that people slow down. As people age, they tend to rely more on the amenities of life (remote controls, cellular telephones, intercoms, single-level homes, riding lawnmowers) that lull a person into sedentary living.

Basal metabolism is related to lean body weight. The more lean tissue, the higher the metabolic rate. As a consequence of sedentary living and less physical activity, the lean component decreases and fat tissue increases. The human body requires a certain amount of oxygen per pound of lean body mass. Given that fat is considered metabolically inert from the point of view of caloric use, the lean tissue uses most of the oxygen, even at rest. As muscle and organ mass (which make up lean body mass) decrease, so do the energy requirements at rest.

> When people crash diet, about half of the weight loss is in the form of lean tissue.

Reductions in lean body mass are common in aging people (primarily because of physical inactivity) and those on severely restricted diets. The loss of lean body mass also may account for a lower metabolic rate and the longer time it takes to kick back up.

Diets with caloric intakes below 1,200 to 1,500 calories cannot guarantee the retention of lean body mass. Even at this intake level, some loss is inevitable, unless the diet is combined with exercise. Despite the claims of many diets that they do not alter the lean component, the simple truth is that, regardless of what

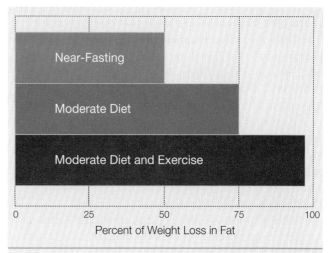

FIGURE 9.3 Effects of three forms of diet on fat loss.

Percent of Weight Loss in Fat

Adapted from R. J. Shephard, *Alive Man: The Physiology of Physical Activity* (Springfield, IL: Charles C Thomas, 1975), 484–488.

nutrients may be added to the diet, severe caloric restrictions always prompt the loss of lean tissue. Too many people go on low-calorie diets constantly. Every time they do, the metabolic rate slows down as more lean tissue is lost.

People in their 40s and older who weigh the same as they did when they were 20 tend to think they are at recommended body weight. During this span of 20 years or more, they may have dieted many times without participating in an exercise program. They regain the weight shortly after they terminate each diet, and most of that gain is in fat. Maybe at age 20 they weighed 150 pounds, of which only 15 percent was fat. Now at age 40, even though they still weigh 150 pounds, they might be 30 percent fat (see Figure 9.4). At recommended body weight, they wonder why they are eating very little and still having trouble staying at that weight.

EXERCISE: THE KEY TO WEIGHT LOSS AND WEIGHT MAINTENANCE

A more effective way to tilt the energy-balancing equation in your favor is by burning calories through physical activity. Exercise also seems to exert control over how much a person weighs.

Starting at age 25, the typical American gains 1 pound of weight per year. This weight gain represents a simple energy surplus of under 10 calories per day.

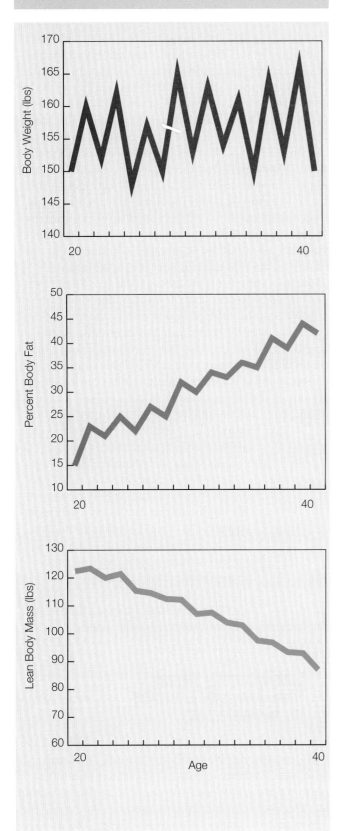

FIGURE 9.4 Effects of frequent dieting without exercise on lean body mass, percent body fat, and body weight.

In most cases, the additional weight accumulated in middle age comes from people becoming less physically active, and not as a result of increased caloric intake. Dr. Jack Wilmore, a leading exercise physiologist and expert weight management researcher, stated:

> Physical inactivity is certainly a major, if not the primary, cause of obesity in the United States today. A certain minimal level of activity might be necessary for us to accurately balance our caloric intake to our caloric expenditure. With too little activity, we appear to lose the fine control we normally have to maintain this incredible balance. This fine balance amounts to less than 10 calories per day, or the equivalent of one potato chip.[13]

Exercise is crucial to losing weight and maintaining weight. Not only will exercise maintain lean tissue, but advocates of the setpoint theory say that exercise resets the fat thermostat to a new, lower level. This change may be rapid, or it may take time. A few overweight individuals have exercised faithfully almost daily, 60 minutes at a time, for a whole year before seeing significant weight change. People with a "sticky" setpoint have to be patient and persistent.

If a person is trying to lose weight, a combination of aerobic and strength-training exercises works best. Aerobic exercise is the best to offset the setpoint, and the continuity and duration of these types of activities cause many calories to be burned in the process. The role of aerobic exercise in successful lifetime weight management cannot be overestimated. Strength training is critical in helping raise the lean component, and thus, the basal metabolic rate.

As illustrated in Figure 9.5, greater weight loss is achieved by combining a diet with an aerobic exercise program.[14] Of even greater significance, only the individuals who participated in an 18-month post-diet aerobic exercise program were able to keep the weight off. Those who discontinued exercise regained weight. Furthermore, of those who initiated or resumed exercise during the 18-month follow-up, all were able to lose weight again. Individuals who only dieted and did not exercise regained 60 percent and 92 percent of their weight loss at the 6- and 18-month follow-ups, respectively.

Weight loss might be more rapid when aerobic exercise is combined with a strength-training program. Each additional pound of muscle tissue can raise the basal metabolic rate by about 35 calories per day.[15] Thus, an individual who adds 5 pounds of muscle tissue as a result of strength training increases the basal metabolic rate by 175 calories per day (35×5), which equals 63,875 calories per year (175×365) or the equivalent of 18.25 pounds of fat ($63,875 \div 3,500$).

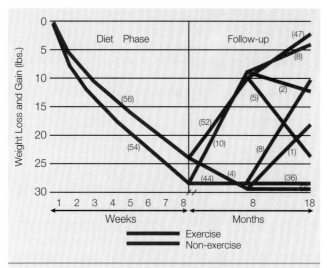

FIGURE 9.5 Aerobic exercise, weight loss, and maintenance in moderately obese individuals.

NOTE: Numbers in parentheses indicate number of participants.

SOURCE: K. N., Pavlou, S. Krey, and W. P. Steffe, "Exercise as an Adjunct to Weight Loss and Maintenance in Moderately Obese Subjects," *American Journal of Clinical Nutrition*, 49 (1989): 1115–1123.

Strength training is suggested especially for people who think they are at their recommended body weight, yet their body fat percentage is higher than recommended. The number of calories burned during a typical hour-long strength-training session is much less than during an hour of aerobic exercise. Because of the high intensity of strength training, the person needs frequent rest intervals to recover from each set of exercise. The average person actually lifts weights only 10 to 12 minutes during each hour of exercise. In the long run, however, the person enjoys the benefits of gains in lean tissue. Guidelines for developing aerobic and strength-training programs are given in Chapters 4 and 5.

Although size (inches) and percent body fat both decrease when sedentary individuals begin an exercise program, body weight often remains the same or may even increase during the first couple of weeks of the program. Exercise helps to increase muscle tissue, connective tissue, blood volume (as much as 500 ml, or the equivalent of 1 pound, following the first week of aerobic exercise), enzymes and other structures within the cell, and glycogen (which binds water). All of these changes lead to a higher functional capacity of the human body. With exercise, most of the weight loss becomes apparent after a few weeks of training, after the lean component has stabilized.

Although we know that a negative caloric balance of 3,500 calories does not always result in a loss of exactly 1 pound of fat, the role of exercise in achieving a negative balance by burning additional calories is significant in weight reduction and maintenance programs. Sadly, some individuals claim that the number of calories burned during exercise is hardly worth the effort. They think that cutting their daily intake by some 300 calories is easier than participating in some sort of exercise that would burn the same amount of calories. The problem is that the willpower to cut those 300 calories lasts only a few weeks, and then the person goes right back to the old eating patterns.

If a person gets into the habit of exercising regularly, say 3 times a week, jogging 3 miles per exercise session (about 300 calories burned), this represents 900 calories in one week, about 3,600 calories in one month, or 46,800 calories per year. This minimal amount of exercise represents as many as 13.5 extra pounds of fat in one year, 27 in two, and so on.

We tend to forget that our weight creeps up gradually over the years, not just overnight. Hardly worth the effort? And we have not even taken into consideration the increase in lean tissue, possible resetting of the setpoint, benefits to the cardiovascular system, and, most important, the improved quality of life. The fundamental reasons for overweight and obesity, few could argue, are sedentary living and lack of physical activity.

In terms of preventing disease, many of the health benefits people try to achieve by losing weight are reaped through exercise alone, even without weight loss. Exercise offers protection against premature morbidity and mortality for everyone, including people who already have risk factors for disease. The lack of physical activity, not the weight problem itself, may be the cause of many of the health risks associated with obesity.

> **Following weight loss, only those people who maintain an exercise program are able to keep the weight off.**

Low-Intensity Versus High-Intensity Exercise for Weight Loss

Some individuals promote low-intensity exercise over high-intensity for weight-loss purposes. As compared with high intensity, a greater proportion of calories burned during low-intensity exercise are derived from fat. The lower the intensity of exercise, the higher the percentage of fat utilization as an energy source. In theory, if you are trying to lose fat, this principle makes sense, but in reality it is misleading. The bottom line when you are trying to lose weight is to burn more calories. When your daily caloric expenditure exceeds your intake, weight is lost. The more calories you burn, the more fat is lost.

During low-intensity exercise, up to 50 percent of the calories burned may be derived from fat (the other 50 percent from glucose [carbohydrates]). With intense exercise, only 30 to 40 percent of the caloric expenditure comes from fat. Overall, however, you can burn twice as many (or more) calories during high-intensity exercise, and, subsequently more fat as well.

Let's look at a practical illustration. If you exercise for 30 minutes at a moderate intensity and burn 200 calories, about 100 of those calories (50 percent) would come from fat. If you exercise at high intensity during those same 30 minutes, you may burn 400 calories—with 120 to 160 of the calories (30 to 40 percent) coming from fat. Thus, if you exercised at a low intensity, you would have to do so twice as long to burn the same number of calories. Another benefit is that the metabolic rate remains at a higher level longer after high-intensity exercise, so you continue to burn more calories following exercise.

Moreover, high-intensity exercise by itself appears to trigger greater fat loss than low-intensity exercise. Research conducted at Laval University in Quebec, Canada, showed that subjects who performed a high-intensity intermittent-training program lost more body fat than participants in a low- to moderate-intensity continuous aerobic endurance group.[16] Even more surprisingly, this finding occurred despite the fact that the high-intensity group burned fewer total calories per exercise session. The results support the notion that vigorous exercise is more conducive to weight loss than low- to moderate-intensity exercise.

Before you start high-intensity exercise sessions, a word of caution is in order. Be sure that it is medically safe for you to participate in such activities and that you build up gradually to that level. If you are cleared to participate in high-intensity exercise, do not attempt to do too much too quickly, because you may suffer injuries and discouragement. You must allow your body a proper conditioning period of 8 to 12 weeks, or even longer for people with a moderate-to-serious weight problem. High intensity also does not mean high impact. High-impact activities are the most common cause of exercise-related injuries. Additional information on these topics is presented in Chapter 4.

The previous discussion on high- versus low-intensity exercise does not mean that low intensity is not effective. Low-intensity exercise provides substantial health benefits, and people who initiate exercise programs may be more willing to participate and stay with low-intensity programs. Low-intensity exercise does promote weight loss, but you will need to exercise longer to obtain the same results.

Healthy Weight Gain

"Skinny" people, too, should realize that the only healthy way to gain weight is through exercise (mainly strength-training exercises) and a slight increase in caloric intake. Attempting to gain weight just by overeating will raise the fat component and not the lean component—which is not the path to better health. Exercise is the best solution to weight (fat) reduction and weight (lean) gain alike.

A strength-training program such as the one outlined in Chapter 5 is the best approach to add body weight. The training program should include at least two exercises of three sets for each major body part. Each set should consist of about 10 repetitions maximum.

Even though the metabolic cost of synthesizing a pound of muscle tissue is still unclear, consuming an estimated 500 additional calories daily, including 15 grams of protein above the RDA, is the recommendation to gain an average of 1 pound of muscle tissue per week. Based on the typical American diet, the extra 15 grams of protein are not necessary. Each day, the average person in the United States already consumes 30 to 60 grams of protein above the RDA. The extra 500 calories should be primarily in the form of complex carbohydrates. If the higher caloric intake is not accompanied by a strength-training program, the increase in body weight will be in the form of fat, not muscle tissue.

Weight-Loss Myths

Cellulite and **spot reducing** are mythical concepts. **Cellulite** is nothing but enlarged fat cells that bulge out from accumulated body fat.

Doing several sets of daily sit-ups will not get rid of fat in the midsection of the body. When fat comes off, it does so throughout the entire body, not just the exercised area. The greatest proportion of fat may

KeyTerms

Spot reducing Fallacious theory that exercising a specific body part will result in significant fat reduction in that area.

Cellulite Term frequently used in reference to fat deposits that "bulge out"; these deposits are nothing but enlarged fat cells from excessive accumulation of body fat.

come off the biggest fat deposits, but the caloric output of a few sets of sit-ups has practically no effect on reducing total body fat. A person has to exercise much longer to really see results.

Other touted means toward quick weight loss—rubberized sweatsuits, steam baths, mechanical vibrators—are misleading. When a person wears a sweatsuit or steps into a sauna, the weight lost is not fat, but merely a significant amount of water. Sure, it looks nice when you step on the scale immediately afterward, but this represents a false loss of weight. As soon as you replace body fluids, you gain back the weight quickly.

Wearing rubberized sweatsuits not only hastens the rate of body fluid loss—fluid that is vital during prolonged exercise—but it raises core temperature at the same time. This combination puts a person in danger of dehydration, which impairs cellular function and, in extreme cases, can even cause death.

Similarly, mechanical vibrators are worthless in a weight-control program. Vibrating belts and turning rollers may feel good, but they require no effort whatsoever. Fat cannot be shaken off. It is lost primarily by burning it, through physical activity, in muscle tissue.

LOSING WEIGHT THE SOUND AND SENSIBLE WAY

Dieting never has been fun and never will be. People who are overweight and are serious about losing weight, however, have to include regular exercise in their life along with proper food management and a sensible reduction in caloric intake.

Some precautions are in order, because excessive body fat is a risk factor for cardiovascular disease. Depending on the extent of the weight problem, a medical examination and possibly a stress ECG (see "Abnormal Electrocardiograms" in Chapter 10) may be a good idea before undertaking the exercise program. A physician should be consulted in this regard.

Significantly overweight individuals also may have to choose activities in which they will not have to support their own body weight but that will still be effective in burning calories. Injuries to joints and muscles are common in overweight individuals who participate in weight-bearing exercises such as walking, jogging, and aerobics.

Swimming may not be a good weight-loss exercise either. More body fat makes a person more buoyant, and most people are not at the skill level to swim fast enough to get the best training effect. They tend to just float along, limiting the number of calories burned as well as the benefits to the cardiorespiratory system.

Some better alternatives are riding a bicycle (either road or stationary), walking in a shallow pool, doing water aerobics, or running in place in deep water (treading water). The latter forms of water exercise are gaining popularity and have proven to be effective in reducing weight without the fear of injuries.

How long should each exercise session last? To develop and maintain cardiorespiratory fitness, 20 to 30 minutes of exercise at the recommended target rate, 3 to 5 times per week, is suggested (see Chapter 4). For weight-loss purposes, many experts recommend exercising at least 45 minutes at a time, 5 to 6 times a week.

A person should not try to do too much too fast. Unconditioned beginners should start with about 15 minutes of aerobic exercise 3 times a week, gradually increasing the duration by

> **For weight-loss purposes, experts recommend exercising at least 45 minutes at a time, most days of the week.**

Regular participation in a lifetime exercise program is the key to successful weight management.

approximately 5 minutes per week and the frequency by 1 day per week during the next 3 to 4 weeks.

One final benefit of long-duration exercise for weight control is that it allows fat to be burned more efficiently. Carbohydrates and fats are both sources of energy. When the glucose levels begin to drop during prolonged exercise, more fat is used as energy substrate.

Equally important is that fat-burning enzymes increase with aerobic training. Fat is lost primarily by burning it in muscle. Therefore, as the concentration of the enzymes increases, so does the ability to burn fat.

In addition to exercise and adequate food management, sensible adjustments in caloric intake are recommended. Most research finds that a negative caloric balance is required to lose weight. Perhaps the only exception is with people who are eating too few calories. A nutrient analysis often reveals that faithful dieters are not consuming enough calories. These people actually need to increase their daily caloric intake (and combine that with an exercise program) to get their metabolism to kick back up to a normal level.

The reasons for prescribing a lower caloric figure to lose weight are as follows:

1. Most people underestimate their caloric intake and are eating more than they should be eating.

2. Developing new behaviors takes time, and some people have trouble changing and adjusting to new eating habits.

3. Many individuals are in such poor physical condition that they take a long time to increase their activity level enough to offset the setpoint and burn enough calories to aid in loss of body fat.

4. Some dieters have difficulty succeeding unless they can count calories.

5. A few people simply will not alter their food selection. For those who will not (which will still increase the risk for chronic diseases), a large increase in physical activity, a negative caloric balance, or a combination of the two is the only solution to lose weight successfully.

You can estimate your daily caloric requirement by consulting Tables 9.2 and 9.3 and completing Figure 9.6 (page 257). Given that this is only an estimated value, individual adjustments related to many of the factors discussed in this chapter may be necessary to establish a more precise value. Nevertheless, the estimated value does offer a beginning guideline for weight control or reduction.

The average daily caloric requirement without exercise is based on typical lifestyle patterns, total

TABLE **9.2** Average Caloric Requirement Per Pound of Body Weight Based on Lifestyle Patterns and Gender		
	Calories Per Pound	
	Men	Women*
Sedentary—limited physical activity	13.0	12.0
Moderate physical activity	15.0	13.5
Hard Labor—strenuous physical effort	17.0	15.0

*Pregnant or lactating women: Add 3 calories to these values.

body weight, and gender. Individuals who hold jobs that require heavy manual labor burn more calories during the day than those who have sedentary jobs (such as working behind a desk). To find your activity level, refer to Table 9.2 and rate yourself accordingly. The number given in Table 9.2 is per pound of body weight, so you multiply your current weight by that number. For example, the typical caloric requirement to maintain body weight for a moderately active male who weighs 160 pounds is 2,400 calories (160 lbs × 15 cal/lb).

To determine the average number of calories you burn daily as a result of exercise, figure out the total number of minutes you exercise weekly, then figure the daily average exercise time. For instance, a person cycling at 13 miles per hour 5 times a week, 30 minutes each time, exercises 150 minutes per week (5 × 30). The average daily exercise time is therefore 21 minutes (150 ÷ 7, rounded off to the lowest unit).

Next, from Table 9.3, find the energy expenditure for the activity (or activities) chosen for the exercise program. In the case of cycling (13 miles per hour), the expenditure is .071 calories per pound of body weight per minute of activity (cal/ lb/min). With a body weight of 160 pounds, this man would burn 11.4 calories each minute (body weight × .071, or 160 × .071). In 21 minutes he burns approximately 240 calories (21 × 11.4).

Now you can obtain the estimated total caloric requirement, with exercise, needed to maintain body weight. To do this, add the typical daily requirement (without exercise) obtained from Table 9.2 and the average calories burned through exercise. In our example, it is 2,640 calories (2,400 + 240).

If a negative caloric balance is recommended to lose weight, this person has to consume fewer than 2,640 calories daily to achieve the objective. Because of the many factors that play a role in weight control, this 2,640-calorie value is only an estimated daily

TABLE 9.3 Caloric Expenditure of Selected Physical Activities

Activity*	Cal/lb/min	Activity*	Cal/lb/min	Activity*	Cal/lb/min
Aero-belt Exercise		Dance		Stairmaster	
Aero-belt jogging/6 mph	0.098	Moderate	0.030	Moderate	0.070
Aero-belt Step-aerobics/8"	0.105	Vigorous	0.055	Vigorous	0.090
Aero-belt walking/4 mph	0.073	Golf	0.030	Stationary Cycling	
Aerobics		Gymnastics		Moderate	0.055
Moderate	0.065	Light	0.030	Vigorous	0.070
Vigorous	0.095	Heavy	0.056	Strength Training	0.050
Step aerobics	0.070	Handball	0.064	Swimming (crawl)	
Archery	0.030	Hiking	0.040	20 yds/min	0.031
Badminton		Judo/Karate	0.086	25 yds/min	0.040
Recreation	0.038	Racquetball	0.065	45 yds/min	0.057
Competition	0.065	Rope Jumping	0.060	50 yds/min	0.070
Baseball	0.031	Rowing (vigorous)	0.090	Table Tennis	0.030
Basketball		Running (on a level surface)		Tennis	
Moderate	0.046	11.0 min/mile	0.070	Moderate	0.045
Competition	0.063	8.5 min/mile	0.090	Competition	0.064
Bowling	0.030	7.0 min/mile	0.102	Volleyball	0.030
Calisthenics	0.033	6.0 min/mile	0.114	Walking	
Cycling (on a level surface)		Deep water**	0.100	4.5 mph	0.045
5.5 mph	0.033	Skating (moderate)	0.038	Shallow pool	0.090
10.0 mph	0.050	Skiing		Water Aerobics	
13.0 mph	0.071	Downhill	0.060	Moderate	0.050
		Level (5 mph)	0.078	Vigorous	0.070
		Soccer	0.059	Wrestling	0.085

Adapted from:

P. E. Allsen, J. M. Harrison, and B. Vance. *Fitness for Life: An Individualized Approach* (Dubuque, IA: Wm. C. Brown, 1989).
C. A. Bucher and W. E. Prentice, *Fitness for College and Life* (St. Louis: Times Mirror/Mosby College Publishing, 1989).
C. F. Consolazio, R. E. Johnson, and L. J. Pecora. *Physiological Measurements of Metabolic Functions in Man* (New York: McGraw-Hill, 1963).
R. V. Hockey, *Physical Fitness: The Pathway to Healthful Living* (St. Louis: Times Mirror/Mosby College Publishing, 1989).
W. W. K. Hoeger et al. Research conducted at Boise State University, 1986–1993.

*Values are for actual time engaged in the activity.   **Treading water

requirement. Furthermore, we cannot predict that you will lose exactly 1 pound of fat in 1 week if you cut your daily intake by 500 calories ($500 \times 7 = 3,500$ calories, or the equivalent of 1 pound of fat).

The estimated daily caloric figure is only a target guideline for weight control. Periodic readjustments are necessary because individuals differ, and the estimated daily cost changes as you lose weight and modify your exercise habits.

To determine the target caloric intake to lose weight, multiply your current weight by 5 and subtract

> **Weight loss should be gradual and not abrupt. One to two pounds per week are recommended in conjunction with permanent behavioral changes that will promote permanent weight management.**

this amount from the total caloric requirement (2,640 in our example) with exercise. For our moderately active male example, this would mean reducing intake to 1,840 calories per day to lose weight ($160 \times 5 = 800$ and $2,640 - 800 = 1,840$ calories).

This final caloric intake to lose weight should never be below 1,200 calories for women or 1,500 for men. If distributed properly over the various food groups, these figures are the lowest caloric intakes that provide the necessary nutrients the body needs. In terms of percentages of total calories, the daily distribution should

The establishment of healthy eating patterns start at a young age.

© Fitness & Wellness, Inc.

TABLE **9.4**	Grams of Fat at 10%, 20%, and 30% of Total Calories for Selected Energy Intakes		
	Grams of Fat		
Caloric Intake	10%	20%	30%
1,200	13	27	40
1,300	14	29	43
1,400	16	31	47
1,500	17	33	50
1,600	18	36	53
1,700	19	38	57
1,800	20	40	60
1,900	21	42	63
2,000	22	44	67
2,100	23	47	70
2,200	24	49	73
2,300	26	51	77
2,400	27	53	80
2,500	28	56	83
2,600	29	58	87
2,700	30	60	90
2,800	31	62	93
2,900	32	64	97
3,000	33	67	100

be approximately 60 percent carbohydrates (mostly complex carbohydrates), less than 30 percent fat, and about 12 percent protein.

Many experts believe a person can take off weight more efficiently by reducing the amount of daily fat intake to 10 to 20 percent of the total daily caloric intake. Because 1 gram of fat supplies more than twice the amount of calories that carbohydrates and protein do, the general tendency when someone eats less fat is to consume fewer calories.

Further, it takes only 3 to 5 percent of ingested calories to store fat as fat, whereas it takes approximately 25 percent of ingested calories to convert carbohydrates to fat. Other research indicates that if people eat the same number of calories as carbohydrate or fat, those on the fat diet will store more fat. Successful weight-loss programs allow only small amounts of fat in the diet.

Many people have trouble adhering to a 10- to 20-percent fat–calorie diet. During weight loss periods, however, you are strongly encouraged to do so. Start with a 20 percent fat–calorie diet. Refer to Table 9.4 to aid you in determining the grams of fat at 10 percent, 20 percent, and 30 percent of the total calories for selected energy intakes. Also, use the form provided in Figure 8.14 (page 215) to monitor your daily fat intake.

The time of day when food is consumed also may play a part in weight reduction. A study conducted at the Aerobics Research Institute in Dallas, Texas, indicated that when a person is on a diet, weight is lost most effectively if the person consumes most of the calories before 1:00 P.M. and not during the evening meal. The institute recommends that, when a person is attempting to lose weight, intake should consist of a minimum of 25 percent of the total daily calories for breakfast, 50 percent for lunch, and 25 percent or less at dinner.

Other experts have reported that, if most of the daily calories are consumed during one meal, the body may perceive that something is wrong and will slow down the metabolism so it can store more calories in the form of fat. Also, eating most of the calories during one meal causes a person to go hungry the rest of the day, making it more difficult to adhere to the diet.

Consuming most of the calories earlier in the day seems helpful in losing weight and also in managing atherosclerosis. The time of day when most of the fats and cholesterol are consumed can influence blood lipids and coronary heart disease. Peak digestion time following a heavy

Successful weight management is accomplished by making a lifetime commitment to physical activity and proper food selection.

meal is about 7 hours after that meal. If most lipids are consumed during the evening meal, digestion peaks while the person is sound asleep, when the metabolism is at its lowest rate. Consequently, the body may not metabolize fats and cholesterol as well, leading to a higher blood lipid count and increasing the risk for atherosclerosis and coronary heart disease.

Before you proceed with the development of a thorough weight-loss program, take a moment to identify in Figure 9.7 your current stage of change as it pertains to your recommended body weight. If applicable—that is, if you are not at recommended weight—list also the processes and techniques for change that you will use to accomplish your goal. In Figure 9.8 you can outline your exercise program for weight management.

Monitoring Your Diet With Daily Food Logs

To help you monitor and adhere to your diet plan, you may use the daily food logs provided in Figures 9.9 to 9.12. Before using any of these forms, make a master copy for your files so you can make future copies as needed. Guidelines are provided for 1,200-, 1,500-, 1,800-, and 2,000-calorie diet plans. These plans have been developed based on the Food Guide Pyramid and the Dietary Guidelines for Americans to meet the Recommended Dietary Allowances.[17] The objective is to meet (not exceed) the number of servings allowed for each diet plan. Each time you eat a serving of a certain food, record it in the appropriate box.

To lose weight, you should use the diet plan that most closely approximates your target caloric intake. The plan is based on the following caloric allowances for each food group:

- Bread, cereal, rice, and pasta group: 80 calories per serving.
- Fruit group: 60 calories per serving.
- Vegetable group: 25 calories per serving.
- Milk, yogurt, and cheese group (use low-fat products): 120 calories per serving.
- Meat, poultry, fish, dry beans, eggs, and nuts group: Use low-fat (300 calories per serving) frozen entrees or an equivalent amount if you prepare your own main dish (see discussion that follows).

As you start your diet plan, pay particular attention to food serving sizes. To find out what counts as one serving, refer to the Food Guide Pyramid (see Figure 8.1, page 193). Take care with cup and glass sizes. A standard cup is 8 ounces, but most glasses

nowadays contain between 12 and 16 ounces. If you drink 12 ounces of fruit juice, in essence you are getting two servings of fruit because a standard serving is 3/4 cup of juice.

Read food labels carefully to compare the caloric value of the serving listed on the label with the caloric guidelines provided previously. Here are some examples:

- One slice of standard white bread has about 80 calories. A plain bagel may have 200 to 350 calories. Although it is low in fat, a 350-calorie bagel is equivalent to almost 4 servings in the bread, cereal, rice, and pasta group.
- The standard serving size listed on the food label for most cereals is 1 cup. As you read the nutrition information, however, you find that for the same cup of cereal, one type of cereal has 120 calories whereas another cereal has 200 calories. Because a standard serving in the bread, cereal, rice and pasta group is 80 calories, the first cereal would be 1¼ servings and the second one 2¼ servings.
- A medium-size fruit usually is considered 1 serving. Large fruits could provide as many as 3 servings.
- In the milk, yogurt, and cheese groups, 1 serving represents 120 calories. A cup of whole milk has about 160 calories, whereas a cup of skim milk contains 88 calories. A cup of whole milk, therefore, would provide 1⅓ servings in this food group.

To be more accurate with caloric intake and to simplify meal preparation, use commercially prepared low-fat frozen entrees as the main dish for lunch and dinner meals (only one entree per day for the 1,200-calorie diet plan—see Figure 9.9). Look for entrees that provide about 300 calories and no more than 6 grams of fat per entree. These two entrees can be used as selections for the meat, poultry, fish, dry beans, eggs, and nuts group and will provide most of the daily protein requirement for the body. Along with each entree, supplement the meal with some of your servings from the other food groups. This diet plan has been used successfully in weight-loss research programs.[18] If you choose not to use these low-fat entrees, prepare a similar meal using 3 ounces (cooked) of lean meat, poultry, or fish with additional vegetables, rice, or pasta, which will provide 300 calories with fewer than 6 grams of fat per dish.

In your daily logs, be sure to record the precise amount in each serving. If you choose to do so, you can run a computerized nutrient analysis to verify your caloric intake and food distribution pattern (percent of total calories from carbohydrate, fat, and protein).

FIGURE 9.6 Computation form for daily caloric requirement.

Name:_____ Date: _____

Course: _____ Section: _____ Gender:_____ Age:_____

I. Computation Form for Daily Caloric Requirement

A. Current body weight in pounds. . . . . [ ]

B. Caloric requirement per pound of body weight (use Table 9.2) . . . . [ ]

C. Typical daily caloric requirement without exercise to maintain body weight (A × B) . . . . [ ]

D. Selected physical activity (e.g., jogging)[a] . . . . [ ]

E. Number of exercise sessions per week . . . . [ ]

F. Duration of exercise session (in minutes) . . . . [ ]

G. Total weekly exercise time in minutes (E × F) . . . . [ ]

H. Average daily exercise time in minutes (G ÷ 7) . . . . [ ]

I. Caloric expenditure per pound per minute (cal/lb/min) of physical activity (use Table 9.3) . . . . [ ]

J. Total calories burned per minute of physical activity (A × I) . . . . [ ]

K. Average daily calories burned as a result of the exercise program (H × J) . . . . [ ]

L. Total daily caloric requirement with exercise to maintain body weight (C + K) . . . . [ ]

M. Number of calories to subtract from daily requirement to achieve a negative caloric balance
(multiply current body weight by 5) . . . . [ ]

N. Target caloric intake to lose weight (L − M)[b] . . . . [ ]

[a] If more than one physical activity is selected, you will need to estimate the average daily calories burned as a result of each additional activity (steps D through K) and add all of these figures to L above.

[b] This figure should never be below 1,200 calories for women or 1,500 calories for men. See Figures 9.9 through 9.12 for the 1,200-, 1,500-, 1,800-, and 2,000-calorie-diet plans.

FIGURE 9.7 Stage of change for recommended body weight.

1. Using Figure 2.4 (page 45) and Table 2.3 (page 43), identify your current stage of change regarding recommended body weight: [ ]

2. How much weight do you want to lose? [ ]   Is it a realistic goal? [ ]

3. Based on the processes and techniques of change discussed in Chapter 2, indicate what you can do to help yourself implement a weight management program.

_____

_____

_____

FIGURE 9.8 Exercise program selection.

Name: _____ Date: _____

Course: _____ Section: _____ Gender: _____ Age: _____

1. How much effort are you willing to put into reaching your weight loss goal?

_____

_____

2. Indicate your feelings about participating in an exercise program.

_____

_____

3. Will you commit to participate in a combined aerobic and strength-training program?*　　Yes ☐　　No ☐

    If your answer is "Yes," proceed to the next question; if you answered "No," please review Chapters 3 through 8 again.

4. List aerobic activities you enjoy or may enjoy doing.

_____

_____

5. Select one or two aerobic activities in which you will participate regularly.

    ┌─────────────────────────┐   ┌─────────────────────────┐
    └─────────────────────────┘   └─────────────────────────┘

6. List facilities available to you where you can carry out the aerobic and strength-training programs.

_____

_____

7. Indicate days and times you will set aside for your aerobic and strength-training program (5 to 6 days per week should be devoted to aerobic exercise and 1 to 3 nonconsecutive days per week to strength training).

    Monday: _____

    Tuesday: _____

    Wednesday: _____

    Thursday: _____

    Friday: _____

    Saturday: _____

    Sunday: A complete day of rest once a week is recommended to allow your body to fully recover from exercise.

conclusion　　Briefly describe whether you think you can meet the goals of your aerobic and strength training program. What obstacles will you have to overcome and how will you overcome them?

_____

_____

_____

* Flexibility programs are necessary for injury prevention, adequate fitness, and good health but do not help with weight loss. Stretching exercises can be conducted regularly during the cool-down phase of your aerobic and strength-training programs (see Chapter 6).

FIGURE 9.9 Daily food intake record: 1,200-calorie diet plan.

Name: _____ Date: _____

Course: _____ Section: _____ Gender: _____ Age: _____

Instructions:

The objective of the diet plan is to meet (not exceed) the number of servings allowed for the food groups listed. Each time you eat a food, record it in the space provided for each group, along with the appropriate serving size. Refer to the Food Guide Pyramid to find out what counts as one serving for each group listed (see Figure 8.1, page 193). Instead of the meat, poultry, fish, dry beans, eggs, and nuts group, you are allowed to have a commercially available low-fat frozen entree for your main meal (this entree should provide no more than 300 calories and less than 6 grams of fat). You can make additional copies of this form as needed.

Bread, Cereal, Rice, Pasta Group (80 calories/serving): 6 servings

1 _____

2 _____

3 _____

4 _____

5 _____

6 _____

Vegetable Group (25 calories/serving): 3 servings

1 _____

2 _____

3 _____

Fruit Group (60 calories/serving): 2 servings

1 _____

2 _____

Milk Group (120 calories/serving, use low-fat milk and low-fat milk products): 2 servings

1 _____

2 _____

Low-fat Frozen Entree (300 calories and less than 6 grams of fat): 1 serving

1 _____

FIGURE 9.10 Daily food intake record: 1,500-calorie diet plan.

Name: _____ Date: _____

Course: _____ Section: _____ Gender: _____ Age: _____

Instructions:

The objective of the diet plan is to meet (not exceed) the number of servings allowed for the food groups listed. Each time that you eat a food, record it in the space provided for each group, along with the appropriate serving size. Refer to the Food Guide Pyramid to find out what counts as one serving for each group listed (see Figure 8.1, page 193). Instead of the meat, poultry, fish, dry beans, eggs, and nuts group, you are allowed to have two commercially available low-fat frozen entrees for two of your meals (these entrees should provide no more than 300 calories and less than 6 grams of fat). You can make additional copies of this form as needed.

Bread, Cereal, Rice, Pasta Group (80 calories/serving): 6 servings

1 _____
2 _____
3 _____
4 _____
5 _____
6 _____

Vegetable Group (25 calories/serving): 3 servings

1 _____
2 _____
3 _____

Fruit Group (60 calories/serving): 2 servings

1 _____
2 _____

Milk Group (120 calories/serving, use low-fat milk and low-fat milk products): 2 servings

1 _____
2 _____

Two Low-fat Frozen Entrees (300 calories and less than 6 grams of fat each): 2 servings

1 _____
2 _____

FIGURE 9.11 Daily food intake record: 1,800-calorie diet plan.

Name:_____ Date: _____

Course: _____ Section: _____ Gender:_____ Age: _____

Instructions:

The objective of the diet plan is to meet (not exceed) the number of servings allowed for the food groups listed. Each time that you eat a food, record it in the space provided for each group, along with the appropriate serving size. Refer to the Food Guide Pyramid to find out what counts as one serving for each group listed (see Figure 8.1, page 193). Instead of the meat, poultry, fish, dry beans, eggs, and nuts group, you are allowed to have two commercially available low-fat frozen entrees for two of your meals (these entrees should provide no more than 300 calories and less than 6 grams of fat). You can make additional copies of this form as needed.

Bread, Cereal, Rice, Pasta Group (80 calories/serving): 8 servings

1	_____	5	_____
2	_____	6	_____
3	_____	7	_____
4	_____	8	_____

Vegetable Group (25 calories/serving): 5 servings

1 _____
2 _____
3 _____
4 _____
5 _____

Fruit Group (60 calories/serving): 3 servings

1 _____
2 _____
3 _____

Milk Group (120 calories/serving, use low-fat milk and low-fat milk products): 2 servings

1 _____
2 _____

Two Low-fat Frozen Entrees (300 calories and less than 6 grams of fat each): 2 servings

1 _____
2 _____

FIGURE 9.12 Daily food intake record: 2,000-calorie diet plan.

Name: _____ Date: _____

Course: _____ Section: _____ Gender: _____ Age: _____

Instructions:

The objective of the diet plan is to meet (not exceed) the number of servings allowed for the food groups listed. Each time that you eat a food, record it in the space provided for each group, along with the appropriate serving size. Refer to the Food Guide Pyramid to find out what counts as one serving for each group listed (see Figure 8.1, page 193). Instead of the meat, poultry, fish, dry beans, eggs, and nuts group, you are allowed to have two commercially available low-fat frozen entrees for two of your meals (these entrees should provide no more than 300 calories and less than 6 grams of fat). You can make additional copies of this form as needed.

Bread, Cereal, Rice, Pasta Group (80 calories/serving): 10 servings

1 _____   6 _____

2 _____   7 _____

3 _____   8 _____

4 _____   9 _____

5 _____   10 _____

Vegetable Group (25 calories/serving): 5 servings

1 _____

2 _____

3 _____

4 _____

5 _____

Fruit Group (60 calories/serving): 4 servings

1 _____

2 _____

3 _____

4 _____

Milk Group (120 calories/serving, use low-fat milk and low-fat milk products): 2 servings

1 _____

2 _____

Two Low-fat Frozen Entrees (300 calories and less than 6 grams of fat each): 2 servings

1 _____

2 _____

BEHAVIOR MODIFICATION AND ADHERENCE TO A WEIGHT MANAGEMENT PROGRAM

Achieving and maintaining recommended body composition is by no means impossible, but it does require desire and commitment. If weight management is to become a priority in life, people must realize that they have to transform their behavior to some extent.

Modifying old habits and developing new, positive behaviors take time. Individuals have applied the following management techniques to change detrimental behavior successfully and adhere to a positive lifetime weight-control program. In developing a retraining program, people are not expected to incorporate all of the strategies listed, but should note the ones that apply to them. The form provided in Figure 9.13 (page 269) will allow you to evaluate and monitor your own weight management behaviors.

> **The desire to lose weight must become more important than the desire to overeat or not exercise.**

- Make a commitment to change. The first necessary ingredient is the desire to modify your behavior. You need to stop precontemplating and contemplating change and get going! The reasons for change must be more compelling than those for continuing your present lifestyle patterns. You must accept that you have a problem and decide by yourself whether you really want to change. If you are sincerely committed, the chances for success are enhanced already.

- Set realistic goals. Most people with a weight problem would like the pounds to melt away, failing to realize that the weight problem developed over several years. A sound weight reduction and maintenance program can be accomplished only by establishing new lifetime eating and exercise habits, both of which take time to develop. In setting a realistic long-term goal, short-term objectives also should be planned. The long-term goal may be to decrease body fat to 20 percent of total body weight. The short-term objective may be a 1 percent decrease in body fat each month. Objectives like these allow for regular evaluation and help maintain motivation and renewed commitment to attain the long-term goal.

- Incorporate exercise into the program. Choosing enjoyable activities, places, times, equipment, and people to work with helps a person adhere to an exercise program. Details on developing a complete exercise program are given in Chapters 4, 5, and 6.

- Differentiate hunger and appetite. Hunger is the actual physical need for food. Appetite is a desire for food, usually triggered by factors such as stress, habit, boredom, depression, availability of food, or just the thought of food itself. People should eat only when they have a physical need. In this regard, developing and sticking to a regular meal pattern help control hunger.

- Eat less fat. Each gram of fat provides 9 calories, and protein and carbohydrates provide only 4.

Exercising with other people and in different places helps maintain exercise adherence.

In essence, you can eat more food on a low-fat diet because you consume fewer calories with each meal.

- Pay attention to calories. Some people think that because a certain food is low in fat, they can eat as much as they want. Entire boxes of fat-free cookies and bags of pretzels have been consumed under this pretense. A homemade chocolate-chip cookie may have 100 calories, whereas a low-fat one may have 50. Simple math will tell you that eating one homemade cookie is better than eating a half dozen low-fat ones. When reading food labels, don't just look at the fat content, but pay attention to calories as well.

- Cut unnecessary items from your diet. Many people regularly drink a 140-calorie can of soda pop (or more) each day. Substituting a glass of water would cut 51,100 (140×365) calories yearly from the diet—the equivalent of 14.6 ($51,000 \div 3,500$) pounds of fat.

- Add foods to your diet that reduce cravings.[19] Many people have a biological imbalance of insulin. Insulin helps the body use and conserve energy. Some people produce so much insulin that their bodies can't use it all. This imbalance leads to an overpowering craving for carbohydrates. As they eat more carbohydrates, even more insulin is released. Foods that reduce cravings include eggs, red meat, fish, poultry, cheese, tofu, oils, fats, and nonstarchy vegetables such as lettuce, green beans, peppers, asparagus, broccoli, mushrooms, and Brussels sprouts. If you watch your portion sizes, eating foods that reduce cravings at regular meals and for snacks helps to decrease the intense desire for carbohydrates, prevent overeating, and aid with weight loss.

- Avoid automatic eating. Many people associate certain daily activities with eating. For example, people may eat while cooking, watching television, or reading. Most of the time the foods consumed in these situations lack nutritional value or are high in sugar and fat.

- Stay busy. People tend to eat more when they sit around and do nothing. Occupying the mind and body with activities not associated with eating helps take away the desire to eat. Some options are walking; cycling; playing sports; gardening; sewing; or visiting a library, a museum, or a park. To break the routine of life, you might develop other skills and interests or try something new and exciting.

Supersized foods create supersized people.

- Plan meals ahead of time. Sensible shopping is necessary to accomplish this objective. Always shop on a full stomach, because hungry shoppers tend to buy unhealthy foods impulsively—and then snack on the way home. The shopping list should include whole-grain breads and cereals, fruits and vegetables, low-fat milk and dairy products, lean meats, fish, and poultry.

- Cook wisely.
  - Use less fat and fewer refined foods in food preparation.
  - Trim all visible fat from meats and remove skin from poultry before cooking.
  - Skim the fat off gravies and soups.
  - Bake, broil, boil, or steam instead of frying.
  - Sparingly use butter, cream, mayonnaise, and salad dressings.
  - Avoid coconut oil, palm oil, and cocoa butter.
  - Prepare plenty of foods that contain fiber.
  - Include whole-grain breads and cereals, vegetables, and legumes in most meals.
  - Eat fruits for dessert.
  - Stay away from soda pop, fruit juices, and fruit-flavored drinks.
  - In addition to using less sugar, cut down on other refined carbohydrates such as corn syrup, malt sugar, dextrose, and fructose.
  - Drink plenty of water—at least six glasses a day.

- Do not serve more food than you should eat. Measure the food in portions and keep serving dishes away from the table. In this way you will eat less, have a harder time getting seconds, and have less appetite because the food is not visible. People should not be forced to eat when they are satisfied (including children after they already have had a healthy, nutritious serving).

- Try "junior size" instead of "super size." Use smaller plates, bowls, cups, and glasses. Try eating half as much food as you commonly eat. Over the years, the sizes of dishes and glasses have gotten bigger. Consequently, people serve and eat a lot more food than they need. If you use a smaller plate, it will look like more food and you'll tend to eat less. Watch for portion sizes at restaurants as well. Plate and portion sizes at restaurants now are so large that people overeat and still end up with leftovers to take home. Similarly, the original bottle of Coca-Cola contained 6.5 ounces. Machines now routinely dispense 20-ounce bottles, and convenience stores sell 64-ounce "buckets" of soda pop (about 750 calories). Supersized foods create supersized people.

- Eat out infrequently. Research indicates that the more often people of all ages eat out, the more body fat they have. People who eat out 6 or more times per week consume an average of about 300 extra calories per day and 30 percent more fat than those who eat out less often.

- Eat slowly and at the table only. Eating is one of the pleasures of life, and we need to take time to enjoy it. Eating on the run is not good because the body doesn't have enough time to "register" nutritive and caloric consumption, and people overeat before the body perceives the fullness signal. Eating at the table also forces people to take time out to eat, and it deters snacking between meals, primarily because of the extra time and effort required to sit down and eat. When people are done eating, they should not sit around the table but, rather, clean up and put away the food to avoid snacking.

- Avoid social binges. Social gatherings tend to entice self-defeating behavior. Visual imagery might help before attending social gatherings. Plan ahead and visualize yourself there. Do not feel pressured to eat or drink and don't rationalize in these situations. Choose low-calorie foods and entertain yourself with other activities, such as dancing and talking.

- Do not raid the refrigerator or the cookie jar. In these tempting situations, take control. Stop and think. Do not bring high-calorie, high-sugar, or high-fat foods into the house. If they are there already, store them where they are hard to get to or see. If they are out of sight or not readily available, the temptation is less. Keeping food in places such as the garage and basement discourages people from taking the time and effort to get them. By no means should you try to eliminate treats entirely, but all things should be done in moderation.

- Avoid evening food raids. Most people with weight problems do really well during the day but then "lose it" at night. Excessive snacking following the evening meal is a common pitfall. Stay busy after your evening meal. Go for a short walk and get to bed earlier. In most cases the intense desire for food that you get during the evening hours disappears following a good night's rest.

- Practice stress-management techniques (discussed in Chapter 12). Many people snack and increase food consumption in stressful situations. Eating is not a stress-releasing activity and, instead, can aggravate the problem if weight control is an issue.

- Get support. People who receive support from friends, relatives, and formal support groups are much more likely to lose weight and maintain weight loss than those without such support. The more support you receive, the better off you will be.

- Monitor changes and reward accomplishments. Feedback on fat loss and lean tissue gain is a reward in itself. Awareness of changes in body composition also helps reinforce new behaviors. Being able to exercise without interruption for 15, 20, 30, or 60 minutes; swimming a certain distance; running a mile—all these accomplishments deserve recognition. Meeting objectives calls for rewards that are not related to eating: new clothing, a tennis racquet, a bicycle, exercise shoes, or something else that is special and you would not have acquired otherwise.

- Prepare for slips. Most people will slip and occasionally splurge. If that happens, do not despair and give up. Reevaluate and continue with your efforts. An occasional slip will not make much difference in the long run.

- Think positive. Avoid negative thoughts about how difficult changing past behaviors might be. Instead, think of the benefits you will reap, such as feeling, looking, and functioning better, plus enjoying better health and improving the quality of life. Avoid negative environments and people who will not be supportive.

IN CONCLUSION

There is no simple and quick way to take off excess body fat and keep it off for good. Weight management is accomplished by making a lifetime commitment to physical activity and proper food selection. When taking part in a weight (fat) reduction program, people also have to decrease their caloric intake moderately and implement strategies to modify unhealthy eating behaviors.

During the process, relapses into past negative behaviors are almost inevitable. The three most common reasons for relapse are the following:

1. Stress-related factors (such as major life changes, depression, job changes, illness).

2. Social reasons (entertaining, eating out, business travel).

3. Self-enticing behaviors (placing yourself in a situation to see how much you can get away with ("One small taste won't hurt," leading to "I'll eat just one slice," and finally, "I haven't done well, so I might as well eat some more").

Making mistakes is human and does not necessarily mean failure. Failure comes to those who give up and do not build upon previous experiences. Success comes with developing skills that will prevent self-defeating behaviors in the future. Where there's a will, there's a way, and those who persist will reap the rewards.

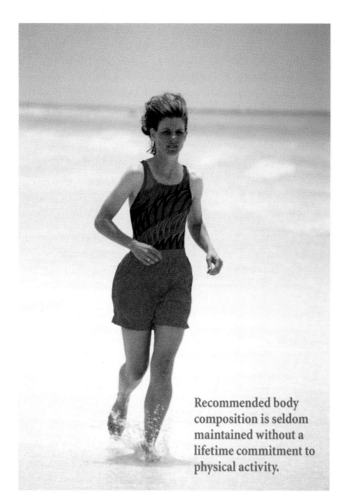

Recommended body composition is seldom maintained without a lifetime commitment to physical activity.

WEB INTERACTIVE

Shape Up America! Maintenance Center

This excellent fitness and weight management site is endorsed by former U.S. Surgeon General C. Everett Koop, M.D., and describes how to select a safe weight loss plan that combines exercise and healthy diet. Also included are suggestions for lifestyle changes such as controlling mood eating, stressors, and binge eating to promote long-term weight management.

http://shapeup.org/support/index.htm

Weight Loss and Control

This site, sponsored by the National Institute of Diabetes & Digestive & Kidney Diseases, features diverse articles on weight loss and control, links to other organizations and bibliographic resources, current research, and statistics.

http://www.niddk.nih.gov/health/nutri/nutri.htm

Obesity Education Initiative: Aim for a Healthy Weight

This site, sponsored by the National Heart, Lung, and Blood Institute, provides an easy-to-read guide to weight management by assessing your risk and providing tips to successfully control your weight.

http://www.wellweb.com/nutri/weight_management.htm

Eating Disorders

This comprehensive site, sponsored by the National Institute of Health, features links to information on clinical trials sponsored by the NIH, news articles, treatments, and other organizations for other research options.

http://www.nlm.nih.gov/medlineplus/eatingdisorders.html

INTERACTIVE SITES:

Count Your Calories Because Your Calories Count

This interactive site, sponsored by Wake Forest University Baptist Medical Center, features a four-step assessment of your diet, including "How's Your Diet?" "Fit or Not Quiz," "Calorie Counter," and "Drive-Thru Diet." There is also an "Eating Disorder Quiz."

http://www.bgsm.edu/nutrition/in.html

The Shape Up America! Nutrition Center

is designed to help you understand nutritional requirements for active people. The Daily Calorie Goal is an interactive assessment that will give you an estimate of the number of calories you need at your current level of activity to maintain your weight. You will also find the percentage of protein, carbohydrate, and fat calories you should have in your diet to maximize your workout. To learn how these percentages translate to foods, you can also visit the Food Guide Pyramid link and even test your knowledge by taking the Food Guide Pyramid quiz.

http://www.shapeup.org/fitness/nutrition/fset3.htm

n*tes

1. A. Must et al., "The Disease Burden Associated with Overweight and Obesity," *Journal of the American Medical Association* 282 (1999): 1523–1529.

2. National Institutes of Health, *Clinical Guidelines on the Identification, Evaluation, and Treatment of Overweight and Obesity in Adults*, NIH Publication No. 98-4083 (Washington, DC: NIH, 1998).

3. K. M. Flegal, M. D. Carrol, R. J. Kuczmarski, and C. L. Johnson, "Overweight and Obesity in the United States: Prevalence and Trends, 1960–1994," *International Journal of Obesity and Related Metabolic Disorders* 22 (1998): 39–47.

4. M. K. Serdula et al., "Prevalence of Attempting Weight Loss and Strategies for Controlling Weight," *Journal of the American Medical Association* 282 (1999): 1353–1358.

5. R. Sturm and K. B. Wells, "Does Obesity Contribute as much to Morbidity as Poverty or Smoking," *Public Health* 115 (2001): 229–235.

6. C. E. Barlow, H. W. Kohl, III, L. W. Gibbons, and S. N. Blair, "Physical Fitness, Mortality, and Obesity," *International Journal of Obesity* 19 (1996): S41–44.

7. Dr. Steven Lichtman and associates, "Discrepancy Between Self-Reported and Actual Caloric Intake and Exercise in Obese Subjects," *New England Journal of Medicine* 327 (1992): 1893–1898.

8. American Psychiatric Association, *Diagnostic and Statistical Manual of Mental Disorders* (Washington, DC: APA, 1994).

9. See note 7.

10. R. L. Leibel, M. Rosenbaum, and J. Hirsh, "Changes in Energy Expenditure Resulting from Altered Body Weight," *New England Journal of Medicine* 332 (1995): 621–628.

11. "Olestra: Just Say No," *University of California at Berkeley Wellness Letter* (Palm Coast, FL: The Editors, February 1996).

12. R. J. Shepard, *Alive Man: The Physiology of Physical Activity* (Springfield, IL: Charles C Thomas, 1975): 484–488.

13. J. H. Wilmore, "Exercise, Obesity, and Weight Control," *Physical Activity and Fitness Research Digest* (Washington DC: President's Council on Physical Fitness & Sports, 1994).

14. K. N. Pavlou, S. Krey, and W. P. Steffe, "Exercise as an Adjunct to Weight Loss and Maintenance in Moderately Obese Subjects," *American Journal of Clinical Nutrition* 49 (1989): 1115–1123.

15. W. W. Campbell, M. C. Crim, V. R. Young, and W. J. Evans, "Increased Energy Requirements and Changes in Body Composition with Resistance Training in Older Adults," *American Journal of Clinical Nutrition* 60 (1994): 167–175.

16. A. Tremblay, J. A. Simoneau, and C. Bouchard. "Impact of Exercise Intensity on Body Fatness and Skeletal Muscle Metabolism." *Metabolism* 43 (1994): 814–818.

17. U. S. Department of Health and Human Services: Department of Agriculture. *Nutrition and Your Health: Dietary Guidelines for Americans*, Home and Garden Bulletin 232 (2000).

U. S. Department of Agriculture, Human Nutrition Information Service, *The Food Guide Pyramid*, Home and Garden Bulletin 252 (Dec. 1992).

National Academy Press, Food and Nutrition Board, *Recommended Dietary Allowances*, (Washington DC: National Academy Press, 1989).

18. W. W. K. Hoeger, C. Harris, E. M. Long, and D. R. Hopkins, "Four-Week Supplementation With a Natural Dietary Compound Produces Favorable Changes in Body Composition," *Advances in Therapy* 15, no. 5 (1998): 305–313.

W. W. K. Hoeger, C. Harris, E. M. Long, R. L. Kjorstad, M. Welch, T. L. Hafner, D. R. Hopkins, "Dietary Supplementation with Chromium Picolinate/L-Carnitine Complex in Combination with Diet and Exercise Enhances Body Composition," *Journal of the American Nutraceutical Association* 2, no. 2 (1999): 40–45.

19. R. Heller and R. Heller, "How The Weight-Loss Scientists Lost Their Weight: You Can, Too," *Bottom Line/Personal Health* 18, no. 11 (1997): 9–10.

 Suggested Readings

▪ American Diabetes Association and American Dietetic Association. *Exchange Lists for Meal Planning.* Chicago: American Dietetic Association and American Diabetes Association, 1995.

▪ Bouchard, C., et al. *Physical Activity, Fitness, and Health.* Champaign, IL: Human Kinetics, 1994.

▪ Bray, G. "The Nutrient Balance Approach to Obesity." *Nutrition Today* 28 (May/June 1993): 13–18.

▪ Broeder, C. E., K. A. Burrhus, L. S. Svanevick, and J. H. Wilmore. "The Effects of Either High-Intensity Resistance or Endurance Training on Resting Metabolic Rate." *American Journal of Clinical Nutrition* 55 (1992): 802–810.

▪ Broeder, C. E., et al. "The Metabolic Consequences of Low and Moderate Intensity Exercise With or Without Feeding in Lean and Borderline Obese Males." *International Journal of Obesity* 15 (1990): 95–104.

▪ Brownell, K. *The Learn Program for Weight Control.* Dallas: American Health Publishing, 1997.

▪ Clark, N. "How to Gain Weight Healthfully." *Physician and Sportsmedicine* 19 (1991): 53.

▪ Clarkson, P. M. "Nutritional Supplements for Weight Gain." *Gatorade Sports Science Institute: Sports Science Exchange* 11 (1998): 68.

▪ Clarkson, P. M. "The Skinny on Weight Loss Supplements and Drugs: Winning the War Against Fat." *ACSM's Health and Fitness Journal* (1998): 18.

▪ Grundy, S. M., et al. "Physical Activity in the Prevention and Treatment of Obesity." *Medicine and Science in Sports and Exercise* 31 (1999): S497–S667.

- Kassirer, J. P., and M. Angell. "Losing Weight—An Ill-fated New Year's Resolution." *New England Journal of Medicine* 338 (1998): 52–54.

- Mokdad, A. H., et al. "The Spread of the Obesity Epidemic in the United States, 1991–1998." *Journal of the American Medical Association* 282 (1999): 1519–1522.

- National Institutes of Health. *Clinical Guidelines on the Identification, Evaluation, and Treatment of Overweight and Obesity in Adults.* NIH Publication No. 98-4083. Washington, DC: NIH, 1998.

- Parr, R. B., and L. Capozzi. "Counseling Patients About Physical Activity." *Journal of the American Academy of Physician Assistants* 10 (1997): 45–49.

- Prentice, A., et al. "Effects of Weight Cycling on Body Composition." *American Journal of Clinical Nutrition* 56 (1992): 209S–216S.

- Robison, J., et al. "Obesity, Weight Loss, and Health." *Journal of the American Dietetic Association* 93 (1993): 445–449.

- Rolls, B., and D. Shide. "The Influence of Dietary Fat on Food Intake and Body Weight." *Nutrition Reviews* 50 (1992): 283–290.

- Rosenbaum, M., R. L. Leibel, and J. Hirsh. "Obesity." *New England Journal of Medicine* 337 (1997): 396–406.

- Sjüdin, A. M., et al. "The Influence of Physical Activity on BMR." *Medicine and Science in Sports and Exercise* 28 (1996): 85–91.

- Stefanick, M. "Exercise and Weight Control." *Exercise and Sport Sciences Review* 21 (1993): 363–396.

- Stunkard, A. J., et al. "An Adoption Study of Human Obesity." *New England Journal of Medicine* 314 (1986): 193–198.

- Wadden, T. A., T. B. Van Itallie, and G. L. Blackburn. "Responsible and Irresponsible Use of Very-Low-Calorie Diets in the Treatment of Obesity." *Journal of the American Medical Association* 263 (1990): 83–85.

- Wilmore, J. "Exercise, Obesity, and Weight Control." *Physical Activity and Fitness Research Digest* 1 (May, 1994): 1–8.

Cardiovascular Disease Prevention

Objectives

Define cardiovascular disease and coronary heart disease.

Understand the importance of a healthy lifestyle in preventing cardiovascular disease.

Understand the major risk factors that lead to the development of coronary heart disease, including physical inactivity, hypertension, smoking, and abnormal cholesterol profile.

Assess your own risk of developing coronary heart disease.

Become acquainted with a comprehensive program for reducing coronary heart disease risk and managing overall risk for cardiovascular disease.

271

The most prevalent degenerative conditions in the United States are **cardiovascular diseases**. About 20 percent of the population have some form of cardiovascular disease. Death rates are higher in men than in women (see Figure 10.1). One in three men and one in ten women will develop a major cardiovascular problem before age 60.[1] Based on 2000 statistics, 38.8 percent of all deaths in the United States were attributable to heart and blood vessel disease.[2]

Some examples of cardiovascular diseases are coronary heart disease, **peripheral vascular disease**, congenital heart disease, rheumatic heart disease, atherosclerosis, strokes, high blood pressure, and congestive heart failure. According to estimates, if all deaths from the major cardiovascular diseases were eliminated, life expectancy in the United States would increase by about 10 years.[3]

The estimated cost of heart and blood vessel disease in the United States exceeded $286 billion in 1998. About 1.1 million people have heart attacks each year, and more than 350,000 of them die as a result. More than half of these deaths occur within 1 hour of the onset of symptoms, before the person reaches the hospital.[4]

Although heart and blood vessel disease is still the number-one health problem in the United States, the

FIGURE 10.2 Incidence of cardiovascular disease in the United States for selected years: 1900–2000.

incidence declined by 28 percent between 1960 and 2000 (see Figure 10.2), in large part because of health education. More people are now aware of the risk factors for cardiovascular disease and are changing their lifestyle to lower their potential risk for these diseases.

The heart and the coronary arteries are illustrated in Figure 10.3. The major form of cardiovascular disease is **coronary heart disease** (CHD), wherein the arteries that supply the heart muscle with oxygen and nutrients are narrowed by fatty deposits such as cholesterol and triglycerides. Narrowing of the coronary arteries diminishes the blood supply to the heart muscle, which can precipitate a heart attack.

CHD is the single leading cause of death in the United States, accounting for approximately 20 percent of all deaths and about half of all cardiovascular deaths[5]. More than half of the people who died suddenly from CHD had no previous symptoms of the disease. Further, approximately 80 percent of deaths from CHD in people under age 65 occur during the first heart attack. The risk of death is also greater in the least-educated segment of the population.[6] Almost all of the risk factors for CHD are preventable and reversible, therefore individuals can reduce their risk by adhering to a healthy lifestyle.

According to the American Heart Association, each year, more than 330,000 coronary bypass operations and 190,000 coronary **angioplasty** procedures are performed in the United States. Health-care costs for a coronary bypass average more than $44,000 and for an angioplasty procedure over $21,000—or about $11 billion per year for coronary heart disease surgery.

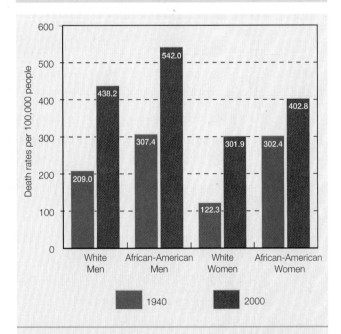

FIGURE 10.1 Death rates for cardiovascular disease in the United States, years 1940 and 2000.

SOURCE: American Heart Association, *Heart and Stroke Facts: 2000* (Statistical Supplement), Dallas: AHA, 1999.

FIGURE **10.3** The heart and its blood vessels.

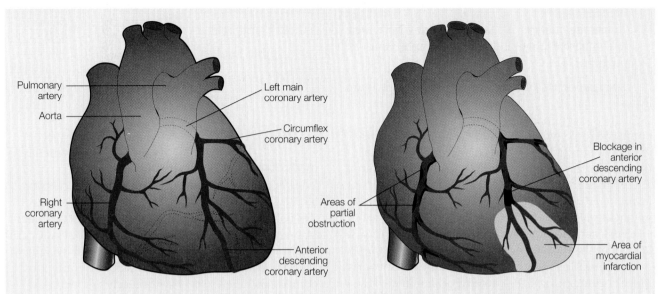

Normal Healthy Heart

Myocardial infarction (heart attack) as a result of acute reduction in blood flow through the anterior descending coronary artery

Signs of heart attack and stroke

These signs or symptoms may not all be present during a heart attack or a stroke. If any start to occur and last longer than a few minutes, do not delay, seek medical attention immediately. Call 911 or the emergency medical service (EMS) for an ambulance. If ambulance service is not available, immediately have someone drive you to the nearest hospital emergency room. Failure to do so may result in death.

Warning Signs of a Heart Attack

- Discomfort, pressure, fullness, squeezing, or pain in the middle of the chest that persists for several minutes. It may go away and return later.
- Pain that radiates to the shoulders, neck, or arms.
- Chest discomfort with lightheadedness, shortness of breath, nausea, sweating, or fainting.

Warning Signs of Stroke

- Sudden numbness or weakness of the face, arm, or leg—particularly on one side of the body.
- Sudden confusion, difficulty in speech or understanding.
- Sudden trouble seeing out of one or both eyes.
- Sudden trouble walking, dizziness, loss of balance or coordination.
- A sudden severe headache of unknown cause.

Adapted from American Heart Association, *Heart Stroke Facts*, Dallas: AHA, 1999.

CORONARY HEART DISEASE RISK PROFILE

Although genetic inheritance plays a role in CHD, the most important determinant is personal lifestyle. CHD risk factor analyses are administered to evaluate the impact of a person's lifestyle and genetic endowment as potential factors contributing to the development of coronary disease. The specific objectives of a CHD risk factor analysis are the following:

- To screen individuals who may be at risk for the disease.

Cardiovascular diseases The array of conditions that affect the heart and the blood vessels.

Peripheral vascular disease Narrowing of the peripheral blood vessels (excludes the cerebral and coronary arteries).

Coronary heart disease (CHD) Condition in which the arteries that supply the heart muscle with oxygen and nutrients are narrowed by fatty deposits, such as cholesterol and triglycerides.

Angioplasty A procedure in which a balloon-tipped catheter is inserted, then inflated, to widen the inner lumen of one or more arteries.

- To educate people regarding the leading risk factors for developing CHD.
- To implement programs aimed at reducing the risks.
- To use the analysis as a starting point with which to compare changes induced by the intervention program.

The leading **risk factors** contributing to CHD are listed in Table 10.1. A self-assessment of risk factors for CHD is given in Figure 10.4. This analysis can be done by people who have little or no medical information about their cardiovascular health, as well as those who have had a thorough medical examination. The guidelines for zero risk are outlined for each factor, making this self-analysis a valuable tool for managing CHD risk factors.

For example, a person who fills out the form will learn that the ideal blood pressure is around 120/80 or lower, that risk is reduced by smoking less or quitting altogether, that HDL-cholesterol should be 45 mg/dl (milligrams per deciliter) or higher for men and 55 mg/dl or higher for women, and that LDL-cholesterol should be less than 170 mg/dl (if unknown, basic nutritional guidelines also are given). (The role of HDL- and LDL-cholesterol in protecting and causing heart disease is discussed later in this chapter.)

> Almost all of the risk factors for coronary heart disease are preventable and reversible, so the individual can reduce the risk of acquiring CHD.

To provide a meaningful score for CHD risk, a weighting system was developed to show the impact of each factor on the risk of developing the disease. This system is based on current research and on the work done at leading preventive medical facilities in the United States. The most significant risk factors are given the heaviest numerical weight.

For example, a poor cholesterol profile seems to be the largest predictor for developing CHD. Up to 12 risk points are assigned to individuals with "very high" LDL-cholesterol levels and "very low" HDL-cholesterol levels. On the other hand, the least heavily weighted risk factor is triglycerides. A maximum of only 2 risk points is assigned to this factor. Each risk factor also is assigned a zero risk level—the level at which it does not appear to increase the risk for disease at all.

Based on actual test results, a person receives a score anywhere from zero to the maximum number of points for each factor. When the risk points from all of the risk factors are totaled, the final number is used to place an individual in one of five overall risk categories for potential development of CHD.

A "very low" CHD risk category designates the group at lowest risk for developing heart disease based on age and gender. "Low" CHD suggests that, even though people in this category are taking good care of their cardiovascular health, they can improve it (unless all of the risk points come from age and family history). "Moderate" CHD risk means that the person can definitely improve his or her lifestyle to lower the risk for disease, or medical treatment may be required. A score in the "high" or "very high" CHD risk category points to a strong probability of developing heart disease within the next few years and calls for immediate implementation of a personal risk-reduction program, including professional medical, nutritional, and exercise intervention.

> A risk factor analysis helps to determine the potential effect of lifestyle in the development of coronary heart disease.

TABLE 10.1 Coronary Heart Disease Risk Factors	
Risk Factors	Maximal Risk Points
Abnormal cholesterol profile	12
Low HDL-cholesterol	6
High LDL-cholesterol	6
Physical inactivity	8
Smoking	8
Hypertension	8
Systolic blood pressure	4
Diastolic blood pressure	4
Personal history of heart disease	8
Abnormal stress electrocardiogram	8
Diabetes	6
High blood glucose	3
Known diabetes	3
Family history of heart disease	6
Elevated homocysteine	4
Age	4
Excessive body fat	3
Tension and stress	3
Abnormal resting electrocardiogram	3
Elevated triglycerides	2

Key Terms

Risk factors Lifestyle and genetic variables that may lead to disease.

FIGURE 10.4 Self-assessment: Risk factor analysis for coronary heart disease.

Name: _____ Date: _____

Course: _____ Section: _____ Gender: _____ Age: _____

1. Physical Activity	Do you participate in a regular aerobic exercise program (brisk walking, jogging, swimming, bicycling, aerobics, etc.) for more than 30 minutes:	Score
	Once a week or less 8	
	Two times per week 3	
	Three or more times per week 0	**8**

2. Resting and Stress Electrocardiograms (ECG)

Add scores for both ECGs

ECG	Resting	Stress	
Normal	(0)	(0)	 0
Equivocal	(1)	(4)	 1–5
Abnormal	(3)	(8)	 3–11

3. HDL-Cholesterol (If unknown, answer question 6)

Men	Women	
≥45	≥55	 0
36–44	46–54	 3
≤35	≤45	 6

4. LDL-Cholesterol (If unknown, answer question 6)

≤129	. . . .	0
130–159	. . . .	3
≥160	. . . .	6

5. Triglycerides (If unknown, answer question 6)

≤125	. . . .	0
126–499	. . . .	1
≥500	. . . .	2

6. Diet (Do not answer if questions 3, 4, and 5 have been answered)

Does your regular diet include (high score if all apply):
One or more daily servings of red meat; 7 or more eggs/week;
daily butter, cheese, whole milk, sweets and alcohol 10–14
Four to six servings of red meat/week, 4–6 eggs per week,
margarine, 1% or 2% milk, some cheese, sweets, and alcohol 4–10
Fish, poultry, red meat less than three times/week,
less than 3 eggs/week, skim milk and skim milk
products, moderate sweets and alcohol 0–3   **4**

7. Homocysteine

Does your daily diet include:
2 and 3 servings of fruits and vegetables respectively 0
less than 2 and 3 servings of fruits and vegetables respectively 4   **4**

8. Diabetes/Glucose

≤120	. . . .	0
121–128	. . . .	1
129–136	. . . .	1.5
137–144	. . . .	2
145–149	. . . .	2.5
>150	. . . .	3
Diabetics add another 3 points	. . . .	3

9. Blood Pressure

Score applies to each reading (e.g., 144/88 score = 4)

Systolic		Diastolic		
≤120	(0)	≤80	(0)	 0
121–130	(1)	81–90	(1)	 1–2
131–140	(2)	91–98	(2)	 2–4
141–150	(3)	99–106	(3)	 3–6
≥151	(4)	≥107	(4)	 4–8

Subtotal Risk Score: _____

(continued)

Score

10. Percent Body Fat		Men	Women		Score
		12–17%	18–22%	0	
		18–22%	23–27%	1	
		23–27%	28–32%	2	
		≥28%	≥33%	3	

11. Smoking		
	Lifetime nonsmoker	0
	Ex-smoker over one year	0
	Ex-smoker less than one year	1
	Smoke less than 1 cigarette/day	1
	Nonsmoker, but live or work in smoking environment	2
	Pipe, cigar smoker, or chew tobacco	2
	Smoke 1–9 cigarettes/day	3
	Smoke 10–19 cigarettes/day	4
	Smoke 20–29 cigarettes/day	5
	Smoke 30–39 cigarettes/day	6
	Smoke 40 or more cigarettes/day	8

Score: (0)

12. Tension and Stress		
	Are you:	
	Sometimes tense	0
	Often tense	1
	Nearly always tense	2
	Always tense	3

Score: (0)

13. Personal History		
	Have you ever had a heart attack, stroke, coronary disease, or any known heart problem:	
	During the last year	8
	1–2 years ago	5
	2–5 years ago	3
	More than 5 years ago	2
	Never suffered from heart disease	0

Score: (0)

14. Family History		
	Have any of your blood relatives (parents, uncles, brothers, sisters, grandparents) suffered from cardiovascular disease (heart attack, strokes, bypass surgery):	
	One or more before age 51	6
	One or more between 51 and 60	3
	One or more after age 60	1
	None have suffered from cardiovascular disease	0

Score: (0)

15. Age		
	29 or younger	0
	30–39	1
	40–49	2
	50–59	3
	≥60	4

Score: (0)

Total Risk Score:

Risk Categories

Very low	5 or less points
Low	Between 6 and 15 points
Moderate	Between 16 and 25 points
High	Between 26 and 35 points
Very high	36 or more points

Using Figure 2.4 (page 45) and Table 2.3 (page 43), fill in your stage of change for cardiovascular disease prevention:

With the exceptions of age, family history of heart disease, and certain electrocardiogram (ECG) abnormalities, the risk factors are preventable and reversible. The leading risk factors for CHD are discussed next, along with the general recommendations for risk reduction.

Physical Inactivity

Physical inactivity is responsible for low levels of cardiorespiratory endurance (the ability of the heart, lungs, and blood vessels to deliver enough oxygen to the cells to meet the demands of prolonged physical activity). The level of cardiorespiratory endurance (or fitness) is given most commonly by the maximal amount of oxygen (in milliliters) that every kilogram (2.2 pounds) of body weight is able to utilize per minute of physical activity (ml/kg/min). As maximal oxygen uptake increases, so does the efficiency of the cardiorespiratory system.

Even though a poor level of fitness has not been assigned the most risk points (8 points for physical inactivity, versus 12 for a poor cholesterol profile—see Table 10.1), improving cardiorespiratory endurance through daily physical activity and aerobic exercise reduces the overall risk for heart disease.

Although specific recommendations can be followed to improve each risk factor, daily physical activity and a regular aerobic exercise program help to control most of the major risk factors that lead to heart disease. Physical activity and aerobic exercise will

- Increase cardiorespiratory endurance.
- Decrease and control blood pressure.
- Reduce body fat.
- Lower blood lipids (cholesterol and triglycerides).
- Improve HDL-cholesterol.
- Help control diabetes.
- Increase and maintain good heart function, sometimes improving certain ECG abnormalities.
- Motivate toward smoking cessation.
- Alleviate tension and stress.
- Counteract a personal history of heart disease.

The significance of physical inactivity in contributing to cardiovascular disease risk was clearly shown in 1992, when the American Heart Association added physical inactivity to the major risk factors for cardiovascular disease. (The other five factors are smoking, a poor cholesterol profile, high blood pressure, diabetes, and obesity.) Based on the overwhelming amount of scientific data in this area, evidence of the benefits of aerobic exercise in reducing heart disease is far too impressive to be ignored.

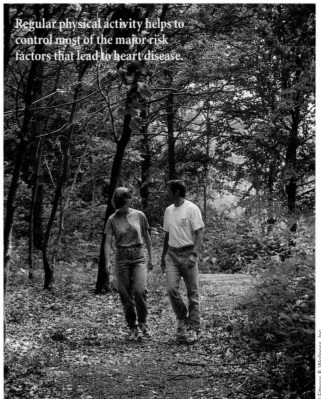

Regular physical activity helps to control most of the major risk factors that lead to heart disease.

© Fitness & Wellness, Inc.

Research at the Aerobics Research Institute in Dallas, Texas, clearly shows the tie between physical activity and mortality, regardless of age and other risk factors.[7] (See Figure 1.7, page 11 and Figures 10.9, page 282, and Figure 10.10, page 290.) A higher level of physical fitness benefits even those who have other risk factors, such as high blood pressure and serum cholesterol, cigarette smoking, and a family history of heart disease. In most cases, unfit people in the study (group 1) without these risk factors had higher death rates than fit people (groups 4 and 5) with these same risk factors.

Although the findings show that the higher the level of cardiorespiratory fitness, the longer the life, the largest drop in premature death is seen between the unfit and the moderately fit groups. Even small improvements in cardiorespiratory endurance greatly decrease the risk for cardiovascular mortality. Most adults who engage in a moderate exercise program can attain these fitness levels easily. The minimum amount of exercise recommended for adults to achieve moderate fitness is presented in Table 10.2. Program 1 is of higher intensity than Program 2, thus only three exercise sessions per week are required for Program 1 (versus five to seven times per week for Program 2).

Subsequent research published in the *New England Journal of Medicine* substantiated the importance of exercise in preventing CHD.[8] Dr. Ralph Paffenbarger and his colleagues indicated that the benefits (to previously inactive adults) of starting a moderate-to-vigorous physical activity program were as important as quitting smoking, managing blood pressure, or controlling cholesterol. In relative risk for death from CHD, the increase in physical activity led to the same decrease as giving up cigarette smoking.

Even though aerobically fit individuals have a lower incidence of cardiovascular disease, regular physical activity and aerobic exercise by themselves do not guarantee a lifetime free of cardiovascular problems. Poor lifestyle habits—such as smoking, eating too many fatty/salty/sweet foods, being overweight, and having high stress levels—increase cardiovascular risk and will not be eliminated completely through an active lifestyle.

Overall management of risk factors is the best guideline to lower the risk for cardiovascular disease. Still, aerobic exercise is one of the most important factors in preventing and reducing cardiovascular problems. The basic principles for cardiorespiratory exercise are given in Chapter 4.

As more research studies are conducted, the addition of strength training is increasingly recommended for good heart function. The American Heart Association recommends it even for individuals who have had a heart attack or have high blood pressure, as long as they do so under a physician's advice. Strength training helps control body weight and blood sugar and lowers cholesterol and blood pressure.

Abnormal Electrocardiograms

The **electrocardiogram (ECG or EKG)** is a valuable measure of the heart's function. The ECG provides a record of the electrical impulses that stimulate the heart to contract (see Figure 10.5). In reading an ECG, doctors interpret five general areas: heart rate, heart rhythm, axis of the heart, enlargement or hypertrophy of the heart, and myocardial infarction.

During a standard 12-lead ECG, 10 electrodes are placed on the person's chest. From these 10 electrodes, the "pictures" (or tracks) of the electrical impulses as they travel through the heart muscle (**myocardium**) can be studied from 12 different positions. By looking at ECG tracings, doctors can identify abnormalities in heart functioning (see Figure 10.6). Based on the findings, the ECG may be interpreted to be normal, equivocal, or abnormal. An ECG will not always identify problems, so a normal tracing is not an absolute guarantee. Conversely, an abnormal tracing does not necessarily signal a serious condition.

TABLE 10.2	Minimum Amount of Walking (Aerobic Activity) Required for Moderate Fitness in Adults		
Program 1	Days/ Week	Distance (miles)	Time (min)
Women	≥3	2	≤30
Men	≥3	2	≤27
Program 2			
Women	5–6	2	30–40
Men	6–7	2	30–40

From S. N. Blair, *Fitness and Mortality* (Dallas: Aerobics Research Center, 1991).

© Brent and Amber Fawson

Lifetime participation in aerobic activities is one of the most important factors in the prevention of cardiovascular disease.

FIGURE **10.5** Normal electrocardiogram.

P wave = atrial depolarization
QRS complex = ventricular depolarization
T wave = ventricular repolarization

Exercise tolerance test with twelve-lead electrocardiographic monitoring (an exercise stress-ECG).

© Fitness & Wellness, Inc.

FIGURE **10.6** Abnormal electrocardiogram showing depressed S-T segment.

S-T Segment

ECGs are taken at rest, during the stress of exercise, and during recovery. A **stress electrocardiogram** is also known as a "graded exercise stress test" or a "maximal exercise tolerance test." Similar to a high-speed test on a car, a stress ECG reveals the tolerance of the heart to increased physical activity. It is a much better test than a resting ECG to discover CHD.

Stress ECGs also are used to assess cardiorespiratory fitness levels, to screen individuals for preventive and cardiac rehabilitation programs, to detect abnormal blood pressure response during exercise, and to establish actual or functional maximal heart rate for exercise prescription. The recovery ECG is another important diagnostic tool to monitor the return of the heart's activity to normal conditions.

> A stress electrocardiogram reveals the tolerance of the heart to increases in physical activity.

Not every adult who wishes to start or continue an exercise program needs a stress ECG. This type of test, however, should be administered to all of the following:

1. Men over age 40 and women over age 50.

2. Anyone with total cholesterol level above 200 mg/dl or an HDL-cholesterol below 35 mg/dl.

3. Hypertensive and diabetic patients.

4. Cigarette smokers.

5. Individuals with a family history of CHD, syncope, or sudden death before age 60.

6. People with an abnormal resting ECG.

7. All individuals with symptoms of chest discomfort, dysrhythmias (abnormal heartbeat), syncope, or chronotropic incompetence (heart rate that increases slowly during exercise and never reaches maximum).

KeyTerms

Electrocardiogram (ECG or EKG) A recording of the electrical activity of the heart.

Myocardium Heart muscle.

Stress electrocardiogram An exercise test during which the workload is gradually increased (until the subject reaches maximal fatigue) with blood pressure and 12-lead electrocardiographic monitoring throughout the test.

At times the stress ECG has been questioned as a reliable predictor of CHD. Nevertheless, it remains the most practical, inexpensive, noninvasive procedure available to diagnose latent (undiagnosed/ unknown) CHD. The test is accurate in diagnosing CHD about 65 percent of the time.

Part of the problem with reliability is that many times those who administer stress ECGs do so without clearly understanding the test's indications and limitations. In any event, sensitivity of the test increases along with the severity of the disease. The test also produces more accurate results in people who are at high risk for cardiovascular disease, in particular men over age 40 and women over age 50 with a poor cholesterol profile, high blood pressure, or a family history of heart disease.

Test protocols, number of leads, electrocardiographic criteria, and the skill of technicians administering the test also affect its sensitivity. In spite of its limitations, it is still a useful tool for identifying people who are at high risk for CHD and exercise-related sudden death.

Abnormal Cholesterol Profile

Blood lipids (fats) are carried in the bloodstream by molecules of protein known as **high-density lipoproteins (HDLs)**, **low-density lipoproteins (LDLs)**, **very low-density lipoproteins (VLDLs)**, and **chylomicrons**. Although subcategories of these lipoproteins have been identified recently, the discussion here focuses primarily on the four major categories.

Cholesterol has received much attention because direct relationships have been established between high total cholesterol, high LDL-cholesterol, low HDL-cholesterol, and the rate of CHD in men and women. An abnormal cholesterol profile contributes to **atherosclerosis**, the build-up of fatty tissue in the walls of the arteries (see Figures 10.7 and 10.8). As the plaque builds up, it blocks the blood vessels that supply the myocardium with oxygen and nutrients (the coronary arteries), and these obstructions can trigger a **myocardial infarction**, or heart attack.

Unfortunately, the heart disguises its problems quite well, and typical symptoms of heart disease, such

FIGURE 10.7 The atherosclerotic process.

Early stage of atherosclerosis

Normal artery

Progression of the atherosclerotic plaque

Advanced stage of atherosclerosis

FIGURE **10.8** Comparison of a normal healthy artery (A) and diseased arteries (B and C).

From *Heart of a Healthy Life*. Courtesy of the American Heart Association, © 1992.

as **angina pectoris**, do not start until the arteries are about 75 percent blocked. In many cases, the first symptom is sudden death.

Based on research conducted at the Aerobics Research Institute in Dallas, Texas, the relative risk for all causes of mortality by physical fitness and total cholesterol levels is given in Figure 10.9. A closer look at this figure shows that a man with high cholesterol (greater than 260 mg/dl) but who is highly fit (groups 4 and 5) or moderately fit (groups 2 and 3) has a lower relative risk of early mortality than an unfit man (group 1) with low cholesterol (less than 200 mg/dl). The data indicate that, at least in men, it is better to be fit with high cholesterol than to be unfit with low cholesterol. The data aren't quite as strong for women, because fewer women have been included in the study. As the number of women studied increases, the data are expected to show a trend similar to men. The lowest mortality rate, of course, is seen in fit people with low total cholesterol levels.

The most recent recommendation released in 2001 by the National Cholesterol Education Program (NCEP) is to keep total cholesterol levels below 200 mg/dl. Other health professionals recommend that total cholesterol in individuals age 30 and younger should not be higher than 180 mg/dl, and for children the level should be below 170 mg/dl. Cholesterol levels between 200 and 239 mg/dl are borderline high, and levels of 240 mg/dl and above indicate high risk for disease (see Table 10.3). The risk for heart attack increases 2 percent for every 1 percent increase in total cholesterol.[9] More than 50 percent, or 100,870,000 U.S. adults, have total cholesterol values of 200 mg/dl or higher, and 40.6 million adults have values at or above 240 mg/dl.[10]

Many preventive medicine practitioners recommend a range between 160 and 180 mg/dl as ideal for total cholesterol. In the Framingham Heart Study (a 50-year ongoing project in the community of Framingham, Massachusetts), not a single individual with a total cholesterol level of 150 mg/dl or lower has had a heart attack. Dr. William Castelli, director of the Framingham Study, recommends a total cholesterol level of less than 150 mg/dl for possible plaque regression in people with atherosclerosis.

KeyTerms

Blood lipids (fats) Cholesterol and triglycerides.

High-density lipoproteins (HDLs) Cholesterol-transporting molecules in the blood that help clear cholesterol from the blood; also called "good" cholesterol.

Low-density lipoproteins (LDLs) Cholesterol-transporting molecules in the blood that tend to increase blood cholesterol; also called "bad" cholesterol.

Very low-density lipoproteins (VLDLs) Triglyceride-, cholesterol-, and phospholipid-transporting molecules in the blood that tend to increase blood cholesterol.

Chylomicron Triglyceride-transporting molecules.

Cholesterol A waxy substance, technically a steroid alcohol, found only in animal fats and oils; used in making cell membranes, as a building block for some hormones, in the fatty sheath around nerve fibers, and in other necessary substances.

Atherosclerosis Fatty cholesterol deposits in the walls of the arteries leading to plaque formation.

Myocardial infarction Heart attack; damage to or death of an area of the heart muscle as a result of an obstructed artery to that area.

Angina pectoris Chest pain associated with coronary heart disease.

FIGURE 10.9 Relative risks of all-cause mortality by physical fitness and serum cholesterol level.

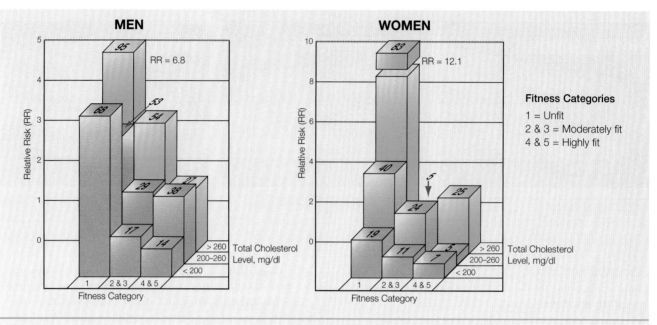

Numbers on top of the bars are all-cause death rates per 10,000 person-years of follow-up for each cell; 1 person-year indicates one person who was followed up one year later.

SOURCE: S. N. Blair, H. W. Kohl III, R. S. Paffenbarger, Jr., D. G. Clark, K. H. Cooper, and L. W. Gibbons, "Physical Fitness and All-Cause Mortality: A Prospective Study of Healthy Men and Women," *Journal of the American Medical Association* 262 (1989): 2395–2401. © American Medical Association. Reproduced by permission.

TABLE 10.3 Cholesterol Guidelines

	Amount	Rating
Total Cholesterol	<200 mg/dl	Desirable
	200–239 mg/dl	Borderline high
	≥240 mg/dl	High risk
LDL-Cholesterol	<100 mg/dl	Optimal
	100–129 mg/dl	Near or above optimal
	130–159 mg/dl	Borderline high
	160–189 mg/dl	High
	≥190 mg/dl	Very high
HDL-Cholesterol	<40 mg/dl	Low (high risk)
	≥60 mg/dl	High (low risk)

From National Cholesterol Education Program.

As important as it is, total cholesterol no longer is the best predictor for cardiovascular risk. Many heart attacks occur in people with only slightly elevated total cholesterol. More significant is the way in which cholesterol is carried in the bloodstream. Cholesterol is transported primarily in the form of high-density lipoprotein (HDL) cholesterol and low-density lipoprotein (LDL) cholesterol.

In a process known as **reverse cholesterol transport**, HDLs act as "scavengers," removing cholesterol from the body and preventing plaque from forming in the arteries. The strength of HDL is in the protein molecules found in its coating. When HDL comes in contact with cholesterol-filled cells, these protein molecules attach to the cells and take their cholesterol.

LDL-cholesterol, on the other hand, tends to release cholesterol, which then may penetrate the lining of the arteries and speed up the process of atherosclerosis. The NCEP guidelines given in Table 10.3 state that an LDL-cholesterol value below 100 mg/dl is optimal, between 130 and 159 mg/dl is borderline high, and 190 mg/dl and above is very high. For people with atherosclerosis, Dr. Castelli recommends an LDL-cholesterol level of 100 mg/dl or lower.[11] A genetic variation of LDL-cholesterol, known as Lp(a), is noteworthy because a high level of these particles leads to an earlier development of atherosclerosis. It is thought that certain substances in the arterial wall interact with Lp(a), leading to premature formation of plaque.

The more HDL-cholesterol (particularly the subcategory HDL$_2$), the better. HDL-cholesterol, the

Habitual aerobic exercise
helps increase HDL-("good") cholesterol.

© Fitness & Wellness, Inc.

"good cholesterol," offers some protection against heart disease. Actually, low levels of HDL-cholesterol could be the best predictor of CHD and may be more significant than the total value. A low level of HDL-cholesterol has the strongest relationship to CHD at all levels of total cholesterol, including levels below 200 mg/dl.[12]

People with low total cholesterol (less than 200 mg/dl) and also low HDL-cholesterol (under 40 mg/dl) may have three times greater risk for heart disease than those with high cholesterol but with good HDL-cholesterol levels. Research, based on 797 patients whose total cholesterol was lower than 200 mg/dl, showed that 60 percent of the patients had heart disease, and almost 75 percent of this group had HDL-cholesterol levels below 40 mg/dl. Data also suggests that for every 1 mg/dl increase in HDL-cholesterol, the risk for CHD drops up to 3 percent in men and 5 percent in women.[13] The recommended HDL-cholesterol values to minimize the risk for CHD are a minimum of 40 mg/dl. HDL-cholesterol levels above 60 mg/dl actually may reduce the risk for CHD.

For the most part, HDL-cholesterol is determined genetically. Generally, women have higher levels than men. The female sex hormone estrogen tends to raise

HDL, so premenopausal women have a much lower incidence of heart disease. African-American children and adult men have higher HDL values than whites. HDL-cholesterol also decreases with age.

Increasing HDL-cholesterol improves the cholesterol profile and lessens the risk for CHD. Habitual aerobic exercise, weight loss, niacin, and quitting smoking help raise HDL-cholesterol.[14] Beta-carotene and drug therapy (see below) may also promote higher HDL-cholesterol levels.[15]

HDL-cholesterol and a regular aerobic exercise program (preferably high intensity, or above 6 METs, for at least 20 minutes three times per week—see Chapter 4) are clearly related. Individual responses to aerobic exercise differ, but, generally, the more you exercise, the higher your HDL-cholesterol level.

Even when more LDL-cholesterol is present than the cells can use, cholesterol seems not to cause a problem until it is oxidized by free radicals. After oxidization, white blood cells invade the arterial wall, take up the cholesterol, and clog the arteries.

The antioxidant effect of vitamins C and E and beta-carotene can also reduce the risk for CHD.[16] Data suggests that a single unstable free radical (an oxygen compound produced during metabolism) can damage LDL particles, accelerating the atherosclerotic process. Vitamin C seems to inactivate free radicals, and vitamin E protects LDL from oxidation. Beta-carotene not only absorbs free radicals, keeping them from causing damage, but it also may help increase HDL levels. One to two medium-size raw carrots per day provide the recommended daily amount of beta-carotene antioxidant nutrients.

Certain cholesterol-lowering drugs also may help raise HDL levels. These agents include colestipol, niacin, cholestyramine, and gemfibrozil.[17] Some experts believe that HDL levels below 35 mg/dl in combination with triglycerides above 160 mg/dl should be treated with medication (see discussion under "Elevated Triglycerides" on page 286).

Many authorities also believe the ratio of LDL-cholesterol to HDL-cholesterol is a strong indicator of potential risk for cardiovascular disease. An LDL-cholesterol to HDL-cholesterol ratio of 3.5 or lower is excellent for men, and 3.0 or lower is best for women. For instance, 50 mg/dl of HDL-cholesterol, as compared with 150 mg/dl of LDL-cholesterol, translates to a ratio of 3.0 ($150 \div 50 = 3.0$).

KeyTerms

Reverse cholesterol transport A process in which HDL molecules attract cholesterol and carry it to the liver, where it is changed to bile and eventually excreted in the stool.

Although the average adult in the United States consumes between 400 and 600 mg of cholesterol daily, the body actually manufactures more than that. Saturated fats raise cholesterol levels more than anything else in the diet. Saturated fats produce approximately 1,000 mg of cholesterol per day.[18] Because of individual differences, some people can have a higher-than-normal intake of saturated fats and still maintain normal levels. Others who have a lower intake can have abnormally high levels.

Saturated fats are found mostly in meats and dairy products and seldom in foods of plant origin (see Table 10.4). Poultry and fish contain less saturated fat than beef does, but should be eaten in moderation (about 3 to 6 ounces per day—see Chapter 8). Unsaturated fats are mainly of plant origin and cannot be converted to cholesterol.

If one's LDL-cholesterol is higher than ideal, it can be lowered by losing body fat, manipulating the diet, taking medication, and participating in a regular aerobic exercise program. Cholesterol-lowering drugs, most notably the statins group, can lower cholesterol by 25 to 50 percent in two to three months. These medications decrease absorption in the intestines or block cholesterol formation by the cells. It is better to lower LDL-cholesterol without medication, because these drugs can cause muscle and joint pain and alter liver enzyme levels. People with heart disease must often take cholesterol-lowering medication, but it is best if medication is combined with lifestyle changes to augment the cholesterol-lowering effect.

To decrease LDL-cholesterol, a diet low in fat, saturated fat, and cholesterol, and high in fiber is recommended. Saturated fat should be replaced with monounsaturated and polyunsaturated fats because the latter tend to decrease LDL-cholesterol (see the section titled "Simple Fats" in Chapter 8). Exercise is important, because dietary manipulation by itself is not as effective in lowering LDL-cholesterol as a combination of diet plus aerobic exercise.[19]

To lower LDL-cholesterol significantly, total daily fiber intake must be in the range of 25 to 30 grams per day (see "Fiber" in Chapter 8), total fat consumption must be significantly lower than the current 30 percent of total daily caloric intake guideline, saturated fat consumption has to be under 7 percent of the total daily caloric intake, and the average cholesterol consumption should be much lower than 200 mg per day.

Most people's fiber intake in the United States averages less than 12 grams per day. Fiber, in particular the soluble type, has been shown to lower cholesterol. Soluble fiber dissolves in water and forms a gel-like substance that encloses food particles. This property helps bind and excrete fats from the body.

TABLE 10.4 Cholesterol and Saturated Fat Content of Selected Foods

Food	Serving Size	Cholesterol (mg)	Sat. Fat (gr)
Avocado	⅛ med.	—	3.2
Bacon	2 slices	30	2.7
Beans (all types)	any	—	—
Beef—lean, fat trimmed off	3 oz	75	6.0
Beef heart (cooked)	3 oz	150	1.6
Beef liver (cooked)	3 oz	255	1.3
Butter	1 tsp	12	0.4
Caviar	1 oz	85	—
Cheese			
American	2 oz	54	11.2
Cheddar	2 oz	60	12.0
Cottage (1% fat)	1 cup	10	0.4
Cottage (4% fat)	1 cup	31	6.0
Cream	2 oz	62	6.0
Muenster	2 oz	54	10.8
Parmesan	2 oz	38	9.3
Swiss	2 oz	52	10.0
Chicken (no skin)	3 oz	45	0.4
Chicken liver	3 oz	472	1.1
Chicken thigh, wing	3 oz	69	3.3
Egg (yolk)	1	250	1.8
Frankfurter	2	90	11.2
Fruits	any	—	—
Grains (all types)	any	—	—
Halibut, flounder	3 oz	43	0.7
Ice cream	½ cup	27	4.4
Lamb	3 oz	60	7.2
Lard	1 tsp	5	1.9
Lobster	3 oz	170	0.5
Margarine (all vegetable)	1 tsp	—	0.7
Mayonnaise	1 tbsp	10	2.1
Milk			
Skim	1 cup	5	0.3
Low fat (2%)	1 cup	18	2.9
Whole	1 cup	34	5.1
Nuts	1 oz	—	1.0
Oysters	3 oz	42	—
Salmon	3 oz	30	0.8
Scallops	3 oz	29	—
Sherbet	½ cup	7	1.2
Shrimp	3 oz	128	0.1
Trout	3 oz	45	2.1
Tuna (canned—drained)	3 oz	55	—
Turkey dark meat	3 oz	60	0.6
Turkey light meat	3 oz	50	0.4
Vegetables (except avocado)	any	—	—

Blood chemistry test guidelines

People who have never had a blood chemistry test should do so to establish a baseline for future reference. The blood test should include total cholesterol, LDL-cholesterol, HDL-cholesterol, triglycerides, and blood glucose.

Following an initial normal baseline test no later than age 20, for a person who adheres to the recommended dietary and exercise guidelines, a blood analysis at least every 5 years prior to age 40 should suffice. Thereafter, a blood lipid test is recommended every year, in conjunction with a regular preventive medicine physical examination.

A single baseline test is not necessarily a valid measure. Cholesterol levels vary from month to month and sometimes even from day to day. If the initial test reveals cholesterol abnormalities, the test should be repeated within a few weeks to confirm the results.

As long as the number of servings is not increased, substituting low-fat for high-fat products in the diet significantly decreases the risk for disease.

The incidence of heart disease is very low in populations where daily fiber intake exceeds 30 grams per day. Further, a 1996 Harvard University Medical School study of 43,000 middle-aged men who were followed for more than 6 years showed that increasing fiber intake to 30 daily grams resulted in a 41 percent reduction in heart attacks.[20]

Research on the effects of a 30 percent–fat diet have shown that it has little or no effect in lowering cholesterol, and that CHD actually continues to progress in people who have the disease. The good news came in a study published in the Archives of Internal Medicine.[21] Men and women in the study lowered their cholesterol by an average of 23 percent in only 3 weeks following a 10 percent or less fat-calorie diet combined with a regular aerobic exercise program, primarily walking. In this diet, cholesterol intake was less than 25 mg/day. The author of the study concluded that the exact percent-fat guideline (10 or 15 percent) is unknown (it also varies from individual to individual), but that 30 percent total fat calories is definitely too much when attempting to lower cholesterol.

A daily 10 percent total–fat diet requires the person to limit fat intake to an absolute minimum. Some health care professionals contend that a diet like this is difficult to follow indefinitely. People with high cholesterol levels, however, may not have to follow that diet indefinitely but should adopt the 10 percent-fat diet while attempting to lower cholesterol. Thereafter, eating a 20 to 30 percent–fat diet may be adequate to maintain recommended cholesterol levels (national data indicate that current fat consumption in the United States averages 34 percent of total calories—see Figure 8.5, page 203).

A drawback of very low-fat diets (less than 25 percent fat) is that they tend to lower HDL-cholesterol and increase triglycerides. If HDL-cholesterol is already low, monounsaturated and polyunsaturated fats should be added to the diet. Olive, canola, corn, and soybean oils and nuts are sample food items that are high in monounsaturated fats and polyunsaturated fats. A specialized nutrition book should be consulted to determine food items that are high in monounsaturated and polyunsaturated fats (also see Figure 8.13, page 213). The 2001 NCEP guidelines for people who are trying to decrease cholesterol allow for a diet with up to 35 percent of calories from fat, as long as less than 7 percent is derived from saturated fats, up to 10 percent from polyunsaturated fats, and up to 20 percent from monounsaturated fats. Carbohydrate intake would be in the range of 50 to 60 percent of calories and protein 15 percent of calories.[22]

Soy protein is also recommended to lower total LDL-cholesterol. Over time, a diet low in saturated fat and cholesterol that includes 25 grams of soy protein a day will lower cholesterol by an additional 5 to 7 percent, compared with the same diet without the soy protein. This benefit is seen primarily in people with total cholesterol levels above 200 mg/dl. Some people may have to consume up to 60 grams a day to see an effect. Additional information on soy foods and their health benefits is given in Chapters 8 and 11.

Margarines and salad dressings that contain stanol ester, a plant-derived compound that lowers cholesterol, are now also on the market. Over the course of several weeks, about 3 grams of margarine or 6 tablespoons of salad dressing containing stanol ester lowers LDL-cholesterol by 14 percent.

To lower LDL-cholesterol levels, the following general dietary guidelines are recommended:

- Consume between 25 and 30 grams of fiber daily, including a minimum of 10 grams of soluble fiber (good sources are oats, fruits, barley, and legumes).
- Do not consume more than 200 mg of dietary cholesterol a day.
- Consume 25 grams of soy protein a day.
- Consume red meats (3 ounces per serving) fewer than three times per week and no organ meats (such as liver and kidneys).
- Do not eat commercially baked foods.
- Increase intake of omega-3 fatty acids (see Chapter 8).
- Avoid foods that contain transfatty acids, hydrogenated fat, or partially hydrogenated vegetable oil.
- Drink low-fat milk (1 percent or less fat, preferably) and low-fat dairy products.
- Do not use coconut oil, palm oil, or cocoa butter.
- Limit egg consumption to less than three eggs per week (this is for people with high cholesterol only; others may consume eggs in moderation).
- Eat fish instead of red meat.
- Bake, broil, grill, poach, or steam food instead of frying.
- Refrigerate cooked meat before adding to other dishes. Remove fat hardened in the refrigerator before mixing the meat with other foods.
- Avoid fatty sauces made with butter, cream, or cheese.
- Maintain recommended body weight.

The combination of a healthy diet, a sound aerobic exercise program, and weight control is the best prescription for controlling blood lipids. If this does not work, a physician can administer a blood test to break down the lipoproteins into their various subcategories. Most U.S. laboratories do not conduct these tests. The American Heart Association, however, has established Lipid Disorder Training Centers that administer comprehensive blood tests. Your local American Heart Association can provide further information.

The NCEP guidelines recommend that people consider drug therapy if, after 6 months on a low-cholesterol, low-fat diet, cholesterol remains unacceptably high. An unacceptable level is an LDL-cholesterol above 190 mg/dl for people with fewer than two risk factors and no signs of heart disease. For people with more than two risk factors and with a history of heart disease, LDL-cholesterol above 160 mg/dl is unacceptable.

ELEVATED TRIGLYCERIDES

Triglycerides are also known as free fatty acids. They make up most of the fat in our diet and most of the fat that circulates in the blood. In combination with cholesterol, triglycerides speed up formation of plaque in the arteries. Triglycerides are carried in the bloodstream primarily by very low-density lipoproteins (VLDLs) and chylomicrons.

> A single cholesterol test may not be a true indicator of a person's regular cholesterol values.

Although they are found in poultry skin, lunch meats, and shellfish, these fatty acids are manufactured mainly in the liver from refined sugars, starches, and alcohol. High intake of alcohol and sugars (honey and fruit juices included) significantly raises triglyceride levels. Triglycerides can be lowered by cutting down on these foods and on overall fat consumption, quitting smoking, reducing weight (if overweight), and doing aerobic exercise. An optimal blood triglyceride level is less than 150 mg/dl (see Table 10.5). For people with cardiovascular problems, this level should be below 100 mg/dl.[23]

Some people consistently have slightly elevated triglyceride levels (above 140 mg/dl) and HDL-cholesterol levels below 35 mg/dl. About 80 percent of these people have a genetic condition called LDL phenotype B (approximately 40 percent of the U.S. population falls in this category). Although the blood lipids may not be notably high, these people are at higher risk for atherosclerosis and CHD.[24]

ELEVATED HOMOCYSTEINE

Clinical data indicating that many heart attack and stroke victims have normal cholesterol levels has led researchers to look for other risk factors that may contribute to atherosclerosis. Although it is not a blood lipid, a high concentration of the amino acid **homocysteine** in the blood is thought to enhance

TABLE 10.5	Triglycerides Guidelines
Amount	**Rating**
<150 mg/dl	Desirable
150–199 mg/dl	Borderline high
200–499 mg/dl	High
≥500 mg/dl	Very high

plaque formation and subsequent blockage of the arteries.[25]

The body uses homocysteine to help build proteins and carry out cellular metabolism. It is an intermediate amino acid in the interconversion of two other amino acids—methionine and cysteine. This interconversion requires the B vitamin folate (folic acid) and vitamins B_6 and B_{12}. Typically, homocysteine is metabolized rapidly, so it does not accumulate in the blood or damage the arteries.

A large number of people, however, have high blood levels of homocysteine. This might result from either a genetic inability to metabolize homocysteine or a deficiency in the vitamins required for its conversion. Homocysteine is typically measured in micromoles per liter (μmol/l). In a 10-year follow-up study of people with high homocysteine levels, the data showed that those individuals with a level above 14.25 μmol/l had almost twice the risk of stroke compared with individuals whose level was below 9.25 μmol/l.[25] It is theorized that homocysteine accumulation is toxic because it may

1. cause damage to the inner lining of the arteries (the initial step in the process of atherosclerosis),
2. stimulate the proliferation of cells that contribute to plaque formation, and
3. encourage clotting, which may completely obstruct an artery and lead to a heart attack or stroke.

Keeping homocysteine from accumulating in the blood seems to be as simple as eating the recommended daily servings of vegetables, fruits, grains, and some meat and legumes: Five servings of fruits and vegetables daily can provide sufficient levels of folate and vitamin B_6 to remove homocysteine from the blood. Vitamin B_{12} is found primarily in animal flesh and animal products, so deficiency is rarely a problem: 1 cup of milk or an egg provides the daily requirement. The body also recycles most of this vitamin; therefore, a deficiency takes years to develop. People who do consume the five daily servings are unlikely to derive extra benefits from a vitamin B complex supplement.

Increasing evidence that folate can prevent heart attacks has led to the recommendation that people (especially women of child-bearing age) consume 400 mcg per day—obtainable from the five daily servings of fruits and vegetables. Unfortunately, estimates indicate that less than 88 percent of Americans get 400 daily mcg of folate.[27]

OTHER APPROACHES

For people who have elevated cholesterol, 500 mg of niacin (also a B vitamin) daily can help lower cholesterol. Niacin supplementation, nonetheless, may produce side effects such as flushing, tingling, and itching. These symptoms usually disappear in a few days but may return if the dose is altered or the supplement is not taken at the same time each day. Supplements, nonetheless, are not a replacement for a diet with ample amounts of fruits, vegetables, and whole grains daily.

Because a large number of people with normal cholesterol have heart attacks, a new test that measures high-sensitivity C-reactive protein (hs-CRP) levels in the blood was recently approved by the FDA. The hs-CRP test measures the probability of plaque rupture within the arterial wall. Ruptured plaque releases clots into the blood stream that can lead a heart attack or stroke. People with high hs-CRP levels are more prone to cardiovascular events.

Diabetes

Diabetes mellitus is a condition in which blood glucose is unable to enter the cells because the pancreas totally stops producing **insulin**, or it does not produce enough to meet the body's needs, or the cells develop **insulin resistance**. The role of insulin is to "unlock" the cells and escort glucose into the cell. Diabetes affects more than 16 million people in the United States and about 800,000 new cases are diagnosed each year. The prevalence of diabetes increased by 33 percent in the last 10 years. The National Institutes of Health estimate the cost of diabetes to be $98 billion annually.

The incidence of cardiovascular disease and death in the diabetic population is quite high. More than 80 percent of people with diabetes mellitus die from cardiovascular disease. People with chronically elevated blood glucose levels may have problems metabolizing fats, which can make them more susceptible to atherosclerosis, coronary heart disease, heart attacks, high blood pressure, and strokes. Diabetics also have lower HDL-cholesterol and higher triglyceride levels.

Key Terms

Triglycerides Fats formed by glycerol and three fatty acids.

Homocysteine An amino acid that, when allowed to accumulate in the blood, may lead to plaque formation and blockage of arteries.

Diabetes mellitus A disease in which the body doesn't produce or utilize insulin properly.

Insulin Hormone secreted by the pancreas; essential for proper metabolism of blood glucose (sugar) and maintenance of blood glucose level.

Insulin resistance The inability of the cells to respond appropriately to insulin.

Chronic high blood sugar can also lead to nerve damage, vision loss, kidney damage, and decreased immune function (making the individual more susceptible to infections). Diabetics are 4 times as likely to become blind and 20 times more likely to develop kidney failure. Nerve damage in the lower extremities decreases the person's awareness of injury and infection. A small, untreated sore can cause severe infection, gangrene, and even lead to an amputation.[28]

> **Adult-onset diabetes is related closely to overeating, obesity, and lack of physical activity.**

An 8-hour fasting blood glucose level above 126 mg/dl on two separate tests confirms a diagnosis of diabetes (see Table 10.6). A level of 126 or higher should be brought to the attention of a physician. (This guideline is a change from previous years. A level above 140 had been used to diagnose diabetes, but this guideline was revised to 126 in 1997.)

Diabetes is of two types: **Type I**, or insulin-dependent diabetes mellitus (IDDM), and **Type II**, or non-insulin–dependent diabetes mellitus (NIDDM). Type I also is called "juvenile diabetes," because it is found mainly in young people. With Type I, the pancreas produces little or no insulin. With Type II, the pancreas either does not produce sufficient insulin or it produces adequate amounts but the cells become insulin-resistant, thereby keeping glucose from entering the cell. Type II accounts for 90 to 95 percent of all diabetes cases.

Although diabetes has a genetic predisposition, Type II, or adult-onset, diabetes is related closely to overeating, obesity, and lack of physical activity. Type II diabetes, once limited primarily to overweight adults, now accounts for almost one-half of the new cases diagnosed in children. More than 80 percent of all Type II diabetics are overweight or have a history of excessive weight. In most cases this condition can be corrected through a special diet, a weight-loss program, and a regular exercise program.

Aerobic exercise helps prevent diabetes in middle-aged men.[29] The protective effect is even greater in those with risk factors such as obesity, high blood pressure, and family propensity. The preventive effect is attributed to less body fat and better sugar and fat metabolism resulting from the regular exercise program. At 3,500 calories per week, the risk was cut in half versus sedentary men. This preventive effect, according to one of the authors of the study, should hold for women, too.

Both moderate-intensity and vigorous physical activity are associated with increased insulin sensitivity

TABLE 10.6 Blood Glucose Guidelines	
Amount	**Rating**
≤126 mg/dl	Desirable
127–149 mg/dl	High
≥150 mg/dl	Very high

and decreased risk for diabetes.[30] The key to increase and maintain proper insulin sensitivity, however, is regularity of the exercise program. Failure to maintain habitual physical activity voids these benefits. A diet high in complex carbohydrates and water-soluble fibers (found in fruits, vegetables, oats, and beans), low in saturated fat, and low in sugar is helpful in treating diabetes. A simple aerobic exercise program (walking, cycling, or swimming four to five times per week) often is prescribed because it increases the body's sensitivity to insulin. Aggressive weight loss, especially if combined with exercise, often allows diabetic patients to normalize their blood sugar level without the use of medication. Individuals who have high blood glucose levels should consult a physician to decide on the best treatment. Exercise guidelines for diabetic patients are discussed in detail in Chapter 4.

Although complex carbohydrates are recommended in the diet, diabetics need to pay careful attention to the glycemic index (explained in Chapter 9 and detailed in Table 9.1). Refined and starchy foods are of a high glycemic index (small-particle carbohydrates, which are quickly digested); whereas grains, fruits, and vegetables are low-glycemic foods. Foods with a high glycemic index cause a rapid increase in blood sugar. A diet that includes many high-glycemic foods increases the risk for cardiovascular disease in people with high insulin resistance and **glucose intolerance**.[31] Combining a moderate amount of high-glycemic foods with low-glycemic index foods or with some fat and protein, however, can bring the average index down.

SYNDROME X

As the cells resist insulin's action, the pancreas releases even more insulin in an attempt to keep blood glucose from rising. A chronic rise in insulin appears to trigger a series of abnormalities referred to as **syndrome X** or **metabolic syndrome**.[32] These abnormal conditions include low HDL-cholesterol, high triglycerides, and an increased blood clotting mechanism. Many individuals with syndrome X also have high blood pressure. All of these conditions increase the risk for CHD and other diabetic-related

Diagnosis of Syndrome X	
Fasting triglycerides	≥ 200 mg/dl
Fasting HDL-cholesterol	≤ 35 mg/dl
Blood pressure	$\geq 145/90$
Fasting blood glucose	≥ 110 mg/dl
Being overweight by	≥ 15 lb

SOURCE: G. M. Reaven, "Syndrome X: The Little Known Cause of Many Heart Attacks," *Bottom Line / Personal Health* 14 (June 2000).

TABLE 10.7 Blood Pressure Guidelines

Rating	Systolic	Diastolic
Optimal	≤ 120	≤ 80
Normal	121–129	81–84
High Normal	130–139	85–89
Stage 1 Hypertension	140–159	90–99
Stage 2 Hypertension	160–179	100–109
Stage 3 Hypertension	≥ 180	≥ 110

SOURCE: National Heart, Lung and Blood Institute.

conditions (blindness, infection, nerve damage, and kidney failure). Approximately 70 million Americans are afflicted by this condition.

People who suffer from syndrome X have an abnormal insulin response to carbohydrates, in particular high-glycemic foods. In contrast with the American Heart Association dietary guidelines, syndrome X researchers indicate that the current low-fat, high-carbohydrate diet may not be the best for the prevention of CHD and could actually increase disease risk in people with high degrees of insulin resistance and glucose intolerance.[33] It might be best for these people to distribute daily caloric intake so that 45 percent of the calories are derived from carbohydrates (primarily low-glycemic), 40 percent from fat, and 15 percent from protein.[34] Of the 40 percent fat calories, most of the fat should come from mono- and poly-unsaturated fats and only 5 to 7 percent should be provided by saturated fat.

Syndrome X patients also benefit from weight loss (if overweight), exercise, and smoking cessation.[35] Insulin resistance drops by about 40 percent in overweight people who lose 20 pounds. Forty-five minutes of daily aerobic exercise enhances insulin efficiency by 25 percent. Smoking, on the other hand, increases insulin resistance.

Hypertension

Some 60,000 miles of blood vessels run through the human body. As the heart forces the blood through these vessels, the fluid is under pressure. **Blood pressure** is measured in milliliters of mercury (mm Hg), usually expressed in two numbers: **Systolic blood pressure** is the higher number and **diastolic blood pressure** is the lower number. Ideal blood pressure is 120/80 or lower (see Table 10.7)

STANDARDS

Statistical evidence indicates that blood pressure readings above 140/90 increase the risk for disease and premature death. Consequently, the American Heart Association considers all blood pressures above

140/90 to be **hypertension**. Based on 2000 estimates, approximately 1 in every 4 people are hypertensive (Figure 10.10). The incidence is higher among African Americans— in fact, it is among the highest in the world. Approximately 30 percent and 20 percent of all deaths in African-American men and women respectively may be caused by high blood pressure.

Even though the threshold for hypertension has been set at 140/90, many experts believe that the lower the blood pressure, the better. Even if the pressure is around 90/50, as long as that person does not

Key Terms

Type I diabetes Insulin-dependent diabetes mellitus (IDDM), a condition in which the pancreas produces little or no insulin. Also known as "juvenile diabetes."

Type II diabetes Non-insulin–dependent diabetes mellitus (NIDDM), a condition in which insulin is not processed properly. Also known as "adult-onset diabetes."

Glucose intolerance A condition characterized by slightly elevated blood glucose levels.

Syndrome X An array of metabolic abnormalities that contribute to the development of atherosclerosis triggered by insulin resistance. These conditions include low HDL-cholesterol, high triglycerides, high blood pressure, and an increased blood clotting mechanism.

Metabolic syndrome *See* Syndrome X.

Blood pressure A measure of the force exerted against the walls of the vessels by the blood flowing through them.

Systolic blood pressure Pressure exerted by blood against walls of arteries during forceful contraction (systole) of the heart; higher of the two numbers in blood pressure readings.

Diastolic blood pressure Pressure exerted by blood against walls of arteries during relaxation phase (diastole) of the heart; lower of the two numbers in blood pressure readings.

Hypertension Chronically elevated blood pressure.

FIGURE **10.10** Incidence of high blood pressure among adults in the United States, Year 2000.

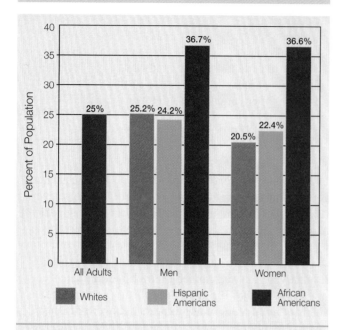

SOURCE: American Heart Association, *Heart and Stroke Facts: 2000* (Statistical Supplement), Dallas: AHA, 1999.

have any symptoms of **hypotension**, he or she need not be concerned. Typical symptoms of hypotension are dizziness, lightheadedness, and fainting.

Blood pressure also may fluctuate during a regular day. Many factors affect blood pressure, and one single reading may not be a true indicator of your real pressure. For example, physical activity and stress increase blood pressure, and rest and relaxation decrease it. Consequently, several measurements should be taken before diagnosing high blood pressure.

INCIDENCE AND PATHOLOGY

Based on 1996 estimates by the American Heart Association, nearly 50 million Americans (age 6 and older) are hypertensive. In 1993, 37,520 Americans died as a result of high blood pressure. Hypertension has been referred to as "the silent killer." It does not hurt; it does not make you feel sick; and, unless you check it, years may go by before you even realize you have a problem. High blood pressure is a risk factor not only for CHD but also for congestive heart failure, strokes, kidney failure, and osteoporosis.

The relative risk for mortality by systolic blood pressure and various fitness levels is shown in Figure 10.11. Similar to the physical fitness and cholesterol data in Figure 10.9, the data here clearly show that, in both men and women, the relative risk of early

mortality is lower in fit people with high systolic blood pressure (140 mm Hg or higher) than in unfit people with an "ideal" systolic blood pressure (120 mm Hg or lower).

All inner walls of arteries are lined by a layer of smooth endothelial cells. Blood lipids cannot penetrate the healthy lining and start to build up on the walls unless damage is done to the cells. High blood pressure is thought to be a leading contributor to destruction of this lining. As blood pressure rises, so does the risk for atherosclerosis. The higher the pressure, the greater the damage to the arterial wall, making the vessels susceptible to fat deposits, especially if serum cholesterol also is high. Blockage of the coronary vessels decreases blood supply to the heart muscle and can lead to heart attacks. When brain arteries are involved, strokes may follow.

A clear example of the connection between high blood pressure and atherosclerosis can be seen by comparing blood vessels in the human body. Even when atherosclerosis is present throughout major arteries, fatty plaques rarely are seen in the pulmonary artery, which goes from the right part of the heart to the lungs. The pressure in this artery is normally below 40 mm Hg, and at such low pressure significant deposits do not occur. This is one of the reasons people with low blood pressure have a lower incidence of cardiovascular disease.

Constantly elevated blood pressure also causes the heart to work much harder. At first the heart does well, but in time this continual strain produces an enlarged heart, followed by congestive heart failure. Furthermore, high blood pressure damages blood vessels to the kidneys and eyes, which can result in kidney failure and loss of vision.

TREATMENT

Of all hypertension, 90 percent has no definite cause. Called "essential hypertension," it is treatable. Aerobic exercise, weight reduction, a low-salt/low-fat and high potassium/high calcium diet, lower alcohol and caffeine intake, smoking cessation, stress management, and antihypertensive medication all have been used effectively to treat essential hypertension.

The remaining 10 percent of hypertensive cases are caused by pathological conditions, such as narrowing of the kidney arteries, glomerulonephritis (a kidney disease), tumors of the adrenal glands, and narrowing of the aortic artery. With this type of hypertension, the pathological cause has to be treated before the blood pressure problem can be corrected.

Antihypertensive medicines often are the first choice of treatment, but they produce many side effects. These include lethargy, sleepiness, sexual difficulties, higher blood cholesterol and glucose levels,

FIGURE **10.11** Relative risks of all-cause mortality by physical fitness and systolic blood pressure.

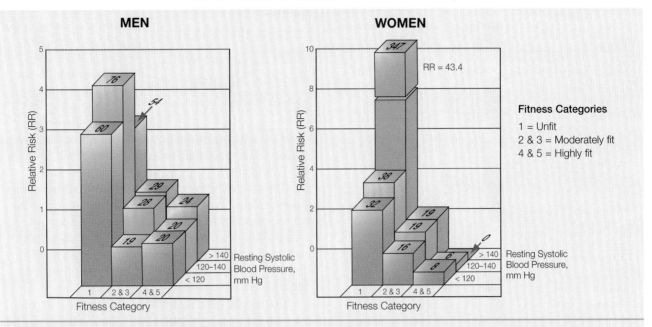

All-cause death rates per 10,000 person-years of follow-up for each cell; 1 person-year indicates one person who was followed up 1 year later. Fitness group 1 is the least fit group; fitness group 5 is the most fit group.

SOURCE: S. N. Blair, H. W. Kohl III, R. S. Paffenbarger, Jr., D. G. Clark, K. H. Cooper, and L. W. Gibbons, "Physical Fitness and All-Cause Mortality: A Prospective Study of Healthy Men and Women," *Journal of the American Medical Association* 262 (1989): 2395–2401. © American Medical Association. Reproduced by permission.

lower potassium levels, and elevated uric acid levels. A physician may end up treating these side effects as often as the hypertension itself. Because of the many side effects, about half of the patients stop taking the medication within the first year of treatment.

Another factor contributing to elevated blood pressure is too much sodium in the diet (salt, or sodium chloride, contains approximately 40 percent sodium). With high sodium intake, the body retains more water, which increases the blood volume and, in turn, drives up the pressure. High intake of potassium seems to regulate water retention and lower the pressure slightly.

Although sodium is essential for normal body functions, the body can function with as little as 200 mg, or a tenth of a teaspoon daily. Even under strenuous conditions of job and sports participation that incite heavy perspiration, the amount of sodium required is seldom more than 3,000 mg per day. Yet, sodium intake in the typical U.S. diet ranges between 6,000 and 20,000 mg per day!

In underdeveloped countries and Native American tribes where no salt is used in cooking or added at the table and the only sodium comes from food in its natural form, daily intake rarely is more than

2,000 mg. Blood pressure in these people does not get higher with age, and hypertension is practically unknown. These findings suggest that the human body may be able to handle 2,000 mg per day, but intakes higher than that over the years may cause a gradual rise in blood pressure.

Where does all the sodium come from? Part of the answer is in Table 10.8. People do not realize the amount of sodium in various foods (the list in Table 10.8 does not include salt added at the table). Unfortunately, most of the sodium in our diets comes from prepared foods, where the consumer does not have control over the ingredients.

When treating high blood pressure (unless it is extremely high), before recommending medication, many sports medicine physicians suggest a combination of aerobic exercise, weight loss, and less sodium in the diet. In most instances this treatment brings blood pressure under control.

The link between hypertension and obesity seems to be quite strong. Not only does blood volume

KeyTerms

Hypotension Low blood pressure.

TABLE 10.8 Sodium and Potassium Levels of Selected Foods

Food	Serving Size	Sodium (mg)	Potassium (gr)
Apple	1 med	1	182
Asparagus	1 cup	2	330
Avocado	1/2	4	680
Banana	1 med	1	440
Bologna	3 oz	1,107	133
Bouillon cube	1	960	4
Cantaloupe	1/4	17	341
Carrot (raw)	1	34	225
Cheese			
American	2 oz	614	93
Cheddar	2 oz	342	56
Muenster	2 oz	356	77
Parmesan	2 oz	1,056	53
Swiss	2 oz	148	64
Chicken (light meat)	6 oz	108	700
Corn (canned)	½ cup	195	80
Corn (natural)	½ cup	3	136
Frankfurter	1	627	136
Haddock	6 oz	300	594
Hamburger (reg)	1	500	321
Lamb (leg)	6 oz	108	700
Milk (whole)	1 cup	120	351
Milk (skim)	1 cup	126	406
Orange	1 med	1	263
Orange juice	1 cup	1	200
Peach	1 med	2	308
Pear	1 med	2	130
Peas (canned)	½ cup	200	82
Peas (boiled-natural)	½ cup	2	178
Pizza			
(cheese—14" diam.)	1/8	456	85
Potato	1 med	6	763
Potato chips	10	150	226
Potato (french fries)	10	5	427
Pork	6 oz	96	438
Roast beef	6 oz	98	448
Salami	3 oz	1,047	170
Salmon (canned)	6 oz	198	756
Salt	1 tsp	2,132	0
Soups			
Chicken noodle	1 cup	979	55
Clam chowder (New England)	1 cup	914	146
Cream of mushroom	1 cup	955	98
Vegetable beef	1 cup	1,046	162
Soy sauce	1 tsp	1,123	22
Spaghetti (tomato sauce and cheese)	6 oz	648	276
Strawberries	1 cup	1	244
Tomato (raw)	1 med	3	444
Tuna (drained)	3 oz	38	255

> **Hypertensive people who are physically active have a lower relative risk of mortality from all causes than inactive individuals with normal blood pressure.**

increase with excess body fat, but every additional pound of fat requires an estimated extra mile of blood vessels to feed this tissue. Furthermore, blood capillaries are constricted by the adipose tissues as these vessels run through them. As a result, the heart muscle must work harder to pump the blood through a longer, constricted network of blood vessels.

The role of regular physical activity in managing blood pressure is becoming more important each day. On the average, fit individuals have lower blood pressure than unfit people do. Further, both aerobic and strength-training exercise have been shown to lower resting systolic and diastolic blood pressure in adults.

Comprehensive reviews on the effects of aerobic exercise on blood pressure found that, in general, an individual can expect exercise-induced reductions of approximately 4 to 5 mm Hg in resting systolic blood pressure and 3 to 4 mm Hg in resting diastolic blood pressure.[36] Although these reductions do not seem

> **Hypertension is practically unknown in populations where daily sodium intake remains below 2,000 mg.**

large, a decrease of about 5 mm Hg in resting diastolic blood pressure has been associated with a 40 percent decrease in the risk for stroke and a 15 percent reduction in the risk for coronary heart disease.[37] Even in the absence of any decrease in resting blood pressure, hypertensive individuals who exercise have a lower risk of all-cause mortality compared with hypertensive/sedentary individuals.[38] The research data also show that exercise, not weight loss, is the major contributor to the lower blood pressure of exercisers. If aerobic exercise is discontinued, these changes are not maintained.

Another extensive review of research studies on the effects of at least 4 weeks of strength training on resting blood pressure yielded similar results.[39] Both systolic and diastolic blood pressures decreased by an average of 3 mm Hg. The participants in these studies, however, were primarily individuals with normal blood pressure. Of greater significance, the results showed that strength training did not cause an increase in resting blood pressure. More research remains to be done on hypertensive subjects.

The effects of long-term participation in exercise could be much more remarkable. An 18-year follow-up study on exercising and nonexercising subjects showed much lower blood pressures in the active group.[40] The exercise group had an average resting blood pressure of 120/78 compared with 150/90 for the nonexercise group (see Table 10.9).

Some health care practitioners recommend that exercise programs for hypertensive patients be of moderate intensity. Training at about 50 percent of heart rate reserve seems to have the same effect in lowering blood pressure as training at a 70 percent heart rate reserve. High-intensity training (above 70 percent) in hypertensive patients may not lower the blood pressure as much as moderate intensity exercise. Even so, a person may be better off being highly fit and having high blood pressure than being unfit and having low blood pressure (see Figure 10.11). The death rates for unfit individuals with low systolic blood pressure are much higher than for highly fit people with high systolic blood pressure.

Most important is a preventive approach. Keeping blood pressure under control is easier than trying to bring it down once it is high. Regardless of your blood pressure history, high or low, you should have it checked routinely. To keep your blood pressure as low as possible, exercise regularly; lose excess weight; eat less salt and sodium-containing foods; do not smoke; practice stress

> **Moderate-intensity exercise lowers high blood pressure more effectively than high-intensity exercise.**

TABLE **10.9**	Effects of a Regular Aerobic Exercise Program on Resting Blood Pressure

	Initial	Final
Exercise Group		
Age	44.6	68.0
Blood Pressure	120/79	120/78
Nonexercise Group		
Age	51.6	69.7
Blood Pressure	135/85	150/90

NOTE: The aerobic exercise program consisted of an average four training sessions per week, each 66 minutes long, at about 76 percent of heart rate reserve.

Based on data from F. W. Kash, J. L. Boyer, S. P. Van Camp, L. S. Verity, and J. P. Wallace, "The Effect of Physical Activity on Aerobic Power in Older Men (A Longitudinal Study)," *The Physician and Sports Medicine* 18, no. 4 (1990): 73–83.

Guidelines to stop hypertension

- Participate in moderate-intensity aerobic exercise program (50% intensity) for 30 to 45 minutes 5 to 7 times per week.
- Participate in a moderate-resistance strength-training program (use 12 to 15 repetitions to near-fatigue on each set) two times per week (seek your physician's approval and advice for this program).
- Lose weight if you are above recommended body weight.
- Eat less salt and sodium-containing foods.
- Do not smoke cigarettes or use tobacco in any other form.
- Practice stress management.
- Do not consume more than two alcoholic beverages a day if you are a man or one if you are a woman.
- Consume more potassium-rich foods.
- Follow the Dietary Approach to Stop Hypertension (DASH Diet):
  - Seven or eight daily servings of grains, bread, cereal, or pasta
  - Eight to ten daily servings of fruits and vegetables.
  - Two or three daily servings of nonfat/low-fat dairy products.
  - Two or less daily servings of meat, poultry, or fish (less than 3 ounces per serving).
  - Four or five servings per week of beans, peas, nuts, or seeds.

management; do not consume more than two alcoholic beverages a day if you are a man, one if you are a woman; and consume more potassium-rich foods such as potatoes, bananas, orange juice, cantaloupe, tomatoes, and beans (see "Guidelines to Stop Hypertension"). The Dietary Approach to Stop Hypertension (DASH)—which emphasizes fruits, vegetables, grains, and dairy products—has shown to lower systolic blood pressure by 11 points and diastolic by 5.5 points.[41]

Those who are taking medication for hypertension should not stop unless the prescribing physician gives the go-ahead. If it is not treated properly, high blood pressure can kill. By combining medication with the other treatments, drug therapy eventually may be reduced or completely eliminated.

Excessive Body Fat

Body composition refers to the ratio of lean body weight to fat weight. If the body contains too much fat, the person is considered overweight or obese (see Table 7.9, page 184).

Although some experts recognize obesity as an independent risk factor for CHD, the risks attributed to obesity may actually be augmented by other risk factors that usually accompany excessive body fat. Risk factors such as high blood lipids, hypertension, and diabetes usually improve with increased physical activity. As discussed in Chapter 9, overweight people who are physically active do not seem to be at increased risk for premature death.

Attaining recommended body composition helps improve some of the CHD risk factors and also helps to reach a better state of health and wellness. People who have a weight problem and want to get down to recommended weight must implement the following:

1. Increase daily physical activity and participate in aerobic and strength-training programs.

2. Follow a diet low in fat and refined sugars and high in complex carbohydrates and fiber.

3. Reduce total caloric intake moderately while getting the necessary nutrients to sustain normal body functions.

Additional recommendations for weight reduction and weight control are discussed in Chapter 9.

SMOKING

More than 47 million adults and 3.5 million adolescents in the United States smoke cigarettes. Smoking is the single largest preventable cause of illness and premature death in the United States. Smoking has been linked to cardiovascular disease, cancer, bronchitis, emphysema, and peptic ulcers. In relation to coronary disease, not only does smoking speed up the process of atherosclerosis, but it also carries a three-fold increase in the risk of sudden death following a myocardial infarction.

According to estimates, about 20 percent of all deaths from cardiovascular diseases are attributable to smoking. Smoking prompts the release of nicotine and some other 1,200 toxic compounds into the bloodstream. As happens with hypertension, many of these substances destroy the inner membrane that protects the walls of the arteries. Once the lining is damaged, cholesterol and triglycerides can be deposited readily in the arterial wall. As the plaque builds up, it obstructs blood flow through the arteries.

Furthermore, smoking encourages the formation of blood clots, which can completely block an artery already narrowed by atherosclerosis. In addition, carbon monoxide, a byproduct of cigarette smoke, decreases the blood's oxygen-carrying capacity. A combination of obstructed arteries, less oxygen, and

nicotine in the heart muscle heightens the risk for a serious heart problem.

Smoking also increases heart rate, raises blood pressure, and irritates the heart, which can trigger fatal cardiac arrhythmias. Another harmful effect is a decrease in HDL-cholesterol, the "good" type that helps control blood lipids. Smoking actually presents a much greater risk of death from heart disease than from lung disease.

Pipe and cigar smoking and chewing tobacco also increase the risk for heart disease. Even if the smoker inhales no smoke, he or she absorbs toxic substances through the membranes of the mouth, and these end up in the bloodstream. Individuals who use tobacco in any of these three forms also have a much greater risk for cancer of the oral cavity.

The risks for both cardiovascular disease and cancer start to decrease the moment you quit smoking. The risk decreases to that of a lifetime nonsmoker 10 years (for CHD) and 15 years (for cancer) after quitting. A more thorough discussion of the harmful effects of cigarette smoking, the benefits of quitting, and a complete program for quitting are detailed in Chapter 13.

Tension and Stress

Tension and stress have become a part of life. Everyone has to deal daily with goals, deadlines, responsibilities, pressures. Almost everything in life (whether positive or negative) can be a source of stress. The stressor itself is not what creates the health hazard but, rather, the individual's response to it.

The human body responds to stress by producing more **catecholamines** to prepare the body for "fight or flight." These hormones increase heart rate, blood pressure, and blood glucose levels, enabling the person to take action. If the person actually fights or flees, the higher levels of catecholamines are metabolized and the body is able to return to a normal state. If, however, a person is under constant stress and unable to take action (as in the death of a close relative or friend, loss of a job, trouble at work, or financial insecurity), the catecholamines remain elevated in the bloodstream.

People who are not able to relax have a constant low-level strain on the cardiovascular system that could manifest itself as heart disease. In addition, when a person is in a stressful situation, the coronary arteries that feed the heart muscle constrict, reducing the oxygen supply to the heart. If the blood vessels are largely blocked by atherosclerosis, **arrhythmias** or even a heart attack may follow.

Individuals who are under a lot of stress and do not cope well with it need to take measures to

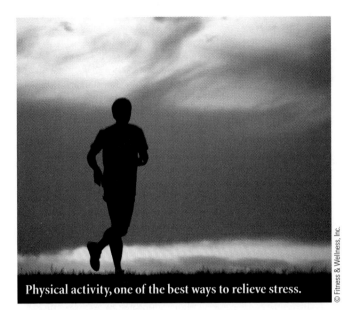

Physical activity, one of the best ways to relieve stress.

© Fitness & Wellness, Inc.

counteract the effects of stress in their lives. One way is to identify the sources of stress and learn how to cope with them. People need to take control of themselves, examine and act upon the things that are most important in their lives, and ignore less-meaningful details.

Physical activity is one of the best ways to relieve stress. When a person takes part in physical activity, the body metabolizes excess catecholamines and is able to return to a normal state. Exercise also steps up muscular activity, which contributes to muscular relaxation after completing the physical activity.

Many executives in large cities are choosing the evening hours for their physical activity programs, stopping after work at the health or fitness club. In doing this, they are able to "burn up" the excess tension accumulated during the day and enjoy the evening hours. This has proven to be one of the best stress management techniques. More information on stress management techniques is presented in Chapter 12.

Personal and Family History

Individuals who have had cardiovascular problems are at higher risk than those who have never had a problem. People with this history should control the other risk factors as much as they can. Most risk factors are reversible, so this will greatly decrease their risk for future problems. The more time that passes since the cardiovascular problem occurred, the lower the risk for recurrence.

Genetic predisposition toward heart disease has been demonstrated clearly. All other factors being equal, a person with blood relatives who now have or did have heart disease run a greater risk than

someone with no such history. Premature CHD is defined as a heart attack before age 55 in a close male relative or before age 65 in a close female relative. The younger the age at which the cardiovascular incident happened to the relative, the greater the risk for the disease.

In some cases there is no way of knowing whether it was a person's genetic predisposition or simply poor lifestyle habits that led to a heart problem. A person may have been physically inactive, been overweight, smoked, and had bad dietary habits—all of which contributed to a heart attack. Regardless, blood relatives fall in the family history category. Because we have no reliable way to differentiate all the factors contributing to cardiovascular disease, a person with a family history should watch all other factors closely and maintain the lowest risk level possible. In addition, the person should have a blood chemistry analysis annually to make sure the body is handling blood lipids properly.

Age

Age is a risk factor because of the higher incidence of heart disease in older people. This tendency may be induced partly by other factors stemming from changes in lifestyle as we get older—less physical activity, poorer nutrition, obesity, and so on.

Young people should not think they are exempt from heart disease. The process begins early in life. Autopsies conducted on American soldiers killed at age 22 and younger revealed that approximately 70 percent had early stages of atherosclerosis. Other studies found elevated blood cholesterol levels in children as young as 10 years old.

Although the aging process cannot be stopped, it certainly can be slowed down. Physiological versus chronological age is important in preventing disease. Some individuals in their 60s or older have the body of a 20-year-old. And 20-year-olds often are in such poor condition and health that they almost seem to have the body of 60-year-olds. Risk factor management and positive lifestyle habits are the best means of slowing down the natural aging process.

Other Factors

Additional evidence points to a few other factors that may be linked to coronary heart disease. One of these

KeyTerms

Catecholamines "Fight-or-flight" hormones, including epinephrine and norepinephrine.

Arrhythmias Irregular heart rhythms.

factors is gum disease. The oral bacteria that builds up with dental plaque can enter the bloodstream and contribute to blood vessel plaque formation, increase blood clots, and thus increase heart attack risk. Daily flossing for 1 to 2 minutes is the best way to prevent gum disease.

Loud snoring has also been linked to cardiovascular disease. People who snore heavily may suffer from sleep apnea, a sleep disorder in which the throat closes for a brief moment, causing breathing to stop. In one study, individuals who snored heavily tripled their risk of a heart attack and quadrupled the risk of a stroke.[42]

Aspirin therapy is also recommended to prevent heart disease. A daily aspirin dose of about 81 mg per day (the equivalent of a baby aspirin) can prevent or dissolve clots that cause heart attack or stroke. The incidence of nonfatal heart attack is decreased by about 32 percent with daily use.[43]

A FINAL WORD ON CORONARY RISK REDUCTION

Most of the risk factors for CHD are reversible and preventable. Having a family history of heart disease, and possibly some of the other risk factors because of neglect in lifestyle, does not mean that you are doomed. A healthier lifestyle—free of cardiovascular problems—is something over which you have great control. Be persistent. Willpower and commitment are required to develop patterns that eventually will turn into healthy habits contributing to total well-being.

WEB INTERACTIVE

Exercise Your Heart: A Guide to Physical Activity

Sponsored by the National Heart, Lung, and Blood Institute, this site discusses the advantages of physical activity, the effects of activity on the heart, practical guidelines for starting and staying on an exercise program, and sample activity programs.

http://nih.gov/health/exercise

The Heart: An Online Exploration

This interesting site, developed by the Franklin Institute of Science, provides an interactive multimedia tour of the heart, as well as statistical information, resources, links, and information on how to monitor your heart's health by becoming aware of your vital signs.

http://www.fi.edu/biosci/heart.html

National Cholesterol Education Program

This comprehensive site features interactive sessions on planning a low-cholesterol diet, information on preventing heart disease, and information for people who already have heart disease. Includes radio messages from the Heart Beat Radio Network. This site is highly recommended.

http://rover.nhlbi.nih.gov/chd

INTERACTIVE SITES:

American Heart Association Health Risk Awareness

Risk factors are your personal characteristics, genetic makeup, and lifestyle behaviors that may increase your chances of having a heart attack or stroke. Some you can't change or control (age, gender, genetics); some you can—by making a few changes in your daily habits. Are you at risk? Find out by taking this short interactive quiz.

http://www.americanheart.org/risk/quiz.html

Create a Diet to Lower your Cholesterol

This interactive site will provide personalized guidelines on how to eat healthy and decrease your risk of heart disease based on your height, weight, age, gender, and activity level.

http://www.nhlbisupport.com/chd1/create.htm

Check your Healthy Heart IQ

This site is sponsored by the National Heart, Lung, and Blood Institute. Test your knowledge about heart disease and its risks (high blood pressure, high blood cholesterol, smoking, lack of exercise, and overweight); learn ways to reduce your risk.

http://www.nhlbi.nih.gov/health/public/heart/other/hh_iq_ab.htm

n*tes

1. American Heart Association, *Heart and Stroke Facts: 2000* (Statistical Supplement) (Dallas: AHA, 1999).
2. U. S. Department of Health and Human Services, Centers for Disease Control and Prevention, National Center for Health Statistics, National Vital Statistics System: *Deaths: Preliminary Data for 2000*, 49, no. 12 (October 10, 2001).
3. American Heart Association, *1999 Heart and Stroke Facts Statistical Update* (Dallas: AHA, 1998).
4. See note 3.
5. See note 2.
6. See note 3.
7. S. N. Blair, H. W. Kohl III, R. S. Paffenbarger, Jr., D. G. Clark, K. H. Cooper, and L. W. Gibbons, "Physical Fitness and All-Cause Mortality: A Prospective Study of Healthy Men and Women," *Journal of the American Medical Association* 262 (1989): 2395–2401.
8. R. S. Paffenbarger, Jr., R. T. Hyde, A. L. Wing, I. Lee, D. L. Jung, and J. B. Kampert, "The Association of Changes in Physical-Activity Level and Other Lifestyle Characteristics with Mortality Among Men," *New England Journal of Medicine* 328 (1993): 538–545.
9. "Lipid Research Clinics Program: The Lipid Research Clinic Coronary Primary Prevention Trial Results," *Journal of the American Medical Association* 251 (1984): 351–364.
10. American Heart Association, *2001 Heart and Stroke Statistical Update* (Dallas: AHA, 2000).
11. W. P. Castelli and K. Anderson, "A Population at Risk: Prevalence of High Cholesterol Levels in Hypertensive Patients in the Framingham Study," *American Journal of Medicine* 80, Supplement 2A (1986): 23–32.
12. P. A. Romm, M. K. Hong, and C. E. Rackley, "High-Density-Lipoprotein Cholesterol and Risk of Coronary Heart Disease," *Practical Cardiology* 16 (1990): 28–40.
13. "HDL on the Rise," *HealthNews* (September 10, 1999).

14. C. J. Gluek, "Nonpharmacologic and Pharmacologic Alteration of High Density Lipoprotein Cholesterol: Therapeutic Approaches to Prevention of Atherosclerosis," *American Heart Journal* 110 (1985): 1107–1115.
15. J. M. Gaziano and C. H. Hennekens, "A New Look at What Can Unclog Your Arteries," *Executive Health Report* 27, no. 8 (1991): 16.
16. See note 15.
17. See note 12.
18. American Heart Association, *Heart and Stroke Facts* (Dallas: AHA, 1999).
19. M. L. Stefanick et al., "Effects of Diet in Men and Postmenopausal Women with Low Levels of HDL Cholesterol and High Levels of LDL Cholesterol," *New England Journal of Medicine* 339 (1998): 12–20.
20. E. B. Rimm, A. Ascherio, E. Giovannucci, D. Spiegelman, M. J. Stampfer, and W. C. Willett, "Vegetable, Fruit, and Cereal Fiber Intake and Risk of Coronary Heart Disease Among Men," *Journal of the American Medical Association* 275 (1996): 447–451.
21. R. J. Barnard, "Effects of Lifestyle Modification on Serum Lipids," *Archives of Internal Medicine* 151 (1991): 1389–1394.
22. National Cholesterol Education Program Expert Panel. "Summary of the Third Report of the National Cholesterol Education Program (NCEP) Expert Panel on Detection, Evaluation, and Treatment of High Blood Cholesterol in Adults (Adult Treatment Panel III)," *Journal of the American Medical Association* 285 (2001): 2486–2497.
23. W. Castelli, "Smart Heart Strategies: Best Ways to Beat Heart Disease," *Bottom Line/Personal Health* 19, no. 4 (1998): 1–3.
24. R. Superko, "Platelets and Lipid Interaction with a Vessel Wall" (paper presented in symposium at American College of Sports Medicine Annual Meeting, 1991).
25. O. Nygard, J. E. Nordreahaug, H. Refsum, P. M. Ueland, M. Farstad, and S. E. Vollset, "Plasma Homocysteine Levels and Mortality in Patients with Coronary Heart Disease," *New England Journal of Medicine* 337 (1997): 230–236.

26. "The Homocysteine-CVD Connection," *HealthNews* (October 25, 1999).
27. C. J. Boushey, S. A. A. Beresford, G. S. Omenn, and A. G. Motulsky, "A Quantitative Assessment of Plasma Homocysteine as a Risk Factor for Vascular Disease," *Journal of the American Medical Association* 274 (1995): 1049–1057.
28. "Diabetes: Weight Control and Exercise May Keep You Off the Road to High Blood Sugar," *Medical Essay*, supplement to *Mayo Clinic Health Letter* (February 1998).
29. S. P. Helmrich, D. R. Ragland, R. W. Leung, and R. S. Paffenbarger, "Physical Activity and Reduced Occurrences of Non-Insulin-Dependent Diabetes Mellitus," *New England Journal of Medicine* 325 (1991): 147–152.
30. E. J. Mayer et al., "Intensity and Amount of Physical Activity in Relation to Insulin Sensitivity," *Journal of the American Medical Association* 279 (1998): 669–674.
31. S. Liu et al., "A Prospective Study of Dietary Glycemic Load, Carbohydrate Intake, and Risk of Coronary Heart Disease in the U.S.," *American Journal of Clinical Nutrition* 71 (2000): 1455–1461.
32. G. M. Reaven, "Syndrome X: The Little Known Cause of Many Heart Attacks," *Bottom Line/Personal Health* 14 (June 2000).
33. See note 30.
34. G. M. Reaven, T. K. Strom, and B. Fox, *Syndrome X: Overcoming the Silent Killer That Can Give You a Heart Attack* (Simon & Schuster, 2000).
35. See note 33.
36. G. Kelley, "Dynamic Resistance Exercise and Resting Blood Pressure in Adults: A Meta-Analysis," *Journal of Applied Physiology* 82 (1997): 1559–1565.

    G. A. Kelley and Z. Tran, "Aerobic Exercise and Normotensive Adults: A Meta-Analysis," *Medicine and Science in Sports and Exercise* 27 (1995): 1371–1377.

    G. Kelley, and P. McClellan, "Antihypertensive Effects of Aerobic Exercise: A Brief Meta-Analytic Review of Randomized Controlled Trials," *American Journal of Hypertension* 7 (1994): 115–119.

37. R. Collins et al., "Blood Pressure, Stroke, and Coronary Heart Disease; Part 2, Short-term Reductions in Blood Pressure: Overview of Randomized Drug Trials in Their Epidemiological Context," *Lancet* 335 (1990): 827–838.

38. S. N. Blair et al., "Influences of Cardiorespiratory Fitness and Other Precursors on Cardiovascular Disease and All-cause Mortality in Men and Women," *Journal of the American Medical Association* 276 (1996): 205–210.

39. G. A. Kelley and K. S. Kelley, "Progressive Resistance Exercise and Resting Blood Pressure: A Meta-Analysis of Randomized Controlled Trials," *Hypertension* 35 (2000): 838–843.

40. F. W. Kash, J. L. Boyer, S. P. Van Camp, L. S. Verity, and J. P. Wallace, "The Effect of Physical Activity on Aerobic Power in Older Men (A Longitudinal Study)," *Physician and Sports Medicine* 18, no. 4 (1990): 73–83.

41. S. G. Sheps, "High Blood Pressure Can Often Be Controlled Without Medication," *Bottom Line/Personal Health* (November, 1999).

42. "Checkup for the New Millennium," *Consumer Reports on Health* (December, 1999).

43. E. Awtry, "Aspirin Helps Prevent Life-Threatening Disease and Chronic Conditions," *Bottom Line/Personal Health* (September, 2000).

Suggested Readings

■ American Heart Association. *2002 Heart and Stroke Facts Statistical Update*. Dallas: AHA, 2001.

■ American Heart Association. *Heart and Stroke Facts*. Dallas: AHA, 2001.

■ Barnard, R. J. "A Carbohydrate Diet to Prevent and Control Coronary Heart Disease." *ACSM's Health and Fitness Journal* 3 (May/June 1999): 23–26.

■ Blair, S. N., et al. "Physical Activity, Nutrition, and Chronic Disease." *Medicine and Science in Sports and Exercise* 28 (1996): 335–349.

■ Gibbons, L. W., S. Blair, K. H. Cooper, and M. Smith. "Association Between Coronary Heart Disease Risk Factors and Physical Fitness in Healthy Adult Women." *Circulation* 5 (1993): 977–983.

■ National Cholesterol Education Program Expert Panel. "Summary of the Third Report of the National Cholesterol Education Program (NCEP) Expert Panel on Detection, Evaluation, and Treatment of High Blood Cholesterol in Adults (Adult Treatment Panel III)." *Journal of the American Medical Association* 285 (2001): 2486–2497.

■ Ornish, D. S., E. Brown, L. W. Scherwitz et al. "Can Lifestyle Changes Reverse Coronary Heart Disease? Lifestyle Heart Trial." *Lancet* 336 (1990): 129–133.

■ Superko, H. R. "New Aspects of Cardiovascular Risk Factors Including Small Dense LDL, Homocysteinemia, and Lp(a)." *Current Opinions in Cardiology* 10 (1995): 347–354.

■ Superko, H. R. "The Most Common Cause of Coronary Heart Disease Can Be Successfully Treated by the Least Expensive Therapy: Exercise." *Certified News* (1998): 1–5.

■ Superko, H. R., R. M. Kraus, and E. M. Alderman. "Diabetics Have Rapid Arteriographic Coronary Disease Progression but Also Arteriographic Benefit from Risk Reduction." *Circulation* 96 (1997): 4289.

■ Whaley, M. H., and S. N. Blair. "Epidemiology of Physical Activity, Physical Fitness and Coronary Heart Disease." *Certified News* 5, no. 2 (1995): 1–7.

Cancer Prevention

Chapter 11

© 2002 EyeWire Collection/Getty Images

Be able to define cancer and understand how it starts and spreads.

Become acquainted with guidelines for preventing cancer.

Become familiar with major risk factors that lead to specific types of cancer.

Assess the risk of developing certain types of cancer.

The human body has approximately 100 trillion cells. Under normal conditions, these cells reproduce themselves in an orderly way. Cell growth (cell reproduction) takes place so old, worn-out tissue can be replaced and injuries can be repaired.

Cell growth is controlled by **deoxyribonucleic acid (DNA)** and **ribonucleic acid (RNA)**, found in the nucleus of each cell. When nuclei lose their ability to regulate and control cell growth, cell division is disrupted and mutant cells can develop (see Figure 11.1). Some of these cells might grow uncontrollably and abnormally, forming a mass of tissue called a "tumor," which can be either **benign** or **malignant**. Benign tumors do not invade other tissues. They can interfere with normal bodily functions, but they rarely cause death. A malignant tumor is a **cancer**. More than 100 types of cancer can develop in any tissue or organ of the human body.

The process of cancer actually begins with an alteration in DNA. Found within DNA are **oncogenes** and tumor **suppressor genes**, which normally work together to repair and replace cells. Defects in these genes—caused by external factors such as radiation, chemicals, and viruses, as well as internal factors such as immune conditions, hormones, and genetic mutations—ultimately allow the cell to grow into a tumor.

A healthy cell may duplicate as many as 100 times in its lifetime. Normally, the DNA molecule is duplicated perfectly during cell division. In the few cases when the DNA molecule is not replicated exactly, specialized enzymes make repairs quickly. Occasionally, however, cells with defective DNA keep dividing and ultimately form a small tumor. As more mutations occur, the altered cells continue to divide and can become malignant. A decade or more can pass between carcinogenic exposure or mutations and the time cancer is diagnosed.

The process of abnormal cell division is related indirectly to chromosome segments called **telomeres** (see Figure 11.2). Each time a cell divides, chromosomes lose some telomeres. After many cell divisions, chromosomes eventually run out of telomeres and the cell then invariably dies.

Scientists have discovered that human tumors make an enzyme known as **telomerase**. In cancer cells, telomerase keeps the chromosome from running out of telomeres entirely. The shortened strand of telomeres (see Figure 11.3) now allows cells to reproduce indefinitely.[1]

FIGURE 11.1 Mutant (cancer) cells.

Illustration courtesy of American Cancer Society (contained in *Youth Looks at Cancer*, New York: American Cancer Society, p. 4, 1982).

FIGURE 11.2 Erosion of chromosome telomeres in normal cells.

Telomeres   * Successive cell divisions   Death of Cell

FIGURE 11.3 Action of the enzyme telomerase.

Telomeres   * Successive cell divisions   Telomerase

Telomerase seems to have another function that is still under investigation: After many cell divisions, by nature cancer cells grow old, but telomerase keeps them from dying. If scientists can confirm that telomerase plays such a crucial role in the formation of tumors, research efforts will be directed to finding a way to block the action of telomerase, thereby making cancerous cells die.

Cancer starts with the abnormal growth of one cell, which then can multiply into billions of cancerous cells. A critical turning point in the development of cancer is when a tumor reaches about 1 million cells. At this stage, it is referred to as **carcinoma in situ**. Such an undetected tumor may go for months or years without any significant growth. While it remains encapsulated, it does not pose a serious threat to human health. However, to grow, the tumor requires more oxygen and nutrients. In time, a few of the cancer cells start producing chemicals that enhance **angiogenesis**, or capillary (blood vessel) formation into the tumor. Angiogenesis is the precursor of **metastasis**. Through the new blood vessels formed by angiogenesis, cancerous cells now can break away from a malignant tumor and migrate to other parts of the body, where they can cause new cancer (Figure 11.4).

Key Terms

Deoxyribonucleic acid (DNA) Genetic substance of which genes are made; molecule that contains cell's genetic code.

Ribonucleic acid (RNA) Genetic material that guides the formation of cell proteins.

Benign Noncancerous.

Malignant Cancerous.

Cancer Group of diseases characterized by uncontrolled growth and spread of abnormal cells.

Oncogenes Genes that initiate cell division.

Suppressor genes Genes that deactivate the process of cell division.

Telomeres A strand of molecules at both ends of a chromosome.

Telomerase An enzyme that allows cells to reproduce indefinitely.

Carcinoma in situ Encapsulated malignant tumor that has not spread.

Angiogenesis Formation of blood vessels (capillaries).

Metastasis The movement of cells from one part of the body to another.

FIGURE 11.4 How cancer starts and spreads.

Most adults have precancerous or cancerous cells in their bodies. By middle age, our bodies contain millions of precancerous cells. Although the immune system and the blood turbulence destroy most cancer cells, it takes only one abnormal cell lodging elsewhere to start a new cancer. These cells grow and multiply uncontrollably, invading and destroying normal tissue. The rate at which cancer cells grow varies from one type to another. Some types grow fast; others take years.

Once cancer cells metastasize, treatment becomes more difficult. Although therapy can kill most cancer cells, a few cells might become resistant to treatment. These cells then can grow into a new tumor that will not respond to the same treatment.

INCIDENCE OF CANCER

According to mortality statistics for 2000 from the National Center for Health Statistics, cancer was the cause of 23.0 percent of all deaths in the United States. It is the second leading cause of death in the country and the leading cause in children between ages 1 and 14.

Cancer will develop in approximately 1 in 2 men and 1 in 3 women in the United States, striking approximately 3 of every 4 families. About 552,200 Americans died from cancer in 2001, and approximately 1,220,100 new cases were diagnosed that same year.[2]

The year 2002 statistical estimates of the incidence of cancer and deaths by sex and site are given in Figure 11.5. These estimates exclude **nonmelanoma skin cancer** and carcinoma in situ.

Like coronary heart disease, cancer is largely preventable. As much as 80 percent of all human cancer is related to lifestyle or environmental factors (including diet and obesity, tobacco use, sedentary lifestyle, excessive use of alcohol, and exposure to occupational hazards—see Figure 11.6). Most of these cancers could be prevented through positive lifestyle habits.

Research sponsored by the American Cancer Society and the National Cancer Institute showed that individuals who have a healthy lifestyle have some of the lowest cancer mortality rates ever reported in scientific studies.[3] A group of about 10,000 members of the Church of Jesus Christ of Latter-Day Saints (commonly referred to as the Mormon church) in California was reported to have only about one-third

FIGURE 11.5 Year 2002 estimated cancer incidence and deaths by site and sex.

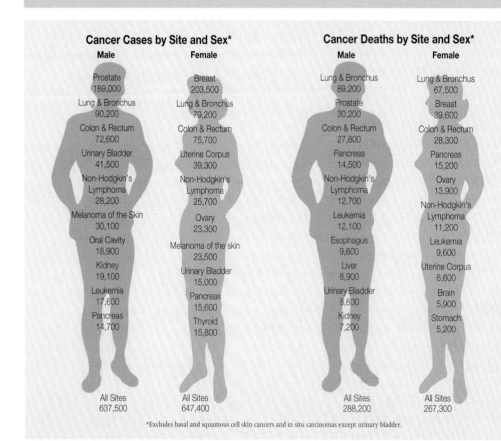

Cancer Cases by Site and Sex*

Male	Female
Prostate 189,000	Breast 203,500
Lung & Bronchus 90,200	Lung & Bronchus 79,200
Colon & Rectum 72,600	Colon & Rectum 75,700
Urinary Bladder 41,500	Uterine Corpus 39,300
Non-Hodgkin's Lymphoma 28,200	Non-Hodgkin's Lymphoma 25,700
Melanoma of the Skin 30,100	Ovary 23,300
Oral Cavity 18,900	Melanoma of the skin 23,500
Kidney 19,100	Urinary Bladder 15,000
Leukemia 17,600	Pancreas 15,600
Pancreas 14,700	Thyroid 15,800
All Sites 637,500	All Sites 647,400

Cancer Deaths by Site and Sex*

Male	Female
Lung & Bronchus 89,200	Lung & Bronchus 67,500
Prostate 30,200	Breast 39,600
Colon & Rectum 27,800	Colon & Rectum 28,300
Pancreas 14,500	Pancreas 15,200
Non-Hodgkin's Lymphoma 12,700	Ovary 13,900
Leukemia 12,100	Non-Hodgkin's Lymphoma 11,200
Esophagus 9,600	Leukemia 9,600
Liver 8,900	Uterine Corpus 6,600
Urinary Bladder 8,600	Brain 5,900
Kidney 7,200	Stomach 5,200
All Sites 288,200	All Sites 267,300

SOURCE: *2002 Cancer Facts and Figures.* American Cancer Society (New York: ACS, 2002).

*Excludes basal and squamous cell skin cancers and in situ carcinomas except urinary bladder.

FIGURE 11.6 Estimate of the relative roles of the major cancer-causing factors.

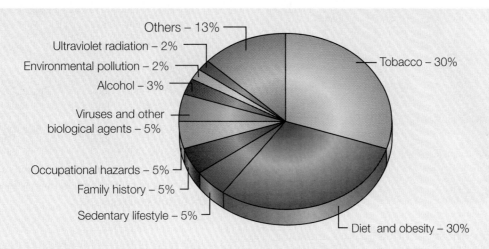

Others – 13%
Ultraviolet radiation – 2%
Environmental pollution – 2%
Alcohol – 3%
Viruses and other biological agents – 5%
Occupational hazards – 5%
Family history – 5%
Sedentary lifestyle – 5%
Tobacco – 30%
Diet and obesity – 30%

SOURCE: Harvard Center for Cancer Prevention. *Causes of Human Cancer*, Harvard Report on Cancer Prevention 1 (1996).

(men) to one-half (women) the rate of cancer mortality of the general white population (Figure 11.7). In this study the investigators looked at three general health habits in the participants: lifetime abstinence from smoking, regular physical activity, and sufficient sleep. In addition, healthy lifestyle guidelines (encouraged by the church since 1833) include abstaining from all forms of tobacco, alcohol, caffeine, and drugs and adhering to a well-balanced diet based on grains, fruits, and vegetables, and moderate amounts of poultry and red meat. Lifestyle is apparently an important factor in cancer risk.

Equally important is that more than 8.4 million Americans with a history of cancer were alive in 2000. Currently, 4 of 10 people diagnosed with cancer are expected to be alive 5 years after the initial diagnosis.[4]

GUIDELINES FOR PREVENTING CANCER

The biggest factor in fighting cancer today is health education. People need to be informed about the risk factors for cancer and the guidelines for early detection. The most effective way to protect against cancer is to change negative lifestyle habits and behaviors. Following are some guidelines for preventing cancer.

Dietary Changes

The American Cancer Society estimates that one-third of all cancers in the United States are related to nutrition. A healthy diet, therefore, is crucial to decrease

FIGURE 11.7 Effects of a healthy lifestyle on cancer mortality rate.

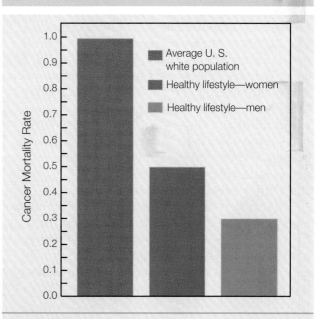

Cancer Mortality Rate

■ Average U. S. white population
■ Healthy lifestyle—women
■ Healthy lifestyle—men

source: "Health Practices and Cancer Mortality Among Active California Mormons," *Journal of the National Cancer Institute* 81 (1989): 1807–1814.

NOTE: Healthy lifestyle factors include proper nutrition, abstinence from cigarette smoking, regular sleep (7–8 hours per night), and regular physical activity.

Key Terms

Nonmelanoma skin cancer Cancer that spreads or grows at the original site but does not metastasize to other regions of the body.

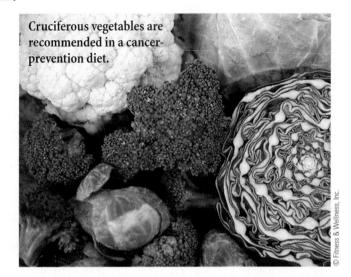

Cruciferous vegetables are recommended in a cancer-prevention diet.

© Fitness & Wellness, Inc.

© Fitness & Wellness, Inc.

Nutrition guidelines for a cancer-prevention program include a diet low in fat and high in fiber, with ample amounts of fruits and vegetables.

the risk for cancer. The diet should be predominately vegetarian, high in fiber, and low in fat (particularly from animal sources). **Cruciferous vegetables**, tea, soy products, calcium, and omega-3 fats are encouraged. Protein intake should be kept within the recommended nutrient guidelines. If alcohol is used, it should be used in moderation. Obesity should be avoided.

Green and dark yellow vegetables, cruciferous vegetables (cauliflower, broccoli, cabbage, Brussels sprouts, and kohlrabi), and beans (legumes) seem to protect against cancer. Folate, found naturally in dark green leafy vegetables, dried beans, and orange juice, may reduce the risk of colon and cervical cancers. Brightly colored fruits and vegetables also contain **carotenoids** and vitamin C. Lycopene, one of the many carotenoids (a phytochemical—see discussion below), has been linked to lower risk of cancers of the prostate, colon, and cervix. Lycopene is especially abundant in cooked tomato products.

Researchers believe the antioxidant effect of vitamins and the mineral selenium help protect the body from oxygen free radicals. As discussed in Chapter 8 (under "Antioxidants", page 220), during normal metabolism most of the oxygen in the human body is converted into stable forms of carbon dioxide and water. A small amount, however, ends up in an unstable form known as "oxygen free radicals," which are thought to attack and damage the cell membrane and DNA, leading to the formation of cancers. Antioxidants absorb free radicals before they can cause damage and also interrupt the sequence of reactions once damage has begun.

A promising horizon in cancer prevention is the discovery of **phytochemicals**. These compounds, found in abundance in fruits and vegetables, seem to prevent cancer by blocking the formation of cancerous tumors and disrupting the process at almost every

step of the way. Phytochemicals exert their protective action in all of the following ways:[5]

- Removing **carcinogens** from cells before they cause damage.
- Activating enzymes that detoxify cancer-causing agents.
- Keeping carcinogens from locking onto cells.
- Preventing carcinogens from binding to DNA.
- Breaking up cancer-causing precursors to benign forms.
- Disrupting the chemical combination of cell molecules that can produce carcinogens.
- Keeping small tumors from accessing capillaries (small blood vessels) to get oxygen and nutrients.

Examples of phytochemicals and their effects are found in Table 11.1.

Although one recent study failed to show an association, many studies have linked low intake of fiber to increased risk for colon cancer. Fiber binds to bile acids in the intestine for excretion from the body in the stools. Bile acids' interaction with intestinal bacteria releases carcinogenic byproducts. Bile acid production increases with higher fat content in the small intestine (created, of course, by higher fat content in the diet).

Daily consumption of 25 to 35 grams of fiber is recommended. Grains are high in fiber and contain vitamins and minerals (folate, selenium, and calcium), which seem to decrease the risk for colon cancer. Selenium also protects against prostate cancer and, possibly, lung cancer. Calcium may also protect against colon cancer by preventing rapid growth of cells in the colon, especially in people with colon polyps.

Polyphenols (phytochemicals) are potent cancer-fighting antioxidants found in fresh fruits and

TABLE **11.1**	Effects and Sources of Selected Phytochemicals	
Phytochemical	**Effect**	**Good Sources**
Sulforaphane	Removes carcinogens from cells	Broccoli
PEITC	Keeps carcinogens from binding to DNA	Broccoli
Genistein	Prevents small tumors from accessing capillaries to get oxygen and nutrients	Soybeans
Flavonoids	Helps keep cancer-causing hormones from locking onto cells	Most fruits and vegetables
p-coumaric and chlorogenic acids	Disrupts the chemical combination of cell molecules that can produce carcinogens	Strawberries, green peppers, tomatoes, pineapple
Capsaicin	Keeps carcinogens from binding to DNA	Hot chili peppers

vegetables, many grains, and regular teas. Green, black, and red tea all appear to provide protection. Evidence also points to certain components in tea that can block the spread of cancers to other parts of the body.

Polyphenols are known to block the formation of **nitrosamines** and quell the activation of carcinogens. Both green and black tea have similar amounts of polyphenols.

Polyphenols are also thought to fight cancer by shutting off the formation of cancer cells, turning up the body's natural detoxification defenses and thereby suppressing progression of the disease.

Green tea seems to be especially helpful in preventing gastrointestinal cancers, including those of the stomach, small intestines, pancreas, and colon. Consumption of green tea also has been linked to a lower incidence of lung, esophageal, and estrogen-related cancers, including most breast cancers. In Japan, where people drink green tea regularly but smoke twice as much as do people in the United States, the incidence of lung cancer is half that of the United States. The antioxidant effect of one of the polyphenols in green tea, epigallocatechin gallate, or EGCG, is at least 25 times more effective than vitamin E and 100 times more effective than vitamin C at protecting cells and the DNA from damage believed to cause cancer, heart disease, and other diseases associated with free radicals.[6] EGCG is also twice as strong as the red wine antioxidant resveratrol in helping prevent heart disease. Other research indicates that phytochemicals in green tea induce cancer cells to self-destruct.[7]

A cancer-prevention diet recommends drinking 2 or more cups of green tea daily. Herbal teas do not provide the same benefits as regular tea.[8]

High fat intake may promote cancer and excessive weight. Some experts recommend that total fat intake should be limited to less than 20 percent of total daily calories.[9] Fat intake should be primarily monounsaturated and omega-3 fats. Omega-3 fats (found in many types of fish, flaxseeds, and flaxseed oil) seem to offer protection against colorectal, pancreatic, breast, oral, esophageal, and stomach cancers. Omega-3 fats block the synthesis of prostaglandins, bodily compounds that promote tumor growth.

Foods high in vitamin C may deter some cancers. Salt-cured, smoked, and nitrite-cured foods have been associated with cancer of the esophagus and stomach. Processed meats should be consumed sparingly and always with orange juice or other vitamin C-rich foods. Vitamin C seems to discourage the formation of nitrosamines. These potentially cancer-causing compounds are formed when nitrites and nitrates, which are used to prevent the growth of harmful bacteria in processed meats, combine with other chemicals in the stomach.

KeyTerms

Cruciferous vegetables Plants that produce cross-shaped leaves (cauliflower, broccoli, cabbage, Brussels sprouts, and kohlrabi); they seem to have a protective effect against cancer.

Carotenoids Pigment substances in plants that are often precursors to vitamin A. Over 600 carotenoids are found in nature and about 50 of them are precursors to vitamin A, the most potent one being beta-carotene.

Phytochemicals Compounds found in fruits and vegetables that block the formation of cancerous tumors and disrupt the progress of cancer.

Carcinogens Substances that contribute to the formation of cancers.

Nitrosamines Potentially cancer-causing compounds formed when nitrites and nitrates, which are used to prevent the growth of harmful bacteria in processed meats, combine with other chemicals in the stomach.

Nutritional guidelines also discourage excessive intake of protein. The daily protein intake for some people is almost twice the amount the human body needs. Too much animal protein seems to decrease blood enzymes that prevent precancerous cells from developing into tumors.

Some research suggests that grilling protein (fat or lean) at high temperatures for a long time increases the formation of carcinogenic substances on the skin or surface of the meat. Microwaving the meat for a couple of minutes before barbecuing decreases the risk, as long as the fluid released by the meat is discarded. Most of the potential carcinogens collect in this solution. Removing the skin before serving and cooking at lower heat to "medium" rather than "well done" also seem to lower the risk.[10]

Soy protein also seems to decrease the formation of carcinogens during cooking of meats.[11] Soy foods may help because soy contains chemicals that prevent cancer. Although further research is merited, isoflavones (phytochemicals) found in soy are structurally similar to estrogen and may prevent breast, prostate, lung, and colon cancers. These isoflavones are frequently referred to as "phytoestrogens" or "plant estrogens." Isoflavones also block angiogenesis. Presently, it is not known if the health benefits of soy are derived from isoflavones by themselves or in combination with other nutrients found in soy.

One drawback of soy was found in animal studies wherein animals with tumors were given very large amounts of soy: The estrogen-like activity of soy isoflavones actually led to the growth of estrogen-dependent tumors. Experts, therefore, caution women with breast cancer or a history of this disease to limit soy intake because it may stimulate cancer cells by closely imitating estrogen's actions.

No specific recommendations are presently available as to the amount of daily soy protein intake for cancer prevention. The FDA allows the health claim that 25 grams per day in conjunction with a diet low in saturated fat and cholesterol lowers the risk for cardiovascular disease (see Chapter 8). Based on the traditional diets of people (including children) in China and Japan who regularly consume soy foods, there doesn't appear to be an unsafe natural level of consumption. Soy protein powder supplementation, however, may elevate soy protein intake to an unnatural (and perhaps unsafe) level.[12]

Tips for a healthy cancer-fighting diet

Increase intake of phytochemicals, fiber, cruciferous vegetables, and more antioxidants by

- Eating a predominantly vegetarian diet
- Eating more fruits and vegetables every day (six to eight servings per day maximize anticancer benefits)
- Increasing the consumption of broccoli, cauliflower, kale, turnips, cabbage, kohlrabi, Brussels sprouts, hot chili peppers, red and green peppers, carrots, sweet potatoes, winter squash, spinach, garlic, onions, strawberries, tomatoes, pineapple, and citrus fruits in your regular diet
- Eating vegetables raw or quickly cooked by steaming or stir-frying
- Substituting tea, fruit, and vegetable juices for coffee and soda
- Eating whole grain breads
- Including calcium in the diet (or from a supplement)
- Including soy products in the diet
- Using whole wheat flour instead of refined white flour in baking
- Using brown (unpolished) rice instead of white (polished) rice

Decrease daily fat intake to 20% of total caloric intake by

- Limiting consumption of beef, poultry, or fish to no more 3 to 6 ounces (about the size of a deck of cards) once or twice a week
- Trimming all visible fat from meat and removing skin from poultry prior to cooking
- Decreasing the amount of fat and oils used in cooking
- Substituting low-fat for high-fat dairy products
- Using salad dressings sparingly
- Using only half to three-quarters the amount of fat required in baking recipes
- Limiting fat intake to mostly monounsaturated (olive oil, canola oil, nuts, and seeds) and omega-3 fats (fish, flaxseed, and flaxseed oil)
- Eating fish once or twice a week
- Including flaxseed oil (or flaxseeds) in the diet

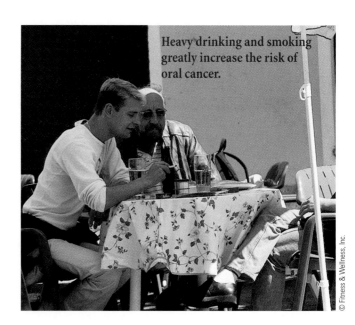

Heavy drinking and smoking greatly increase the risk of oral cancer.

Alcohol should be consumed in moderation, because too much alcohol raises the risk for developing certain cancers, especially when it is combined with tobacco smoking or smokeless tobacco. In combination, these substances significantly increase the risk for cancers of the mouth, larynx, throat, esophagus, and liver. Approximately 17,000 deaths from cancer yearly are attributed to excessive use of alcohol, often in combination with smoking. The combined action of heavy alcohol and tobacco use can increase odds of developing cancer of the oral cavity fifteenfold.

Maintaining recommended body weight also is encouraged. Obesity may be associated with cancers of the colon, rectum, breast, prostate, endometrium, and kidney.

Abstaining from Tobacco

Cigarette smoking by itself is a major health hazard. If we include all related deaths, smoking is responsible for more than 400,000 unnecessary deaths in the United States each year. The World Health Organization estimates that smoking causes 3 million deaths worldwide annually. The average life expectancy for a chronic smoker is about 15 years shorter than for a nonsmoker.[13]

The biggest carcinogenic exposure in the workplace is cigarette smoke. Of all cancers, at least 28 percent are tied to smoking, and 87 percent of lung cancers are tied to smoking. Use of smokeless tobacco also can lead to nicotine addiction and dependence as well as increased risk for mouth, larynx, throat, and esophageal cancers.[14]

Avoiding Excessive Sun Exposure

Too much exposure to ultraviolet radiation (both UVB and UVA rays) is a major contributor to skin cancer. The most common sites of skin cancer are those areas exposed to the sun most often (face, neck, and back of the hands).

The three types of skin cancer are

1. Basal cell carcinoma
2. Squamous cell carcinoma
3. Malignant melanoma

Nearly 90 percent of the almost 1 million cases of basal cell or squamous cell skin cancers reported yearly in the United States could have been prevented by protecting the skin from the sun's rays. **Melanoma** is the most deadly, causing approximately 7,700 deaths in 2000. One in every six Americans will develop some type of skin cancer eventually. Nothing is healthy

Tanning poses a risk for skin cancer from overexposure to ultraviolet rays.

about a "healthy tan." Tanning of the skin is the body's natural reaction to permanent and irreversible damage from too much exposure to the sun. Even small doses of sunlight add up to a greater risk for skin cancer and premature aging. The tan fades at the end of the summer season, but the underlying skin damage does not disappear. People with sensitive skin in particular should avoid sun exposure between 10:00 A.M. and 4:00 P.M.

The stinging sunburn comes from **ultraviolet B rays (UVB)**, which also are thought to be the main cause of premature wrinkling and skin aging, roughened/leathery/sagging skin, and skin cancer. Unfortunately, the damage may not become evident until up to 20 years later. In comparison, skin that has not been overexposed to the sun remains smooth and unblemished, and, over time, shows less evidence of aging.

Sun lamps and tanning parlors provide mainly ultraviolet A rays (UVA). Once thought to be safe, they are now known to be damaging and have been linked to melanoma, the most serious form of skin cancer. As little as 15 to 30 minutes of exposure to UVA can be as dangerous as a day spent in the sun.[15]

Sunscreen lotion should be applied about 30 minutes before lengthy exposure to the sun because the

KeyTerms

Melanoma The most virulent, rapidly spreading form of skin cancer.

Ultraviolet B rays (UVB) Portion of sunlight that causes sunburn and encourages skin cancers.

skin takes that long to absorb the protective ingredients. A **sun protection factor (SPF)** of at least 15 is recommended. SPF 15 means that the skin takes 15 times longer to burn than with no lotion. If you ordinarily get a mild sunburn after 20 minutes of noonday sun, an SPF 15 allows you to remain in the sun about 300 minutes before burning. The higher the number, the stronger the protection. When swimming or sweating, you should reapply waterproof sunscreens more often because all sunscreens lose strength when they are diluted.

Monitoring Estrogen, Radiation Exposure, and Potential Occupational Hazards

Intake of estrogen has been linked to endometrial cancer in some studies, but other evidence contradicts those findings. And, although exposure to radiation increases the risk for cancer, the benefits of X rays may outweigh the risk involved, and most medical facilities use the lowest dose possible to keep the risk to a minimum. Occupational hazards —such as asbestos fibers, nickel and uranium dusts, chromium compounds, vinyl chloride, and bischlormethyl ether —increase the risk for cancer. Cigarette smoking magnifies the risk from occupational hazards.

Engaging in Physical Activity

An active lifestyle seems to have a protective effect against cancer. Although the mechanism is not clear, physical fitness and cancer mortality in men and women may have a graded and consistent inverse relationship[16] (see Figure 11.8). A daily 30-minute moderate-intensity exercise program lowers the risk for colon cancer and may lower the risk for cancers of the breast and reproductive system. Research has shown that regular exercise lowers the risk for breast cancer in women by 20 to 30 percent. In addition, growing evidence suggests that the body's autoimmune system may play a role in preventing cancer. Moderate exercise improves the autoimmune system.[17]

Early Detection

Fortunately, many cancers can be controlled or cured through early detection. The real problem comes when cancerous cells spread, because they become more difficult to destroy. Therefore, effective prevention, or at least early detection, is crucial. Herein lies the importance of periodic screening. Once a month, women should practice breast self-examination (BSE) (see Figure 11.14, page 317) and men testicular self-examination (TSE) (see Figure 11.15, page 320). Men should pick a regular day each month (for example, the first day of each month) to practice TSE, and

FIGURE 11.8 Association between physical fitness and cancer mortality.

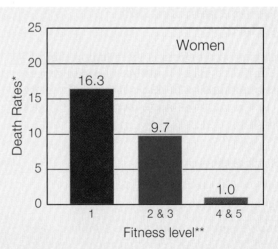

*Age-adjusted per 10,000 person-years at follow-up
**1 = lowest fitness, 5 = highest fitness

SOURCE: S. N. Blair, H. W. Kohl III, R. S. Paffenbarger, Jr., D. G. Clark, K. H. Cooper, and L. W. Gibbons, "Physical Fitness and All-Cause Mortality: A Prospective Study of Healthy Men and Women," *Journal of the American Medical Association* 262 (1989): 2395–2401.

Cancer promoters

- Physical inactivity
- Being more than 10 pounds overweight
- Frequent consumption of red meat
- A diet high in fat
- Charred/burned foods
- Frequent consumption of nitrate/nitrite-cured, salt-cured, or smoked foods
- Alcohol consumption
- Excessive sun exposure

women should perform BSE 2 or 3 days after the menstrual period is over.

Other Factors

The contribution of many of the other much-publicized factors is not as significant as those just pointed out. Intentional food additives, saccharin, processing agents, pesticides, and packaging materials currently used in the United States and other developed countries seem to have minimal consequences. High levels of tension and stress and poor coping may affect the autoimmune system negatively and render the body less effective in dealing with the various cancers. In the workplace, the biggest carcinogenic exposure is that to cigarette smoke.

Genetics plays a role in susceptibility in about 10 percent of all cancers. Most of the effect is seen in the early childhood years. Some cancers are a combination of genetic and environmental liability: Genetics may add to the environmental risk of certain types of cancers. "Environment," however, means more than pollution and smoke. It incorporates diet, lifestyle-related events, viruses, and physical agents such as X rays and exposure to the sun.

WARNING SIGNALS OF CANCER

Everyone should become familiar with the following seven warning signals for cancer and bring them to a physician's attention if any are present:

1. Change in bowel or bladder habits.
2. Sore that does not heal.
3. Unusual bleeding or discharge.
4. Thickening or lump in breast or elsewhere.
5. Indigestion or difficulty in swallowing.
6. Obvious change in wart or mole.
7. Nagging cough or hoarseness.

The recommendations for early detection of cancer in asymptomatic people by the American Cancer Society, outlined in Table 11.2, should be heeded in regular physical examinations as part of a cancer-prevention program. In Figure 11.9 you will be able to determine how well you are doing in terms of cancer prevention. Figure 11.10 provides a questionnaire developed by the American Medical Association to alert people to symptoms that may indicate a serious health problem. Although in most cases nothing serious will be found, any of the symptoms calls for a physician's attention as soon as possible. Scientific evidence and testing procedures for prevention and early detection of cancer do change. Studies continue to provide new information. The intent of cancer-prevention programs is to educate and guide individuals toward a lifestyle that will help prevent cancer and enable early detection of malignancy.

Treatment of cancer should always be left to specialized physicians and cancer clinics. Current treatment modalities include surgery, radiation, radioactive substances, chemotherapy, hormones, and immunotherapy.

CANCER QUESTIONNAIRE: ASSESSING YOUR RISKS

The Texas Division of the American Cancer Society designed a simple self-testing questionnaire, shown in Figure 11.11, to help people assess their risk for cancer. These are the major risk factors for specific cancer sites and by no means represent the only ones that might be involved. Both men and women should complete the questions for lung, colon-rectum, and skin cancer. Three additional cancer types are included for women: breast, cervical, and endometrial.

Check your status against the factors contained in this questionnaire, total your scores, and then locate your "Total Risk" in the sections below. Individual numbers for specific questions are not to be interpreted as a precise measure of relative risk, but the totals for a given site should give you a general indication of your risk. Explanations of the risk factors for each type of cancer follows. If you are at higher risk, you are advised to discuss the results with your physician.

To assess your own risk levels, fill out the questionnaire in Figure 11.11, total the points, and then

KeyTerms

Sun protection factor (SPF) Degree of protection offered by ingredients in sunscreen lotion; at least SPF 15 is recommended.

TABLE 11.2 Summary of Recommendations for Early Detection of Cancer in Asymptomatic People

Cancer-related Checkup	A cancer-related checkup is recommended every 3 years for people aged 20–40 and every year for people age 40 and older. This exam should include health counseling and, depending on a person's age, might include examinations for cancers of the thyroid, oral cavity, skin, lymph nodes, testes, and ovaries, as well as for some nonmalignant diseases.
Breast	Women 40 and older should have an annual mammogram, an annual clinical breast examination (CBE) by a health-care professional, and should perform monthly breast self-examination (BSE). The CBE should be conducted close to and preferably before the scheduled mammogram. Women aged 20–39 should have a clinical breast examination by a health-care professional every three years and should perform monthly BSE.
Colon & Rectum	Beginning at age 50, men and women at average risk should follow one of the examination schedules below: • Fecal occult blood test (FOBT) every year, or • Flexible sigmoidoscopy every five years,* or • FOBT every year and flexible sigmoidoscopy every 5 years,* or • Double-contrast barium enema every 5 years,* or • Colonoscopy every 10 years.* Of these 3 options, the American Cancer Society prefers the third option, annual FOBT and flexible sigmoidoscopy every 5 years. * A digital rectal exam should be done at the same time as sigmoidoscopy, colonoscopy, or double-contrast barium enema. People who are at increased or high risk for colorectal cancer should talk with a doctor about a different testing schedule.
Prostate	Beginning at age 50, the prostate-specific antigen (PSA) test and the digital rectal exam should be offered annually to men who have a life expectancy of at least 10 years. Men at high risk (African-American men and men who have a first-degree relative who was diagnosed with prostate cancer at a young age) should begin testing at age 45. Patients should be given information about the benefits and limitations of tests so they can make an informed decision.
Uterus	**Cervix:** All women who are or have been sexually active or who are 18 and older should have an annual Pap test and pelvic examination. After three or more consecutive satisfactory examinations with normal findings, the Pap test may be performed less frequently. Discuss the matter with your physician. **Endometrium:** Beginning at age 35, women with or at risk for hereditary non-polyposis colon cancer should be offered endometrial biopsy annually to screen for endometrial cancer.

"Cancer Facts and Figures." © 2001, American Cancer Society, Inc. Used by permission.

locate your risk levels in the following section. Record your risk level totals for each cancer site in Figure 11.16, page 325, and in Appendix A.]

Lung Cancer

RISK FACTORS

1. Gender. Men have a higher risk for developing lung cancer than women do, equating them for type, amount, and duration of smoking. However, because more women are smoking cigarettes for a longer duration than previously, their incidence of lung and upper respiratory tract (mouth, tongue, and larynx) cancer is increasing. Lung cancer is now number one in mortality for women by type of cancer.

2. Age. The occurrence of lung and upper respiratory tract cancers increases with age.

3. Smoking status. Cigarette smokers have up to 20 times or even greater risk than nonsmokers. The rates of ex-smokers who have not smoked for 10 years, however, approach those of nonsmokers.

4. Type of smoking. Pipe and cigar smokers are at a higher risk for lung cancer than nonsmokers. Cigarette smokers are at a much higher risk than nonsmokers or pipe and cigar smokers. All forms of tobacco, including chewing, markedly increase the user's risk of developing cancer of the mouth.

5. Number of cigarettes smoked per day. Male smokers of less than one-half pack per day have 5 times higher lung cancer rates than nonsmokers. Male smokers of one to two packs per day have 15 times

FIGURE 11.9 Cancer prevention questionnaire.

Name:_____ Date: _____

Course: _____ Section: _____ Gender:_____ Age: _____

I. Cancer Prevention: Are You Taking Control?

Today, scientists think most cancers may be related to lifestyle and environment—what you eat and drink, whether you smoke, and where you work and play. The good news, then, is that you can help reduce your own cancer risk by taking control of things in your daily life.

10 Steps to a Healthier Life and Reduced Cancer Risk

	Yes	No
1. **Are you eating more cabbage-family vegetables?** They include broccoli, cauliflower, Brussels sprouts, all cabbages, and kale.	☐	☐
2. **Are high-fiber foods included in your diet?** Fiber is found in whole grains, fruits, and vegetables including peaches, strawberries, potatoes, spinach, tomatoes, wheat and bran cereals, rice, popcorn, and whole-wheat bread.	☐	☐
3. **Do you choose foods with vitamin A?** Fresh foods with beta-carotene, including carrots, peaches, apricots, squash, and broccoli are the best source—not vitamin pills.	☐	☐
4. **Is vitamin C included in your diet?** You'll find it naturally in lots of fresh fruits and vegetables including grapefruit, cantaloupe, oranges, strawberries, red and green peppers, broccoli, and tomatoes.	☐	☐
5. **Do you exercise and monitor calorie intake to avoid weight gain?** Walking is ideal exercise for many people.	☐	☐
6. **Are you cutting overall fat intake?** This is done by eating lean meat, fish, skinned poultry, and low-fat dairy products.	☐	☐
7. **Do you limit salt-cured, smoked, nitrite-cured foods?** Choose bacon, ham, hot dogs or salt-cured fish only occasionally if you like them a lot.	☐	☐
8. **If you smoke, have you tried quitting?**	☐	☐
9. **If you drink alcohol, are you moderate in your intake?**	☐	☐
10. **Do you respect the sun's rays?** Protect yourself with sunscreen (at least SPE 15) and wear long sleeves and a hat, especially during midday hours—10 A.M. to 2 P.M.	☐	☐
11. **Do you have a family history of any type of cancer? If so, have you brought this to the attention of your personal physician?**	☐	☐
12. **Are you familiar with the seven warning signals for cancer?**	☐	☐

If you answered "yes" to most of these questions, **congratulations**. You are taking control of simple lifestyle factors that will help you feel better and reduce your risk for cancer.

II. Stage of Change for Cancer Prevention

Using Figure 2.4 (page 45) and Table 2.3 (page 43), identify your current stage of change for participation in a cancer-prevention program:

Adapted from the American Cancer Society, Texas Division.

FIGURE 11.10 Early warning signs of possible serious illness.

Name: _____ Date: _____

Course: _____ Section: _____ Gender: _____ Age: _____

Many serious illnesses begin with apparently minor or localized symptoms that, if recognized early, can alert you to act in time for the disease to be cured or controlled. In most cases, nothing is seriously wrong. **If you experience any of the following symptoms, discuss the problem with your physician without delay.** Check only conditions that apply.

- [ ] 1. Rapid loss of weight—more than about 4 kg (10 lbs) in 10 weeks—without apparent cause.
- [ ] 2. A sore, scab, or ulcer, either in the mouth or on the body, that fails to heal within about 3 weeks.
- [ ] 3. A skin blemish or mole that begins to bleed or itch or that changes color, size, or shape.
- [ ] 4. Severe headaches that develop for no obvious reason.
- [ ] 5. Sudden attacks of vomiting, without preceding nausea.
- [ ] 6. Fainting spells for no apparent reason.
- [ ] 7. Visual problems such as seeing "haloes" around lights or intermittently blurred vision, especially in dim light.
- [ ] 8. Increasing difficulty with swallowing.
- [ ] 9. Hoarseness without apparent cause that lasts for a week or more.
- [ ] 10. A "smoker's cough" or any other nagging cough that has been getting worse.
- [ ] 11. Blood in coughed-up phlegm, or sputum.
- [ ] 12. Constantly swollen ankles.
- [ ] 13. A bluish tinge to the lips, the insides of the eyelids, or the nailbeds.
- [ ] 14. Extreme shortness of breath for no apparent reason.
- [ ] 15. Vomiting of blood or a substance that resembles coffee grounds.
- [ ] 16. Persistent indigestion or abdominal pain.
- [ ] 17. A marked change in normal bowel habits, such as alternating attacks of diarrhea and constipation.
- [ ] 18. Bowel movements that look black and tarry.
- [ ] 19. Rectal bleeding.
- [ ] 20. Unusually cloudy, pink, red, or smoky-looking urine.
- [ ] 21. In men, discomfort or difficulty when urinating.
- [ ] 22. In men, discharge from the tip of the penis.
- [ ] 23. In women, a lump or unusual thickening of a breast or any alteration in breast shape such as flattening, bulging, or puckering of skin.
- [ ] 24. In women, bleeding or unusual discharge from the nipple.
- [ ] 25. In women, vaginal bleeding or "spotting" that occurs between usual menstrual periods or after menopause.

Reproduced with permission from *Family Medical Guide* by American Medical Association (New York: Random House, 1982).

FIGURE 11.11 Cancer questionnaire: Assessing your risks.

Name: _Duncan Brown_   Date: _1-29-03_

Course: _LF117_ Section: _02_ Gender: _M_ Age: _19_

Assessing Your Risks for Cancer

Read each question concerning each site and its specific risk factors. Be honest in your responses. Place the number in parentheses (risk points) in the box provided to the left of each question. For example, Question #2 on lung cancer: If you are 53 years old (age 50 to 59), then enter 5 (risk points) as your score on the left. At the end of each site, total your number of points for that site. Record the final number of points in Figure 11.16, page 325 and in Appendix A.

Lung Cancer

[2] 1. Gender
   a. Male (2)
   b. Female (1)

[1] 2. Age
   a. 39 or less (1)
   b. 40–49 (2)
   c. 50–59 (5)
   d. 60+ (7)

[1] 3. Smoking status
   a. Smoker (8)
   b. Nonsmoker (1)

[ ] 4. Type of smoking
   a. Cigarettes or little cigars (10)
   b. Pipe and/or cigar, but not cigarettes (3)
   c. Ex-cigarette smoker (2)

[1] 5. Amount of cigarettes smoked per day
   a. 0 cigarettes (1)
   b. Less than 1 pack per day (5)
   c. 1 pack (9)
   d. 1–2 packs (15)
   e. 2+ packs (20)

[1] 6. Type of cigarette
   a. High tar/nicotine (10)
   b. Medium T/N (9)
   c. Low T/N (7)
   d. Nonsmoker (1)

[1] 7. Duration of smoking
   a. Never smoked (1)
   b. Ex-smoker (3)
   c. Up to 15 years (5)
   d. 15–25 years (10)
   e. 25+ years (20)

[ ] 8. Type of industrial work
   a. Mining (3)
   b. Asbestos (7)
   c. Uranium and radio-active products (5)

[7] Total

Colon/Rectum Cancer

[10] 1. Age
   a. 39 or less (10)
   b. 40–59 (20)
   c. 60+ (50)

[1] 2. Has anyone in your immediate family ever had
   a. Colon cancer (20)
   b. One or more polyps of the colon (10)
   c. Neither (1)

[1] 3. Have you ever had
   a. Colon cancer (100)
   b. One or more polyps of the colon (40)
   c. Ulcerative colitis (20)
   d. Cancer of the breast or uterus (10)
   e. None (1)

[1] 4. Bleeding from the rectum (other than obvious hemorrhoids or piles)
   a. Yes (75)
   b. No (1)

[13] Total

Skin Cancer

[1] 1. Frequent work or play in the sun:
   a. Yes (10)
   b. No (1)

[1] 2. Work in mines, around coal tars, or around radioactivity:
   a. Yes (10)
   b. No (1)

[10] 3. Complexion—fair and/or light skin:
   a. Yes (10)
   b. No (1)

[12] Total

(Figure 11.11 Cancer questionnaire: Assessing your risks—continued)

Breast Cancer

1. Age group
   a. 20–34 (10)
   b. 35–49 (40)
   c. 50+ (90)

2. Race group
   a. Asian American (5)
   b. African American (20)
   c. White (25)
   d. Hispanic American (10)

3. Family history
   a. Mother, sister, aunt, or grandmother with breast cancer (30)
   b. None (10)

4. Your history
   a. Previous lumps or cysts (25)
   b. No breast disease (10)
   c. Previous breast cancer (100)

5. Maternity
   a. First pregnancy before 25 (10)
   b. First pregnancy after 25 (15)
   c. No pregnancies (20)

   Total

Cervical Cancer

(Lower portion of uterus. These questions do not apply to a woman who has had a total hysterectomy.)

1. Age group
   a. Less than 25 (10)
   b. 25–39 (20)
   c. 40–54 (30)
   d. 55+ (30)

2. Race
   a. Oriental (10)
   b. Puerto Rican (20)
   c. African American (20)
   d. White (10)
   e. Hispanic American (20)

3. Number of pregnancies
   a. 0 (10)
   b. 1–3 (20)
   c. 4 and over (30)

4. Viral infections
   a. Herpes and other viral infections or ulcer formations on the vagina (10)
   b. Never (1)

5. Age at first intercourse
   a. Before 15 (40)
   b. 15–19 (30)
   c. 20–24 (20)
   d. 25 and over (10)
   e. Never (5)

6. Bleeding between periods or after intercourse
   a. Yes (40)
   b. No (1)

   Total

Endometrial Cancer

(Body of uterus. These questions do not apply to a woman who has had a total hysterectomy.)

1. Age group
   a. 39 or less (5)
   b. 40–49 (20)
   c. 50+ (60)

2. Race
   a. Asian American (10)
   b. African American (10)
   c. White (20)
   d. Hispanic American (10)

3. Births
   a. None (15)
   b. 1 to 4 (7)
   c. 5 or more (5)

4. Weight
   a. 50 or more pounds overweight (50)
   b. 20–49 pounds overweight (15)
   c. Underweight for height (10)
   d. Normal (10)

5. Diabetes (elevated blood sugar)
   a. Yes (3)
   b. No (1)

6. Estrogen hormone intake
   a. Yes, regularly (15)
   b. Yes, occasionally (12)
   c. None (10)

7. Abnormal uterine bleeding
   a. Yes (40)
   b. No (1)

8. Hypertension (high blood pressure)
   a. Yes (3)
   b. No (1)

   Total

source: Adapted from the Texas Division of the American Cancer Society. Reproduced with permission.

higher lung cancer rates than nonsmokers. Smokers of more than two packs per day are 20 times more likely to develop lung cancer than nonsmokers.

6. Type of cigarette. Smokers of low-tar/nicotine cigarettes have slightly lower lung cancer rates.

7. Duration of smoking. The frequency of lung and upper respiratory tract cancer increases with the length of time people have smoked.

8. Type of industrial work. Exposure to materials used in the industries mentioned in Figure 11.11 (Question 8) have been demonstrated to be associated with lung cancer. Exposure to materials in other industries also carry a higher risk. Smokers who work in these industries have greatly increased risks. Exposure to arsenic, radon, radiation from occupational/medical/environmental sources, and air pollution increase the risk of lung cancer.

TOTAL RISK

24 or less	You have a low risk for lung cancer (low-risk category).
25–49	You may be a light smoker and would have a good chance of kicking the habit (light risk).
50–74	As a moderate smoker, your risks of lung and upper respiratory tract cancers are increased. If you stop smoking now, these risks will decrease (moderate risk).
75 or over	As a heavy cigarette smoker, your chances of getting cancer of the lung and upper respiratory tract are greatly increased. Your best bet is to stop smoking now—for the health of it. See your doctor if you have a nagging cough, hoarseness, persistent pain, or a sore in the mouth or throat (high risk).

Colon/Rectum Cancer

RISK FACTORS

1. Age. Colon cancer occurs more frequently after 50 years of age.

2. Family predisposition. Colon cancer is more common in families that have a previous history of this disease.

3. Personal history. Polyps and bowel diseases are associated with colon cancer.

4. Rectal bleeding. Rectal bleeding may be a sign of colorectal cancer.

TOTAL RISK:

29 or less	You are at low risk for colon/rectum cancer.

30–69	This is a moderate-risk category. Testing by your physician may be indicated.
70 or over	This is a high-risk category. You should see your physician for the following tests: digital rectal exam, guaiac (stool) slide test, and proctoscopic exam.

In addition to the risk factors mentioned in the questionnaire, a diet high in fat and low in fiber, inadequate consumption of fruits and vegetables, physical inactivity, a history of breast or endometrial cancer, and inflammatory bowel disease also increase the risk for colon or rectum cancer.

Skin Cancer

RISK FACTORS

1. Sun exposure. Excessive ultraviolet light is a culprit in skin cancer. Protect yourself with a sunscreen medication.

2. Work environment. Working in mines, around coal tar, or around radioactive materials can cause cancer of the skin.

3. Complexion. Individuals with light complexions need more protection than others.

TOTAL RISK:

Numerical risks for skin cancer are difficult to state. For instance, a person with a dark complexion can work longer in the sun and be less likely to develop cancer than a light-skinned person. Furthermore, a person wearing a long-sleeved shirt and a wide-brimmed hat who spends hours working in the sun has less risk than a person wearing a swimsuit who sunbathes for only a short period. The risk increases greatly with age, and family history also plays a role.

If you answer "yes" to any question, you need to protect your skin from the sun or any other toxic material. Changes in moles, warts, or skin sores are important and should be evaluated by your doctor (see Figure 11.12).

SKIN SELF-EXAM

One of the easiest and quickest self-exams is a brief survey to detect possible skin cancers (see Figure 11.13). A simple skin self-exam can reduce deaths from melanoma by as much as 63 percent, saving as many as 4,500 lives in the United States each year.

- Make a drawing of yourself. Include a full front view, a full back view, and close-up views of your head (both sides), the soles of your feet, the tops of your feet, and the backs of your hands.

FIGURE 11.12 Warning signs of melanoma: ABCD Rule.

A. *Asymmetry:* One half of a mole or lesion doesn't look like the other half.

B. *Border:* A mole has an irregular, scalloped, or not clearly defined border.

C. *Color:* The color varies or is not uniform from one area of a mole or lesion to another, whether the color is tan, brown, black, white, red, or blue.

D. *Diameter:* The lesion is larger than 6 millimeters (¼ inch) or larger than a pencil eraser.

Adapted from *FDA Consumer*, May 1991.

- After you get out of the bath or shower, examine yourself closely in a full-length mirror. On your sketch make note of any moles, warts, or other skin marks you find anywhere on your body. Pay particular attention to areas that are exposed to the sun constantly, such as your face, the tops of your ears, and your hands.
- Briefly describe each mark on your sketch: its size, color, texture, and so on.
- Repeat the exam about once a month. Watch for changes in the size, texture, or color of moles, wart, or other skin mark. If you notice any difference, contact your physician. You also should contact a doctor if you have a sore that does not heal.

Breast Cancer

RISK FACTORS

1. Age. The risk for breast cancer increases significantly after 50 years of age.
2. Race. Breast cancer occurs more frequently in white women than any other group.

FIGURE 11.13 Self-exam for skin cancer.

1 Examine your face, especially the nose, lips, mouth, and ears —front and back. Use one or both mirrors to get a clear view.

2 Thoroughly inspect your scalp, using a blow dryer and mirror to expose each section to view. Get a friend or family member to help, if you can.

3 Check your hands carefully: palms and backs, between the fingers, and under the fingernails. Continue up the wrists to examine both front and back of your forearms.

4 Standing in front of a full-length mirror, begin at the elbows and scan all sides of your upper arms. Don't forget the underarms.

5 Next focus on the neck, chest, and torso. Women should lift breasts to view the underside.

6 With your back to the full-length mirror, use the hand mirror to inspect the back of your neck, shoulders, upper back, and any part of the back of your upper arms you could not view in step 4.

7 Still using both mirrors, scan your lower back, buttocks, and backs of both legs.

8 Sit down; prop each leg in turn on another stool or chair. Use the hand mirror to examine the genitals. Check front and sides of both legs, thigh to shin; ankles, tops of feet, between toes, and under toenails. Examine soles of feet and heels.

Reprinted with permission from *Family Practice Recertification* 14, no. 3 (March 1992).

3. Family history. The risk for breast cancer is higher in women with a family history of this type of cancer. The risk is even higher if more than one family member has developed breast cancer and is further enhanced by the closeness of the relationship of family member(s) (e.g., a mother or sister with breast cancer indicates a higher risk than a cousin with breast cancer).

4. Personal history. A previous history of breast or ovarian cancer would indicate a greater risk.

5. Maternity. The risk is higher in women who never have had children and in women who bear children after 30 years of age.

TOTAL RISK:

Under 100 Low-risk women should practice monthly breast self-examination (BSE —see Figure 11.14) and have their breasts examined by a doctor as a part of a cancer-related check-up.

100–199 Moderate-risk women should practice monthly BSE and have their breasts examined by a doctor as part of a cancer-related check-up. Periodic **mammograms** (see below) should be included as recommended.

FIGURE 11.14 Breast self-examination.

Why do the breast self-exam?

There are many good reasons for doing a breast self-exam each month. One reason is that it is easy to do and the more you do it, the better you will get at it. When you get to know how your breasts normally feel, you will quickly be able to feel any change, and early detection is the key to successful treatment.

Remember: A breast self-exam could save your breast—and save your life. Most breast lumps are found by women themselves, but in fact, most lumps in the breast are not cancer. Be safe, be sure.

When to do breast self-exam

The best time to do breast self-exam is right after your period, when breasts are not tender or swollen. If you do not have regular periods or sometimes skip a month, do it on the same day every month.

SOURCE: How to Do Breast Self-Examination. © 1998, American Cancer Society, Inc. Used by permission.

How to do breast self-exam

1. Lie down and put a pillow under your right shoulder. Place your right arm behind your head.
2. Use the finger pads of your three middle fingers on your left hand to feel for lumps or thickening. Your finger pads are the top third of each finger.

3. Press firmly enough to know how your breast feels. If you're not sure how hard to press, ask your health care provider. Or try to copy the way your health care provider uses the finger pads during a breast exam. Learn what your breast feels like most of the time. A firm ridge in the lower curve of each breast is normal.
4. Move around the breast in a set way. You can choose either the circle (A), the up and down (B), or the wedge (C). Do it the same way every time. It will help you to make sure that you've gone over the entire breast area, and to remember how your breast feels.

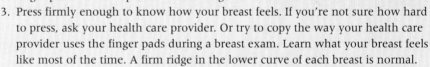

A   **B**   **C**

5. Now examine your left breast using right-hand finger pads.
6. Repeat the examination of both breasts while standing, with one arm behind your head. The upright position makes it easier to check the upper and outer part of the breasts (toward your armpit). You may want to do the standing part of the BSE while you are in the shower. Some breast changes can be felt more easily when your skin is wet and soapy.

For added safety, you can also check your breasts for any dimpling of the skin, changes in the nipple, redness, or swelling while standing in front of a mirror right after your BSE each month.

200 or over   High-risk women should practice monthly BSE and have the above examinations more often. See your doctor for the recommended examinations (including mammograms and physical exam of breasts) related to you.

Clinical breast exams by a physician are recommended every three years for women between ages 20 and 40 and every year for women over 40. The American Cancer Society also recommends an annual mammogram for women over 40. The latter is still an area of debate among health care practitioners, and personal risk factors should be considered to determine the frequency of mammograms.

Other possible risk factors for breast cancer not listed in the questionnaire are a long menstrual history (onset of menstruation prior to age 13 and ending later in life), recent use of oral contraceptives or postmenopausal estrogens, drinking two or more alcoholic beverages per day, chronic cystic disease, and ionizing radiation. A diet high in fat has also been viewed as a predisposing factor, although recent research has questioned its link to breast cancer.

> **An annual mammogram is recommended for all women after the age of 40.**

Cervical Cancer

RISK FACTORS

1. Age. The highest occurrence is in the 40 and over age group. The score numbers in the questionnaire represent the relative rates of cancer for different age groups—that is, a 45-year-old woman has a risk 3 times greater than a 20-year-old.
2. Race. Puerto Ricans, African Americans, and Hispanic Americans have higher rates of cervical cancer.
3. Number of pregnancies. Women who have delivered more children have a higher occurrence.
4. Viral infections. Viral infections of the cervix and vagina are associated with cervical cancer.
5. Age at first intercourse. Women with earlier intercourse and with more sexual partners are at a higher risk.
6. Bleeding. Irregular bleeding may be a sign of uterine cancer.

TOTAL RISK:

40–69   This is a low-risk group. Ask your doctor for a Pap test. You will be advised how often you should be tested after your first test.

70–99   In this moderate-risk group, more frequent Pap tests may be required.

100 or over   You are in a high-risk group and should have a Pap test (and pelvic exam) as advised by your doctor.

Early detection through a Pap test during a pelvic exam should be performed annually in women who are or have been sexually active or who have reached the age of 18. Following three normal tests during three consecutive years, the Pap test may be done less frequently, at the discretion of the physician.

Endometrial Cancer

RISK FACTORS

1. Age. Endometrial cancer is seen in older age groups. The scoring numbers by the age groups represent relative rates of endometrial cancer at different ages—that is, a 50-year-old woman has a risk 12 times higher than that of a 35-year-old woman.
2. Race. White women have a higher occurrence.
3. Births. The fewer children one has delivered, the greater is the risk of endometrial cancer.
4. Weight. Women who are overweight are at greater risk.
5. Diabetes. Cancer of the endometrium is associated with diabetes.
6. Estrogen use. Cancer of the endometrium may be associated with prolonged continuous estrogen hormone intake. This occurs in only a small number of women. Hormone replacement therapy (progesterone plus estrogen) is thought to offset the increased risk related to estrogen use. You should consult your physician before starting or stopping any estrogen medication.
7. Abnormal bleeding. Women who do not have cyclic menstrual periods are at greater risk.
8. Hypertension. Cancer of the endometrium is associated with high blood pressure.

TOTAL RISK:

49–59   You are at low risk for developing endometrial cancer.

60–99   Your risks are slightly higher (moderate risk). Report any abnormal bleeding immediately to your doctor. Tissue sampling at menopause is recommended.

100 or over Your risks are much greater (high risk). See your doctor for tests as appropriate.

Additional risk factors that may be associated with endometrial cancer, not included in the questionnaire, are infertility, a prolonged history of failure to ovulate, and menopause after age 55. Women over 40 should have a yearly pelvic exam by a physician.

Other Cancer Sites

Following are other types of cancers whose risk factors are not as clearly defined as those in Figure 11.11. Risk factors and prevention techniques for these types of cancer have been outlined in "The Causes of Cancer,"[18] published by the American Cancer Society, as well as in a series of pamphlets titled "Facts on Cancer," also available at the American Cancer Society. These types of cancer are presented with the risk factors associated with each type and preventive techniques to decrease risk. No numeric weights for the different risk factors have been assigned. As you read the information, however, rate yourself on a scale from 1 to 3 (1 for low risk, 2 for moderate risk, 3 for high risk) for each cancer site and record your results in Figure 11.16.

Prostate Cancer

The prostate gland is actually a cluster of smaller glands that encircles the top section of the urethra (urinary channel) at the point where it leaves the bladder. Although the function of the prostate is not entirely clear, the muscles of these small glands help squeeze prostatic secretions into the urethra.

RISK FACTORS

1. Advancing age. The highest incidence of prostate cancer is found in men over 65 (75 percent of cases). The incidence is also higher among African Americans than whites, and more married men than single men develop this type of cancer.
2. A family history.
3. Race. African Americans have the highest rate in the world.
4. Diet. A diet high in fat.

PREVENTION AND WARNING SIGNALS

Prostate cancer is difficult to detect and control because the causes are not known. Death rates can be lowered through early detection and awareness of the warning signals. Detection is done by a digital rectal exam of the gland and a prostate-specific antigen (PSA) blood test once a year after the age of 50. Possible warning signals include difficulties in urination (especially at night), painful urination, blood in the urine, and constant pain in the lower back or hip area.

Testicular Cancer

Testicular cancer accounts for only 1 percent of all male cancers, but it is the most common type of cancer seen in men between ages 25 and 35. The incidence is slightly higher in whites than in African Americans, and it is rarely seen in middle-aged and older men. The malignancy rate of testicular tumors is 96 percent, but if it is diagnosed early, this type of cancer is highly curable.

RISK FACTORS

1. Undescended testicle not corrected before age 6.
2. Atrophy of the testicle following mumps or virus infection.
3. Family history of testicular cancer.
4. Recurring injury to the testicle.
5. Abnormalities of the endocrine system (e.g., high hormone levels of pituitary gonadotropin or androgens).
6. Incomplete testicular development.

PREVENTION AND WARNING SIGNALS

The incidence of testicular cancer is quite high in males born with an undescended testicle. Therefore, this condition should be corrected early in life. Parents of infant males need to make sure that the child is checked by a physician to ensure that the testes have descended into the scrotum. Testicular self-examination (TSE) once a month following a warm bath or shower (when the scrotal skin is relaxed) is recommended. Guidelines for performing a TSE are given in Figure 11.15.

Some of the warning signs associated with testicular cancer are a small lump on the testicle, slight enlargement (usually painless) and change in consistency of the testis, sudden build-up of blood or fluid in the scrotum, pain in the groin and lower abdomen or discomfort accompanied by a sensation of dragging and heaviness, breast enlargement or tenderness, and enlarged lymph glands.

Key Terms

Mammogram Low-dose X rays of the breasts used as a screening technique for the early detection of breast cancer.

FIGURE 11.15 Testicular self-examination.

How to Examine the Testicles

You can increase your chances of early detection of testicular cancer by regularly performing a testicular self examination (TSE). The following procedure is recommended:

- Perform the self-exam once a month. Select an easy day to remember such as the first day or first Sunday of the month.

- Learn how your testicle feels normally so that it will be easier to identify changes. A normal testicle should feel oval, smooth, and uniformly firm, like a hard-boiled egg.

- Perform TSE following a warm shower or bath, when the scrotum is relaxed.

- Gently roll each testicle between your thumb and the first three fingers until you have felt the entire surface. Pay particular attention to any lumps, change in size or texture, pain, or a dragging or heavy sensation since your last self-exam. Do not confuse the epididymis at the rear of the testicle for an abnormality.

- Bring any changes to the attention of your physician. A change does not necessarily indicate a malignancy, but only a physician is able to determine that.

Early diagnosis of testicular cancer is essential, because this type of cancer spreads rapidly to other parts of the body. Because in most cases no early symptoms or pain are associated with testicular cancer, most people do not see a physician for months after discovering a lump or a slightly enlarged testis. Unfortunately, this delay allows almost 90 percent of testicular cancer to metastasize (spread) before a diagnosis is made.

Pancreatic Cancer

The pancreas is a thin gland that lies behind the stomach. This gland releases insulin and pancreatic juice. Insulin regulates blood sugar, and pancreatic juice contains enzymes that aid in food digestion.

POSSIBLE RISK FACTORS

1. Increased incidence between ages 35 and 70, but significantly higher around age 55.
2. Cigarette smoking.
3. Chronic pancreatitis.
4. Cirrhosis.
5. Diabetes.
6. High-fat diet.

PREVENTION AND WARNING SIGNALS

Detection of pancreatic cancer is difficult because (a) no symptoms are evoked in the early stages, and (b) advanced disease symptoms are similar to those of other diseases. Only a biopsy can provide a definite diagnosis, but because it is primarily a "silent" disease, the need for a biopsy is only apparent when the disease is already in an advanced stage. Warning signals that may be related to pancreatic cancer include pain in the abdomen or lower back, jaundice, loss of weight and appetite, nausea, weakness, agitated depression, loss of energy and feeling weary, dizziness, chills, muscles spasms, double vision, and coma.

Kidney and Bladder Cancer

The kidneys are the organs that filter the urine, and the bladder stores and empties the urine. Most of these two types of cancer are caused by environmental factors. Bladder cancer occurs most frequently between the ages of 50 and 70. Of all bladder cancers, 80 percent are seen in men, and the incidence among white males is twice that among African-American males.

POSSIBLE RISK FACTORS

1. Heavy cigarette smoking. Smoking is responsible for almost half of all bladder cancer deaths in men and one-third in women.
2. Congenital (inborn) abnormalities of either organ (these conditions are detected by a physician).
3. Exposure to certain chemical compounds such as aniline dyes, naphthalenes, or benzidines.
4. History of schistosomiasis (a parasitic bladder infection).

5. Frequent urinary tract infections, particularly after age 50.

PREVENTION AND WARNING SIGNALS

Avoiding cigarette smoking and occupational exposure to cancer-causing chemicals is important to decrease risk. Bloody urine, especially in repeated occurrences, is always a warning sign and requires immediate evaluation. Bladder cancer is diagnosed through urine analysis and examination of the bladder with a cysto-scope (a small tube that is inserted into the tract through the urethra).

Oral Cancer

Oral cancer includes the mouth, lips, tongue, salivary glands, pharynx, larynx, and floor of the mouth. Most of these cancers seem to be related to cigarette smoking and excessive consumption of alcohol.

RISK FACTORS

1. Heavy use of tobacco (cigarette, cigar, pipe, or smokeless) and/or alcohol drinking.

2. Broken or ill-fitting dentures.

3. Broken tooth that irritates the inside of the mouth.

4. Excessive sun exposure (lip cancer).

PREVENTION AND WARNING SIGNALS

Regular examinations and good dental hygiene help in prevention and early detection of oral cancer. Warning signals include a sore that doesn't heal or a white patch in the mouth, a lump, problems with chewing and swallowing, a constant feeling of having "something" in the throat. A person with any of these conditions should be evaluated by a physician or dentist. A tissue biopsy normally is conducted to diagnose the presence of cancer.

Esophageal and Stomach Cancer

The incidence of gastric cancer in the United States has dropped about 40 percent in the last 30 years. Cancer experts attribute this drastic decrease to changes in dietary habits and refrigeration. This type of cancer is more common in men, and the incidence is higher in African-American males than in white males.

RISK FACTORS

1. A diet high in starch and low in fresh fruits and vegetables.

2. High consumption of salt-cured, smoked, and nitrate-cured foods.

3. Imbalance in stomach acid.

4. History of pernicious anemia.

5. Chronic gastritis or gastric polyps.

6. Family history of these types of cancer.

PREVENTION AND WARNING SIGNALS

Prevention is accomplished primarily by increasing dietary intake of complex carbohydrates and fiber and decreasing the intake of salt-cured, smoked, and nitrate-cured foods. In addition, regular guaiac testing for occult blood (hemoccult test) is recommended. Warning signals for this type of cancer include indigestion for two weeks or longer, blood in the stools, vomiting, and rapid weight loss.

Ovarian Cancer

The ovaries are part of the female reproductive system that produces and releases the egg and the hormone estrogen. Ovarian cancer develops more frequently after menopause, and the highest incidence is seen between ages 55 and 64.

RISK FACTORS

1. Age. Risk increases with age and peaks in the eighth decade of life.

2. History of ovarian problems.

3. Extensive history of menstrual irregularities.

4. Family history of breast or ovarian cancer.

5. Personal history of breast, bowel, or endometrial cancer.

6. Nulliparity (no pregnancies).

7. Hereditary non-polyposis colon cancer.

PREVENTION AND WARNING SIGNALS

In most cases, ovarian cancer has no signs or symptoms. Therefore, regular pelvic examinations to detect signs of enlargement or other abnormalities are highly recommended. Some warning signals may be an enlarged abdomen, abnormal vaginal bleeding, unexplained digestive disturbances in women over age 40, and "normal" size (premenopause size) ovaries after menopause.

Thyroid Cancer

The thyroid gland, located in the lower portion of the front of the neck, helps regulate growth and metabolism. Thyroid cancer occurs almost twice as often in women as in men. The incidence also is higher in whites than African Americans.

RISK FACTORS

1. Aging.
2. Radiation therapy of the head and neck region received in childhood or adolescence.
3. Family history of thyroid cancer.

PREVENTION AND WARNING SIGNALS

Regular inspection for thyroid tumors is done by palpating the gland and surrounding areas during a physical examination. Thyroid cancer is slow-growing; therefore, it is highly treatable. Nevertheless, any unusual lumps in front of the neck should be reported promptly to a physician. Although thyroid cancer does not have many warning signals (besides a lump), these may include difficulty swallowing, choking, labored breathing, and persistent hoarseness.

Liver Cancer

The incidence of liver cancer in the United States is low. Men are more prone to liver cancer, and the disease is more common after age 60.

RISK FACTORS

1. History of cirrhosis of the liver.
2. History of hepatitis B virus.
3. Exposure to vinyl chloride (industrial gas used in plastics manufacturing) and aflatoxin (natural food contaminant).

PREVENTION AND WARNING SIGNALS

Prevention consists primarily of avoiding the risk factors and being aware of warning signals. Possible signs and symptoms are a lump or pain in the upper right abdomen (which may radiate into the back and the shoulder), fever, nausea, rapidly deteriorating health, jaundice, and liver tenderness.

Leukemia

Leukemia is a type of cancer that interferes with blood-forming tissues (bone marrow, lymph nodes, and spleen) by producing too many immature white blood cells. People who have leukemia cannot fight infection very well. The causes of leukemia are mostly unknown, although suspected risk factors have been identified.

POSSIBLE RISK FACTORS

1. Inherited susceptibility, but not directly transmitted from parent to child.
2. Greater incidence in children with Down syndrome (mongolism) and a few other genetic abnormalities.
3. Excessive exposure to ionizing radiation.
4. Environmental exposure to chemicals such as benzene.

PREVENTION AND WARNING SIGNALS

Detection is not easy because early symptoms can be associated with other serious ailments. When leukemia is suspected, the diagnosis is made through blood tests and a bone marrow biopsy. Early warning signals include fatigue, pallor, weight loss, easy bruising, nose bleeds, paleness, loss of appetite, repeated infections, hemorrhages, night sweats, bone and joint pain, and fever. At a more advanced stage, fatigue increases, hemorrhages become more severe, pain and high fever continue, the gums swell, and various skin disorders occur.

Lymphoma

Lymphomas are cancers of the lymphatic system. The lymphatic system consists of lymph nodes found throughout the body and a network of vessels that link these nodes. The lymphatic system participates in the body's immune reaction to foreign cells, substances, and infectious agents.

POSSIBLE RISK FACTORS

As with leukemia, the causes of lymphomas are unknown. People who have received organ transplants are at higher risk. Some researchers suspect that a form of herpes virus (called "Epstein-Barr virus") is active in the initial stages of lymphosarcomas. Risk of non-Hodgkin's lymphoma is higher in people who carry the human immunodeficiency virus (HIV) and human T-cell leukemia/lymphoma virus-I (HTLV-I) virus. Other researchers suggest that certain external factors may alter the immune system, making it more susceptible to the development and multiplication of cancer cells.

PREVENTION AND WARNING SIGNALS

Prevention of lymphoma is limited because little is known about its causes. Enlargement of a lymph node or a cluster of lymph nodes is the first sign of lymphoma. Other signs and symptoms are an enlarged spleen or liver, weakness, fever, back or abdominal pain, nausea/vomiting, unexplained weight loss, unexplained itching and sweating, and fever at night that lasts for a long time.

WHAT CAN YOU DO?

If you are at high risk for any form of cancer, you are advised to discuss this with your physician. An ounce of prevention is worth a pound of cure. Although cardiovascular disease is the number-one killer in the country, cancer is the number-one fear. Of all cancers, 60 to 80 percent are preventable, and about 50 percent are curable. Most cancers are lifestyle-related, so being aware of the risk factors and following the screening guidelines (Table 11.2, page 310) and basic recommendations for cancer prevention will greatly decrease your risk of developing cancer.

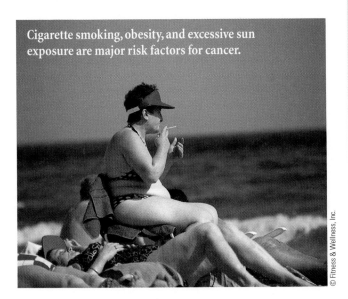

Cigarette smoking, obesity, and excessive sun exposure are major risk factors for cancer.

© Fitness & Wellness, Inc.

WEB INTERACTIVE

American Cancer Society

This comprehensive site features information and fact sheets on a variety of cancer types. The site explores treatment options, including alternative or complementary therapies. It features the popular cancer profiler for personalized cancer treatment information, the cancer survivors' network, and a search engine for local resources.

http://www.cancer.org

Cancer: Causes, Screening, and Prevention

This site, from the University of Pennsylvania Cancer Center, features information about cancer and diet, genetics, hormones, environment, drugs, smoking, and cancer epidemiology.

http://www.oncolink.upenn.edu/causeprevent

Psychosocial Support and Personal Experiences with Cancer

This excellent site, from the University of Pennsylvania Cancer Center, discusses issues such as coping with cancer and with loss/grief. It provides information for family and friends and other excellent links.

http://www.oncolink.upenn.edu/psychosocial

INTERACTIVE SITES:

Breast Cancer Interactive

This excellent site, sponsored by Health Net, features an excellent personal breast cancer risk analysis, as well as several multimedia links to a self-exam video, a clinical exam video, and a mammogram video. The site also contains teaching aids and resources.

http://www.tricaresw.af.mil/breastcd/index.html

Cancer Profilers

This excellent site for current cancer information contains top news stories in the fields of cancer research, prevention, and treatment. It also features separate resources for both consumers and physicians. An excellent feature of the site is the Cancer Profiler, which enables you to obtain information about treatment and clinical trials on melanoma and on breast, cervical, colorectal, kidney, ovarian, prostate, and uterine cancers. You will create your personalized treatment summary, which discusses the impact of cancer and its treatments and will become a resource for making informed treatment decisions.

http://cancerfacts.com

n*tes

1. G. Cowley, "The Secrets of a Cancer Cell's Success," *Newsweek* (April 25, 1994): 48–49.
2. American Cancer Society, *Cancer Facts & Figures—2000* (New York: ACS, 2000).
3. J. E. Enstrom, "Health Practices and Cancer Mortality Among Active California Mormons," *Journal of the National Cancer Institute* 81 (1989): 1807–1814.
4. See note 2.
5. "Antioxidant Vitamins: Are They the Only Cancer-Phyters?" *Cancer Smart* 1, no. 3 (1995): 4–5.
6. L. Mitscher and V. Dolby, *The Green Tea Book—China's Fountain of Youth* (New York: Avery Press, 1997).
7. N. Ahmad et al., "Green Tea Constituent Epigallocatechin-3-Gallate and Induction of Apoptosis and Cell Cycle Arrest in Human Carcinoma Cells," *Journal of the National Cancer Institute* 89 (1997): 1881–1886.
8. "Green, Black, and Red: The Teatotal Evidence," *University of California Berkeley Wellness Letter* 16, no. 6 (2000): 1–2.
9. J. H. Weisburger and G. M. Williams, "Causes of Cancer," *American Cancer Society Textbook of Clinical Oncology* (Atlanta: ACS, 1995): 10–39.
10. "Your Barbecue Grill: A Smoking Gun?" *Cancer Smart*, 1, no. 2 (1995): 4–5.
11. See note 9.
12. D. F. Birt, "The Straight Story on Soy," *American Institute for Cancer Research Newsletter* (Spring 2000): 5.
13. American Cancer Society, *1995 Cancer Facts and Figures* (New York: ACS, 1995).
14. See note 2.
15. "Questions & Answers," *Cancer Smart* 4 (1998): 12.
16. S. N. Blair, H. W. Kohl III, R. S. Paffenbarger, Jr., D. G. Clark, K. H. Cooper, and L. W. Gibbons, "Physical Fitness and All-Cause Mortality: A Prospective Study of Healthy Men and Women," *Journal of the American Medical Association* 262 (1989): 2395–2401.
17. I-Min Lee, "Exercise and Physical Health: Cancer and Immune Function," *Research Quarterly for Exercise and Sport* 66 (1995): 286–291.
18. See note 9.

Suggested Readings

■ American Cancer Society. *Cancer Facts & Figures—2001*. New York: ACS, 2001.

■ American Cancer Society. *Textbook of Clinical Oncology*. Atlanta: ACS, 1995.

■ Feng, J., et al. "The RNA Component of Human Telomerase." *Science* 269 (1995): 1236–1241.

■ "Physical Activity and Cancer." *Physical Activity and Fitness Research Digest*. Washington, DC: President's Council on Physical Fitness and Sport, June 1995.

FIGURE 11.16 Cancer profile.

Name:_____ Date:_____

Course: _____ Section: _____ Gender:_____ Age:_____

I. Risk assessment

Cancer Site	Total Points		Risk Category
	Men	**Women**	
Lung	7		
Colon/Rectum	13		
Skin	12		
Breast			
Cervical			
Endometrial			
Prostate			
Testicular			
Pancreatic			
Kidney and Bladder			
Oral			
Esophageal and Stomach			
Ovarian			
Thyroid			
Liver			
Leukemia			
Lymphomas			

(continued)

(Figure 11.16 Cancer profile—continued)

II. Personal Interpretation

In the space provided below, discuss your results for the various cancer sites. State your feelings about cancer and comment on any experiences that you may have had with cancer patients.

_____

_____

_____

_____

_____

_____

_____

_____

_____

_____

_____

conclusion

III. Cancer Prevention

Discuss lifestyle habits that you should eliminate and habits that you need to adopt to reduce your own risk of cancer. Also indicate how you can best implement and adhere to these changes.

_____

_____

_____

_____

_____

_____

_____

_____

_____

_____

_____

_____

Stress Assessment and Management Techniques

objectives

Define stress, eustress, and distress.

Explain the role of stress in maintaining health and optimal performance.

Identify the major sources of stress in life.

Define the two major types of behavior patterns.

Learn to lower your vulnerability to stress.

Develop time management skills.

Define the role of physical exercise in reducing stress.

Learn to use various stress management techniques.

© 2002 D. C. Lowe/Stone/Getty Images

Learning to live and get ahead today is nearly impossible without **stress**. To succeed in an unpredictable world that changes with every new day, working under pressure has become the rule rather than the exception for most people. As a result, stress has become one of the most common problems we face. Current estimates indicate that the annual cost of stress and stress-related diseases in the United States exceeds $100 billion, a direct result of health care costs, lost productivity, and absenteeism.

Most people have accepted stress as a normal part of daily life and, even though everyone has to deal with it, few seem to understand it or know how to cope effectively. Stress should not be avoided entirely, because a certain amount is necessary for optimum health, performance, and well-being. It is difficult to succeed and have fun in life without "hits, runs, and errors." The good news is that stress can be self-controlled.

Just what is stress? Dr. Hans Selye, one of the foremost authorities on stress, defined it as "the nonspecific response of the human organism to any demand that is placed upon it."[1] "Nonspecific" indicates that the body reacts in a similar fashion regardless of the nature of the event that leads to the stress response. In simpler terms, stress is the body's mental, emotional, and physiological response to any situation that is new, threatening, frightening, or exciting.

The body's response to stress has been the same ever since humans were first put on the earth. Stress prepares the organism to react to the stress-causing event, also called the **stressor**. The problem, though, is the way in which we react to stress. Many people thrive under stress; others under similar circumstances are unable to handle it. An individual's reaction to a stress-causing agent determines whether stress is positive or negative.

Dr. Selye defined the ways in which we react to stress as either eustress or distress. In both cases, the nonspecific response is almost the same. In the case of **eustress**, health and performance continue to improve even as stress increases. On the other hand, **distress** refers to the unpleasant or harmful stress under which health and performance begin to deteriorate. The relationship between stress and performance is illustrated in Figure 12.1.

Stress is a fact of modern life, and every person does need an optimal level of stress that is most conducive to adequate health and performance. When stress levels reach mental, emotional, and physiological limits, however, stress becomes distress and the person no longer functions effectively.

Chronic distress raises the risk for many health disorders—including coronary heart disease, hypertension, eating disorders, ulcers, diabetes, asthma, depression, migraine headaches, sleep disorders, and chronic fatigue—and may even play a role in the development of certain types of cancers. Recognizing this and overcoming the problem quickly and efficiently are crucial in maintaining emotional and physiological stability.

FIGURE 12.1 Relationship between stress and health and performance.

SOURCES OF STRESS

Several instruments have been developed to assess sources of stress in life. The most practical instrument is the **Life Experiences Survey**, presented in Figure 12.2, page 331. This survey identifies a person's life changes within the last 12 months that may have an impact on that person's physical and psychological well-being.

The Life Experiences Survey is divided into two sections. Section 1, to be completed by all respondents, contains a list of 47 life events plus three blank spaces for other events experienced but not listed in the survey. Section 2 contains an additional 10 questions designed for students only (students should fill out both sections).

The survey requires the person to rate the extent to which the life events he or she experienced had a positive or negative impact on his or her life at the time these events occurred. The ratings are on a 7-point scale. A rating of –3 indicates an extremely undesirable impact. A rating of zero (0) suggests neither a positive nor a negative impact. A rating of + 3 indicates an extremely desirable impact.

After the subject determines the life events that have taken place, the negative and the positive points are totaled separately. Both scores are expressed as positive numbers (for example, positive ratings of 2, 1, 3, and 3 = 9 points positive score; negative ratings of –3, –2, –2, –1, and –2 = 10 points negative score). A final "total life change" score can be obtained by adding the positive score and the negative score together as positive numbers (total life change score: 9 + 10 = 19 points).

Because negative and positive changes alike can produce nonspecific responses, the total life change score is a good indicator of total life stress. Most research in this area, however, suggests that the negative change score is a better predictor of potential physical and psychological illness than the total change score. More research is necessary to establish the role of total change and the role of the ratio of positive to negative stress. Therefore, only the negative score is used as part of the stress profile.

Behavior Patterns

Common life events are not the only source of stress in life. All too often individuals bring on stress as a result of their own behavior patterns. The two main types of behavior patterns, Type A and Type B, were originally based on several observable characteristics: **Type A** behavior characterizes a primarily hard-driving, overambitious, aggressive, at times hostile

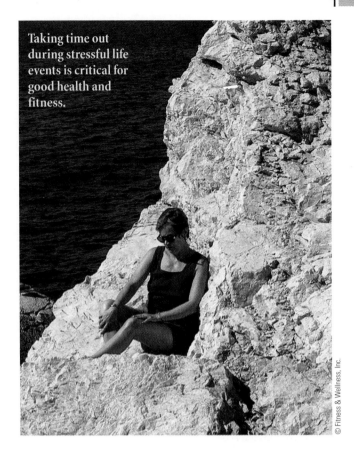

Taking time out during stressful life events is critical for good health and fitness.

© Fitness & Wellness, Inc.

and overly competitive person. Type A individuals often set their own goals, are self-motivated, try to accomplish many tasks at the same time, are excessively achievement-oriented, and have a high degree of time urgency. In contrast, **Type B** behavior is characteristic of calm, casual, relaxed, easy-going individuals. Type B people take one thing at a time, do not feel pressured or hurried, and seldom set their own deadlines.

Key Terms

Stress The mental, emotional, and physiological response of the body to any situation that is new, threatening, frightening, or exciting.

Stressor Stress-causing event.

Eustress Positive stress: Health and performance continue to improve, even as stress increases.

Distress Negative stress: Unpleasant or harmful stress, under which health and performance begin to deteriorate.

Life Experiences Survey A questionnaire used to assess sources of stress in life.

Type A Behavior pattern characteristic of a hard-driving, overambitious, aggressive, at times hostile and overly competitive person.

Type B Behavior pattern characteristic of a calm, casual, relaxed, and easy-going individual.

Changing a Type A personality

- Make a contract with yourself to slow down and take it easy. Put it in writing. Post it in a conspicuous spot, then stick to the terms you set up. Be specific. Abstract statements ("I'm going to be less uptight") don't work.

- Work on only one or two things at a time. Wait until you change one habit before you tackle the next one.

- Eat more slowly and eat only when you are relaxed and sitting down.

- If you smoke, quit.

- Cut down on your caffeine intake, because it increases the tendency to become irritated and agitated.

- Take regular breaks throughout the day, even as brief as 5 or 10 minutes, when you totally change what you're doing. Get up, stretch, get a drink of cool water, walk around for a few minutes.

- Work on fighting your impatience. If you're standing in line at the grocery store, study the interesting things people have in their carts instead of getting upset.

- Work on controlling hostility. Keep a written log. When do you flare up? What causes it? How do you feel at the time? What preceded it? Look for patterns and figure out what sets you off. Then do something about it. Either avoid the situations that cause you hostility or practice reacting to them in different ways.

- Plan some activities just for the fun of it. Load a picnic basket in the car and drive to the country with a friend. After a stressful physics class, stop at a theater and see a good comedy.

- Choose a role model, someone you know and admire who does not have a Type A personality. Observe the person carefully, then try out some techniques the person demonstrates.

- Simplify your life so you can learn to relax a little bit. Figure out which activities or commitments you can eliminate right now, then get rid of them.

- If morning is a problem time for you and you get too hurried, set your alarm clock half an hour earlier.

- Take time out during even the most hectic day to do something truly relaxing. Because you won't be used to it, you may have to work at it at first. Begin by listing things you'd really enjoy that would calm you. Include some things that take only a few minutes: Watch a sunset, lie out on the lawn at night and look at the stars, call an old friend and catch up on news, take a nap, sauté a pan of mushrooms and savor them slowly.

- If you're under a deadline, take short breaks. Stop and talk to someone for 5 minutes, take a short walk, or lie down with a cool cloth over your eyes for 10 minutes.

- Pay attention to what your own body clock is saying. You've probably noticed that every 90 minutes or so, you lose the ability to concentrate, get a little sleepy, and have a tendency to daydream. Instead of fighting the urge, put down your work and let your mind wander for a few minutes. Use the time to imagine and let your creativity run wild.

- Learn to treasure unplanned surprises: a friend dropping by unannounced, a hummingbird outside your window, a child's tightly clutched bouquet of wildflowers.

- Savor your relationships. Think about the people in your life. Relax with them and give yourself to them. Give up trying to control others and resist the urge to end relationships that don't always go as you'd like them to.

From W. W. K. Hoeger, L. W. Turner, and B. Q. Hafen, *Wellness: Guidelines for a Healthy Lifestyle* (Belmont, CA: Wadsworth/Thomson Learning, 2002), 30.

Several attempts have been made to develop an objective scale to identify Type A individuals properly, but questionnaires are not as valid and reliable as researchers would like them to be. Consequently, the main assessment tool to determine behavioral type is still the **structured interview**, during which a person is asked to reply to several questions that describe Type A and Type B behavior patterns. The interviewer notes not only the responses to the questions but also mental, emotional, and physical behaviors the individual exhibits as he or she replies to each question.

Based on the answers and the associated behaviors, the interviewer rates the person along a continuum, ranging from Type A to Type B. Along

> **A Type A person is usually a hard-driving, overambitious, aggressive, at times hostile and overly competitive person.**

this continuum behavioral patterns are classified into five categories: A-1, A-2, X (a mix of Type A and Type B), B-3, and B-4. The Type A-1 exhibits all of the Type A characteristics, and the B-4 shows a relative absence of Type A behaviors. The Type A-2 does not exhibit a complete Type A pattern, and the Type B-3 exhibits only a few Type A characteristics.

KeyTerms

Structured interview An assessment tool used to determine behavioral patterns that define Type A and B personalities.

FIGURE 12.2 Life experiences survey.

Name: _Duncan Brown_   Date: _1-29-03_

Course: _LF117_   Section: _02_   Gender: _M_   Age: _19_

Section I

1. Marriage	−3	−2	−1	(0)	+1	+2	+3
2. Detention in jail or comparable institution	−3	−2	−1	(0)	+1	+2	+3
3. Death of spouse	−3	−2	−1	(0)	+1	+2	+3
4. Major change in sleeping habits (much more or much less sleep)	−3	−2	−1	(0)	+1	+2	+3
5. Death of close family member:							
a. mother	−3	−2	−1	(0)	+1	+2	+3
b. father	−3	−2	−1	(0)	+1	+2	+3
c. brother	−3	−2	−1	(0)	+1	+2	+3
d. sister	−3	−2	−1	(0)	+1	+2	+3
e. grandmother	−3	−2	−1	(0)	+1	+2	+3
f. grandfather	−3	−2	−1	(0)	+1	+2	+3
g. other (specify)	−3	−2	−1	(0)	+1	+2	+3
6. Major change in eating habits (much more or much less food intake)	−3	−2	−1	(0)	+1	+2	+3
7. Foreclosure on mortgage or loan	−3	−2	−1	(0)	+1	+2	+3
8. Death of close friend	−3	−2	−1	(0)	+1	+2	+3
9. Outstanding personal achievement	−3	−2	−1	(0)	+1	+2	+3
10. Minor law violations (traffic tickets, disturbing the peace, etc.)	−3	−2	(−1)	0	+1	+2	+3
11. Male: Wife/girlfriend's pregnancy	−3	−2	−1	(0)	+1	+2	+3
12. Female: Pregnancy	−3	−2	−1	(0)	+1	+2	+3
13. Changed work situation (different work responsibility, major change in working conditions, working hours, etc.)	−3	−2	−1	(0)	+1	+2	+3
14. New job	−3	−2	−1	(0)	+1	+2	+3
15. Serious illness or injury of close family member:							
a. father	−3	−2	−1	(0)	+1	+2	+3
b. mother	−3	−2	−1	(0)	+1	+2	+3
c. sister	−3	−2	−1	(0)	+1	+2	+3
d. brother	−3	−2	−1	(0)	+1	+2	+3
e. grandfather	−3	−2	−1	(0)	+1	+2	+3
f. grandmother	−3	−2	−1	(0)	+1	+2	+3
g. spouse	−3	−2	−1	(0)	+1	+2	+3
h. other (specify)	−3	−2	−1	(0)	+1	+2	+3
16. Sexual difficulties	−3	−2	−1	(0)	+1	+2	+3
17. Trouble with employer (in danger of losing job, being suspended, demoted, etc.)	−3	−2	−1	(0)	+1	+2	+3
18. Trouble with in-laws	−3	−2	−1	(0)	+1	+2	+3
19. Major change in financial status (a lot better off or a lot worse off)	−3	−2	−1	(0)	+1	+2	+3
20. Major change in closeness of family members (increased or decreased closeness)	−3	−2	−1	(0)	+1	+2	+3
21. Gaining a new family member (through birth, adoption, family member moving in, etc.)	−3	−2	−1	(0)	+1	+2	+3
22. Change of residence	−3	−2	−1	(0)	+1	+2	+3
23. Marital separation from mate (because of conflict)	−3	−2	−1	(0)	+1	+2	+3
24. Major change in church activities (increased or decreased attendance)	−3	−2	−1	(0)	+1	+2	+3
25. Marital reconciliation with mate	−3	−2	−1	(0)	+1	+2	+3
26. Major change in number of arguments with spouse (a lot more or a lot less arguments)	−3	−2	−1	(0)	+1	+2	+3
27. Married Male: Change in wife's work outside the home (beginning work, ceasing work, changing to a new job, etc.)	−3	−2	−1	(0)	+1	+2	+3

(continued)

From I. G. Sarason, "Assessing the Impact of Life Changes: Development of the Life Experiences Survey," *Journal of Consulting and Clinical Psychology* 46 (1978): 932–946. Copyright © 1978 by American Psychological Association. Reprinted by permission of the publisher and the author.

(Figure 12.2 Life experiences survey—continued)

28. Married Female: Change in husband's work (loss of job, beginning new job, retirement, etc.)	−3	−2	−1	⓪	+1	+2	+3
29. Major change in usual type and/or amount of recreation	−3	−2	−1	⓪	+1	+2	+3
30. Borrowing more than $10,000 (buying home, business, etc.)	−3	−2	−1	⓪	+1	+2	+3
31. Borrowing less than $10,000 (buying car, TV, getting school loan, etc.)	−3	−2	−1	⓪	+1	+2	+3
32. Being fired from job	−3	−2	−1	⓪	+1	+2	+3
33. Male: Wife/girlfriend having abortion	−3	−2	−1	⓪	+1	+2	+3
34. Female: Having abortion	−3	−2	−1	⓪	+1	+2	+3
35. Major personal illness or injury	−3	−2	−1	⓪	+1	+2	+3
36. Major change in social activities, e.g., parties, movies, visiting (increased or decreased participation)	−3	−2	−1	⓪	+1	+2	+3
37. Major change in living conditions of family (building new home, remodeling, deterioration of home or neighborhood, etc.)	−3	−2	−1	⓪	+1	+2	+3
38. Divorce	−3	−2	−1	⓪	+1	+2	+3
39. Serious injury or illness of close friend	−3	−2	−1	⓪	+1	+2	+3
40. Retirement from work	−3	−2	−1	⓪	+1	+2	+3
41. Son or daughter leaving home (because of marriage, college, etc.)	−3	−2	−1	⓪	+1	+2	+3
42. End of formal schooling	−3	−2	−1	⓪	+1	+2	+3
43. Separation from spouse (because of work, travel, etc.)	−3	−2	−1	⓪	+1	+2	+3
44. Engagement	−3	−2	−1	⓪	+1	+2	+3
45. Breaking up with boyfriend/girlfriend	−3	−2	−1	⓪	+1	+2	+3
46. Leaving home for the first time	−3	−2	−1	⓪	+1	+2	+3
47. Reconciliation with boyfriend/girlfriend	−3	−2	−1	⓪	+1	+2	+3
48. Others	−3	−2	−1	⓪	+1	+2	+3
49.	−3	−2	−1	⓪	+1	+2	+3
50.	−3	−2	−1	⓪	+1	+2	+3

Section 2

51. Beginning a new school experience at a higher academic level (college, graduate school, professional school, etc.)	−3	−2	−1	0	(+1)	+2	+3
52. Changing to a new school at the same academic level (undergraduate, graduate, etc.)	−3	−2	−1	⓪	+1	+2	+3
53. Academic probation	−3	−2	−1	⓪	+1	+2	+3
54. Being dismissed from dormitory or other residence	−3	−2	−1	⓪	+1	+2	+3
55. Failing an important exam	−3	−2	−1	⓪	+1	+2	+3
56. Changing a major	−3	−2	−1	⓪	+1	+2	+3
57. Failing a course	−3	−2	−1	⓪	+1	+2	+3
58. Dropping a course	−3	−2	−1	⓪	+1	+2	+3
59. Joining a fraternity/sorority	−3	−2	−1	⓪	+1	+2	+3
60. Financial problems concerning school (in danger of not having sufficient money to continue)	−3	−2	−1	⓪	+1	+2	+3

Total Negative Points: 1

Total Positive Points: 1

Total Score (Points): 2

Category	Negative Score		Total Score	
	Men	Women	Men	Women
Poor	≥13	≥15	≥27	≥27
Fair	7–12	8–14	17–26	18–26
Average	6	7	16	17
Good	1–5	1–6	5–15	6–16
Excellent	0	0	1–4	1–5

Over the years, experts have indicated that individuals classified as Type A are under too much stress and have a significantly higher incidence of coronary heart disease. Based on these findings, Type A individuals have been counseled to lower their stress level by modifying many of their Type A behaviors.

> **A Type B person is usually calm, casual, relaxed, and easy-going.**

Many of the Type A characteristics are learned behaviors. Consequently, if people can learn to identify the sources of stress and make changes in their behavioral responses, they can move along the continuum and respond more like Type Bs. The debate, however, has centered on which Type A behaviors should be changed, because not all of them are undesirable.

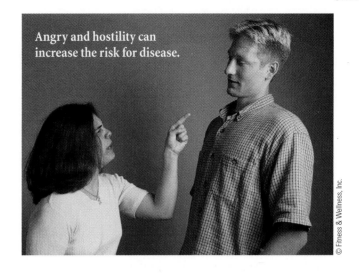

Angry and hostility can increase the risk for disease.

© Fitness & Wellness, Inc.

We also know that many individuals perform well under pressure. They typically are classified as Type A but do not demonstrate any of the detrimental effects of stress. Drs. Robert and Marilyn Kriegel came up with the term Type C to characterize people with these behaviors.[2]

Type C individuals are just as highly stressed as Type As but do not seem to be at higher risk for disease than Type Bs. The keys to successful Type C performance seem to be commitment, confidence, and control. Type C people are highly committed to what they are doing, have a great deal of confidence in their ability to do their work, and are in constant control of their actions. In addition, they enjoy their work and maintain themselves in top physical condition to be able to meet the mental and physical demands of their work.

> **Type C people usually are highly committed to what they are doing, have a great deal of confidence in their ability, and are in control.**

Type A behavior by itself is no longer viewed as a major risk factor for coronary heart disease. Type A individuals who commonly express anger and hostility are the ones at higher risk. Therefore, many behavioral modification counselors now work on changing the latter behaviors to prevent disease.

Anger increases heart rate and blood pressure, and leads to constriction of blood vessels. Over time, these changes are thought to cause damage to the

Common symptoms of stress

- headaches
- muscular aches (mainly in neck, shoulders, and back)
- grinding teeth
- nervous tick, finger tapping, toe tapping
- increased sweating
- increase in or loss of appetite
- insomnia
- nightmares
- fatigue
- dry mouth
- stuttering
- high blood pressure
- tightness or pain in the chest
- impotence
- hives
- dizziness
- depression
- irritation
- anger
- hostility
- fear, panic, anxiety
- stomach pain, flutters
- nausea
- cold, clammy hands
- poor concentration
- pacing
- restlessness
- rapid heart rate
- low-grade infection
- loss of sex drive
- rash or acne

KeyTerms

Type C Behavior pattern of individuals who are just as highly stressed as the Type A but do not seem to be at higher risk for disease than the Type B.

arteries and eventually lead to a heart attack. Several studies indicate that chronically angry people have up to a threefold increased risk for CHD and are seven times more likely to suffer a fatal heart attack by age 50.

Many experts also believe that emotional stress is far more likely than physical stress to trigger a heart attack. People who are impatient and readily annoyed when they have to wait for someone or something—an employee, a traffic light, a table in a restaurant—are especially vulnerable.

> **When you "feel like strangling" someone for what they have done to you, consider that anger is most likely strangling you.**

Research also is focusing on individuals who have anxiety, depression, and feelings of helplessness when they encounter setbacks and failures in life. People who lose control of their lives or who give up on their dreams in life, knowing that they could and should be doing better, probably are more likely to have heart attacks than hard-driving people who enjoy their work.

Vulnerability to Stress

Researchers have identified a number of factors that can affect the way in which people handle stress. How people deal with these factors actually can increase or decrease vulnerability to stress. The questionnaire provided in Figure 12.3 lists these factors so you can determine your vulnerability rating. Many of the items on this questionnaire are related to health, social support, self-worth, and nurturance (sense of being needed). All of the factors are crucial to a person's physical, social, mental, and emotional well-being. The questionnaire will help you identify specific areas in which you can make improvements to help you cope more efficiently.

The health benefits of physical fitness have already been discussed extensively. Further, social support, self-worth, and nurturance are essential to cope effectively with stressful life events. All of these factors play a supportive and protective role in people's lives. The more integrated people are in society, the less vulnerable they are to stress and illness.

Positive correlations have been found between social support and health outcomes. People can draw upon social support to weather crises. Knowing

> **Positive correlations have been found between social support and health outcomes.**

that someone else cares, that people are there to lean on, that support is out there, is valuable for survival (or growth) in times of need.

As you take the questionnaire, you will notice that many of the items describe situations and behaviors that are within your own control. To make yourself less vulnerable to stress, you will want to improve the behaviors that make you more vulnerable to stress. You should start by modifying the behaviors that are easiest to change before undertaking some of the most difficult ones. After completing the questionnaires, record the results in Figure 12.4 and in your fitness and wellness profile in Appendix A.

TIME MANAGEMENT

The present "hurry-up" style of life of the American people is not conducive to wellness. The hassles involved in getting through a routine day often lead to stress-related illnesses. People who do not manage their time properly will quickly experience chronic stress, fatigue, despair, discouragement, and illness.

Although Benjamin Franklin believed that "Time is the stuff life is made of," current surveys indicate that almost 80 percent of Americans reported that time moves too fast for them, and more than 50 percent felt they had to get everything done. The

---

Tips to manage anger

- Commit to change and gain control over the behavior.
- Remind yourself that chronic anger leads to illness and disease and may eventually kill you.
- Recognize when feelings of anger are developing and ask yourself the following questions:
  - Is the matter really that important?
  - Is the anger justified?
  - Can I change the situation without getting angry?
  - Is it worth risking my health over it?
  - How will I feel about the situation in a few hours?
- Tell yourself, "Stop, my health is worth it" every time you start to feel anger.
- Prepare for a positive response: Ask for an explanation or clarification of the situation, walk away and evaluate the situation, exercise, or use appropriate stress management techniques (breathing, meditation, imagery) before you become angry and hostile.
- Manage anger at once, do not let it build up.
- Never attack anyone verbally or physically.
- Keep a journal and ponder the situations that cause you to be angry.
- Seek professional help if you are unable to overcome anger by yourself: You are worth it.

FIGURE **12.3** Stress vulnerability questionnaire.

Name:_____ Date: _____

Course: _____ Section: _____ Gender:_____ Age: _____

Item	Strongly Agree	Mildly Agree	Mildly Disagree	Strongly Disagree
1. I try to incorporate as much physical activity* as possible in my daily schedule.	1	2	3	(4)
2. I exercise aerobically 20 minutes or more at least three times per week.	1	2	3	(4)
3. I regularly sleep 7 to 8 hours per night.	1	(2)	3	4
4. I take my time eating at least one hot, balanced meal a day.	1	(2)	3	4
5. I drink fewer than two cups of coffee (or equivalent) per day.	(1)	2	3	4
6. I am at recommended body weight.	1	2	3	4
7. I enjoy good health.	(1)	2	3	4
8 I do not use tobacco in any form.	(1)	2	3	4
9. I limit my alcohol intake to no more than one drink per day.	(1)	2	3	4
10. I do not use hard drugs.	(1)	2	3	4
11. I have someone I love, trust, and can rely on for help if I have a problem or need to make an essential decision.	(1)	2	3	4
12. There is love in my family.	(1)	2	3	4
13. I routinely give and receive affection.	1	2	(3)	4
14. I have close personal relationships with other people who provide me with a sense of emotional security.	(1)	2	3	4
15. There are people close by whom I can turn to for guidance in time of stress.	(1)	2	3	4
16. I can speak openly about feelings, emotions, and problems with people I trust.	(1)	2	3	4
17. Other people rely on me for help.	1	2	(3)	4
18. I am able to keep my feelings of anger and hostility under control.	(1)	2	3	4
19. I have a network of friends who enjoy the same social activities I do.	1	2	3	(4)
20. I take time to do something fun at least once a week.	(1)	2	3	4
21. My religious beliefs provide guidance and strength to my life.	1	2	3	(4)
22. I often provide service to others.	1	(2)	3	4
23. I enjoy my job (major or school).	1	(2)	3	4
24. I am a competent worker.	1	(2)	3	4
25. I get along well with co-workers (or students).	(1)	2	3	4
26. My income is sufficient for my needs.	1	(2)	3	4
27. I manage time adequately.	1	2	(3)	4
28. I have learned to say "no" to additional commitments when I am already pressed for time.	(1)	2	3	4
29. I take daily quiet time for myself.	(1)	2	3	4
30. I practice stress management as needed.	1	2	(3)	4

Total Points: 55

Scoring:

    0–30 points . . . . Excellent (great resistance to stress)

    31–40 points . . . . Good (little vulnerability to stress)

    41–50 points . . . . Average (somewhat vulnerable to stress)

    51–60 points . . . . Fair (vulnerable to stress)

    ≥61 points . . . . Poor (highly vulnerable to stress)

*Walk instead of driving, avoid escalators and elevators, or walk to neighboring offices, homes, and stores.

FIGURE 12.4 Stress profile.

Name: _____ Date: _____

Course: _____ Section: _____ Gender:_____ Age: _____

I. Assessments

Date: [   ]   [   ]   [   ]

Life Experiences Survey

    Score (negative)   [   ]   [   ]   [   ]

    Stress Rating   [   ]   [   ]   [   ]

Stress Vulnerability Questionnaire

    Score   [   ]   [   ]   [   ]

    Rating   [   ]   [   ]   [   ]

Stress Management
Technique(s) to be used   [   ]   [   ]   [   ]

II. In your own words, express how life stresses and your personality affect you in daily life.

_____

_____

_____

_____

_____

III. In the space provided below, list, in order of priority, behaviors that you would like to change to help you decrease your vulnerability to stress. Also, briefly outline how you intend to accomplish these changes.

Behavior(s)

_____

_____

How to accomplish the change(s)

_____

_____

_____

younger the respondents, the more they struggled with lack of time. Almost half wished they had more time for exercise, recreation, hobbies, and family.

Healthy and successful people are good time managers, able to maintain a pace of life within their comfort zone. In a survey of 1954 Harvard graduates from the school of business, only 27 percent had reached the goals they established in college. Every one of this group had rated him- or herself a superior time manager, and only 8 percent of the remaining graduates perceived themselves to be superior time managers. The successful graduates attributed their success to "smart work," not necessarily "hard work."

Five Steps to Time Management

Trying to achieve one or more goals in a limited time can create a tremendous amount of stress. Many people just don't seem to have enough hours in the day to accomplish their tasks. The greatest demands on our time, nonetheless, are frequently self-imposed: trying to do too much, too fast, too soon.

Some time killers, such as eating, sleeping, and recreation, are necessary for health and wellness, but, in excess, they'll lead to stress in life. You can follow five basic steps to make better use of your time:

1. Find the time killers. Many people do not know how they spend each part of the day. Keep a 4- to 7-day log and record at half-hour intervals the activities you do. A form is provided in Figure 12.5 (page 339) to do this (make as many copies as the number of days that you wish to evaluate). Record the activities as you go through your typical day, so you will remember all of them. At the end of each day, decide when you wasted time. You may be shocked by the amount of time you spent on the phone, on the Internet, sleeping (more than 8 hours per night), or watching television.

2. Set long-range and short-range goals. Setting goals requires some in-depth thinking and helps put your life and daily tasks in perspective. What do I want out of life? Where do I want to be 10 years from now? Next year? Next week? Tomorrow? You can use Figure 12.6 (page 340) to list these goals.

3. Identify your immediate goals and prioritize them for today and this week (Use Figure 12.7, page 341 —make as many copies as necessary). Each day sit down and determine what you need to accomplish that day and that week. Rank your "today" and "this week" tasks in four categories: (a) top-priority, (b) medium-priority, (c) low-priority, and (d) trash.

    Top-priority tasks are the most important ones. If you were to reap most of your productivity from

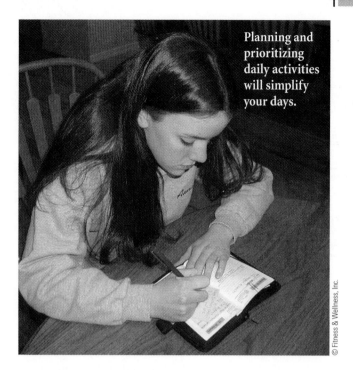

Planning and prioritizing daily activities will simplify your days.

© Fitness & Wellness, Inc.

30 percent of your activities, which would they be? Medium-priority activities are those that must be done but can wait a day or two. Low-priority activities are those to be done only upon completing all top- and middle-priority activities. Trash activities are not worth your time (for example, cruising the hallways, channel-surfing).

4. Use a daily planner to help you organize and simplify your day. In this way you can access your priority list, appointments, notes, references, names, places, phone numbers, and addresses conveniently from your coat pocket or purse. Many individuals think that planning daily and weekly activities is a waste of time. A few minutes to schedule your time each day, however, may pay off in hours saved.

    As you plan your day, be realistic and find your comfort zone. Determine what is the best way to organize your day. Which is the most productive time for work, study, errands? Are you a morning person, or are you getting most of your work done when people are quitting for the day? Pick your best hours for top-priority activities. Be sure to schedule enough time for exercise and relaxation. Recreation is not necessarily wasted time. You need to take care of your physical and emotional well-being. Otherwise your life will be seriously imbalanced.

5. Conduct nightly audits. Take 10 minutes each night to figure out how well you accomplished your goals that day. Successful time managers evaluate themselves daily. This simple task will help

you see the entire picture. Cross off the goals you accomplished and carry over to the next day those you did not get done. You also may realize that some goals can be moved down to low-priority or be trashed.

Time Management Skills

In addition to the five major steps, the following can help you make better use of your time:

- Delegate. If possible, delegate activities that someone else can do for you. Having another person type your paper while you prepare for an exam might be well worth the expense and your time.

- Say "no." Learn to say no to activities that keep you from getting your top priorities done. You can do only so much in a single day. Nobody has enough time to do everything he or she would like to get done. Don't overload either. Many people are afraid to say no because they feel guilty if they do. Think ahead, and think of the consequences. Are you doing it to please others? What will it do to your well-being? Can you handle one more task? At some point you have to balance your activities and look at life and time realistically.

- Protect against boredom. Doing nothing can be a source of stress. People need to feel that they are contributing and that they are productive members of society. It also is good for self-esteem and self-worth. Set realistic goals and work toward them each day.

- Plan ahead for disruptions. Even a careful plan of action can be disrupted. An unexpected phone call or visitor can ruin your schedule. Planning your response ahead will help you deal with these saboteurs.

- Get it done. Select only one task at a time, concentrate on it, and see it through. Many people do a little here, do a little there, then do something else. In the end, nothing gets done. An exception to working on just one task at a time is when you are doing a difficult task. Rather than "killing yourself" in one lengthy work session, interchange with another activity that is not as hard.

- Eliminate distractions. If you have trouble adhering to a set plan, remove distractions and trash activities from your eyesight. Television, radio, magazines, open doors, or studying in a park might distract you and become time killers.

- Set aside "overtimes." Regularly schedule time you did not think you would need as overtime to complete unfinished projects. Most people underschedule rather than overschedule time. The result is usually late-night burnout! If you schedule overtimes and get your tasks done, enjoy some leisure time, get ahead on another project, or work on some of your trash activities.

- Plan time for you. Set aside special time for yourself daily. Life is not meant to be all work. Use your time to walk, read, or listen to your favorite music.

- Reward yourself. As with any other healthy behavior, positive change or a job well done deserves a reward. We often overlook the value of rewards, even if they are self-given. People practice behaviors that are rewarded and discontinue those that are not.

One more activity that you should perform weekly is to go through the list of strategies in Figure 12.8 (page 342) to determine if you are becoming a good time manager. Provide a yes or no answer to each statement. If you are able to answer yes to most questions, congratulations. You are becoming a good time manager.

COPING WITH STRESS

The ways in which people perceive and cope with stress seem to be more important in the development of disease than the amount and type of stress itself. If individuals perceive stress as a definite problem in their lives or if it interferes with optimal level of health and performance, several excellent stress management techniques exist to help them cope more effectively.

First, of course, the person must recognize that a problem exists. Many people either do not want to believe they are under too much stress or they fail to recognize some of the typical symptoms of distress. Noting some of the stress-related symptoms (see box on page 333) will help a person respond more objectively and initiate an adequate coping response.

> The ways in which people perceive and cope with stress seem to be more important in the development of disease than the amount and type of stress itself.

When people have stress-related symptoms, they should first try to identify and remove the stressor or stress-causing agent. This is not as simple as it may seem, because in some situations eliminating the stressor is not possible, or a person may not even know the exact causing agent. If the cause is unknown, keeping a log of the time and days when

FIGURE 12.5 Finding the time killers.

Name: _____ Date: _____

Course: _____ Section: _____ Gender: _____ Age: _____

Keep a 4- to 7-day log and record at half-hour intervals the activities you do (make additional copies of this form as needed). Record the activities as you go through your typical day, so you will remember them all. At the end of each day, decide when you wasted time. Using a highlighter, identify the time killers on this form and plan necessary changes for the next day.

6:00	
6:30	
7:00	
7:30	
8:00	
8:30	
9:00	
9:30	
10:00	
10:30	
11:00	
11:30	
12:00	
12:30	
1:00	
1:30	
2:00	
2:30	
3:00	
3:30	
4:00	
4:30	
5:00	
5:30	
6:00	
6:30	
7:00	
7:30	
8:00	
8:30	
9:00	
9:30	
10:00	
10:30	
11:00	
11:30	
12:00	

FIGURE 12.6 Planning your long- and short-range goals.

Name: _____ Date: _____

Course: _____ Section: _____ Gender:_____ Age: _____

In the spaces provided below, list your goals as indicated. You may want to keep this form and review it in years to come.

I. List three goals you wish to accomplish in this life:

   1. _____

   2. _____

   3. _____

II. List three goals you wish to see accomplished 10 years from now:

   1. _____

   2. _____

   3. _____

III. List three goals you wish to accomplish this year:

   1. _____

   2. _____

   3. _____

IV. List three goals you wish to accomplish this month:

   1. _____

   2. _____

   3. _____

V. List three goals you wish to accomplish this week:

   1. _____

   2. _____

   3. _____

Signature: _____ Date: _____

FIGURE 12.7 My daily and weekly goals and priorities.

Take 10 minutes each morning and write down the goals or tasks you wish to accomplish that day. Rank them as top, medium, low, or trash priorities (make as many copies of this form as needed). At the end of the day, evaluate how well you accomplished your tasks for the day. Cross off the goals you accomplished and carry over to the next day those you did not get done.

Date: _____ Day of the Week: _____

Top-Priority Goals

1. _____
2. _____
3. _____
4. _____

Medium-Priority Goals

1. _____
2. _____
3. _____
4. _____

Low-Priority Goals

1. _____
2. _____
3. _____
4. _____

Trash (do only after all other goals have been accomplished)

1. _____
2. _____
3. _____
4. _____

Take a few minutes each Sunday night and write down the goals or tasks you wish to accomplish during the upcoming week. As with your daily goals, rank them as top, medium, low, or trash priorities (make as many copies of this form as needed). At the end of the week, evaluate how well you accomplished your goals. Cross off the goals you accomplished and carry over to the next week those you did not get done.

Week: _____/_____/200____ to _____/_____/200____

Top-Priority Goals

1. _____
2. _____
3. _____
4. _____

Medium-Priority Goals

1. _____
2. _____
3. _____
4. _____

Low-Priority Goals

1. _____
2. _____
3. _____
4. _____

Trash (do only after all other goals have been accomplished)

1. _____
2. _____
3. _____
4. _____

FIGURE 12.8 Evaluation of my time management skills.

Name: _____ Date: _____

Course: _____ Section: _____ Gender: _____ Age: _____

Weekly, go through the list of strategies below and write a "yes" or "no" in response to each statement. If you are able to answer "yes" to most questions, congratulations. You are becoming a good time manager.

Strategy — Date:																
1. I evaluate my time killers periodically.																
2. I have written down my long-range goals.																
3. I have written down my short-range goals.																
4. I use a daily planner.																
5. I conduct nightly audits.																
6. I conduct weekly audits.																
7. I delegate activities that others can do.																
8. I have learned to say no to additional tasks when I'm already in overload.																
9. I plan activities to avoid boredom.																
10. I plan ahead for distractions.																
11. I work on one task at a time until it's done.																
12. I have removed distractions from my work.																
13. I set aside "overtimes."																
14. I set aside special time for myself daily.																
15. I reward myself for a job well done.																

the symptoms occur, as well as the events preceding and following the onset of symptoms, may be helpful.

For instance, a couple noted that every afternoon around 6 o'clock, the wife became nauseated and had abdominal pain. After seeking professional help, both were instructed to keep a log of daily events. It soon became clear that the symptoms did not occur on weekends but always started just before the husband came home from work during the week. Following some personal interviews with the couple, it was determined that the wife felt a lack of attention from her husband and responded subconsciously by becoming ill to the point at which she required personal care and affection from her husband. Once the stressor was identified, appropriate behavior changes were initiated to correct the situation.

In many instances, however, the stressor cannot be removed. Examples of such situations are the death of a close family member, the first year on the job, an intolerable boss, or a change in work responsibility. Nevertheless, stress can be managed through relaxation techniques.

The body responds to stress by activating the **fight-or-flight** mechanism, which prepares a person to take action by stimulating the vital defense systems. This stimulation originates in the hypothalamus and the pituitary gland in the brain. The hypothalamus activates the sympathetic nervous system, and the pituitary activates the release of catecholamines (hormones) from the adrenal glands.

These hormonal changes increase heart rate, blood pressure, blood flow to active muscles and the brain, glucose levels, oxygen consumption, and strength—all necessary for the body to fight or flee. For the body to relax, one of these actions must take place. However, if the person is unable to take action, the muscles tense up and tighten (see Figure 12.9). This increased tension and tightening can be dissipated effectively through some coping techniques.

Physical Activity

Physical activity is one of the simplest tools to control stress. The value of exercise in reducing stress is related to several factors, the main one being a decrease in muscular tension. For example, a person can be distressed because he or she has had a miserable 8 hours of work in a smoke-filled room with an intolerable boss. To make matters

> You cannot hit your boss or the car in front of you, but you can certainly "hit" the swimming pool, the tennis ball, the weights, or the jogging trail.

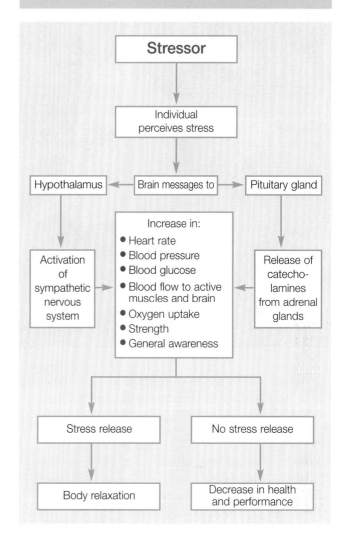

FIGURE 12.9 Physiological response to stress: fight-or-flight mechanism.

Stressor
↓
Individual perceives stress
↓
Hypothalamus ← Brain messages to → Pituitary gland

Activation of sympathetic nervous system

Increase in:
- Heart rate
- Blood pressure
- Blood glucose
- Blood flow to active muscles and brain
- Oxygen uptake
- Strength
- General awareness

Release of catecholamines from adrenal glands

Stress release → Body relaxation

No stress release → Decrease in health and performance

worse, it is late and, on the way home, the car in front is going much slower than the speed limit. The fight-or-flight mechanism is activated, catecholamines rise, heart rate and blood pressure shoot up, breathing quickens and deepens, muscles tense up, and all systems say "go." No action can be initiated or stress dissipated, though, because the person cannot just hit the boss or the car in front.

A real remedy would be to take action by "hitting" the swimming pool, the tennis ball, the weights, or the jogging trail. By engaging in physical activity, a person is able to reduce the muscular tension and

Fight or flight Physiological response of the body to stress that prepares the individual to take action by stimulating the vital defense systems.

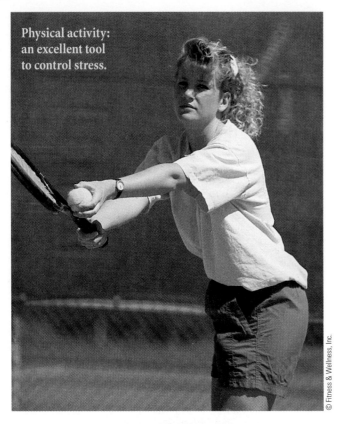

Physical activity: an excellent tool to control stress.

© Fitness & Wellness, Inc.

metabolize the increased catecholamines that brought about the physiological changes triggering the fight-or-flight mechanism. Although exercise does not solve problems at work or take care of slow drivers, it certainly can help a person cope with stress and can prevent stress from becoming a chronic problem.

The early evening hours are becoming the most popular time to exercise for many highly stressed executives. On the way home from work, they stop at the health club or the fitness center. Exercising at this time helps them to dissipate the stress accumulated during the day. Not only does evening exercise help to get rid of the stress, but it also provides an opportunity to enjoy the evening more. At home, the family will appreciate Dad or Mom coming home more relaxed, leaving work problems behind, and being able to dedicate all energy to family activities.

Most people can relate to exercise as a means of managing stress by remembering how good they felt the last time they concluded a strenuous exercise session after a long, difficult day at the office. A fatigued muscle is a relaxed muscle. For this reason, many people have said that the best part of exercise is the shower afterward.

Research has also shown that physical exercise requiring continuous and rhythmic muscular activity, such as aerobic exercise, stimulates alpha-wave activity in the brain. These are the same wave patterns seen commonly during meditation and relaxation.

Further, during vigorous aerobic exercise lasting 30 minutes or longer, morphine-like substances referred to as **endorphins** are thought to be released from the pituitary gland in the brain. These substances not only act as painkillers but also seem to induce the soothing, calming effect often associated with aerobic exercise.

Another way that exercise helps lower stress is by deliberately diverting stress to various body systems. Dr. Hans Selye explains in his book *Stress Without Distress* that, when one specific task becomes difficult, a change in activity can be as good or better than rest itself. For example, if a person is having trouble with a task and does not seem to be getting anywhere, jogging or swimming for a while is better than sitting around and getting frustrated. In this way the mental strain is diverted to the working muscles, and one system helps the other to relax.[3]

Other psychologists indicate that, when muscular tension is removed from the emotional strain, the emotional strain disappears. In many cases, the change of activity suddenly clears the mind and helps put the pieces together.

Researchers have found that physical exercise gives people a psychological boost because exercise does all the following:

- Lessens feelings of anxiety, depression, frustration, aggression, anger, and hostility.
- Alleviates insomnia.
- Provides an opportunity to meet social needs and develop new friendships.
- Allows the person to share common interests and problems.
- Develops discipline.
- Provides the opportunity to do something enjoyable and constructive that will lead to better health and total well-being.

Beyond the short-term benefits of exercise in lessening stress, another benefit of a regular aerobic exercise program is in actually strengthening the cardiorespiratory system itself. Because the cardiorespiratory system seems to be affected seriously by stress, a stronger system should be able to cope more effectively. For instance, good cardiorespiratory endurance has been shown to lower resting heart rate and blood pressure. Because both heart rate and blood pressure rise in stressful situations, initiating the stress response at a lower baseline will counteract the negative effects of stress. People who have a fit cardiorespiratory system can cope more effectively and are less affected by the stresses of daily living.

Relaxation Techniques

Although benefits are reaped immediately after engaging in any of the several relaxation techniques, several months of regular practice may be necessary for total mastery. The relaxation exercises that follow should not be considered cure-alls. If these exercises do not prove to be effective, more specialized textbooks and professional help are called for. In some instances a person's symptoms may not be caused by stress but rather may be related to a different medical disorder.

BIOFEEDBACK

Clinical application of **biofeedback** to treat various medical disorders has become popular in the last few years. Besides its successful application in managing stress, it is commonly used to treat medical disorders such as essential hypertension, asthma, heart rhythm and rate disturbances, cardiac neurosis, eczematous dermatitis, fecal incontinence, insomnia, and stuttering. Biofeedback as a treatment modality has been defined as

> A process in which a person learns to reliably influence physiological responses of two kinds: either responses which are not ordinarily under voluntary control or responses which ordinarily are easily regulated but for which regulation has broken down due to trauma or disease.[4]

In simpler terms, biofeedback is the interaction with the interior self. This interaction allows a person to learn the relationship between the mind and the biological response. The person actually can "feel" how thought processes influence biological responses (such as heart rate, blood pressure, body temperature, and muscle tension) and how biological responses influence the thought process.

As an illustration of this process, consider the association between a strange noise in the middle of a dark, quiet night and the heart rate response. At first the heart rate shoots up because of the stress the unknown noise induces. The individual may even feel the heart palpitating in the chest and, although still uncertain about the noise, may attempt not to panic to prevent an even faster heart rate. Upon realizing that all is well, the person resumes control and influences the heart rate to come down. The mind now is able to exert almost complete control over the biological response.

Complex electronic instruments are required to conduct biofeedback. The process itself entails a three-stage, closed-loop feedback system:

1. A biological response to a stressor is detected and amplified.

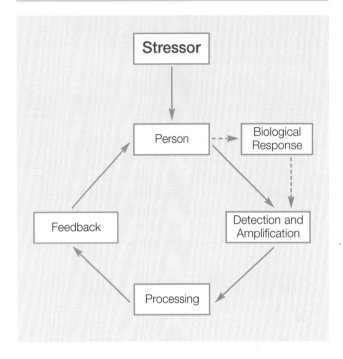

FIGURE 12.10 Biofeedback mechanism.

2. The response is processed.
3. Results of the response are fed back to the individual immediately.

The person uses this new input and attempts to change the physiological response voluntarily—this attempt, in turn, is detected, amplified, and processed. The results are then fed back to the person. The process continues with the intent of teaching the person to reliably influence the physiological response for the better (see Figure 12.10). The most common physiological parameters measured are heart rate, finger temperature, and blood pressure; electromyograms and electroencephalograms are also used.

Although biofeedback has significant applications in treating various medical disorders, including stress, it requires adequately trained personnel and, in many

Key Terms

Endorphins Morphine-like substances released from the pituitary gland during prolonged aerobic exercise. They are thought to induce feelings of euphoria and natural well-being.

Biofeedback A stress management technique in which a person learns to reliably influence physiological responses of two kinds: either responses that are not ordinarily under voluntary control or responses that ordinarily are easily regulated but for which regulation has broken down because of trauma or disease.

cases, costly equipment. Therefore, several alternative methods that yield similar results are frequently substituted for biofeedback. For example, research has shown that physical exercise and progressive muscle relaxation, used successfully in stress management, seem to be just as effective as biofeedback in treating essential hypertension.

PROGRESSIVE MUSCLE RELAXATION

Progressive muscle relaxation was developed by Dr. Edmund Jacobsen in the 1930s. This technique enables individuals to relearn the sensation of deep relaxation. The technique involves progressively contracting and relaxing muscle groups throughout the body. Because chronic stress leads to high levels of muscular tension, acute awareness of how progressively tightening and relaxing the muscles feels can release the tension on the muscles and teach the body to relax at will.

Feeling the tension during the exercises also helps the person to be more alert to signs of distress, because this tension is similar to that experienced in stressful situations. In everyday life, these feelings then can cue the person to do relaxation exercises.

Relaxation exercises should be done in a quiet, warm, well-ventilated room. The recommended exercises and the duration of the routine vary from one person to the next. Most important is that the individual pay attention to the sensation he or she feels each time the muscles are tensed and relaxed.

The exercises should encompass all muscle groups of the body. Following is an example of a sequence of progressive muscle relaxation exercises. The instructions for these exercises can be read to the person, memorized, or tape-recorded. At least 20 minutes should be set aside to complete the entire sequence. Doing the exercises any faster will defeat their purpose. Ideally, the sequence should be done twice a day.

Example Relaxation Routine The individual performing the exercises stretches out comfortably on the floor, face up, with a pillow under the knees, and assumes a passive attitude, allowing the body to relax as much as possible. Each muscle group is to be contracted in sequence, taking care to avoid any strain. Muscles should be tightened to only about 70 percent of the total possible tension to avoid cramping or injury to the muscle itself.

To produce the relaxation effects, the person must pay attention to the sensation of tensing up and relaxing. The person holds each contraction about 5 seconds and then allows the muscles to go totally limp. The person should take enough time to contract and

Practicing progressive muscle relaxation on a regular basis helps to reduce stress.

© Fitness & Wellness, Inc.

relax each muscle group before going on to the next. An example of a complete progressive muscle relaxation sequence is as follows:

1. Point your feet, curling the toes downward. Study the tension in the arches and the top of the feet. Hold, continue to note the tension, then relax. Repeat once.

2. Flex the feet upward toward the face and note the tension in your feet and calves. Hold and relax. Repeat once.

3. Push your heels down against the floor as if burying them in the sand. Hold and note the tension at the back of the thigh. Relax. Repeat once.

4. Contract the right thigh by straightening the leg, gently raising the leg off the floor. Hold and study the tension. Relax. Repeat with the left leg. Hold and relax. Repeat each leg.

5. Tense the buttocks by raising your hips ever so slightly off the floor. Hold and note the tension. Relax. Repeat once.

6. Contract the abdominal muscles. Hold them tight and note the tension. Relax. Repeat once.

7. Suck in your stomach. Try to make it reach your spine. Flatten your lower back to the floor. Hold and feel the tension in the stomach and lower back. Relax. Repeat once.

8. Take a deep breath and hold it, then exhale. Repeat. Note your breathing becoming slower and more relaxed.

9. Place your arms at the sides of your body and clench both fists. Hold, study the tension, and relax. Repeat.

10. Flex the elbow by bringing both hands to the shoulders. Hold tight and study the tension in the biceps. Relax. Repeat.

11. Place your arms flat on the floor, palms up, and push the forearms hard against the floor. Note the tension on the triceps. Hold, and relax. Repeat.

12. Shrug your shoulders, raising them as high as possible. Hold and note the tension. Relax. Repeat.

13. Gently push your head backward. Note the tension in the back of the neck. Hold, relax. Repeat.

14. Gently bring the head against the chest, push forward, hold, and note the tension in the neck. Relax. Repeat.

15. Press your tongue toward the roof of your mouth. Hold, study the tension, and relax. Repeat.

16. Press your teeth together. Hold, and study the tension. Relax. Repeat.

17. Close your eyes tightly. Hold them closed and note the tension. Relax, leaving your eyes closed. Do this one more time.

18. Wrinkle your forehead and note the tension. Hold and relax. Repeat.

When time is a factor during the daily routine and an individual is not able to go through the entire sequence, he or she may do only the exercises specific to the area that feels most tense. Performing a partial sequence is better than not doing the exercises at all. Completing the entire sequence, of course, yields the best results.

BREATHING TECHNIQUES FOR RELAXATION

Breathing exercises also can be an antidote to stress. These exercises have been used for centuries in the Orient and India to improve mental, physical, and emotional stamina. In breathing exercises, the person concentrates on "breathing away" the tension and inhaling a large amount of air with each breath. Breathing exercises can be learned in only a few minutes and require considerably less time than the progressive muscle relaxation exercises.

As with any other relaxation technique, these exercises should be done in a quiet, pleasant, well-ventilated room. Any of the three examples of breathing exercises presented here will help relieve tension induced by stress.

1. Deep breathing. Lie with your back flat against the floor and place a pillow under your knees. Feet are slightly separated, with toes pointing outward. (The exercise may also be done while sitting up in a chair or standing erect.) Place one hand on your abdomen and the other hand on your chest.

    Slowly breathe in and out so the hand on your abdomen rises when you inhale and falls as you exhale (also referred to as "diaphragmatic breathing"). The hand on the chest should not move much at all. Repeat the exercise about 10 times. Next, scan your body for tension and compare your present tension with the tension you felt at the beginning of the exercise. Repeat the entire process once or twice.

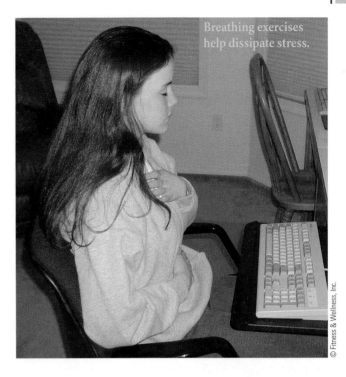

Breathing exercises help dissipate stress.

© Fitness & Wellness, Inc.

2. Sighing. Using the abdominal breathing technique, breathe in through your nose to a specific count (e.g., 4, 5, or 6). Now exhale through pursed lips to double the intake count (e.g., 8, 10, or 12). Repeat the exercise eight to ten times whenever you feel tense.

3. Complete natural breathing. Sit in an upright position or stand straight up. Breathing through your nose, gradually fill your lungs from the bottom up. Hold your breath for several seconds. Now exhale slowly by allowing your chest and abdomen to relax completely. Repeat the exercise eight to ten times.

VISUAL IMAGERY

Visual or mental **imagery** has been used as a healing technique for centuries in various cultures around the world. In Western medicine the practice of imagery is relatively new and not widely accepted among health

Key Terms

Progressive muscle relaxation A stress management technique that uses progressive contraction and relaxation of muscle groups throughout the body.

Breathing exercise A stress management technique wherein the individual concentrates on "breathing away" the tension and inhaling fresh air to the entire body.

Imagery Mental visualization of relaxing images and scenes to induce body relaxation in times of stress or as an aid in the treatment of certain medical conditions such as cancer, hypertension, asthma, chronic pain, and obesity.

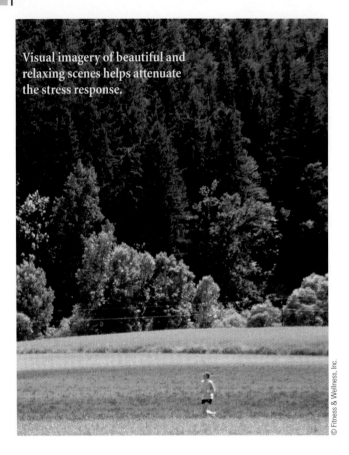

Visual imagery of beautiful and relaxing scenes helps attenuate the stress response.

© Fitness & Wellness, Inc.

care professionals. Research is now being done to study the effects of imagery on the treatment of conditions such as cancer, hypertension, asthma, chronic pain, and obesity.

Visual imagery involves the creation of relaxing visual images and scenes in times of stress to elicit body and mind relaxation. Imagery works by offsetting the stressor with the visualization of relaxing scenes such as a sunny beach, a beautiful meadow, a quiet mountaintop, or some other peaceful setting. Imagery can also be used in conjunction with breathing exercises, meditation, or yoga.

As with other stress management techniques, imagery should be performed in a quiet and comfortable environment. You can either sit or lie down for the exercise. If you lie down, use a soft surface and place a pillow under your knees. Be sure that your clothes are loose and that you are as comfortable as you can be.

To start the exercise, close your eyes and take a few breaths using one of the breathing techniques previously described. You can then proceed to visualize one of your favorite scenes in nature. You may place yourself right into the scene and visualize yourself moving about and experiencing nature to its fullest. Enjoy the people, the animals, the colors, the sounds, the smells, and even the temperature in your scene. After 10 to 20 minutes of visualization, open

your eyes and compare the tension in your body and mind at this point with how you felt prior to the exercise. You can repeat this exercise as often as you deem necessary when you are feeling tension or stress.

You may not always be able to use a quiet, comfortable setting or to sit or lie down for 10 to 20 minutes. If you feel that imagery works for you, you can perform this technique while standing or sitting in an active setting. If you are able, close your eyes and disregard your surroundings for a short moment and visualize one of your favorite scenes. Once you feel that you have regained some control over the stressor, open your eyes and continue with your assigned tasks.

AUTOGENIC TRAINING

Autogenic training is a form of self-suggestion in which people are able to place themselves in an auto-hypnotic state by repeating and concentrating on feelings of heaviness and warmth in the extremities. This technique was developed by Johannes Schultz, a German psychiatrist who noted that hypnotized individuals developed sensations of warmth and heaviness in the limbs and torso. The sensation of warmth is caused by dilation of blood vessels, which increases blood flow to the limbs. Muscular relaxation produces the feeling of heaviness.

In this technique the person lies down or sits in a comfortable position with eyes closed, then says (or thinks) the following. During this process, the person concentrates progressively on the six fundamental stages.

1. Heaviness

   "My right arm is heavy.
   My left arm is heavy.
   Both arms are heavy.
   My right leg is heavy.
   My left leg is heavy.
   Both legs are heavy.
   My arms and legs are heavy."

2. Warmth

   "My right (left) arm is warm.
   Both arms are warm.
   My right (left) leg is warm.
   Both legs are warm.
   My arms and legs are warm."

3. Heart

   "My heartbeat is calm and regular." (Repeat four or five times.)

4. Respiration

   "My body breathes itself." (Repeat four or five times.)

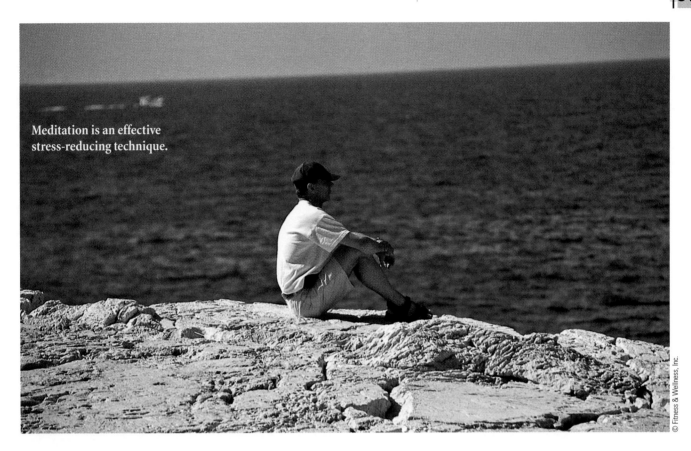

Meditation is an effective stress-reducing technique.

© Fitness & Wellness, Inc.

5. Abdomen

   "My abdomen is warm." (Repeat four or five times.)

6. Forehead

   "My forehead is cool." (Repeat four or five times.)

   The autogenic training technique is more difficult to master than any of those mentioned previously. The person should not move too fast through the entire exercise, because this actually may interfere with learning and relaxation. Each stage must be mastered before proceeding to the next.

MEDITATION

Meditation is a mental exercise that can bring about psychological and physical benefits. The objective of meditation is to gain control over one's attention by clearing the mind and blocking out the stressor(s) responsible for the higher tension. This technique can be learned rather quickly and can be used frequently during times of increased tension and stress.

   Initially the person who is learning to meditate should choose a place or room that is comfortable, quiet, and free of all disturbances (including telephones). After learning the technique, the person will be able to meditate just about anywhere. A time block of approximately 15 minutes, twice a day, is needed to meditate.

1. Sit in a chair in an upright position with the hands resting either in your lap or on the arms of the chair. Close your eyes and focus on your breathing. Allow your body to relax as much as possible. Do not try to consciously relax, because trying means work. Rather, assume a passive attitude and concentrate on your breathing.

2. Allow the body to breathe regularly, at its own rhythm. Repeat in your mind the word "one" every time you inhale and the word "two" every time you exhale. Paying attention to these two words keeps distressing thoughts from entering into your mind.

3. Continue to breathe in this way about 15 minutes. Because the objective of meditation is to bring

KeyTerms

Autogenic training Stress management technique using a form of self-suggestion, wherein an individual is able to place him/herself in an autohypnotic state by repeating and concentrating on feelings of heaviness and warmth in the extremities.

Meditation A stress management technique used to gain control over one's attention by clearing the mind and blocking out the stressor(s) responsible for the increased tension.

about a hypometabolic state leading to body relaxation, do not use an alarm clock to remind you that the 15 minutes have expired. The alarm will only trigger your stress response again, defeating the purpose of the exercise. Opening your eyes once in a while to keep track of the time is fine, but do not rush or anticipate the end of the 15 minutes. This time has been set aside for meditation, and you need to relax, take your time, and enjoy the exercise.

YOGA

Yoga is a school of thought in the Hindu religion that seeks to help the individual attain a higher level of spirituality and peace of mind. Practitioners adhere to a specific code of ethics and a system of mental and physical exercises that promote control of the mind and the body. In Western countries, many people are mainly familiar with the exercise portion of yoga. This system of exercises (postures) can be used as a relaxation technique for stress management. The exercises include a combination of postures, diaphragmatic breathing, muscle relaxation, and meditation that help buffer the biological effects of stress.

Western interest in yoga exercises gradually developed over the last century, particularly since the 1970s. People pursue yoga exercises for their potential to dispel stress by raising self-esteem, clearing the mind, slowing respiration, promoting neuromuscular relaxation, and increasing body awareness. Additionally, the exercises help control involuntary body functions like heart rate, blood pressure, oxygen consumption, and metabolic rate. The practice of yoga exercises can help increase muscular flexibility, muscular strength and endurance, and balance.

Additionally, yoga exercises have been used to help treat chemical dependency, insomnia, and prevent injury. New research on patients with coronary heart disease who practiced yoga (among other lifestyle changes) has shown that it slows down or even reverses atherosclerosis. These patients were compared with others who did not use yoga as one of the lifestyle changes.[5]

There are many different styles of yoga. Classes vary according to their emphasis. Some styles of yoga are athletic; others are passive in nature. The most popular variety in the Western world is hatha yoga, which incorporates a series of static-stretching postures performed in a specific sequence, also known as "asanas," that helps induce the relaxation response. The postures are held for several seconds while participants concentrate on breathing patterns, meditation, and body awareness. Many of the typical stretches

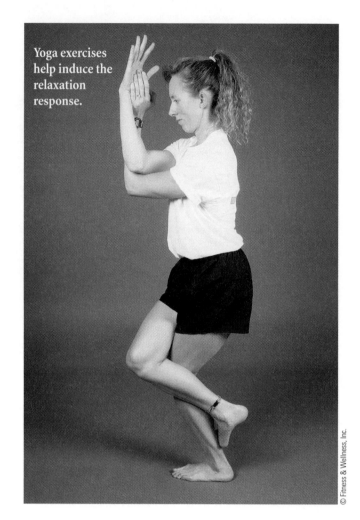

Yoga exercises help induce the relaxation response.

used in flexibility exercises today have been adapted from hatha yoga.

As with flexibility exercises, the stretches in hatha yoga should not be performed to the point of discomfort. Instructors should not push participants beyond their physical limitations. Similar to other stress management techniques, yoga exercises are best performed in a quiet place for about 15 to 60 minutes per session. Many yoga participants like to perform the exercises on a daily basis.

To appreciate yoga exercises, a person needs to experience them. This section, nonetheless, serves only as an introduction. Although yoga exercises can be practiced with the instruction of a book or video, most participants take classes. The postures are difficult and complex, and few individuals can master the entire sequence in the first few weeks.

Individuals interested in yoga exercises should initially pursue its practice under qualified instruction. Many universities offer yoga courses and you can also check the phone book for a listing of yoga instructors or classes. Yoga courses are offered at many health clubs and recreation centers. Because instructors and yoga styles vary, you may want to sit in on a class before enrolling. The most important thing is to look for is an instructor whose views on wellness parallel your own. There are no national certification standards for instructors. If you are new to yoga, you are encouraged to compare a couple of instructors before you select a class.

Which Technique Is Best?

Each person reacts to stress differently. Therefore, the best coping strategy depends mostly on the individual. Which technique is used does not really matter as long as it works. An individual may want to experiment with all of them to find out which works best. A combination of two or more works best for many people.

All of the coping strategies discussed here help to block out stressors and promote mental and physical relaxation by diverting the attention to a different, nonthreatening action. Some of the techniques are easier to learn and may take less time per session. As a part of your class experience, you may participate in a stress management session (see Figure 12.11, page 353). Regardless of which technique you select, the time spent doing stress management exercises (several times a day, as needed) is well worth the effort when stress becomes a significant problem in life.

People need to learn to relax and take time out for themselves. Stress is not what makes people ill but, rather, the way they react to the stress-causing agent. Individuals who learn to be diligent and start taking control of themselves find that they can enjoy a better, happier, and healthier life.

WEB INTERACTIVE

Stress Management: A Review of Principles

Presented by Wesley E. Sime, Ph.D., MPS, professor of Health and Human Performance at the University of Nebraska—Lincoln. This online series of lectures on stress management education features information on the psychobiology of stress and relaxation as well as pathophysiology of stress.

http://www.une.edu/stress/mgmt

Stress: Who Has Time For It?

A visually appealing site that describes the symptoms of stress and how to manage it.

http://www.health4teens.org/stress

Biofeedback

The basics of biofeedback are presented in this site along with links to other alternative forms of therapy for stress.

http://www.thriveonline.com/serenity/stress/smq.index.html

INTERACTIVE SITES

Stress Assess

This three-part online educational tool was developed by the National Wellness Institute at the University of Wisconsin—Steven's Point. The questionnaire, designed to increase your knowledge about stress, features separate evaluations for stress sources, distress symptoms, and stress-balancing strategies. Based on these results, you will learn healthy ways to better manage your specific stressors.

http://www.uwsp.edu/Health_Service/services/stress

Are You Under Stress?

Take this comprehensive stress questionnaire to find out how well you are handling stress in your life. This tool assesses eight key stress warning signs: anger, perfectionism, time-urgency, disappointment, negative mood, underachievement, tension, and physical problems.

http://www.thriveonline.com/serenity/stress/smq.index.html

Key Terms

Yoga A school of thought in the Hindu religion that seeks to help the individual attain a higher level of spirituality and peace of mind.

n*tes

1. H. Selye, *Stress Without Distress* (New York: Signet, 1974).

2. R. J. Kriegel and M. H. Kriegel, *The C Zone: Peak Performance Under Stress* (Garden City, NY: Anchor Press/ Doubleday, 1984).

3. See note 1.

4. E. B. Blanchard and L. H. Epstein, *A Biofeedback Primer* (Reading, MA: Addison-Wesley, 1978).

5. S. C. Manchanda, et al., "Retardation of Coronary Atherosclerosis With Yoga Lifestyle Intervention," *Journal of the Association of Physicians of India* 48 (2000): 687–694.

 Suggested Readings

■ Andrasik, F., D. Coleman, and L. H. Epstein. "Biofeedback: Clinical and Research Considerations." In *Behavioral Medicine: Assessment and Treatment Strategies*, edited by D. M. Doleys, R. L. Meredith, and A. R. Ciminero. New York: Plenum Press, 1982.

■ Chesney, M. A., J. R. Eagleston, and R. H. Roseman. "Type A Assessment and Intervention." In *Medical Psychology: Contributions to Behavioral Medicine*, edited by C. K. Prokop and L. A. Bradley. New York: Academic Press, 1981.

■ Gauron, E. F. *Mental Training for Peak Performance*. Lansing, NY: Sport Science Associates, 1984.

■ Girdano, D., and G. Everly. *Controlling Stress and Tension: A Holistic Approach*. Englewood Cliffs, NJ: Prentice Hall, 1996.

■ Greenberg, J. S. *Comprehensive Stress Management*. Dubuque, IA: Wm. C. Brown, 1993.

■ Luthe, W. "Autogenic Training: Method, Research and Applications in Medicine." *American Journal of Psychotherapy* 17 (1963): 174–195.

■ Schafer, W. *Stress Management for Wellness*. Fort Worth: HBJ College Publishers, 1995.

■ Selye, H. *The Stress of Life*. New York: McGraw-Hill, 1978.

■ Smith, J. S. *Creative Stress Management: The 1-2-3 Cope System*. Englewood Cliffs, NJ: Prentice Hall, 1993.

FIGURE 12.11 Sample stress management program.

Name: _____ Date: _____

Course: _____ Section: _____ Gender: _____ Age: _____

I. Stage of Change for Stress Management

Using Figure 2.4 (page 45) and Table 2.3 (page 43), identify your current stage of change for a stress management program:

[   ]

II. Stress Management

Instructions: The class should be divided into groups of about five students per group. Each group should select and go through a minimum of two of the following stress management techniques outlined in this chapter:

1. Progressive Muscle Relaxation   3. Visual Imagery   5. Meditation
2. Breathing Techniques for Relaxation   4. Autogenic Training

A group leader is chosen who will lead the exercise according to the instructions provided for each relaxation technique in this chapter. Be sure this experience is conducted in a comfortable room that is as free of noise as possible. If trained personnel or a tape-recording for progressive muscle relaxation exercises or visual imagery is available, the entire class may participate in this experience at once. Institutions that have biofeedback equipment may use it in this laboratory as well. After completing this lab, answer the four questions given below.

1. Indicate the two relaxation techniques used in your class:

A. [   ]   B. [   ]

2. In your own words, relate your feelings as you were going through exercises A and B above:

Exercise A: _____

_____

Exercise B: _____

_____

3. Indicate how you felt mentally, emotionally, and physically after participating in this experience:

_____

_____

4. Are there situations in your daily life in which you think you would benefit from practicing the selected stress management exercises?

_____

_____

(continued)

(Figure 12.11 Sample stress management program—continued)

III. Self-Assessment Stress Evaluation

1. Do you currently perceive stress to be a problem in your life? ☐ Yes ☐ No

2. Do you experience any of the typical stress symptoms listed in the box on page 333? If so, which ones?

3. Indicate any specific events in your life that trigger a stress response.

4. Write specific objectives to either avoid or help you manage the various stress-inducing events listed above, including one or more stress-management techniques.

5. Do you have any behavior patterns you would like to modify? List those you would like to change.

6. List specific techniques of change you will use to change undesirable behaviors (see Table 2.2, page 42).

Freedom from Addictive Behavior

objectives

Address the detrimental effects of addictive substances, including marijuana, cocaine, methamphetamine, ecstasy, heroin, and alcohol.

Understand the detrimental health effects of tobacco use in general.

Recognize cigarette smoking as the largest preventable cause of premature illness and death in the United States.

Learn the fundamental reasons people smoke.

Understand the benefits and the significance of a smoking cessation program.

Learn how to implement a smoking cessation program, either for yourself (if you smoke), or to help others go through the quitting process.

As we begin the 21st century, one of the most serious health problems that continues to afflict society is that of chemical dependency. Substance abuse is an extremely destructive behavior that has ruined and ended millions of lives. Perhaps more than with any other unhealthy behavior, education is critical when addictive behaviors are at issue. The time to make healthy choices is now. The information in this chapter will help you make informed decisions. Education concerning these subjects may assist in the search for answers, treatment, and a more productive and happier life.

ADDICTION

When people think of **addiction**, most probably think of dark and dirty alleys, an addict shooting drugs into the veins, or a wino passed out next to a garbage can after having spent an evening with alcohol. Jacquelyn Small, psychotherapist and author, has described addiction as a problem of imbalance or unease within the body and mind.

Almost anything can be addicting, but some addictive behaviors are more detrimental than others. The most serious type of addiction is chemical dependency on drugs such as tobacco, coffee, alcohol, cocaine, methamphetamine, MDMA (ecstasy), heroin, marijuana, and prescription drugs. Less serious addictions are to work, shopping, and even exercise.

People who are addicted to food eat to release stress or boredom or to reward themselves for every small personal achievement. Many people are addicted to television or the Internet. Others become so addicted to their jobs that all they think about is work. Although work may start out as an enjoyable activity, when it totally consumes a person's life, work can become an unhealthy behavior. If you find that you are readily irritated, moody, grouchy, constantly tired, not as alert as you used to be, or making more mistakes than usual, you may be becoming a workaholic and need to slow down or take time off work.

Even though exercise has enhanced the health and quality of life of millions of people, a relatively small number become obsessed with exercise, which has the potential for overuse and addiction. Compulsive exercisers feel guilty and uncomfortable when they miss a day's workout. Often they continue to exercise even when they have injuries and sickness that require proper rest for adequate recovery. People who exceed the recommended guidelines for development and maintenance of fitness (see Chapters 4, 5, and 6) are exercising for reasons other than health—including addiction.

Addiction to caffeine can produce undesirable side effects. Caffeine doses in excess of 200 to 500 mg can produce an abnormally rapid heart rate, abnormal heart rhythms, higher blood pressure, higher body temperature, and increased secretion of gastric acids leading to stomach problems, as well as birth defects in offspring. It may also induce symptoms of anxiety, depression, nervousness, and dizziness. The caffeine content of drinks varies according to the product. In 6 ounces of coffee, for example, the content varies from 65 mg in instant coffee to as high as 180 mg in drip coffee. Soft drinks, mainly colas, range in caffeine content from about 30 to 70 mg per 12-ounce can.

The previous examples, as well as more serious forms of chemical dependency, are by no means the only types of addiction but are used here to illustrate addictive behaviors. Other addictions are gambling, pornography, sex, people, places, and on and on.

Recognizing that all forms of addiction are unhealthy, this chapter focuses on some of the most self-destructive addictive substances in our society: marijuana, cocaine, methamphetamine, MDMA, heroin, alcohol, and tobacco. About a half a million Americans die each year from tobacco, alcohol, and illegal drug use.

DRUGS AND DEPENDENCE

A drug is any substance that alters the user's ability to function. Drugs encompass over-the-counter drugs, prescription medications, and illegal substances. Many drugs lead to physical and psychological dependence.

Any drug can be misused and abused. Drug misuse implies the intentional or inappropriate use of over-the-counter or prescribed medications.[1] Examples of drug misuse include the intake of a greater amount of a medication than prescribed, mixing drugs, not following prescription instructions, or discontinuing a drug prior to a physicians' approval.

Drug abuse is the intentional and inappropriate use of a drug resulting in physical, emotional, financial, intellectual, or social consequences for their use.[2] Many substances, if used in the wrong manner, can be abused.

When drugs are used regularly, they integrate into the body's chemistry, increasing tolerance to the drug and forcing the user to constantly increase the dosage to obtain similar results. Drug abuse leads to serious health problems, and more than half of all adolescent suicides are drug-related. Often, drug abuse also opens the gate to other illegal activities. According to U.S. Department of Justice, the majority of convicted criminals—about 70 percent of federal inmates and 80 percent of state inmates—have abused drugs.

Approximately 60 percent of the world's production of illegal drugs is consumed in the United States. Each year Americans spend more than $100 billion on illegal drugs, an amount that surpasses the total dollars taken in from all crops by U.S. farmers. According to the U.S. Department of Education, today's drugs are stronger and more addictive, and they pose a greater risk than ever before. If you are uncertain about addictive behavior(s) in your life, the questionnaire "Could You Be an Addict?" in Figure 13.4 (page 368) can help you identify a potential problem. Some of the most commonly abused drugs in our society are discussed next.

> **Americans spend more than $100 billion annually on illegal drugs.**

The flowering top of *Cannabis sativa*.

U.S. Department of Justice, Drug Enforcement Administration

Marijuana

Marijuana (pot or grass, as it is commonly called) is the most widely used illegal drug in the United States. Estimates by the Office of National Drug Control Policy indicate that 46 percent of Americans between ages 18 and 25 and 42 percent of those age 26 and older have smoked marijuana. Approximately 31 million people in the United States use marijuana regularly. Most users smoke loose marijuana that has been rolled into a joint or packed into a pipe. A few users will bake it into foods such as brownies.

In small doses, marijuana has a sedative effect. Larger doses produce physical and psychic changes. Studies in the 1960s indicated that the potential effects of marijuana were exaggerated and that the drug was relatively harmless. The drug used today, however, is as much as 10 times stronger than when the initial studies were conducted. Most of the research today shows marijuana to be dangerous and harmful.

The main, and most active, psychoactive and mind-altering ingredient in marijuana is thought to be delta-9-tetrahydrocannabinol (THC). In the 1960s, THC content in marijuana ranged from .02 to 2 percent. Users called the latter "real good grass." Today's THC content averages 4 to 6 percent, although it has been reported as high as 20 percent. The THC content in sinsemilla, a variety of high-potency marijuana grown from the seedless female cannabis plant, is approximately 7 percent THC.

THC reaches the brain within a few seconds after marijuana smoke is inhaled, and the psychic and physical changes reach their peak in about 2 or 3 minutes. THC then is metabolized in the liver to waste metabolites, but 30 percent of it remains in the body a week after the marijuana was smoked. THC is not completely eliminated until 30 days or longer after an initial dose of the drug. The drug always remains in the system of regular users.

Some of the short-term effects of marijuana are **tachycardia**, dryness of the mouth, reddened eyes, stronger appetite, decrease in coordination and tracking (following a moving stimulus), difficulty in concentration, intermittent confusion, impairment of short-term memory and continuity of speech, interference with the physical and mental learning process during periods of intoxication, and increased risk of a heart attack for a full day after smoking the drug. Another common effect is the **amotivational syndrome**. This syndrome persists after periods of intoxication but usually disappears a few weeks after the individual stops using the drug. Long-term harmful effects include atrophy of the brain (leading to irreversible brain damage), less resistance to infectious diseases, chronic bronchitis, lung cancer (marijuana smoke may contain as much as 50 percent more cancer-producing hydrocarbons than cigarette smoke), and possible sterility and impotence.

Key Terms

Addiction Compulsive and uncontrollable behavior(s) or use of substance(s).

Marijuana A psychoactive drug prepared from a mixture of crushed leaves, flowers, small branches, stems, and seeds from the hemp plant *Cannabis sativa*.

Tachycardia Faster-than-normal heart rate.

Amotivational syndrome A condition characterized by loss of motivation, dullness, apathy, and lack of interest in the future.

One of the most common myths about marijuana use is that it is not addictive. This myth has grown recently among young people as lobbyists work to convince the federal government to legalize marijuana for medical purposes. Ample scientific evidence clearly shows that regular users of marijuana do develop physical and psychological dependence. As with cigarette smokers, when regular users go without the drug, they crave the substance, go through mood changes, are irritable and nervous, and develop an obsession to get more.

Cocaine

Similar to marijuana, **cocaine** was thought for many years to be relatively harmless. This misconception came to an abrupt halt in the mid-1980s when two well-known athletes (Len Bias, a basketball player, and Don Rogers, a football player) died suddenly following cocaine overdoses. Between 1 and 1.5 million Americans use cocaine, 96 percent of whom had used marijuana previously. Over the years it has been given several different names including, among others, coke, C, snow, blow, toot, flake, Peruvian lady, white girl, and happy dust. This drug can be sniffed or snorted, smoked, or injected.

When cocaine is snorted, it is absorbed quickly through the mucous membranes of the nose into the bloodstream. The drug is usually arranged in fine powder lines 1 to 2 inches long. Each line stimulates the autonomic nervous system for about 30 minutes. When cocaine is injected intravenously, larger amounts of cocaine can enter the body in less time. The popularity of cocaine is based on the almost universal guarantee that users will find themselves in an immediate state of euphoria and well-being. It's an expensive drug: Some users pay more than $4,800 per ounce for cocaine. Cocaine used in medical therapy sells for about $100 per ounce. The addiction begins with a desire to get high, often at social gatherings, and usually with the assurance that "occasional use is harmless." About 1 in 5 of these first-time users will continue to use the drug now and then, and for some it is the beginning of a lifetime nightmare.

Crack cocaine is a smokable form of cocaine that has become more popular in the past decade. It is many times more potent than cocaine and is highly addictive; two-thirds of users in the United States who are addicted to cocaine use crack. Because they are so potent, crack doses are smaller and therefore less expensive, at a price of $10 to $30 each, although

Powdered cocaine.

U.S. Department of Justice, Drug Enforcement Administration

users will still spend hundreds of dollars a day to support their addiction.

Crack is often made by boiling cocaine hydrochloride in a solution of baking soda, then letting the solution dry. The residue is then broken up to be smoked in a pipe. The high from crack comes within seconds, faster than the high from injected cocaine. The crack high lasts about 12 minutes, which is shorter than the high from snorted or injected cocaine. Choosing to use cocaine in this form heightens the risk for emphysema and heart attack.

Cocaine seems to alleviate fatigue and raise energy levels, as well as lessen the need for food and sleep. Following the high comes a "crash," a state of physiological and psychological depression, often leaving the user with the desire to get more. This can lead to a constant craving for the drug. Similar to alcoholics, cocaine users recover only by abstaining from the drug completely. A single "backslide" can result in renewed addiction.

Light-to-moderate cocaine use is commonly associated with feelings of pleasure and well-being. Sustained cocaine snorting can lead to a constant runny nose, nasal congestion and inflammation, and perforation of the nasal septum. Long-term consequences of cocaine use include loss of appetite, digestive disorders, weight loss, malnutrition, insomnia, confusion, anxiety, and cocaine psychosis, characterized by paranoia and hallucinations. In one type of hallucination, referred to as "formication" or "coke bugs," the chronic user perceives imaginary insects or snakes crawling on or underneath the skin.

High doses of cocaine can cause nervousness, dizziness, blurred vision, vomiting, tremors, seizures,

> **Cocaine hallucinations include "coke bugs" or imaginary insects and snakes crawling on or underneath the skin.**

strokes, angina, cardiac arrhythmias, and high blood pressure. As with smoking marijuana, the increased risk of having a heart attack following cocaine use is immediate. The user's risk may be 24 times higher than normal for up to 3 hours following cocaine use. Almost one-third of cocaine users who suffered a heart attack had no symptoms of heart disease prior to taking cocaine. Intravenous users are also at risk for hepatitis, HIV, and other infectious diseases.

Large overdoses of cocaine can precipitate sudden death from respiratory paralysis, cardiac arrhythmias, and severe convulsions. If individuals lack an enzyme used in metabolizing cocaine, as few as two to three lines of cocaine may be fatal.

Chronic users who constantly crave the drug often turn to crime, including murder, to sustain their habit. Some users view suicide as the only solution to this sad syndrome.

Methamphetamine

Methamphetamine, or "meth," is a more potent form of **amphetamine** that has become the fastest-growing drug threat in the United States. Amphetamines in general are part of a large group of synthetic agents used to stimulate the central nervous system. Amphetamines were widely given to soldiers during World War II to help them overcome fatigue, improve endurance, enhance battlefield ferocity, heighten mood, and keep the soldiers going. During the Vietnam War, U.S. soldiers used a greater amount of amphetamines than soldiers from all countries combined during World War II.

Methamphetamine is a powerfully addictive drug. It falls under the same category of psychostimulant drugs as amphetamines and cocaine. It is also known as a "club drug," a group of illegal substances used at dance clubs, rock concerts, and raves (all-night dance parties). Other club drugs include MDMA, LSD, GHB, Rohypnol, and ketamine.

Methamphetamine is typically a white, odorless, and bitter-tasting powder that dissolves readily in water or alcohol. The drug is a potent central nervous system stimulant that produces a general feeling of well-being, decreases appetite, increases motor activity, and decreases fatigue and the need for sleep.

Based on 1996 estimates by the National Institute on Drug Abuse (NIDA), 4.7 million Americans have tried methamphetamines. Unlike most other drugs, methamphetamine use reaches rural and urban populations alike. Young people especially prefer methamphetamines because of its low cost and the long-lasting effects of the drug, up to 12 hours following use.

"Ice," so named for its appearance, is a smokable form of methamphetamine.

U.S. Department of Justice, Drug Enforcement Administration

Methamphetamine is easily manufactured with over-the-counter ingredients in clandestine "meth labs." These labs can be set up almost anywhere, including garages, basements, or hotel rooms. The abundance of potential meth lab sites makes it difficult for drug enforcement agencies to locate many of these facilities. The risk of injury in a meth lab, however, is high, because potentially explosive environmental contaminants are discarded during the production of the drug.

Methamphetamines can be snorted, swallowed, smoked, or injected. It is commonly referred to as "speed" or "crystal" when snorted or taken orally, "ice" or "glass" when smoked, and "crank" when injected. Depending on how it is taken, methamphetamines affect the body differently.

Smoked or injected methamphetamines provide an immediate intense, pleasurable rush that lasts only a few minutes. Negative effects, nonetheless, can continue for several hours. When the drug is snorted or taken orally, the user does not experience a rush, but develops a feeling of euphoria that lasts up to 16 hours.

Methamphetamine users experience increases in body temperature, blood pressure, heart rate, and breathing rate; a decrease in appetite; hyperactivity;

KeyTerms

Cocaine 2-beta-carbomethoxy-3-betabenozoxytropane, the primary psychoactive ingredient derived from coca plant leaves.

Methamphetamine A more potent form of amphetamine.

Amphetamine Powerful central nervous system stimulant.

tremors; and violent behavior. High doses produce irritability, paranoia, irreversible damage to blood vessels in the brain (causing strokes), and risk of sudden death from hypothermia and convulsions if not treated at once.

Chronic abusers experience insomnia, confusion, hallucinations, inflammation to the heart lining, schizophrenia-like mental disorder, and brain cell damage similar to that caused by strokes. Physical changes to the brain may last months or perhaps permanently. Over time, methamphetamine use may reduce brain levels of **dopamine**, which can lead to symptoms similar to those of Parkinson's disease. Additionally, users are frequently involved in violent crime, homicide, and suicide. Using methamphetamines during pregnancy may cause prenatal complications, premature delivery, and abnormal physical and emotional development of the child.

Similar to other stimulants, methamphetamines are often used in a binge cycle. Addiction develops very quickly because tolerance to methamphetamines is developed within minutes of initial use. The high disappears long before drug blood levels drop significantly. The user then attempts to maintain the pleasurable feelings by taking in more of the drug, and a binge cycle ensues.

The binge cycle can last for a couple of weeks and consists of several stages. The initial rush lasts five to 30 minutes. During this stage heart rate, blood pressure, and metabolism increase along with a great sense of pleasure. The high follows, lasting up to 16 hours; during this stage, users becomes aggressively smarter and more argumentative. The binge stage sets in next: It lasts between 2 and 14 days. Addicts continue to use the drug in an attempt to maintain the high for as long as possible.

When addicts can no longer achieve a satisfying high, they enter the tweaking stage, the most dangerous stage of the cycle. At this point users may have gone without food for several days and without sleep anywhere from 3 to 15 days. They become paranoid, irritable, and violent. Tweakers crave more of the drug, but no amount of amphetamines will restore the pleasurable, euphoric feelings achieved during the high. Thus the addicts become increasingly frustrated, unpredictable, and dangerous to those around them (including police officers, medical personnel, and even to themselves). Once they finally crash, they are no longer dangerous. The user now becomes lethargic and sleeps for 1 to 3 days.

Following the crash, addicts fall into a 1- to 3-month period of withdrawal. During this stage they can be paranoid, aggressive, fatigued, depressed, suicidal, and filled with an intense craving for another high. Reuse of the drug relieves these feelings, thus the incidence of relapse in users who seek treatment is high.

MDMA (Ecstasy)

MDMA, also known as "**ecstasy**," became popular among teenagers and young adults in the United States in the mid-1980s when it evolved into the most common club drug. Although its use was already a serious drug problem in Europe, MDMA was not illegal in the United states until 1985. Prior to 1985, few Americans abused this drug. In the 1970s, MDMA was used as a tool by some therapists to help patients open up and feel at ease. MDMA is named for its chemical structure: 3,4-methylenedioxymethamphetamine. Besides ecstasy, other street names for the drug are X-TC, E, Adam, and love drug.

Year 2000 statistics from the National Institute on Drug Abuse found that 1 in 23 eighth graders had tried MDMA at least once, and 1 in 9 high school seniors had used the drug. These numbers were significantly higher than reports from previous years. Emergency room mentions of MDMA in the United States also increased significantly: from 253 in 1994 to 4,511 in 2000.

Most users of MDMA are Hispanic American or white and are middle or high in socioeconomic rank. Typically, dealers are workers at nightclubs or raves. They push the drug as a way to increase energy, pleasure, and self-confidence. Some clubs have made an effort to protect their public image by hiring private ambulances to quickly treat and remove victims of overdose. Unfortunately, MDMA is now being pushed in new venues, including high schools and popular gathering places for teenagers and young adults.

MDMA is usually swallowed in the form of one or two pills in doses of 50–240 mg, but it can also be smoked, snorted, or occasionally injected. Because the drug is often prepared with other substances, users have no way of knowing the exact potency of the drug or additional substances found in each pill. Further, many users combine MDMA with alcohol, marijuana, or other drugs that makes its use more dangerous.

MDMA shares characteristics with stimulants and hallucinogens. Its chemical structure closely parallels the hallucinogen **MDA** (methylenedioxyamphetamine) and methamphetamine, both manmade stimulants that damage the brain. Its addictive properties and stimulation of hyperactivity have been compared to stimulants like amphetamines and cocaine. MDMA's chemical structure and its appeal, however, are similar to hallucinogens, but with milder psychedelic effects.

MDMA has a reputation among young people for being fun and harmless as long as it is used sensibly. MDMA, however, is not a harmless drug. Current research is uncovering many negative side effects to its use. MDMA's pleasurable effects peak about an hour after a pill is swallowed and last for 2 to 6 hours. MDMA's appeal is that users claim to feel enlightened and introspective, accepting of themselves and trustful of others. Because they tend to act and feel closer to or more intimate with the people around them, some believe this drug to be an aphrodisiac—even though MDMA actually hampers sexual ability. MDMA also acts as a stimulant by increasing brain activity and making users feel more energetic.

MDMA users may experience rapid eye movement, faintness, blurred vision, chills, sweating, nausea, muscle tension, and teeth-grinding. Users often bring infant pacifiers to raves to combat the latter side effect. Individuals with heart, liver, or kidney disease or high blood pressure are especially at risk because MDMA increases blood pressure, heart rate, and body temperature; thus it may lead to kidney failure, a heart attack, a stroke, and seizures. The hot, crowded atmosphere at raves and dance clubs also heightens the user's risk. Deaths are more likely to occur when water is unavailable because the crowded atmosphere, combined with MDMA's stimulant effects, causes dehydration (bottled water is often sold at inflated prices at raves). Other evidence suggests that a pregnant woman using MDMA may find lasting learning and memory difficulties in her child. Like most addictive drugs, MDMA's effects are said to diminish with each use.

Long-term side effects, lasting for weeks after use, include confusion, depression, sleep disorders, anxiety, aggression, paranoia, and impulsive behavior. Questions still remain about other potential long-term effects. Verbal and visual memory may be significantly impaired for years after prolonged use. Researchers are now focusing on these lasting side effects, which may be the result of depleted serotonin, a neurotransmitter that is released with each dose of MDMA (increased brain activity is the short-term effect of serotonin release). Serotonin helps to regulate sleep cycles, pain, emotion, and appetite. MDMA may damage the neurons that release serotonin, thus, long-term effects could be dangerous.

Advocates of MDMA are attempting to get approval to study medical uses of the drug. For example, MDMA could relieve suffering in terminally ill cancer patients. It could also help people in therapy for marital problems by encouraging introspection and conversation. Because MDMA is heralded as an instant antidepressant, it may help people who are in mourning. Opponents, meanwhile, question MDMA's

value as an effective treatment modality because its effects diminish with continued use.

Heroin

For the first time in decades, **heroin** use is on the increase, and its use is again being publicized by pop culture. Heroin started to make a comeback in 1991. It became increasingly stylish in 1995 following the arrests and deaths of prominent rock stars who abused the drug. According to the National Institute on Drug Abuse, some 600,000 Americans are currently addicted to heroin. Although the most common users are suburban middle-class people and lower-income populations, its use is starting to appear in more affluent communities as well.

Common nicknames for heroin include diesel, dope, dynamite, white death, nasty boy, China white, H. Harry, gumball, junk, brown sugar, smack, Tootsie Roll, black tar, and chasing the dragon. Heroin is classified as a narcotic drug. It is synthesized from morphine, a natural substance found in the seed pod of several types of poppy plants. In its purest form, heroin is a white powder, but on the streets it is typically available in yellow or brown powders. The latter colors are attained when pure heroin is combined with other drugs or substances such as sugar, cornstarch, chalk, brick dust, or laundry soap. Heroin is also sold in a hardened or solid form (black tar), which is usually dissolved with other liquids for use in injectable form. Many users combine heroin with cocaine, a risky process called "speedballing."

Today's heroin is more pure, powerful, and affordable than ever before. The average price has dropped by two-thirds over the last 10 years, which partially accounts for the increased popularity of the drug. For $100, drug users can get about 300 mg of heroin, an amount that will provide several doses, or "hits."

Heroin is a very dangerous drug. A significant health threat to users today is that they have no way of determining the strength of the drug purchased on

Dopamine A neurotransmitter that affects emotional, mental, and motor functions.

MDMA A synthetic hallucinogen drug with a chemical structure that closely resembles MDA and methamphetamine. It is also known as "ecstasy."

Ecstasy *See* MDMA.

MDA A hallucinogenic drug that is structurally similar to amphetamines.

Heroin A potent drug that is a derivative of opium.

the street, thus placing them at a constant risk for overdose and death. Based on a 1999 report from the Drug Abuse Warning Network, an estimated 15 percent of all drug-related hospital emergency room cases that year involved heroin use.

Heroin can be injected intravenously or intramuscularly, sniffed, snorted, or smoked. Although injection is the predominant method of heroin use, users are turning away from intravenous injections because of the risk for HIV infection. The availability of relatively low-priced, high-purity heroin further contributes to the number of people who smoke or snort the drug. Some users also have the misconception that heroin is less addictive when snorted or smoked. Whether injected, snorted, or smoked, heroin is an extremely addictive drug and both physical and psychological dependence develop very rapidly. Drug tolerance sets in quickly and, each time the drug is used, a higher dose is required to produce the same effects.

Heroin use induces a state of euphoria that comes within seconds of intravenous injection or within 5 to 15 minutes when other methods of administration are used. The drug is a sedative, so during the initial rush, the person has a sense of relaxation and does not feel any pain. In users who inhale the drug, however, the rush may be accompanied by nausea, vomiting, intense itching, and at times severe asthma attacks. As the rush wears off, users experience drowsiness, confusion, slowed cardiac function, and decreased breathing rate.

A heroin overdose can cause convulsions, coma, and death. During an overdose, heart rate, breathing, blood pressure, and body temperature drop dramatically. These physiological responses can induce vomiting or tightening of muscles and cause breathing to stop. Death is often the result of lack of oxygen or choking to death on vomit.

About 4 to 5 hours after the drug is taken, withdrawal sets in. Heroin withdrawal is painful and usually lasts up to 2 weeks—but could go on for several months.

Short-term use symptoms include red, raw nostrils; bone and muscle pains; muscle spasms and cramps; sweating; hot and cold flashes; runny nose and eyes; drowsiness; sluggishness; slurred speech; loss of appetite; nausea; diarrhea; restlessness and violent yawning. Heroin use can also kill a developing fetus or cause a spontaneous abortion.

Symptoms of long-term heroin use include hallucinations, nightmares, constipation, sexual difficulties, impaired vision, reduced fertility, boils, collapsed veins, and a significantly elevated risk for lung, liver, and cardiovascular diseases, including bacterial infections in blood vessels and heart valves. The additives

used in street heroin can clog vital blood vessels because they do not dissolve in the body, leading to infections and death of cells in vital organs. Sudden infant death syndrome (SIDS) is also more frequently seen in children born to addicted mothers.

Heroin addiction is treated with behavioral therapies and pharmaceutical agents. The use of medication helps suppress withdrawal symptoms, which makes it easier for patients to stop heroin use. The combination of these two treatment modalities helps the individual learn to lead a more stable, productive, and drug-free lifestyle.

Alcohol

Drinking **alcohol** has been a socially acceptable behavior for centuries. Alcohol is an accepted accompaniment at parties, ceremonies, dinners, sport contests, the establishment of kingdoms or governments, and the signing of treaties between nations. Alcohol also has been used for medical reasons as a mild sedative or as a painkiller for surgery.

For a short period of 14 years, from 1920 to 1933, by constitutional amendment, the sale and use of alcohol were declared illegal in the United States. This amendment was repealed because drinkers and non-drinkers alike questioned the right of government to pass judgment on individual moral standards. In addition, organized crime activities to smuggle and sell alcohol illegally expanded enormously during this period.

Alcohol is the cause of one of the most significant health-related drug problems in the United States today. An estimated 6 in 10 adults—more than 100

The sale of alcohol was illegal in the United States between 1920 and 1933.

million people 18 years and older—are drinkers. More than 13.8 million of them will develop a drinking problem, including **alcoholism**, in their lifetime. Another 10.4 million teenagers are thought to have a drinking problem.

The addiction to alcohol develops slowly. Most people think they are in control of their drinking habits and do not realize they have a problem until they become alcoholics, when they find themselves physically and emotionally dependent on the drug. This addiction is characterized by excessive use of and constant preoccupation with drinking. Alcohol abuse, in turn, leads to mental, emotional, physical, and social problems.

Alcohol intake impedes peripheral vision, lowers visual and hearing acuity, decreases reaction time, impairs concentration and motor performance (including increased swaying), and causes impaired judgment of distance and speed of moving objects. Further, it alleviates fear, increases risk-taking, stimulates urination, and induces sleep.

A single large dose of alcohol also may decrease sexual function.

One of the most unpleasant, dangerous, and life-threatening effects of drinking is the **synergistic action** of alcohol when combined with other drugs,

particularly central nervous system depressants. Each person reacts to a combination of alcohol and other drugs in a different way. The effects range from loss of consciousness to death.

Long-term effects of alcohol abuse are serious and often life-threatening (see Figure 13.1). Some of these detrimental effects are lower resistance to disease; **cirrhosis** of the liver; higher risk for oral, esophageal, stomach, and liver cancer; **cardiomyopathy**; irregular heartbeat; elevated blood pressure; greater risk for strokes; inflammation of the esophagus, stomach, small intestine, and pancreas; stomach ulcers; sexual

Key Terms

Alcohol (ethyl alcohol) A depressant drug that affects the brain and slows down central nervous system activity; has strong addictive properties.

Alcoholism Disease in which an individual loses control over drinking alcoholic beverages.

Synergistic action The effect of mixing two or more drugs, which can be much greater than the sum of the same drugs acting by themselves.

Cirrhosis A disease characterized by scarring of the liver.

Cardiomyopathy A disease affecting the heart muscle.

FIGURE 13.1 Long-term risks associated with alcohol abuse.

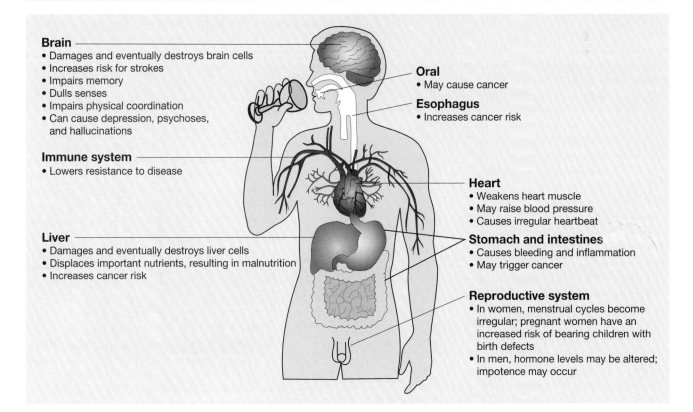

Brain
- Damages and eventually destroys brain cells
- Increases risk for strokes
- Impairs memory
- Dulls senses
- Impairs physical coordination
- Can cause depression, psychoses, and hallucinations

Immune system
- Lowers resistance to disease

Liver
- Damages and eventually destroys liver cells
- Displaces important nutrients, resulting in malnutrition
- Increases cancer risk

Oral
- May cause cancer

Esophagus
- Increases cancer risk

Heart
- Weakens heart muscle
- May raise blood pressure
- Causes irregular heartbeat

Stomach and intestines
- Causes bleeding and inflammation
- May trigger cancer

Reproductive system
- In women, menstrual cycles become irregular; pregnant women have an increased risk of bearing children with birth defects
- In men, hormone levels may be altered; impotence may occur

Approximately 14 million Americans will develop a drinking problem during their lifetime.

© Fitness & Wellness, Inc.

impotence; birth defects; malnutrition; damage to brain cells leading to loss of memory; depression; psychosis; and hallucinations.

ALCOHOL ON CAMPUSES

Alcohol is the number-one drug problem among college students. According to national surveys, about 66 percent of college students reported using alcohol, and 43 percent of college students had engaged in binge drinking (5 or more drinks in a row) at least once in the 2 weeks preceding the survey. Alcohol is a factor in about 28 percent of all college dropouts, costing the federal government more than $3 billion in taxes. Today's student spends more on alcohol than on books.

Another survey involving 56,000 college students showed that grade point average (GPA) is related to average number of drinks per week (see Figure 13.2). Students with a "D" or "F" GPA reported a weekly consumption of almost 11 drinks. Students with "A" GPAs consumed about 3.5 drinks per week. Furthermore, 30 percent of all academic problems result from alcohol misuse. Of greater concern is that 36 percent of the surveyed students admitted driving while intoxicated. Of the 12 million college students in the United States, between 2 and 3 percent will die from alcohol-related causes. This represents more students than those who will receive advanced degrees (master's and doctorate degrees combined).

Another major concern is that more than half of college students participate in games that involve heavy drinking (6 to 10 drinks) in a short time. Often students take part because of peer pressure and fear of rejection. Up to 48 percent report getting drunk at least once a month. Excessive drinking can precipitate unplanned and unprotected sex (risking HIV infection) or date rape.

HOW TO CUT DOWN ON DRINKING

To find out if drinking is a problem in your life, refer to the questionnaire "Alcohol Abuse: Are You Drinking Too Much?," in Figure 13.3, developed by the American Medical Association. If you respond "yes" twice or more on this questionnaire, you may be jeopardizing your health.

If a person is determined to control the problem, it is not that difficult. The first and most important

FIGURE 13.2 Average number of drinks by college students per week by GPA.

When your date drinks ...

- **Don't** make excuses for his/her behavior, no matter how embarrassing.
- **Don't** allow embarrassment to put you in a situation with which you are uncomfortable.
- **Do** be sure that body language and tone of voice match verbal messages you send.
- **Do** leave as quickly as you can, without your date. **Don't** stop to argue. Intoxicated people can't listen to reason.
- **Do** call a cab, a friend, or your parents. Don't ride home with your date.

For Women:

- **Do** make your position clear. "No!" is much more effective than "Please stop!" or "Don't!"
- **Do** make it clear that you will call the police if rape is attempted.

SOURCE: "Sexuality Under the Influence of Alcohol." *Human Sexuality Supplement to Current Health* 2 (October 1990): 3.

step is to want to cut down. If you want to do this but you cannot, you had better accept the probability that alcohol is becoming a serious problem for you, and you should seek guidance from your physician or from an organization such as Alcoholics Anonymous. The next few suggestions may help you cut down alcohol intake:

1. Set reasonable limits for yourself. Decide not to exceed a certain number of drinks on a given occasion and stick to your decision. No more than two beers or two cocktails a day is a reasonable limit. If you set a target such as this and consistently do not exceed it, you have proven to yourself that you can control your drinking.

2. Learn to say no. Many people have "just one more" drink because others in the group are drinking or because someone puts pressure on them, not because they really want a drink. When you reach the sensible limit you have set for yourself, politely but firmly refuse to exceed it. If you are being the generous host, pour yourself a glass of water or juice over ice ("on the rocks"). Nobody will notice the difference.

3. Drink slowly. Don't gulp down a drink. Choose your drinks for their flavor, not their kick, and savor the taste of each sip.

4. Dilute your drinks. If you prefer cocktails to beer, try having "long" drinks: Instead of downing gin or whiskey neat or nearly so, drink it diluted with a mixer such as tonic water or soda water in a tall glass. That way you can enjoy both the flavor and the act of drinking but you will take longer to finish each drink. Also, you can make your two-drink limit last all evening or switch to the mixer by itself.

5. Do not drink on your own. Confine your drinking to social gatherings. You may have a hard time resisting the urge to pour yourself a relaxing drink at the end of a hard day, but many formerly heavy drinkers have found that a soft drink satisfies the need as well as alcohol did. What may help you really unwind, even with no drink at all, is a comfortable chair, loosened clothing, and perhaps a soothing audiotape, television program, or good book to read.

TREATMENT OF ADDICTION

Recovery from alcoholism and other drug addictions is more likely to be successful with professional guidance and support. The first step is to recognize the reality of the problem. The questionnaire "Could You Be an Addict?" in Figure 13.4 will help you recognize possible addictive behavior in yourself or someone you know. If the answers to more than half of these questions are positive, a problem may exist—and you should contact a physician, your institution's counseling center, or the local mental health clinic for a referral (see the Yellow Pages in your phone book).

A person may also contact the National Center for Substance Abuse Treatment at 1-800-662-HELP (1-800-662-4357) for 24-hour substance abuse treatment centers in their local area. The national center

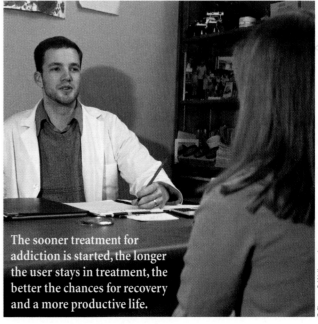

The sooner treatment for addiction is started, the longer the user stays in treatment, the better the chances for recovery and a more productive life.

also provides printed information on drug abuse and addictive behavior. All information discussed during a phone call to this center is kept strictly confidential.

About 5 million Americans have received treatment for addictive behavior.[3] An additional 7 million people are estimated to need treatment for substance abuse.[4] Treatment programs for addiction include a variety of intervention modalities, including psychotherapy, medical care, and behavior modification. If addiction is a problem in your life, you need to act upon it without delay. Addicts do not have to resign themselves to a lifetime of addiction. The sooner you start, and the longer you stay in treatment, the better your chances for recovery and a healthier and more productive life.

TOBACCO USE

People throughout the world have used tobacco for hundreds of years. Before the 18th century, they smoked tobacco primarily in pipes or cigars. Cigarette smoking per se did not become popular until the mid-1800s, and its use started to increase dramatically in the 20th century.

In 1900, people in the United States consumed 2.5 billion cigarettes, compared to 640 billion in 1981. This figure dropped to 487 billion in 1995. Nonetheless, more than 47 million Americans over age 18 still smoked in 1995.

The harmful effects of cigarette smoking and tobacco use in general were not exactly known until the early 1960s, when research began to show a link between tobacco use and disease. In 1964, the U.S. Surgeon General issued the first major report presenting scientific evidence that cigarettes were indeed a major health hazard in our society.

Tobacco use in all its forms is considered a significant threat to life. World Health Organization estimates indicate that 10 percent of the 5 billion people presently living will die as a result of smoking-related illnesses, which kill approximately 4 million people each year. At the present rate of escalation, this figure is expected to climb to 10 million annual deaths by the year 2025. Tobacco will kill 150 million people in the first quarter of this century and another 300 million in the second quarter.

Morbidity and Mortality

Overdoses of illegal drugs kill about 17,500 people per year in the United States. Drug felonies and drug-related murders kill another 1,600 people each year. This brings drug-related deaths to a grand total of 19,100. Citizens and the government have mounted a tremendous campaign to eradicate illegal drug use in America. Cigarettes, however, a legal drug, kill about 26 times as many people as all illegal drugs combined.

Cigarette smoking is the largest preventable cause of illness and premature death in the United States. When we consider all related deaths, smoking is responsible for about 430,000 unnecessary deaths each year—enough deaths to wipe out the entire population of Miami and Miami Beach in a single year.

Death rates from heart disease, cancer, stroke, aortic aneurysm, chronic bronchitis, emphysema, and peptic ulcers have increased. Figure 13.5 illustrates normal and diseased **alveoli**. Cigarette smoking by pregnant women has been linked to retarded fetal growth, higher risk for spontaneous abortion (miscarriage), and prenatal death. Smoking also is the most prevalent cause of injury and death from fire. The average life expectancy for a chronic smoker is as much as 18 years shorter than for a nonsmoker, and the death rate among chronic smokers during the most productive years of life, between ages 25 and 65, is twice the national average.

Based on a 1993 report by U.S. government physicians, each cigarette shortens life by 7 minutes. This figure represents 5 million years of potential life that Americans lose to smoking each year. According to estimates by the American Heart Association, more than 30 percent of fatal heart attacks—or 120,000 in the United States annually—result from smoking.

> **Cigarettes, a legal drug, kill about 26 times as many people as all illegal drugs combined.**

The risk of heart attack is 50 to 100 percent higher for smokers than for nonsmokers. The mortality rate following heart attacks also is higher for smokers, because their attacks usually are more severe and their risk for deadly arrhythmias is much greater.

Cigarette smoking affects the cardiovascular system by increasing heart rate, blood pressure, and susceptibility to atherosclerosis, blood clots, coronary artery spasm, cardiac arrhythmia, and arteriosclerotic peripheral vascular disease. Evidence also indicates that smoking decreases high-density lipoprotein (HDL) cholesterol, the "good" cholesterol that lowers the risk for heart disease. Smoking further increases the amount of fatty acids,

KeyTerms

Alveoli Air sacs in the lungs where exchange of gases (oxygen and carbon dioxide) takes place.

FIGURE **13.3** American Medical Association questionnaire on drinking.

Alcohol abuse: Are you drinking too much?

1. When you are holding an empty glass at a party, do you always actively look for a refill instead of waiting to be offered one?

2. If given the chance, do you frequently pour out a more generous drink for yourself than seems to be the "going" amount for others?

3. Do you often have a drink or two when you are alone, either at home or in a bar?

4. Is your drinking ever the direct cause of a family quarrel, or do quarrels often seem to occur, if only by coincidence, when you have had a drink or two?

5. Do you feel that you must have a drink at a specific time every day—right after work, for instance?

6. When worried or under unusual stress, do you almost automatically take a stiff drink to "settle your nerves?"

7. Are you untruthful about how much you have had to drink when questioned on the subject?

8. Does drinking ever cause you to take time off work or to miss scheduled meetings or appointments?

9. Do you feel physically deprived if you cannot have at least one drink every day?

10. Do you sometimes crave a drink in the morning?

11. Do you sometimes have "mornings after" when you cannot remember what happened the night before?

Evaluation

You should regard a "yes" answer to any one of the above questions as a warning sign. Do not increase your consumption of alcohol. Two "yes" answers suggest that you already may be becoming dependent on alcohol. Three or more "yes" answers indicate that you may have a serious problem, and you should get professional help.

FIGURE 13.4 Questionnaire on addiction.

Could you be an addict?

I. Recognizing Addictive Behavior*

Instructions The following test, designed by Dr. Lawrence J. Hatterer, is not a way to diagnose whether you are in the early, middle, or chronic stage of addictive disease. It is meant merely to help you understand addictive behavior better so you can recognize it in yourself or perhaps in people you know.

1. I am a person of excesses. I can't regulate what I do for pleasure and often use a substance or indulge in an activity heavily to get high.
2. I am an extremely self-involved person. People tell me I am into myself too much.
3. I am compulsive. I must have what I want when I want it, regardless of the consequences.
4. I am excessively dependent on or independent of others.
5. I am preoccupied. I spend a lot of time thinking or fantasizing about a particular activity or substance. Also, I will work my day around doing it or go to pains to make sure it's available.
6. I deny that I do this and lie about it to others who ask me.
7. I have been involved in this behavior for at least a year.
8. I've told myself I could easily stop, even though I've shown no signs of slowing down.
9. Once I start indulging in this behavior or substance, I find I have trouble stopping.
10. One or more members of my family are also involved in some kind of excessive behavior or substance abuse.
11. I find I gravitate mostly toward people who have the same behavior or take the same substance as I do.
12. I seem to be developing a tolerance of the behavior or substance. I have had a need to steadily increase the amounts I take or the time I spend doing it.
13. I have found that my excessive use of highs has, in fact, only made my problems worse.
14. If someone tries to keep me from obtaining the substance or practicing the activity, I get angry and reject or abuse that person.
15. I experience withdrawal symptoms if I cannot indulge in the substance or activity.
16. This has gotten in the way of my functioning. I have missed something important—days at work or time with my friends, family, children—because of it.
17. The substance/activity is destroying my home life. I know I am hurting those closest to me.
18. I have failed in many goals in life, lost money, given up many social and occupational contacts, all because of my excessive behavior.
19. I have tried to stop or cut down on my excesses but have been unsuccessful.
20. I have physically endangered myself or others in accidents that were a direct result of my excessive behavior.

Evaluation If you answer "yes" to half or more of the questions, you may have a problem with addictive disease and should seek immediate professional help. For a referral, contact your local mental health clinic (look in the Yellow Pages) or speak to your doctor.

II. Stage of Change for Addictive Behavior

If chemical dependency is a problem in your life, use Figure 2.4 (page 45) and Table 2.3 (page 43) to identify your current stage of change for participation in a treatment program for addictive behavior.

III. Changing Addictive Behavior

On a separate sheet of paper indicate the steps that you are going to take to correct addictive behavior(s) and identify people or organizations that you will contact to help you get started.

*Used by permission from *McCall's* magazine. Copyright © 1986 by the McCall Publishing Company.

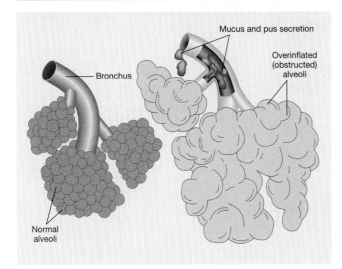

FIGURE 13.5 Normal and diseased alveoli in lungs.

Mucus and pus secretion

Overinflated (obstructed) alveoli

Bronchus

Normal alveoli

glucose, and various hormones in the blood. The carbon monoxide in smoke hinders the capacity of the blood to carry oxygen to body tissues. Both carbon monoxide and **nicotine** can damage the inner walls of the arteries and thus encourage the buildup of fat on these walls. Smoking also increases adhesiveness and clustering of platelets in the blood, decreases platelet survival and clotting time, and increases blood thickness. All of these effects can precipitate a heart attack.

The American Cancer Society reports that 87 percent of lung cancer is attributable to smoking. Lung cancer is the leading cancer killer, accounting for approximately 157,000 deaths in the United States in the year 2000, or about 28 percent of all deaths from cancer.[5] Cigarette smoking also leads to chronic obstructive pulmonary disease, the fourth leading cause of death in the United States (also see Chapter 1).

The most common carcinogenic exposure in the workplace is to cigarette smoke. Both fatal and nonfatal cardiac events are increased greatly in people who are exposed to passive smoke. Secondhand smoke is ranked behind active smoking and alcohol as the third leading preventable cause of death in the United States.[6] About 3,000 people die each year from lung cancer because of secondhand smoke. Passive smoke is also a significant risk factor for heart disease in children and adults alike. It causes an estimated 35,000 to 40,000 yearly deaths from heart disease in nonsmokers.[7]

Although half of all cancers are now curable, the 5-year survival rate for lung cancer is less than 13 percent. Cigarette smoking is also responsible for most cancers of the oral cavity, larynx, and esophagus (see Figure 13.6). Tobacco use also is related to the development of and deaths from bladder, pancreas, and kidney, and cervical cancers.

Even though many tobacco users are aware of the health consequences of cigarette smoking, they may fail to realize the risk of pipe smoking, cigar smoking, and tobacco chewing. As a group, pipe and cigar smokers have lower risks for heart disease and lung cancer. Nevertheless, blood nicotine levels in pipe and cigar smokers have been shown to approach those of cigarette smokers, because nicotine is still absorbed through the membranes of the mouth. Therefore, these tobacco users still have a higher risk for heart disease than nonsmokers do.

> Approximately 430,000 people die each year in the United States from smoking-related conditions.

Cigarette smokers who substitute pipe or cigar smoking for cigarettes usually continue to inhale the smoke, which actually results in more nicotine and **tar** being brought into the lungs. Consequently, the risk for disease is even higher if pipe or cigar smoke is inhaled. The risk and mortality rates for lip, mouth, and larynx cancer for pipe smoking, cigar smoking, and tobacco chewing are actually higher than for cigarette smoking.

Economic Impact

The economic impact of cigarette smoking on the health care system is staggering. In 1992, the Surgeon General calculated the lifetime excess medical care costs for smokers and former smokers at $501 billion above that of nonsmokers. Other estimates indicate that in the United States people pay more than $130 billion annually for tobacco-related health care costs and lost productivity.[8] Each pack of cigarettes sold represents about $5.10 in smoking-related expenses.

Heavy smokers use the health care system, especially hospitals, twice as much as nonsmokers do. The yearly cost to a given company has been estimated to be between $624 and $4,611 per smoking employee. These costs include employee health care; absenteeism; additional health insurance; morbidity, disability,

KeyTerms

Nicotine Addictive compound found in tobacco leaves.

Tar Chemical compound that forms during the burning of tobacco leaves.

FIGURE 13.6 The health effects of smoking.

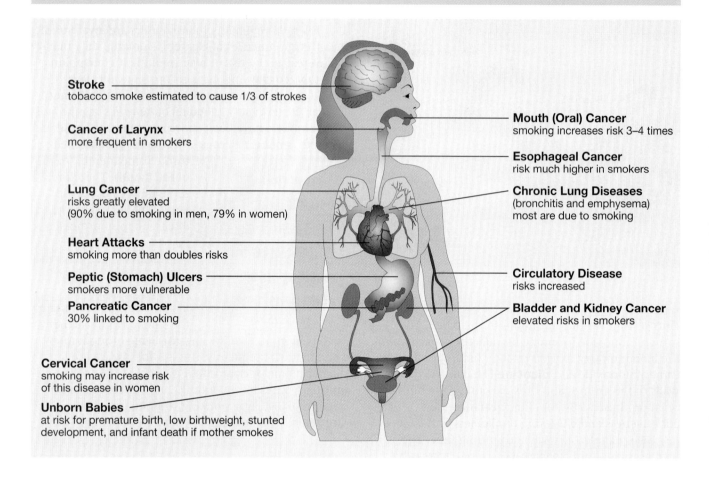

Stroke
tobacco smoke estimated to cause 1/3 of strokes

Cancer of Larynx
more frequent in smokers

Lung Cancer
risks greatly elevated
(90% due to smoking in men, 79% in women)

Heart Attacks
smoking more than doubles risks

Peptic (Stomach) Ulcers
smokers more vulnerable

Pancreatic Cancer
30% linked to smoking

Cervical Cancer
smoking may increase risk
of this disease in women

Unborn Babies
at risk for premature birth, low birthweight, stunted
development, and infant death if mother smokes

Mouth (Oral) Cancer
smoking increases risk 3–4 times

Esophageal Cancer
risk much higher in smokers

Chronic Lung Diseases
(bronchitis and emphysema)
most are due to smoking

Circulatory Disease
risks increased

Bladder and Kidney Cancer
elevated risks in smokers

Cigarette smoking is the single largest preventable cause of illness and premature death in the United States.

© Fitness & Wellness, Inc.

and early mortality; on-the-job time lost; property damage, maintenance, and depreciation; worker compensation; and the impact of secondhand smoke.

Every day more than 1,200 Americans die from smoking-related illnesses.[9] Smoking kills more

Americans in a single year than those who died in battle during World War II and the Vietnam War combined. Think of the public outrage if 430,000 Americans were to die annually from, say, an over-the-counter drug? What if a single nonprescription drug caused more than 138,000 deaths from cancer and 120,000 fatal heart attacks each year? The U.S. public would not tolerate these situations. We probably would mount an intense fight to prevent the deaths.

Yet, are we not committing slow suicide by smoking cigarettes? Isn't tobacco a nonprescription drug available to almost anyone who wishes to smoke, killing more than 400,000 people each year? If cigarettes were invented today, the tobacco industry would be put on trial for mass murder.

Trends

The fight against all forms of tobacco use has been gaining momentum in the last few years. This was not always the case. It has been difficult to fight an industry that has such immense financial and political influence as the tobacco industry has in the United States. Tobacco is the sixth largest cash crop in the United States, producing 2.5 percent of the gross national product. It has influenced elections cleverly by emphasizing the individual's right to smoke, avoiding the fact that so many people die because of its use.

In 1990, Philip Morris, one of the largest tobacco-producing companies in the world, ranked seventh among Fortune 500 companies. Nearly 70 percent of its profits came from the sale of cigarettes. In 1992, Philip Morris donated about $17 million to several prominent organizations, so they no longer question the detrimental effects of tobacco use. Among the organizations receiving donations from Philip Morris in 1992 were United Way, YMCA, Salvation Army, Pediatric AIDS Foundation, Red Cross, Cystic Fibrosis Foundation, March of Dimes, Easter Seals, Muscular Dystrophy Association, Multiple Sclerosis Society, Hemophilia Foundation, United Cerebral Palsy, American Civil Liberties Union, American Bar Association, Task Force for Battered Women, Boy Scouts, Boys and Girls Club, and Big Brothers and Big Sisters. We call Colombian drug-runners unprincipled scum (responsible for about 19,100 illegal drug-related deaths per year), yet we welcome Philip Morris with glee and call it civic pride.[10]

Tobacco was socially accepted for many years. In the 1980s, however, cigarette smoking no longer was acceptable in many social circles. Nonsmokers and ex-smokers alike are fighting for their rights to clean air and health. If every smoker were to give up cigarettes, in one year alone sick time would drop by approximately 90 million days, heart conditions would decrease by 280,000, chronic bronchitis and emphysema would number 1 million fewer cases, and total death rates from cardiovascular disease, cancer, and peptic ulcers would fall off drastically.

Many smokers are unaware of, or simply do not care to realize, how much cigarette smoke bothers nonsmokers. Smokers sometimes think that blowing the smoke off to the side is enough to get it out of the way. As a matter of fact, it is not enough. Smokers do not comprehend this until they quit and later find themselves in that situation. Suddenly, they realize why cigarette smoke is so unpleasant and undesirable to most people.

In recent years, the Food and Drug Administration (FDA) Drug Abuse Advisory Committee has taken a strong stance against the use of all forms of tobacco products. Although the American

> **Each cigarette smoked shortens a person's life by 7 minutes.**

Heart Association (AHA) commends the work initiated by the FDA, the AHA has further stated that the FDA and the federal government have an obligation to take regulatory action against the national problem of nicotine addiction and abuse of cigarettes and tobacco products in general. In a statement before the FDA Drug Abuse Advisory Committee, the AHA commented that it is a national health travesty that a product [tobacco] that accounts for over 430,000 deaths in the United States each year has escaped regulation under every major health and safety law enacted by Congress to protect the public health.[11]

Smokeless Tobacco

Smokeless tobacco often is promoted as a safe alternative to cigarette smoking. According to the Advisory Committee to the U.S. Surgeon General, smokeless tobacco represents a significant health risk and is just as addictive as cigarette smoking.

Unlike smoking, the use of smokeless tobacco has increased during the last 15 years. Currently, some 15 million Americans use tobacco in this form. The greatest concern is the increase in use of "spit" tobacco, especially by young people. More than 2 million people under age 25 use spit tobacco, including nearly 20 percent of all males in grades 9 through 12. One-third of those who use spit tobacco started at age 5, and the average starting age was 9. Spit tobacco contains 2.5 times as much nicotine as a similarly priced pack of cigarettes.

Using smokeless tobacco can lead to gingivitis and periodontitis. It carries a fourfold increase in oral cancer, and in some cases even premature death. People who chew or dip also have a higher rate of cavities, sore gums, bad breath, and stained teeth. Their senses of smell and taste diminish; consequently, they tend to add more sugar and salt to food. These

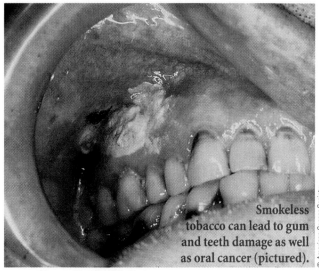

Smokeless tobacco can lead to gum and teeth damage as well as oral cancer (pictured).

© American Cancer Society

practices alone increase the risk for being overweight and having high blood pressure.

Nicotine addiction and its related health risks also hold true for smokeless tobacco users. Nicotine blood levels approach those of cigarette smokers, increasing the risk for diseases of the cardiovascular system. Further, research has revealed changes in heart rate and blood pressure similar to those of cigarette smokers.

Using tobacco in any form can be addictive and poses a serious threat to health and well-being. Completely eliminating its use is the single most important lifestyle change a tobacco user can make to improve health, quality of life, and longevity.

Why People Smoke

People typically begin to smoke without realizing its detrimental effects on their health and life in general. Although people start to smoke for many different reasons, the three fundamental instigators are peer pressure, the desire to appear "grown up," and rebellion against authority. Smoking only three packs of cigarettes can lead to physiological addiction, turning smoking into a nasty habit that has become the most widespread example of drug dependency in the United States.

> **More than 1,200 toxic chemicals have been found in tobacco smoke.**

When tobacco leaves are burned, hot air and gases containing tar (chemical compounds) and nicotine are released in the smoke. More than 1,200 toxic chemicals have been found in tobacco smoke. Tar contains about 60 chemical compounds that are proven carcinogens.

SMOKING ADDICTION

The drug nicotine has strong addictive properties. Within seconds of inhalation, nicotine affects the central nervous system and can act simultaneously as a tranquilizer and a stimulant. The stimulating effect produces strong physiological and psychological dependency. The physical addiction to nicotine is six to eight times more powerful than the addiction to alcohol, and most likely greater than for some of the hard drugs currently used.

SMOKING DEPENDENCY

The psychological dependency develops over a longer time. People smoke to help themselves relax, and they also gain a certain amount of pleasure from the ritual of smoking. Smokers automatically associate many activities of daily life with cigarettes. Typical associated activities are coffee drinking, alcohol drinking, being part of a social gathering, relaxing after a meal, talking on the telephone, driving, reading, watching television. In many cases the social rituals of smoking are the most difficult to eliminate. The dependency is so strong that, years after people have stopped smoking, they may still crave cigarettes when they engage in particular social activities.

Most of the remaining information in this chapter is written directly to smokers. Nonsmokers, however, will gain a better understanding of smokers by reading it. The following material also provides valuable information so you can help others implement a smoking cessation program.

"Why Do You Smoke?" Test

Most people smoke for a variety of reasons. To find out why people smoke, the National Clearinghouse for Smoking and Health developed a simple "Why-Do-You-Smoke?" Test. This test, contained in Figure 13.7, lists some statements by people describing what they get out of smoking cigarettes. Smokers are asked to indicate how often they have the feelings described in each statement when they are smoking.

The scores obtained on this test rate each of six factors that describe people's feelings when they smoke. The first three highlight the positive feelings people derive from smoking. The fourth factor relates to reducing tension and relaxing. The fifth reveals the extent of dependence on cigarettes. The sixth factor differentiates habit smoking and purely automatic smoking. Each of the remaining factors fits one of the six reasons for smoking, discussed next. A score of 11 or above on any factor indicates that smoking is an important source of satisfaction for you. The higher you score (15 is the highest), the more important a given factor is in your smoking and the more useful the discussion of that factor can be in your attempt to quit.

If you do not score high on any of the six factors, chances are that you do not smoke much or have not been smoking for very many years. If so, giving up smoking, and staying off, should be fairly easy.

1. Stimulation. If you score high or fairly high on the stimulation factor, you are one of those smokers who is stimulated by the cigarette. You think it helps wake you up, organize your energies, and keep you going. If you try to give up smoking, you may want a safe substitute—a brisk walk or moderate exercise, for example—whenever you feel the urge to smoke.

2. Handling. Handling things can be satisfying, but you can keep your hands busy in many ways without lighting up or playing with a cigarette.

Why not toy with a pen or pencil? Try doodling. Play with a coin, a piece of jewelry, or some other harmless object.

3. **Accentuation of pleasure/pleasurable relaxation.** Distinguishing between whether you use the cigarette to feel good—get real, honest pleasure from smoking (Factor 3)—or to keep from feeling bad (Factor 4) is not always easy. About two-thirds of smokers score high or fairly high on accentuation of pleasure, and about half of those score as high or higher on reduction of negative feelings. Those who do get real pleasure from smoking often find that honest consideration of the harmful effects of their habit is enough to help them quit. They substitute social and physical activities and find they do not seriously miss cigarettes.

4. **Reduction of negative feelings, or "crutch."** Many smokers use cigarettes as a kind of crutch during moments of stress or discomfort. Ironically, the heavy smoker—the person who tries to handle severe personal problems by smoking many times a day—is apt to discover that cigarettes do not help deal with problems effectively. This kind of smoker may stop smoking readily when everything is going well but may be tempted to start again in a time of crisis. Again, physical exertion or social activity may be a useful substitute for cigarettes, especially in times of tension.

5. **Craving or dependence.** Quitting smoking is difficult for people who score high on this factor. The craving for a cigarette begins to build the moment the previous cigarette is put out, so tapering off is not likely to work. This smoker must go **cold turkey**. If you are dependent on cigarettes, you may try smoking more than usual for a day or two to spoil your taste for cigarettes, then isolating yourself completely from cigarettes until the craving is gone.

6. **Habit.** If you are smoking from habit, you no longer get much satisfaction from the cigarettes. You light them frequently without even realizing you are doing it. You may have an easy time quitting and staying off if you can break the habitual patterns you have built up. Cutting down gradually may be effective if you change the way you smoke cigarettes and the conditions under which you smoke them. The key to success is to become aware of each cigarette you smoke. You can do this by asking yourself, "Do I really want this cigarette?" You may be surprised at how many you do not want.

SMOKING CESSATION

If you are contemplating or preparing to stop cigarette smoking, you need to know that quitting smoking is not easy. Annually, only about 20 percent of smokers who try to quit the first time succeed. The addictive properties of nicotine and smoke make quitting difficult.

The American Psychiatric Association and the National Institute on Drug Abuse have indicated that nicotine is perhaps the most addictive drug known to humans. The 1988 Surgeon General's Report on Nicotine Addiction concluded that

- Cigarettes and other forms of tobacco are addicting.
- Nicotine is the drug responsible for the addictive behavior.
- Pharmacological and behavioral traits that determine addiction to tobacco are similar to those that determine addiction to drugs such as heroin and cocaine.[12]

Smokers develop a tolerance to nicotine and other ingredients of tobacco smoke. They become dependent on both and get physical and psychological withdrawal symptoms when they stop smoking. Even though giving up smoking can be extremely difficult, it is by no means impossible, as attested by the many people who have quit.

During the last three decades, cigarette smoking in the United States has been declining gradually among smokers of all ages with the exception of young women. Surveys have shown that between 75 and 90 percent of all smokers would like to quit. Forty percent of the adult population—53 percent of men and 32 percent of women—smoked in 1964 when the U. S. Surgeon General first reported the link between smoking and increased risk for disease and mortality. By 1995, only 25 percent, or 47 million adults, smoked. Among men, 25 million (28.2 percent) were smokers, and 22 million (23.1 percent) women smoked. More than 38 million Americans have given up cigarettes. More than 40 percent of all adults who have ever smoked have quit since 1964.

> Nicotine is perhaps the most addictive drug known to humans.

More than 95 percent of successful ex-smokers have been able to do it on their own, either by

Key Terms

Cold turkey Eliminating a negative behavior all at once.

quitting cold turkey or by using self-help kits available from organizations such as the American Cancer Society, the American Heart Association, and the American Lung Association. Only 3 percent of ex-smokers have done so as a result of formal cessation programs. Smokers' information and treatment centers are listed in the Yellow Pages of the telephone book.

"Do You Want To Quit?" Test

The most important factor in quitting cigarette smoking is the person's sincere desire to do so. Although some smokers can simply quit, this is not usually the case. Those who can quit easily are primarily light or casual smokers. They realize that the pleasure of an occasional cigarette is not worth the added risk of disease and premature death. For heavy smokers, quitting most likely will be a difficult battle. Even though many do not succeed the first time around, the odds of quitting are much better for those who try to stop repeatedly.

If you are a smoker and want to evaluate your readiness to quit, the "Do You Want To Quit?" test, contained in Figure 13.8 and developed by the National Clearinghouse for Smoking and Health, will measure your attitude toward the four primary reasons you want to quit smoking. The results give an indication of whether you are ready to start the program. On this test, the higher you score in any category, say the Health category, the more important that reason is to you. A score of 9 or above in one of these categories indicates that this is one of the most important reasons you may want to quit.

1. Health. Knowing the harmful consequences of cigarettes, many people have stopped smoking and many others are considering doing so. If your score on the Health factor is 9 or above, the health hazards of smoking may be enough to make you want to quit now. If your score on this factor is low (6 or below), consider the hazards of smoking. You may be lacking important information or may even have incorrect information. If so, health considerations are not playing the role they should be in your decision to keep smoking or to quit.

2. Example. Some people stop smoking because they want to set a good example for others. Parents quit to make it easier for their children to resist starting to smoke. Doctors quit to be role models for their patients. Teachers quit to discourage their students from smoking. Sports stars want to set an example for their young fans. Husbands quit to influence their wives to quit, and vice versa. Examples have

a significant influence on our behavior. Surveys show that almost twice as many high school students smoke if both parents are smokers, compared with those whose parents are nonsmokers or former smokers.

If your score is low (6 or lower), you might not be interested in giving up smoking to set an example for others. Perhaps you do not realize how important your example could be.

3. Aesthetics. People who score high (9 or above) in this category recognize and are disturbed by some of the unpleasant aspects of smoking. The smell of stale smoke on their clothing, bad breath, and stains on their fingers and teeth might be reason enough to consider quitting.

4. Mastery. If you score 9 or above on this factor, you are bothered by knowing that you cannot control your desire to smoke. You are not your own master. Awareness of this challenge to your self-control may make you want to quit.

Breaking the Habit

The following seven-step plan has been developed as a guide to help you quit smoking. The total program should be completed in 4 weeks or less. Steps One through Four combined should take no longer than 2 weeks. A maximum of 2 additional weeks is allowed for the rest of the program.

STEP ONE

Decide positively that you want to quit. Avoid negative thoughts of how difficult this can be. Think positive. You can do it.

Now prepare a list of the reasons you smoke and why you want to quit (see Figure 13.9). Make several copies of the list and keep them in places where you commonly smoke. Frequently review the reasons for quitting, because this will motivate and prepare you psychologically to quit.

Giving up one pack of cigarettes a day is the equivalent of losing between 50 and 75 pounds of excess body fat!

When the reasons for quitting outweigh the reasons for smoking, you will have an easier time quitting. Try to read as much information as possible on the detrimental effects of tobacco and the benefits of quitting.

STEP TWO

Initiate a personal diet and exercise program. About one-third of the people who quit smoking gain weight.

FIGURE 13.7 "Why do you smoke?" test.

Name: _____ Date: _____

Course: _____ Section: _____ Gender: _____ Age: _____

	Always	Fre-quently	Occa-sionally	Seldom	Never
A. I smoke cigarettes to keep myself from slowing down.	5	4	3	2	1
B. Handling a cigarette is part of the enjoyment of smoking it.	5	4	3	2	1
C. Smoking cigarettes is pleasant and relaxing.	5	4	3	2	1
D. I light up a cigarette when I feel angry about something.	5	4	3	2	1
E. When I have run out of cigarettes, I find it almost unbearable until I can get them.	5	4	3	2	1
F. I smoke cigarettes automatically without even being aware of it.	5	4	3	2	1
G. I smoke cigarettes for the stimulation, to perk myself up.	5	4	3	2	1
H. Part of the enjoyment of smoking a cigarette comes from the steps I take to light up.	5	4	3	2	1
I. I find cigarettes pleasurable.	5	4	3	2	1
J. When I feel uncomfortable or upset about something, I light up a cigarette.	5	4	3	2	1
K. I am very much aware of the fact when I am not smoking a cigarette.	5	4	3	2	1
L. I light up a cigarette without realizing I still have one burning in the ashtray.	5	4	3	2	1
M. I smoke cigarettes to give me a "lift."	5	4	3	2	1
N. When I smoke a cigarette, part of the enjoyment is watching the smoke as I exhale it.	5	4	3	2	1
O. I want a cigarette most when I am comfortable and relaxed.	5	4	3	2	1
P. When I feel "blue" or want to take my mind off cares and worries, I smoke cigarettes.	5	4	3	2	1
Q. I get a real gnawing hunger for a cigarette when I haven't smoked for a while.	5	4	3	2	1
R. I've found a cigarette in my mouth and didn't remember putting it there.	5	4	3	2	1

Scoring Your Test:

Enter the numbers you have circled on the test questions in the spaces provided below, putting the number you circled for question A on line A, for question B on line B, etc. Add the three scores on each line to get a total for each factor. For example, the sum of your scores for lines A, G, and M gives you your score on "Stimulation," lines B, H, and N give the score on "Handling," etc. Scores can vary from 3 to 15. Any score 11 and above is high; any score 7 and below is low.

A _____ + G _____ + M _____ = _____ Stimulation
B _____ + H _____ + N _____ = _____ Handling
C _____ + I _____ + O _____ = _____ Pleasure/Relaxation
D _____ + J _____ + P _____ = _____ Crutch: Tension Reduction
E _____ + K _____ + Q _____ = _____ Craving: Psychological Addiction
F _____ + L _____ + R _____ = _____ Habit

From *A Self-Test for Smokers* (Washington, DC: U.S. Department of Health and Human Services, 1983).

FIGURE 13.8 "Do you want to quit?" test.

Name:_____ Date: _____

Course: _____ Section: _____ Gender:_____ Age: _____

	Strongly Agree	Mildly Agree	Mildly Disagree	Strongly Disagree
A. Cigarette smoking might give me a serious illness.	4	3	2	1
B. My cigarette smoking sets a bad example for others.	4	3	2	1
C. I find cigarette smoking to be a messy kind of habit.	4	3	2	1
D. Controlling my cigarette smoking is a challenge to me.	4	3	2	1
E. Smoking causes shortness of breath.	4	3	2	1
F. If I quit smoking cigarettes, it might influence others to stop.	4	3	2	1
G. Cigarettes damage clothing and other personal property.	4	3	2	1
H. Quitting smoking would show that I have willpower.	4	3	2	1
I. My cigarette smoking will have a harmful effect on my health.	4	3	2	1
J. My cigarette smoking influences others close to me to take up or continue smoking.	4	3	2	1
K. If I quit smoking, my sense of taste or smell would improve.	4	3	2	1
L. I do not like the idea of feeling dependent on smoking.	4	3	2	1

Scoring Your Test:

Write the number you have circled after each statement on the test in the corresponding space to the right. Add the scores on each line to get your totals. For example, the sum of your scores A, E, I gives you your score for the Health factor. Scores can vary from 3 to 12. Any score of 9 or over is high, and a score of 6 or under is low.

A _____ + E _____ + I _____ = _____ Health
B _____ + F _____ + J _____ = _____ Example
C _____ + G _____ + K _____ = _____ Aesthetics
D _____ + H _____ + L _____ = _____ Mastery

From National Clearinghouse for Smoking and Health, *A Self-Test for Smokers* (Washington, DC: U.S. Department of Health and Human Services, 1983).

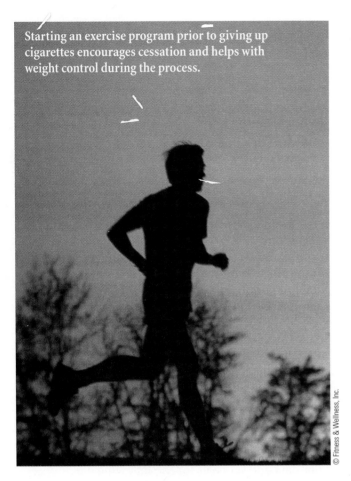

Starting an exercise program prior to giving up cigarettes encourages cessation and helps with weight control during the process.

© Fitness & Wellness, Inc.

This could be caused by one or a combination of the following reasons:

1. Food becomes a substitute for cigarettes.
2. Appetite increases.
3. Basal metabolism may slow down.

If you start an exercise and weight-control program prior to quitting smoking, weight gain should not be a problem. If anything, exercise and lower body weight create more awareness of healthy living and strengthen the motivation for giving up cigarettes.

Even if you gain some weight, the harmful effects of cigarette smoking are much more detrimental to human health than a few extra pounds of body weight. Experts have indicated that, as far as the extra load on the heart is concerned, giving up one pack of cigarettes a day is the equivalent of losing between 50 and 75 pounds of excess body fat!

STEP THREE

Decide on the approach you will use to stop smoking. You may quit cold turkey or gradually cut down the number of cigarettes you smoke daily. Base your decision on your scores obtained on the "Why Do You Smoke?" test. If you scored 11 points or higher in either the "Crutch: Tension Reduction" or the

"Craving: Psychological Addiction" categories, your best chance for success is quitting cold turkey. If you scored high in any of the other four categories, you may choose either approach.

People still argue about which approach is more effective. Quitting cold turkey may cause fewer withdrawal symptoms than tapering off gradually. When you are cutting down slowly, the fewer cigarettes you smoke, the more important each one becomes. Therefore, you have a greater chance for relapse and returning to the original number of cigarettes smoked. However, when the cutting-down approach is accompanied by a definite target date for quitting, the technique has been shown to be quite effective. Smokers who taper off without a target date for quitting are the most likely to relapse.

STEP FOUR

Keep a daily log of your smoking habit for a few days. This will help you understand the situations in which you smoke. To assist you in doing this, make copies of Figure 13.10, or develop your own form. Keep this form with you and, every time you smoke, record the required information. Keep track of the number of cigarettes you smoke, times of day you smoke them, events associated with smoking, amount of each cigarette smoked, and a rating of how badly you needed that cigarette. Rate each cigarette from 1 to 3. A 1 means "desperately needed," a 2 means "moderately needed," and a 3 means "no real need." This daily log will assist you in three ways:

1. You will get to know your habit.
2. It will help you eliminate cigarettes you really do not crave.
3. It will help you find positive substitutes for situations that trigger your desire to smoke.

STEP FIVE

Set the target date for quitting. If you are going to taper off gradually, read the instructions under the "Cutting Down Gradually" (on page 378) before you proceed to Step Six. In setting the target date, a special date may add a little extra incentive. An upcoming birthday, anniversary, vacation, graduation, family reunion—all are examples of good dates to free yourself from smoking. Dates when you are going to be away from events and environments that trigger your desire to smoke may be especially helpful. Once you have set the date, do not change it. Do not let anyone or anything interfere with this date.

Let your friends and relatives know of your intentions and ask for their support. Consider asking someone else to quit with you. That way, you can support each other in your efforts to stop. Avoid anyone who will not support you in your effort to quit. When you are attempting to quit, other people can be a prime obstacle. Many smokers are intolerable when they first stop smoking, so some friends and relatives prefer that the person continue to smoke.

STEP SIX

Stock up on low-calorie foods—carrots, broccoli, cauliflower, celery, popcorn (butter- and salt-free), fruits, sunflower seeds (in the shell), sugarless gum— and drink plenty of water. Keep the food handy on the day you stop and the first few days following cessation. Substitute this food for a cigarette when you want one.

STEP SEVEN

On your quit day and the first few days thereafter, do not keep cigarettes handy. Stay away from friends and events that trigger your desire to smoke and drink a lot of water and fruit juices. To replace the old behavior with new behavior, replace smoking time with new, positive substitutes that will make smoking difficult or impossible.

When you want a cigarette, take a few deep breaths and then occupy yourself by doing any of a number of things such as talking to someone else, washing your hands, brushing your teeth, eating a healthy snack, chewing on a straw, doing dishes, playing sports, going for a walk or a bike ride, going swimming, and so on. Engage in activities that require the use of your hands. Try gardening, sewing, writing letters, drawing, doing household chores, or washing the car. Visit nonsmoking places such as libraries, museums, stores, and theaters. Plan an outing or a trip away from home. Any of these activities can keep your mind off cigarettes. Record your choice of activity or substitute under the "Remarks/Substitutes" column in Figure 13.10.

Quitting Cold Turkey

Many people have found that quitting all at once is the easiest way to do it. Most smokers have tried this approach at least once. Even though it might not work the first time, they do not allow themselves to get discouraged, and they eventually succeed. Many people report that, after several attempts, all of a sudden they were able to overcome smoking without too much difficulty.

On the average, as few as three smokeless days are sufficient to break the physiological addiction to nicotine. The psychological addiction may linger for years but will get weaker as time goes by.

Cutting Down Gradually

Tapering off cigarettes can be done in several ways.

1. Eliminate cigarettes you do not strongly crave (those ranked numbers 3 and 2 on your daily log from Figure 13.10).
2. Switch to a brand lower in nicotine and tar every few days.
3. Smoke less of each cigarette.
4. Smoke fewer cigarettes each day.

Most people prefer a combination of these four suggestions.

Before you start cutting down, set a target date for quitting. Once the date is set, don't change it. The total time until your quit date should be no longer than 2 weeks. Reduce the total number of cigarettes you smoke each day by 10 to 25 percent. As you smoke less, be careful not to take more puffs or inhale more deeply as you smoke, because this would offset the principle of cutting down.

As an aid in tapering off, make several copies of Figure 13.10. (By now you should have already completed the first daily log of your smoking habit— see Step Four under "Breaking the Habit" on page 377.) Start a new daily log and, every night, review your data and set goals for the following day.

Decide which cigarettes will be easiest to give up, what brand you will smoke, the total number of cigarettes to be smoked, and how much of each you will smoke. Write down any comments or situations you want to avoid, as well as any substitutes you could use to help you in the program. For example, if you always smoke while drinking coffee, substitute juice for coffee. If you smoke while driving, arrange for a ride or take a bus to work. If you smoke with a certain friend at lunch, avoid having lunch with that friend for a week or so. Continue using this log until you have stopped smoking completely.

Nicotine Substitution Products

Nicotine substitution drug products such as nicotine transdermal patches and nicotine gum have been developed to help people kick the tobacco habit. These products are most effective when they are used in a physician-supervised cessation program. As with tapering off, these products gradually decrease the amount of nicotine used until the person no longer craves the drug.

Nicotine patches are used to supply a steady dose of nicotine through the skin. These patches are available in various dosages, delivering anywhere from about 5 to 21 mg of nicotine in a 24-hour period. A

FIGURE 13.9 Reasons for smoking versus quitting.

Name: _____ Date: _____

Course: _____ Section: _____ Gender: _____ Age: _____

Reasons for Smoking Cigarettes

1. _____
2. _____
3. _____
4. _____
5. _____
6. _____
7. _____
8. _____
9. _____
10. _____

Reasons for Quitting Cigarette Smoking

1. _____
2. _____
3. _____
4. _____
5. _____
6. _____
7. _____
8. _____
9. _____
10. _____

FIGURE 13.10 Daily cigarette smoking log.

Name:_____

       Course: _____ Section: _____ Gender:_____ Age: _____

Today's Date: _____ Quit Date: _____ Decision Date:_____

Cigarettes to be Smoked Today: ____ Brand:_____

No.	Time	Activity	Amount Smoked[a]	Rating[b]	Remarks/Substitutes
1.					
2.					
3.					
4.					
5.					
6.					
7.					
8.					
9.					
10.					
11.					
12.					
13.					
14.					
15.					
16.					
17.					
18.					
19.					
20.					

Additional comments, list of friends, and/or activities to avoid

_____

_____

_____

_____

[a] Amount smoked: entire cigarette, two-thirds, half, etc.
[b] Rating: 1 = desperately needed, 2 = moderately needed, 3 = no real need

typical program lasts between 3 and 10 weeks with an average weekly cost to the consumer of about $35. Sales of nicotine patches approximate $1 billion per year.

Public safety concerns regarding the use of nicotine patches, including indications, precautions, warnings, contra-indications, potential for abuse, and marketing and labeling issues are monitored and regulated by the FDA. People contemplating their use should pay careful attention to contraindications and potential side effects. Pregnant and lactating women and people with heart disease, high blood pressure, or who have had a recent heart attack should check with their physician prior to using nicotine substitution products. Skin redness, swelling, or rashes are sometimes associated with the use of nicotine patches. Other undesirable side effects are listed on the label and should be monitored closely.

> **About three smokeless days are sufficient to break the physiological addiction to nicotine.**

LIFE AFTER CIGARETTES

During the first few days after you quit smoking, you can expect a series of withdrawal symptoms; among them are lower heart rate and blood pressure, head-aches, gastrointestinal discomfort, mood changes, irritability, aggressiveness, and difficulty sleeping.

The physiological addiction to nicotine is broken only 3 days following your last cigarette. Thereafter, you should not crave cigarettes as much. For the habitual smoker, the psychological dependency could be the most difficult to break. The first few days probably will not be as difficult as the first few months. Any of the activities of daily life that have been asso-ciated with smoking—either stress or relaxation, joy or unhappiness—may trigger a relapse even months or, at times, years after quitting.

Ex-smokers should realize that, even though some harm may have been done already, it is never too late to quit. The greatest early benefit is a lower risk for sudden death. Furthermore, the risk for illness starts to decrease the moment you stop smoking. You will have fewer sore throats and sores in the mouth, less hoarseness, no more cigarette cough, and lower risk for peptic ulcers.

Circulation to the hands and feet will improve, as will gastrointestinal and kidney and bladder functions. Everything will taste and smell better. You will have more energy, and you will gain a sense of freedom, pride, and well-being. You will no longer have to worry whether you have enough cigarettes to last through a day, a party, a meeting, a weekend, a trip.

When you first quit and you think how tough it is and how miserable you feel because you cannot have a cigarette, try the opposite: Think of the benefits and how great it is not to smoke! The ex-smoker's risk for heart disease approaches that of a lifetime non-smoker 10 years following cessation, and for cancer, 15 years after cessation.

If you have been successful and stopped smoking, a lot of events can still trigger your urge to smoke. When confronted with these events, some people rationalize and think, "One cigarette won't hurt. I've been off for months (years in some cases)" or, "I can handle it. I'll smoke just today." It won't work! Before you know it, you will be back to the regular nasty habit. Be prepared to take action in those situations. Find substitutes. In addition to the many things that have been discussed in this chapter, the tips given in Figure 13.11 should help you retrain yourself to live without cigarettes.

Start thinking of yourself as a nonsmoker—no "butts" about it. Remind yourself how difficult it has been and how long it has taken you to get to this point. If you have come this far, you certainly can resist brief moments of temptation. It will get easier rather than harder as time goes on.

The simple pleasures of life, such as taste and smell, improve with smoking cessation.

WEB INTERACTIVE

Web of Addictions

This site features comprehensive, factual information on a variety of addictions, including that of alcohol and other drugs.

http://www.well.com/user/woa

National Institute on Alcohol Abuse and Alcoholism

This site, sponsored by the U.S. Government, features information on alcohol use and abuse.

http://www.niaaa.nih.gov

CDC Page on Smoking and Health: Tobacco Information and Prevention Source

A comprehensive site featuring education information, research, a report from the U.S. Surgeon General, tips on how to quit, and much more.

http://www.cdc.gov/tobacco

Club Drugs

Information from the National Institute of Drug Abuse concerning these drugs: Alcohol, LSD (acid), MDMA (Ecstasy),

GHB, GBL, Ketamine (Special-K), Fentanyl, Rohypnol, amphetamines, and methamphetamine.

http://www.nida.nih.gov/drugpages/clubdrugs.html

INTERACTIVE SITES:

Why Do I Smoke? Quiz

An interactive self-assessment from the *American Family Physician* journal.

http://www.familydoctor.org/handouts/296.html

Facts on Tap: Alcohol and Your College Experience

This excellent site, geared to college students, features links to the following topics:

Risky Relationship: Alcohol and Sex
College Experience: Alcohol and Student Life
The Naked Truth: Alcohol and Your Body
When Someone Else's Drinking Gives You a Hangover

http://www.factsontap.org

n*tes

1. R. Goldberg, *Drugs Across the Spectrum* (Belmont, CA: Wadsworth/Thomson Learning, 2000).
2. See note 1.
3. *National Drug Control Strategy* (Washington, DC: U.S. Government Printing Office, 1998).
4. Join Together, *Results of the Fourth National Survey on Community Efforts to Reduce Substance Abuse and Gun Violence* (Boston: Join Together, 1999).
5. American Cancer Society, *Cancer Facts & Figures—2000* (New York: ACS, 2000).
6. S. A. Glantz and W. W. Parmley, "Passive Smoking and Heart Disease," *Journal of the American Medical Association* 273 (1995): 1047–1053.
7. See note 5.
8. American Heart Association, *2001 Heart and Stroke Statistical Update* (Dallas: AHA, 2000).
9. "Wellness Facts," *University of California Berkeley Wellness Letter* 14 (1998): 1.
10. American Cancer Society, *World Smoking & Health* (Atlanta: ACS, 1993).
11. American Heart Association, *AHA Public Affairs/Coalition on Smoking: Health Position* (Dallas: AHA, 1996).
12. U.S. Department of Health and Human Services, *Nicotine Addiction: A Report of the Surgeon General* (Atlanta: U.S. Department of Health and Human Services, Centers for Disease Control and Prevention, National Center for Chronic Disease Prevention and Health Promotion, 1988).

 Suggested Readings

- American Cancer Society. *Fifty Most Often Asked Questions About Smoking and Health and the Answers.* New York: ACS, 1982.
- American Cancer Society. *1998 Cancer Facts & Figures.* New York: ACS, 1998.
- American Heart Association. *How to Quit.* Dallas: AHA, 1984.
- American Heart Association. *The Good Life: A Guide to Becoming a Nonsmoker.* Dallas: AHA, 1984.
- Goldberg, R. *Drugs Across the Spectrum.* Belmont, CA: Wadsworth/Thomson Learning, 2000.
- Hodgson, R. J., and P. Miller. *Self-Watching: Addictions, Habits, Compulsions—What to Do.* New York: Facts on File, 1982.
- U.S. Office on Smoking and Health. *Smoking and Health: A Report of the Surgeon General.* Washington, DC: U.S. Department of Health, Education and Welfare, 1979.
- U.S. Public Health Service. *Smoking Tobacco and Health: A Fact Book.* Rockville, MD: U.S. Department of Health and Human Services, 1981.
- U.S. Public Health Service. *Why People Smoke Cigarettes.* Rockville, MD: U.S. Department of Health and Human Services, 1982.
- U.S. Public Health Service. *A Self-Test for Smokers.* Rockville, MD: U.S. Department of Health and Human Services, 1983.
- U.S. Public Health Service. *Chronic Obstructive Lung Disease: A Report of the Surgeon General.* Rockville, MD: U.S. Department of Health and Human Services, 1984.

FIGURE 13.11 Tips to help stop smoking.

The following are different ways smokers retrained themselves to live without cigarettes. Any one or several of these methods in combination might be helpful to you. Check the ones you like and from these develop your own retraining program.

☐ Before you quit smoking, try wrapping your cigarettes with a sheet of paper like a Christmas present. Every time you want a cigarette, unwrap the pack and write down what you are doing, how you feel, and how important this cigarette is to you. Do this for 2 weeks and you'll have cut down as well as developed new insights into your smoking.

☐ If cigarettes give you an energy boost, try gum, modest exercise, a brisk walk, or a new hobby. Avoid eating new foods that are high in calories.

☐ If cigarettes help you relax, try eating, drinking new beverages, or social activities within reasonable bounds.

☐ Try smoking an excess of cigarettes for a day or two before you quit so the taste of cigarettes is spoiled. Another opportune time to quit is when you are ill with a cold or flu and have lost your taste for cigarettes.

☐ On a 3" × 5" card, list what you like and dislike about smoking. Add to it and read it daily.

☐ Make up a short list of luxuries you have wanted or items you would like to purchase for a loved one. Next to each item, write down the cost. Now convert the cost to "packs of cigarettes." If you save the money each day from packs of cigarettes, you will be able to purchase these items. Use a special "piggy bank" for saving your money, or start a "Christmas Club" account at your bank.

☐ Don't smoke after you get a craving for a cigarette until 3 minutes have passed since you got the urge. During those 3 minutes, change your thinking or activity.

☐ Telephone an ex-smoker or somebody you can talk to until the craving subsides.

☐ Plan a memorable day for stopping. You might choose your vacation, New Year's Day, your birthday, a holiday, the birthday of your child, your anniversary. But don't make the date so distant that you lose momentum.

☐ If you smoke under stress at work, pick a date for stopping when you will be away from your work.

☐ Decide whether you are going to stop suddenly or gradually. If it is to be gradual, work out a tapering-off system so you have intermediate goals.

☐ Don't store cigarettes. Never buy a carton. Wait until one pack is finished before you buy another.

☐ Never carry cigarettes with you at home or at work. Keep your cigarettes as far from you as possible. Leave them with someone or lock them up.

☐ Until you quit, make yourself a "smoking corner" that is far from anything interesting. If you like to smoke with others, always smoke alone. If you like to smoke alone, always smoke with others, preferably if they are nonsmokers. Never smoke while watching television.

☐ Never carry matches or a lighter with you.

☐ Put away your ashtrays or fill them with objects so they cannot be used for ashes. Plant flowers in them or fill them with walnuts. The latter will give you something to do with your hands.

☐ Change your brand of cigarettes weekly so you always are smoking a brand of lower tar and nicotine content than the week before.

☐ Never say, "I quit smoking," because your resolution is broken if you have a cigarette. Better to say, "I don't want to smoke." This way you maintain your resolution even if you accidentally have a cigarette.

☐ Try to help someone else quit smoking, particularly your mate.

☐ Always ask yourself, "Do I need this cigarette or is this just a reflex?"

☐ Each day try to put off lighting your first cigarette.

☐ Decide arbitrarily that you will smoke only on even- or odd-numbered hours of the clock.

☐ Try going to bed early and rising a half hour earlier than usual to avoid hurrying through breakfast and rushing to work.

☐ Keep your hands occupied. Try playing a musical instrument, knitting, or fiddling with hand puzzles.

(continued)

(Figure 13.11 Tips to help stop smoking—continued)

☐ Take a shower. You cannot smoke in the shower.

☐ Brush your teeth frequently to get rid of the tobacco taste and stains.

☐ If you have a sudden craving for a cigarette, take 10 deep breaths, holding the last breath while you strike a match. Exhale slowly, blowing out the match. Pretend the match was a cigarette by crushing it out in an ashtray. Now immediately get busy on some work or activity.

☐ Smoke only half a cigarette.

☐ After you quit, start using your lungs. Increase your activities and indulge in moderate exercise, such as short walks before or after a meal.

☐ Bet with someone that you can quit. Put the cigarette money in a jar each morning and forfeit it if you smoke. Keep the money if you don't smoke by the end of the week. Try to extend this period for a month.

☐ If you gain weight because you are not smoking, wait until you get over the craving before you diet. Dieting is easier then.

☐ If you are depressed or have physical symptoms that might be related to your smoking, relieve your mind by discussing this with your physician. It is easier to quit when you know your health status.

☐ After you quit, visit your dentist and have your teeth cleaned to get rid of the tobacco stains.

☐ If the cost of cigarettes is your motivation for quitting, purchase a money order equivalent to a year's supply of cigarettes. Give it to a friend. If you smoke in the next year, he or she cashes the money order and keeps the money. If you don't smoke, he or she gives back the money order at the end of the year.

☐ After you quit, redirect the temptation to smoke by calling or visiting someone.

☐ When you feel irritable or tense, shut your eyes and count backward from 10 to zero as you imagine yourself descending a flight of stairs, or imagine that you are looking at the horizon as the sun sets in the west.

☐ Get out of your old habits. Seek new activities or perform old activities in a new way. Don't rely on the old ways of solving problems. Do things differently.

☐ If you are a "kitchen smoker" in the morning, volunteer your services to a school or nonprofit organization to get you out of the house.

☐ Stock up on light reading materials, crossword puzzles, and vacation brochures that you can read during your coffee breaks.

☐ Frequent places where you can't smoke, such as libraries, buses, theaters, swimming pools, department stores.

☐ Give yourself time to think and get fit by walking one-half hour each day. If you have a dog, take it for a walk with you.

Excerpted from TIPS, American Cancer Society, Texas Division. Used by permission.

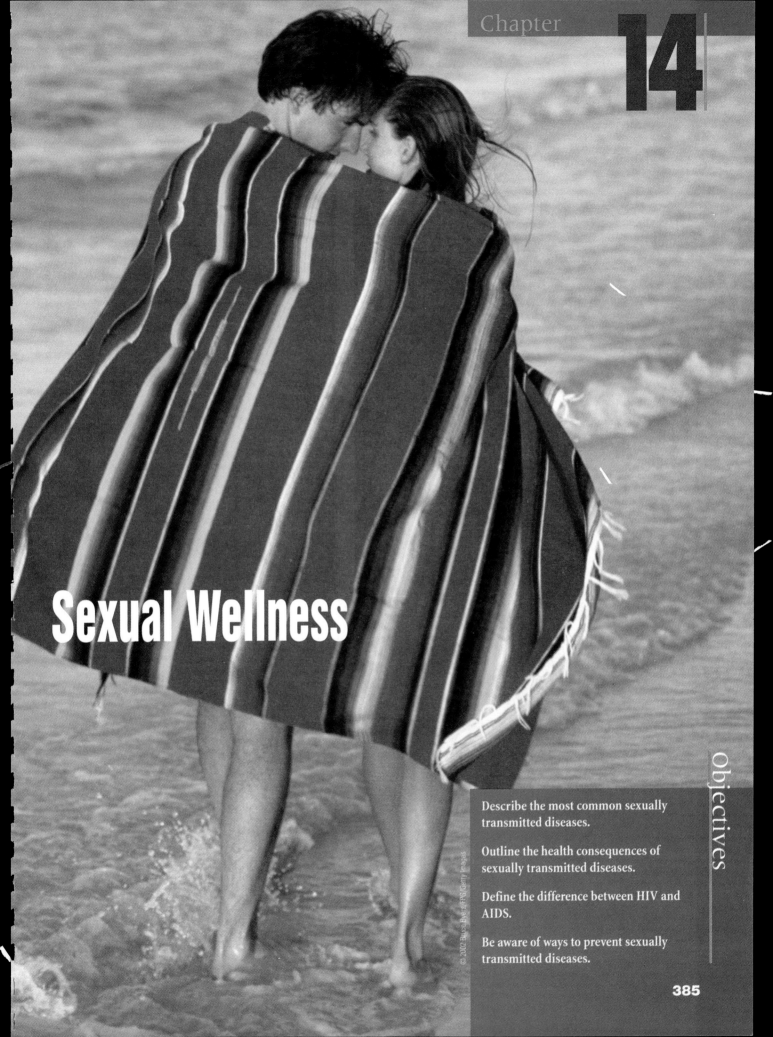

Sexual Wellness

objectives

Describe the most common sexually transmitted diseases.

Outline the health consequences of sexually transmitted diseases.

Define the difference between HIV and AIDS.

Be aware of ways to prevent sexually transmitted diseases.

Sexually transmitted diseases (STDs) have reached epidemic proportions in the United States. Of the more than 25 known STDs, some are still incurable. Based on estimates by the World Health Organization, world wide, 1 million people are infected daily with STDs not including HIV. The American Social Health Association stated that 25 percent of all Americans will acquire at least one STD in their lifetime. Each year, more than 15 million people in the United States are newly infected with STDs, and more than 68 million Americans have an incurable STD.[1] These infections include more than 4 million cases of chlamydia, 800,000 cases of gonorrhea, between one-half and 1 million cases of genital warts, half a million cases of herpes, and nearly 15,000 cases of syphilis. Attracting most of the attention because of its life-threatening potential is HIV infection, which leads to AIDS.

> Each year, more than 15 million people in the United States are newly infected with sexually transmitted diseases.

More than 25 diseases are spread through sexual contact. About 1 in 4 adults in the United States has a sexually transmitted disease.

© Fitness & Wellness, Inc.

CHLAMYDIA

Chlamydia is a bacterial infection that spreads during vaginal, anal, or oral sex, or from the vagina to a newborn baby during childbirth. Chlamydia can damage the reproductive system seriously. This disease is considered to be a major factor in male and female infertility. Because it may have no symptoms, 3 of 4 people don't know they're infected until the disease has become quite serious. Each year, 3 million new cases of chlamydia are reported in the United States.[2] Furthermore, according to the U.S. Centers for Disease Control and Prevention (CDC), 15- to 19-year-old girls represent 46 percent of infections, and 20- to 24-year-old women represent another 33 percent.[3]

When symptoms are present, they tend to mimic other STDs, so the disease can be mistreated. Symptoms of serious infection include abdominal pain, fever, nausea, vaginal bleeding, and arthritis. Chlamydia can be treated successfully with oral antibiotics, but its damage to the reproductive system is irreversible.

GONORRHEA

One of the oldest STDs, **gonorrhea** is also caused by a bacterial infection. Gonorrhea is transmitted through vaginal, anal, and oral sex.

Typical symptoms in men include a pus-like secretion from the penis and painful urination. Most infected women don't have any symptoms until the infection has become fairly serious. At this stage, women develop fever, severe abdominal pain, and pelvic inflammatory disease (see below).

If untreated, gonorrhea can produce infertility, widespread bacterial infection, heart damage, and arthritis in men and women and blindness in children born to infected women. Gonorrhea is treated successfully with penicillin and other antibiotics.

PELVIC INFLAMMATORY DISEASE

Each year more than 1 million women in the United States develop a condition known under the umbrella term **pelvic inflammatory disease (PID)**.[4] It usually results from chlamydia or gonorrhea infection.

Typical symptoms of PID are fever, nausea, vomiting, chills, spotting between menstrual periods, heavy bleeding during periods, and pain in the lower abdomen during sexual intercourse, between menstrual periods, or urination. However, many women do not know they have PID because these symptoms are not always present.

PID often develops when the STD spreads to the fallopian tubes, uterus, and ovaries. If the woman becomes pregnant, she could have an ectopic (or tubal) pregnancy, which destroys the embryo and can kill the woman.

PID is treated with antibiotics, bed rest, and sexual abstinence. Further, surgery may be required to remove infected or scarred tissue or to repair or remove the fallopian tubes or uterus.

GENITAL WARTS

Genital warts are caused by viral infection. They show up anywhere from 1 to 8 months after exposure. These warts may be flat or raised and usually are found on the penis or around the vulva and the vagina. They also can appear in the mouth, throat, rectum, on the cervix, or around the anus.

Based on data from the CDC, as many as one million new cases of this STD are diagnosed in the United States each year. In some cities, nearly half of all sexually active teenagers have genital warts. Similar to chlamydia, the virus is spread through vaginal, anal, or oral sex, or from the vagina to a newborn baby.

Health problems associated with genital warts include increased risk for cancers of the cervix, vulva, and penis, and enlargement and spread of the warts, leading to obstruction of the urethra, vagina, and anus. Babies born to infected mothers commonly develop warts over their bodies; therefore, Cesarean sections are recommended.

Treatment requires completely removing all warts. This can be done by freezing them with liquid nitrogen, dissolving them with chemicals, or removing them through electro-surgery or laser surgery. Infected patients may have to be treated more than once, because genital warts can recur.

> **Treatment of genital warts requires completely removing all warts by freezing them with liquid nitrogen, dissolving them with chemicals, or removing them through electro-surgery or laser surgery.**

GENITAL HERPES

Genital herpes, one of the most common STDs, is caused by the herpes simplex virus (HSV). The several types of HSV produce different ailments, including genital herpes, oral (lip) herpes, shingles, and chicken pox. The two most common forms of HSV are Types I and II. Type I is the HSV most often known to cause oral herpes—cold sores or fever blisters that appear on the lips and mouth. HSV Type II is better known as the virus that causes genital herpes.

HSV is a highly contagious virus. Victims are most contagious during an outbreak, and HSV spreads by contact with an active sore. The disease can also be spread through virus-containing secretions from the vagina or penis. A few days following infection, sores appear on the infected areas, most notably the mouth, genitals, and rectum, but may also surface on other parts of the body. In conjunction with the sores, victims usually have mild fever, swollen glands, and headaches. The symptoms usually disappear within a few weeks, causing some people to believe they are cured. Herpes is presently incurable, though, and its victims do remain infected. The virus can remain dormant for extended periods of time, but repeated outbreaks are common. Excessive stress and illness can precipitate new outbreaks.

Both HSV Type I and II can cause oral and genital sores. People who have an outbreak of oral herpes should not touch their genitals or someone else's after touching the oral cold sores; doing so can lead to herpes infection of the genitals. Oral sex can also cause transmission of the HSV from the lips to the genitals and vice versa. People with cold sores on the lips or mouth should exercise care not to touch these sores. Hands should be carefully washed with soap following contact with cold or herpes sores.

> **People who have an outbreak of oral herpes should not touch their genitals or someone else's after touching the oral cold sores; doing so can lead to herpes infection of the genitals.**

Key Terms

Sexually transmitted diseases (STDs) Communicable diseases spread through sexual contact.

Chlamydia A sexually transmitted disease, caused by a bacterial infection, that can cause significant damage to the reproductive system.

Gonorrhea Sexually transmitted disease caused by a bacterial infection.

Pelvic inflammatory disease (PID) An overall designation referring to the effects of other STDs, primarily chlamydia and gonorrhea.

Genital warts A sexually transmitted disease caused by a viral infection.

Genital herpes A sexually transmitted disease caused by a viral infection of the herpes simplex virus Types I and II. The virus can attack different areas of the body, but commonly causes blisters on the genitals.

SYPHILIS

Another common type of STD, also caused by bacterial infection, is **syphilis**. Approximately 3 weeks after infection, a painless sore appears where the bacteria entered the body. This sore disappears on its own in a few weeks. If untreated, more sores may appear within 6 months of the initial outbreak but again will disappear by themselves.

A latent stage, during which the victim is not contagious, may last up to 30 years, lulling victims into thinking they are healed. During the last stage of the disease, some people develop paralysis, crippling, blindness, heart disease, brain damage and insanity, and they even can die as a direct result of the disease. One of the oldest known STDs, syphilis once killed its victims. Penicillin and other antibiotics now are used to treat it.

VANESSA WAS IN A FATAL CAR ACCIDENT LAST NIGHT. ONLY SHE DOESN'T KNOW IT YET.

Photo courtesy of the National Institute on Drug Abuse, U.S. Department of Health & Human Services

Drug and alcohol use can make people more willing to have unplanned and unprotected sex, thereby risking HIV infection.

HIV AND AIDS

AIDS is the most frightening of all STDs because it is fatal and has no known cure. AIDS—which stands for **acquired immunodeficiency syndrome (AIDS)**—is the end stage of infection by the **human immunodeficiency virus (HIV)**.

HIV is a chronic infectious disease that spreads among individuals who engage in risky behavior such as having unprotected sex or sharing hypodermic needles. When a person becomes infected with HIV, the virus multiplies and attacks and destroys white blood cells. These cells are part of the immune system, and their function is to fight off infections and diseases in the body.

As the number of white blood cells killed increases, the body's immune system gradually breaks down or may be destroyed completely. Without the immune system, a person becomes susceptible to various **opportunistic diseases** and to cancers.

HIV is a progressive disease. At first, people who become infected with HIV might not know they are infected. An incubation period of weeks, months, or years may pass during which no symptoms appear. The virus may live in the body 10 years or longer before symptoms emerge.

As the infection progresses to the point at which certain diseases develop, the person is said to have AIDS. HIV itself doesn't kill. Nor do people die of AIDS. "AIDS" is the term designating the final stage of HIV infection. Death is caused by a weakened immune system that is unable to fight off these opportunistic diseases.

Earliest symptoms of AIDS include unexplained weight loss, constant fatigue, mild fever, swollen lymph glands, diarrhea, and sore throat. Advanced symptoms include loss of appetite, skin diseases, night sweats, and deterioration of mucous membranes.

Most of the illnesses that AIDS patients develop are harmless and rare in the general population but are fatal to AIDS victims. The two most common fatal conditions in AIDS patients are pneumocystis carinii pneumonia (a parasitic infection of the lungs) and Kaposi's sarcoma (a type of skin cancer). The AIDS virus also may attack the nervous system, causing damage to the brain and spinal cord.

On the average, the individual develops the symptoms that fit the case definition of AIDS about 9 to 10 years following infection. From that point on, the person might live another 3 years or so. In essence, from the point of infection, the individual might endure a chronic disease for about 12 years.

> **On the average, the symptoms that fit the case definition of AIDS appear about 9 to 10 years following HIV infection.**

The only means to determine whether someone has HIV is through an HIV antibody test. Being HIV-positive does not necessarily mean the person has AIDS. Several years can go by before the person develops the diseases that fit the case definition of AIDS.

Upon HIV infection, the immune system forms antibodies that bind to the virus. HIV antibodies can be detected in the blood as early as 25 days following infection. According to the CDC, all except 5 percent of infected individuals will show these antibodies within 12 to 14 weeks of infection. In some cases, they are not detectable until after 6 months or longer.

If HIV infection is suspected, a person should wait 6 months to be tested, when the test is believed to be almost 100 percent accurate. During this time, and from then on, individuals should refrain from further endangering themselves and others through risky behaviors. Some people are tested to reassure themselves that their risky behaviors are acceptable. Even if the test turns up negative for HIV, this does not represent a license to continue risky behaviors.

No one has to become infected with HIV. At present, once infected, a person cannot become un-infected. There is no second chance. Everyone must protect himself or herself against this chronic disease. People who are so ignorant as to believe that it can never happen to them are putting themselves and their partners at risk.

New therapies are preventing AIDS from developing in a growing number of HIV-infected persons. Professionals, however, disagree as to how many HIV carriers actually will develop AIDS. Even if individuals have not developed AIDS, they can pass on the virus to others, who easily could then develop AIDS.

Transmission of HIV

HIV is transmitted by the exchange of cellular body fluids including blood, semen, vaginal secretions, and maternal milk. These fluids can be exchanged during sexual intercourse, by using hypodermic needles that infected individuals have used previously, between a pregnant woman and her developing fetus, by infection of babies from the mother during childbirth, less frequently during breast feeding, and, rarely, from a blood transfusion or organ transplant. The primary modes of HIV transmission in reported U.S. AIDS cases are presented in Table 14.1.

Today, the risk of being infected with HIV from a blood transfusion is slight. Prior to 1985, several cases of HIV infection came from blood transfusions because the blood was donated by HIV-infected individuals. Now, all individuals who donate blood are first tested for HIV. To be absolutely safe, people who are planning to have surgery might consider storing their own blood in advance so safe blood will be available if a transfusion becomes necessary.

A myth regarding HIV is that it can be transmitted by donating blood. People cannot

> **People do not get HIV because of who they are but, rather, because of what they do.**

get HIV from giving blood. Health professionals use a brand-new needle every time they withdraw blood from a person. They use these needles only once and destroy them immediately after each person has donated blood.

People do not get HIV because of who they are but, rather, because of what they do. HIV and AIDS can threaten anyone, anywhere: men, women, children, teenagers, young people, older adults, whites, African Americans, Hispanic Americans, Asian Americans, Native Americans, Africans, Europeans, homosexuals, heterosexuals, bisexuals, druggies. Nobody is immune to HIV.

HIV can be transmitted between males, between females, from male to female, or from female to male. Although HIV and AIDS are preventable, almost all of the people who get HIV do so because they engage in risky behaviors.

TABLE 14.1	Primary Modes of HIV Transmission in Adults Based on Reported U.S. and Estimated Worldwide AIDS Cases		
	U.S. Men	U.S. Women	Worldwide
Same-gender sexual contact	45%		10%
Heterosexual contact	7	38%	75
Sharing hypodermic needles	21	29	10
Unidentified cause	20	32	
Blood transfusion		1	5

SOURCES: "The HIV/AIDS Epidemic in the U.S." Kaiser Family Foundation, June 1999. UNAIDS: Joint United Nations Programme on HIV/AIDS, United Nations, 2000.

Key Terms

Syphilis A sexually transmitted disease caused by a bacterial infection.

Acquired immunodeficiency syndrome (AIDS) Any of a number of diseases that arise when the body's immune system is compromised by HIV.

Human immunodeficiency virus (HIV) Virus that leads to acquired immunodeficiency syndrome (AIDS).

Opportunistic diseases Diseases that arise in the absence of a healthy immune system, which would fight them off in healthy people.

Risky Behaviors

You cannot tell if people are infected with HIV or have AIDS by simply looking at them or taking their word. Not you, not a nurse, not even a doctor can tell without an HIV antibody test. Therefore, every time you engage in risky behavior, you run the risk of contracting HIV. The two most basic risky behaviors are the following:

1. Having unprotected vaginal, anal, or oral sex with an HIV-infected person. Unprotected sex means having sex without using a condom properly. A person should select only latex (rubber or prophylactic) condoms that state "disease prevention" on the package. Although you might have unprotected sex with an infected person and not get the virus, you can also get it by having unprotected sex only once with an infected individual.

   Rubbing during sexual intercourse often damages mucous membranes and causes unseen bleeding (even in the mouth). During vaginal, anal, or oral sexual contact, infected blood, semen, or vaginal fluids can penetrate the mucous membranes that line the vagina, the penis, the rectum, the mouth, or the throat. From the membrane, HIV then travels into the previously uninfected person's blood.

   Health experts believe that unprotected anal sex is the riskiest type of sex. Even though bleeding is not visible in most cases, anal sex almost always causes tiny tears and bleeding in the rectum. This happens because the rectum does not stretch easily, the mucous membrane is quite thin, and small blood vessels lie directly beneath the membrane. Condoms also are more likely to break during anal intercourse because of the greater friction produced in a smaller cavity. All of these factors greatly enhance the risk of transmitting HIV.

   Although latex condoms, if used correctly, provide for safer sex, they are not 100 percent foolproof. Abstaining from sex is the only 100 percent sure way to protect yourself from HIV infection and other STDs.

2. Sharing hypodermic needles or other drug paraphernalia with someone who is infected. Following an injection, a small amount of blood remains in the needle, and sometimes in the syringe itself. If the person who used the syringe is infected with HIV and someone else uses that same syringe to shoot up, regardless of the drug used (legal or illegal),

> **Unprotected sex means having sex without using a condom properly.**

> **Latex condoms, if used correctly, provide for safer sex, they are not 100 percent foolproof.**

that small amount of blood is sufficient to spread the virus. All used syringes should be destroyed and disposed of immediately.

In addition, a person must be cautious when getting acupuncture, getting a tattoo, or having the ears or other body parts pierced. If the needle used was used previously on someone who is HIV-infected and the needle was not disinfected properly, the person risks getting HIV.

Otherwise prudent people often act irrationally and engage in risky behaviors when they are under the influence of drugs. Getting high can make you willing to have sex when you really didn't plan to—thereby running the risk of contracting HIV.

Small concentrations of the virus have been found in saliva and teardrops. In principle, if both people have open cuts in the lips, mouth, or gums, HIV could be transmitted through open-mouthed kissing, but these cases are rare.

The virus cannot be transmitted through perspiration. Sporting activities with no physical contact pose no risk to uninfected individuals unless they both have open wounds through which blood from an infected person can come in direct contact with the open wound of the uninfected person. The skin is an excellent line of defense against HIV. Blood from an infected person cannot penetrate the skin except through an opening in the skin. As an extra precaution, a person should use vinyl or latex gloves when performing work that requires direct contact with someone else's blood or open wound.

Some people fear getting HIV from health care professionals. The chances of getting infected during physical or medical procedures are practically nil. Health-care workers take extra care to protect themselves and their patients from HIV.

With the advent of the Internet, people now search for sex partners online. Use of the Internet to find sexual partners may further increase the risk of contracting an STD. A recent study showed that those who seek sex partners over the Internet are at a greater risk of contracting an STD. Such people are also more likely to have behavioral characteristics that increase their chances of transmitting STDs.[5]

HIV is not transmitted through casual contact. HIV cannot be caught by spending time with, shaking hands with, or hugging an infected person; from a toilet seat, dishes, or silverware used by an HIV patient; or by sharing a drink, food, a towel, or clothes with a person who has HIV.

What about dating? Dating and getting to know other people are normal aspects of life. Dating, however, does not mean the same thing as having sex. Sexual intercourse as a part of dating can be risky, and one of the risks is AIDS. You can't tell if someone you are dating or would like to date has been exposed to HIV. The good news is that as long as you avoid sexual activity and don't share drug needles, it doesn't matter whom you date.

Another myth regarding HIV transmission is that you can get it from insects or animals. The H in HIV stands for "human." You cannot catch HIV from insects or animals. Animals do not get infected with HIV.

HIV and AIDS Statistics

Based on estimates by the National Institute on Drug Abuse, more than 34.3 million people around the world are infected with HIV, and about 18.8 million have died from AIDS since the epidemic began. Estimates by the CDC indicate that between 300,000 and 900,000 people in the United States are infected with HIV. One in every 300 Americans is presently infected, and about 23 percent of the newly reported cases are women. Through the end of 1998, a cumulative total of 688,200 AIDS cases had been diagnosed in the United States (see Figure 14.1), and 410,800 people had died from the diseases caused by HIV.

Most of the people who die (71.6 percent) are in the 25- to 44-year-old age group.

Although initially more than half of all AIDS cases in the United States occurred in homosexual or bisexual men, HIV infection is now spreading at a faster rate in heterosexuals. Many heterosexuals practice unprotected sex because they don't believe it can happen to their segment of the population. HIV is an epidemic that does not discriminate by sexual orientation. Worldwide, up to 80 percent of the AIDS cases have been reported in heterosexuals.[6]

AIDS experts are turning their attention to the population of sub-Saharan Africa, where 70 percent of the world's HIV victims live. Within 10 years, life expectancy is predicted to hit its lowest point in a century in this part of the world, and the number of AIDS orphans will accelerate dramatically. The AIDS epidemic could also ruin the economies of these already impoverished countries. The medications used to treat victims in Western countries are unaffordable in sub-Saharan Africa. Public awareness programs may be the only answer to the HIV epidemic there.

As with any other serious illness, HIV infected people and AIDS patients deserve respect, understanding, and support. Rejection and discrimination are traits of immature, hateful, and ignorant people. Education, knowledge, and responsible behaviors are the best ways to minimize fear and discrimination.

FIGURE 14.1 AIDS cases reported in the United States between 1985 and 1999.

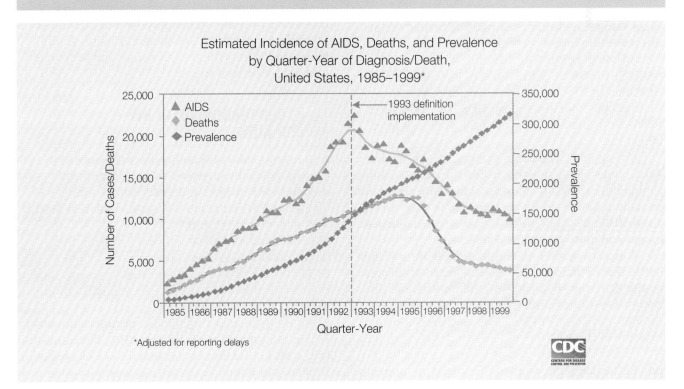

Estimated Incidence of AIDS, Deaths, and Prevalence by Quarter-Year of Diagnosis/Death, United States, 1985–1999*

*Adjusted for reporting delays

HIV Testing

A person can be tested for HIV in several ways. You may look up your local Public Health Department or AIDS Information Service (or related names) in the phone book. Testing is usually free of charge, and the results are kept confidential.

> As with any other serious illness, HIV-infected people and AIDS patients deserve respect, understanding, and support.

Many states also conduct anonymous testing. Your name is never recorded. You can call several toll-free hotlines for more information on anonymous testing, treatment programs, support services, HIV and AIDS information, and STDs in general. All information discussed during a phone call to these hotlines is kept strictly confidential. The numbers to call are

- National AIDS Hotline: 1-800-342-AIDS (1-800-342-2437) or La Linea Nacional de SIDA: 1-800-344-SIDA (1-800-344-7432), for Spanish-speaking people.
- STD Hotline: 1-800-227-8922.

HIV Treatment

Even though several drugs are being tested to treat and slow the disease process, AIDS has no known cure. Approximately 40 different approaches to an AIDS vaccine are being explored. The best advice at this point is to take a preventive approach.

Although HIV has no cure, medications are available that delay the progress of infection, allow HIV-infected patients to live longer, and even keep some people from developing AIDS. The sooner the treatment is initiated, the better the prognosis for a longer life.

Developing a vaccine to prevent HIV infection or AIDS seems highly unlikely within the decade. People should not expect a medical breakthrough. Treatment modalities, however, should continue to improve and allow HIV-infected persons and AIDS patients to live longer and more productive lives.

Presently, several AIDS clinical trials are available in the United States. These projects are co-sponsored by the CDC, the Food and Drug Administration, the National Institute of Allergy and Infectious Diseases, the National Library of Medicine, and the National Institute of Health. The purpose of AIDS clinical trials is to evaluate experimental drugs and various therapies for people at all stages of HIV infection. Interested

A monogamous sexual relationship almost completely removes people from risk of HIV infection and the danger of contracting other sexual transmitted diseases.

© Fitness & Wellness, Inc.

individuals can call 1-800-TRIALS-A. As with all HIV testing, calls are completely confidential. Eligibility to participate in an AIDS clinical trial varies, and all applicants are evaluated individually. By calling the telephone number given, an interested person will receive information on the purpose and location of the trials (studies) that are open, eligibility requirements, exclusion criteria, and names and telephone numbers of persons to contact.

Economic Impact of HIV and AIDS

Federal government spending for AIDS-related projects gradually increased to more than $900 million between 1982 and 1988. Costs continued to escalate to $1.3 billion in 1989, $4.3 billion in 1992, $5.7 billion in 1997, and $9.7 billion in 1999. The CDC National Aids Clearinghouse estimates the direct-treatment cost per AIDS victim at about $133,500 over 8.3 years of life. This represents more than $41.2 billion to treat the 308,933 AIDS cases reported as of June 1999.

If the estimated 1 million people infected with HIV in the United States develop AIDS, direct health-care costs for the disease will equal $121.383 billion. To place this figure in perspective, a person would have to spend $1 million per day for the next 332.5 years to spend the $121.383 billion—a sobering amount for a preventable disease. Everyone in the United States will help pay for these costs through taxes and a more expensive health-care system.

GUIDELINES FOR PREVENTING SEXUALLY TRANSMITTED DISEASES

The good news is that you can do things to prevent the spread of STDs and take precautions to keep yourself from becoming a victim. The facts are in: The best prevention technique is a mutually **monogamous** sexual relationship. This one behavior will remove you almost completely from any risk for developing an STD.

Unfortunately, in today's society, trust is elusive. You may be led to believe you are in a monogamous relationship when your partner actually (a) may cheat on you and get infected, (b) has a one-night stand with someone who is infected, (c) got the virus several years ago before the current relationship and still doesn't know about the infection, (d) may choose not to tell you about the infection, or (e) shoots up drugs and becomes infected. In any of these cases, HIV can be passed on to you.

> **The best prevention technique is a mutually monogamous sexual relationship.**

Because your future and your life are at stake, and because you may never know if your partner is infected, you should give serious and careful consideration to postponing sex until you believe you have found an uninfected person with whom you can have a lifetime monogamous relationship. In doing so, you will not have to live with the fear of catching HIV or other STDs or deal with an unplanned pregnancy.

As strange as this may seem to some, many people postpone sexual activity until they are married. This is the best guarantee against HIV. Young people should understand that married life will provide plenty of time for fulfilling and rewarding sex.

If you choose to delay sex, do not let peers pressure you into having sex. Some people would have you believe that you are not a "real" man or woman if you don't

> **Manhood and womanhood are not proven during sexual intercourse but, instead, through mature, responsible, and healthy choices.**

have sex. Manhood and womanhood are not proven during sexual intercourse but, instead, through mature, responsible, and healthy choices.

Other people lead you to believe that love doesn't exist without sex. Sex in the early stages of a relationship is not the product of love. It is simply the fulfillment of a physical, and often selfish, drive. A loving relationship develops over a long time with mutual respect for each other.

Teenagers are especially susceptible to peer pressure leading to premature sexual intercourse. The result: more than a million teen pregnancies per year and a 43 percent pregnancy rate for all girls at least once as a teenager.

> **Sex lasts a few minutes, parenthood lasts a lifetime.**

Presently, the U.S. teen pregnancy rate is the highest of any industrialized nation. Too many young people wish they had postponed sex and silently admire those who do. Sex lasts only a few minutes. The consequences of irresponsible sex may last a lifetime. And in some cases, they are fatal!

Then there are those who enjoy bragging about their sexual conquests and mock people who choose to wait. Many of these conquests are only fantasies expounded in an attempt to gain popularity with peers.

Sexual promiscuity never leads to a trusting, loving, and lasting relationship. Mature people respect others' choices. If someone does not respect your choice to wait, he or she certainly does not deserve your friendship or, for that matter, anything else.

There is no greater sex than that between two loving and responsible individuals who mutually trust, admire, and love each other. Contrary to many beliefs, these relationships are possible. They are built upon unselfish attitudes and behaviors.

As you look around, you will find that many people hold these values. Seek them out and build your friendships and future around people who respect you for who you are and what you believe. You don't have to compromise your choices or values. In the end, you will reap the greater rewards of a lasting relationship free of AIDS and other STDs.

Also, be prepared so that you will know your course of action before you get into an intimate situation. Look for common interests and work together toward them. Express your feelings openly: "I'm not ready for sex; I just want to have fun, and

Key Terms

Monogamous A sexual relationship in which two people have sexual relations only with each other.

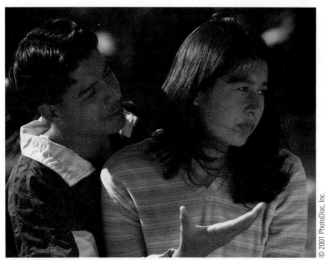

© 2001 PhotoDisc, Inc.

If someone does not respect your choice to wait, he or she certainly does not deserve your friendship, or for that matter, anything else.

kissing is fine with me." If your friend does not accept your answer and is not willing to stop the advances, be prepared with a strong response. Statements like "Please stop" or "Don't!" are for the most part ineffective. Use a firm statement such as, "No, I'm not willing to have sex" or "I've already thought about this and I'm not going to have sex." If this still does not work, label the behavior what it is—rape—and say, "This is rape, and I'm going to call the police."

Reducing the Risk for STDs

What about those who do not have—or do not desire—a monogamous relationship? Some other things can be done to lower, but not completely eliminate, the risk for developing STDs in general:

1. Plan before you get into a sexual situation. Determine the conditions under which you will allow sex to take place. Take a few moments now and ask yourself: "Am I willing to have sex with this person?" If you decide to have sex, practice safer sex. There is no reason to accept anything else. You will feel better about yourself.

2. Know your partner. The days are gone when anonymous bathhouse or singles-bar sex is safe. Limit your sexual relationships and always practice safer sex.

3. Discuss STDs with the person you are contemplating having sex with before you do so. Even though talking about STDs might be awkward, the short-lived embarrassment of addressing intimate questions can keep you from contracting or spreading disease. If you do not know the person well enough to address this issue or you

are uncertain about the answers, do not have sex with this individual.

4. Limit the number of sexual partners you have. Having one partner lowers your chances of becoming infected. The more partners you have, the greater your chance for infection.

5. If you are sexually promiscuous, consider having periodic physical check-ups. You can easily get exposed to an STD from a person who does not have any symptoms and who is unaware of the infection. Sexually promiscuous men and women between ages 15 and 35 are considered a particularly high-risk group for developing STDs.

6. Use barrier methods of contraception to help prevent the disease from spreading. Condoms, diaphragms, and spermicidal suppositories, foams, and jellies can all deter the spread of certain STDs. Spermicidal agents may act as a disinfectant as well. Many physicians are encouraging promiscuous teenagers especially to use condoms. Traditionally, teenagers do not use birth-control methods at all and remain at high risk for STDs. Take a few minutes at this time and list at least three ways you might bring up the subject of condom use with your partner. Also, think of ways you might convince a person to use one. If your partner refuses to use a condom, your answer should be quite simple: "No condom, no sex."

7. Negotiate safer sex. Focus on the problem and not the person. Describe your feelings about the problem, using "I" instead of "you." For example, you might say, "I'm feeling awkward and uncomfortable. The only way I can feel comfortable is by using a condom." You also can offer options and provide alternative solutions to your partner. You might indicate: "We can work this out together. Let's go for a drive and get a condom with a spermicide agent. We'll feel better about what we're doing."

8. Be responsible enough to abstain from sexual activity if you know you have an infection. Go to a physician or a clinic for treatment, and ask your doctor when you can safely resume sexual activity. Abstain until it is safe. Just as you want to be protected in a sexual relationship, you should want to protect your partner as well.

   If you are diagnosed with an STD and you believe you know the person who gave it to you, think of ways you could bring up the subject of STDs with this person. You need to take responsibility and discuss this matter with your partner. As a result of your conversation, medical treatment can be initiated, and other people can be protected from infection as well.

9. Urinate immediately following sexual intercourse. Although this is not an entirely reliable method, it may help flush bacteria and viruses from the urinary tract.

10. Thoroughly wash immediately after sexual activity. Although washing with hot, soapy water will not guarantee safety against STDs, it can prevent you from spreading certain germs on your fingers and may wash away bacteria and viruses that have not entered the body yet.

11. If you suspect that your partner is infected with an STD, ask. He or she may not even be aware of the infection, so look for signs of infection, such as sores, redness, inflammation, a rash, growths, warts, or a discharge. If you are unsure, abstain.

12. Consider abstaining from sexual relations if you have any kind of an illness or disease, even a common cold. Any kind of illness makes you more susceptible to other illnesses, and lower immunity can make you more vulnerable to STDs. The same holds true for times when you are under extreme stress, when you are fatigued, and when you are overworked. Drugs and alcohol also can lower your resistance to disease.

13. Wear loose-fitting clothes made from natural fibers. Tight-fitting clothing made from synthetic fibers (especially underwear and nylon pantyhose) can create conditions that encourage the growth of bacteria and actually can aggravate STDs.

Reducing the Risks for HIV

Based upon recommendations from health experts, observing the following precautions can reduce your risk for getting HIV and, subsequently, AIDS:

1. Postpone sex until you and your uninfected partner are prepared to enter into a lifetime monogamous relationship.

2. Unless you are in a monogamous relationship and you know your partner is not infected (which you may never know for sure), practice safer sex every time you have sex. This means you should use a latex condom from start to finish for each sexual act. If you think your partner should use a condom but refuses to do so, say "No" to sex with that person.

   Many experts believe that greater protection can be obtained by placing a small amount of the spermicide nonoxynol-9 inside the condom at its tip and then lubricating the outside with additional spermicide. Nonoxynol-9 is used to kill the man's sperm for birth-control purposes. In test tubes, it has been shown to kill STD germs and HIV. This spermicide, however, should not be used in place of a condom, because it will not offer the same protection as the condom does by itself.

3. Don't have multiple and anonymous sexual partners. Keep in mind that anyone you have sex with could be infected with HIV.

4. Don't have sexual contact with anyone who doesn't practice safer sex.

5. Avoid sexual contact with anyone who has had sex with people at risk for getting HIV, even if they are now practicing safer sex.

6. Don't have sex with prostitutes.

7. If you do have sex with someone who might be infected with HIV or whose history is unknown to you, avoid exchange of body fluids.

8. Don't share toothbrushes, razors, or other implements that could become contaminated with blood with anyone who is, or who might be, infected with HIV.

9. Be cautious regarding procedures (such as acupuncture, tattooing, and ear piercing) in which needles or other nonsterile instruments may be used again and again to pierce the skin or mucous membranes. These procedures are safe if proper sterilization methods are followed or disposable needles are used. Before undergoing the procedure, ask what precautions are being taken.

10. If you are planning to undergo artificial insemination, insist on frozen sperm obtained from a laboratory that tests all donors for infection with HIV. Donors should be tested twice before the lab accepts the sperm—once at the time of donation and again a few months later.

11. If you know you will be having surgery in the near future, and if you are able, consider donating blood for your own use. This will eliminate completely the already small risk of contracting HIV through a blood transfusion. It also will eliminate the more substantial risk for contracting other bloodborne diseases, such as hepatitis, from a transfusion.

Avoiding risky behaviors that destroy quality of life and life itself is crucial to a healthy lifestyle. Learning the facts and acting upon your personal values, so you can make responsible choices, can protect you and those around you from painful, embarrassing, startling, unexpected, or fatal conditions.

WEB INTERACTIVE

The Body: Safer Sex and Prevention

This site features information for consumers, gay men, and health care professionals on a variety of disease-prevention issues, including safer sex and general preventive guidelines, condoms, sexual communication skills, sexual and non-sexual disease prevention, effective education programs, treatment, and research.

http://www.thebody.com/safesex.html

American Social Health Association

This site features information on a variety of sexually transmitted diseases, a comprehensive frequently-asked-questions section, and lists of STD hotlines. It also features a link to iwannaknow.org, the ASHA's STD prevention Web site for teens.

http://www.ashastd.org

CDC National Center for HIV, STD, and TB Prevention

This comprehensive site features a variety of links to information regarding HIV/AIDS prevention. Also includes the latest statistics.

http://www.cdc.gov/hiv/pubs/facts.htm

Sexual Communication

This site, from Duke University Student Health Service, provides excellent guidelines to help discuss sex (or abstinence) with your partner as well as information about sexual dysfunction, rape and sexual assault. It also provides information concerning gay, lesbian, and bisexual issues. In addition, there is a page that suggests 101 alternatives to having sex.

http://www.healthydevil.stuaff.duke.edu/info/sex/sex/html

INTERACTIVE SITES:

Assess Your Risk for HIV and Other Sexually Transmitted Diseases

By completing this simple 24-item multiple-choice questionnaire, you will obtain an accurate portrayal of your personal risk of acquiring HIV and other sexually transmitted diseases.

http://www.thebody.com/surveys/sexsurvey.html

Sexuality Information from Columbia University Health Education Department: "Go Ask Alice"

This site features a series of questions and answers on sexual intercourse, abstinence, kissing, and genital wonderings.

http://www.goaskalice.columbia.edu/Cat6/html

1. Tanne, J. H., "US Has Epidemic of Sexually Transmitted Disease," *British Medical Journal* 317 (1998): 1616.
2. See note 2.
3. Unless otherwise indicated, all the statistics regarding STDs are from the U. S. Centers for Disease Control and Prevention, Atlanta.
4. Igra, V., "Pelvic Inflammatory Disease in Adolescents," *AIDS Patient Care & STDs* (February 1998): 109–124.
5. McFarlane, M., S. S. Bull, and C. A. Rietmeijer, "The Internet as a Newly Emerging Risk Environment for Sexually Transmitted Diseases," *Journal of the American Medical Association* 284 (2000): 443–446.
6. Philpott, P., "Heterosexual Transmission Studies," *Reappraising AIDS* 6, no. 1 (1998): 1.

Suggested Readings

■ W. W. K. Hoeger, L. W. Turner, and B. Q. Hafen. *Wellness: Guidelines for a Healthy Lifestyle*. Belmont, CA: Wadsworth/ Thomson Learning, 2002.

■ Institute of Medicine. *The Hidden Epidemic: Confronting Sexually Transmitted Diseases*. Washington, DC: National Academy Press, 1997.

Healthy Lifestyle Issues and Wellness Guidelines for the Future

Understand the effects of a healthy lifestyle on longevity.

Learn to differentiate between physiological and chronological age.

Estimate your life expectancy and determine your real physiological age.

Learn about complementary and alternative medicine practices.

Learn guidelines for preventing consumer fraud.

Understand factors to consider when selecting a health/fitness club.

Know how to select appropriate exercise equipment.

Review health/fitness accomplishments and chart a wellness program for the future.

Better health, higher quality of life, and increased longevity are the three most important benefits derived from a lifetime fitness and wellness program. You have learned that physical fitness in itself does not always lower the risk for chronic diseases and ensure better health. Thus implementation of healthy behaviors is one means to attain your highest potential for complete well-being. The real challenge will come now that you are about to finish this course: a lifetime commitment to fitness and wellness. Adhering to a program in a structured setting is a lot easier, but from now on, you will be on your own.

This chapter will help you evaluate how well you are adhering to health-promoting behaviors and the impact that these behaviors may have on your **physiological age** and length of life. You will also learn how to chart a personal wellness program for the future.

Research data indicates that healthy (and unhealthy) lifestyle actions you take today will have an impact on health and quality of life in middle and advanced age. Whereas most young people don't seem to worry much about health and longevity, you may want to take a closer look at the quality of life of your parents or other middle-aged and older friends and relatives that you know. Though you may have a difficult time envisioning yourself at that age, their health status and **functional capacity** may help you determine how you would like to live when you reach your fourth, fifth, and sixth decade of life.

Although previous research has documented declines in physiologic function and motor capacity as a result of aging, no hard evidence at present proves that large declines in physical work capacity are related primarily to aging alone. Lack of physical activity—a common phenomenon seen in our society as people age—is accompanied by decreases in physical work capacity that are greater by far than the effects of aging itself.

> **Sedentary people often stop living at age 60 but choose to be buried at age 70!**

Data on individuals who have taken part in systematic physical activity throughout life indicate that these people maintain a higher level of functional capacity and do not experience the typical declines in later years. From a functional point of view, typical sedentary people in the United States are about 25 years older than their **chronological age** indicates. Thus, an active 60-year-old person can have a physical work capacity similar to that of a sedentary 35-year-old person.

Unhealthy behaviors precipitate premature aging. For sedentary people, any type of physical activity is seriously impaired by age 40 and productive life ends before age 60. Most of these people hope to live to be

Good physical fitness provides freedom to enjoy many of life's recreational and leisure activities.

Chuck Scheer, Boise State University

FIGURE **15.1** Relationships between physical work capacity, aging, and lifestyle habits.

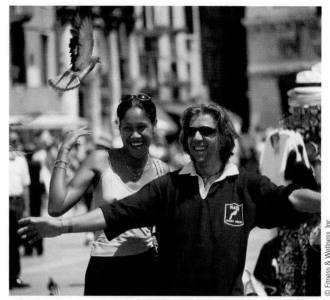

A healthy lifestyle enhances functional capacity and quality of life.

age 65 or 70 and often must cope with serious physical ailments. These people "stop living at age 60 but choose to be buried at age 70" (see the theoretical model in Figure 15.1).

Scientists believe that a healthy lifestyle allows people to live a vibrant life—a physically, intellectually, emotionally, socially active, and functionally independent existence—to age 95. Such are the rewards of a wellness way of life. When death comes to active people, it usually is rather quick and not as a result of prolonged illness: In Figure 15.1, note the low, longer slope of the "unhealthy lifestyle" before death.

LIFE EXPECTANCY AND PHYSIOLOGICAL AGE

Aging is a natural process, but some people seem to age better than others. Most likely you know someone who looks much younger than their chronological age indicates, or vice versa: They appear much older than their chronological age indicates. For example, you may have an instructor who you would have guessed was about 40, but in reality is 52 years old. On the other hand, you may have a relative who looks 60, but who is actually 50 years old. Why the differences?

During the aging process, natural biological changes occur within the body. Although no one measurement can predict how long you will live, the rate at which aging changes take place depends on a combination of genetic and lifestyle factors. Your lifestyle habits will determine to a great extent how your genes will affect your aging process. Hundreds of research studies now point to critical lifestyle behaviors that will determine your statistical chances of dying at a younger age or living a longer life. Research also shows that lifestyle behaviors have a far greater impact on health and longevity than your genes alone.

Throughout this book, you have studied many of these factors. The question that you now need to ask yourself is: Are your lifestyle habits accelerating or decelerating the rate at which your body is aging? To help you determine how long and how well you may live the rest of your life, the **Life Expectancy** and Physiological Age Questionnaire, provided in Figure 15.2, can help answer this question. By looking at 46 critical genetic and lifestyle factors, you will be able to

KeyTerms

Physiological age The biological and functional capacity of the body as it should be in relation to the person's maximal potential at any given age of the lifespan.

Functional capacity The ability to perform ordinary and unusual demands of daily living without limitations and excessive fatigue or injury.

Chronological age Calendar age.

Life expectancy How many years a person is expected to live.

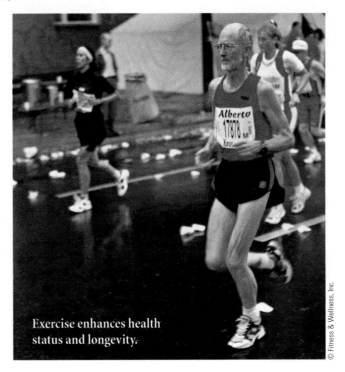

Exercise enhances health status and longevity.

estimate your life expectancy and your real physiological age. Of greater importance, most of these factors are under your own control, and you can do something to make them work for you instead of against you.

As you fill out the questionnaire, you must be completely honest with yourself. Your life expectancy and physiological age prediction is based on your present lifestyle habits, should you continue those habits for life. Using the questionnaire, you will review factors that you can modify or implement in daily living and that may add years and health to your life. Please note that the questionnaire is not a precise scientific instrument, but rather an estimated life expectancy analysis according to the impact of lifestyle factors on health and longevity. Also, the questionnaire is not intended to be a substitute for advice and tests conducted by medical and health care practitioners.

COMPLEMENTARY AND ALTERNATIVE MEDICINE

Conventional Western medicine, also known as "**allopathic medicine**," has seen major advances in care and treatment modalities during the last few decades. Conventional medicine is based on scientifically proven methods, wherein medical treatments are tested through rigorous scientific trials. In addition to a **primary care physician** (medical doctor), people seek advice from other practitioners of conventional medicine, including **osteopaths, dentists, oral surgeons, orthodontists, ophthalmologists, optometrists, physician assistants**, and **nurses**.

In spite of modern-day technological and scientific advancements, many medical treatments either do not improve the patient's condition or create other ailments caused by the treatment itself. Only about 20 percent of conventional treatments have been proven to be clinically effective in scientific trials.[1] Thus, millions of consumers are turning to **complementary and alternative medicine** (also called "unconventional" or "nonallopathic") in search of answers to their health problems.

The reasons for seeking complementary and alternative treatments are diverse. Lack of progress in curing illnesses and disease, frustration and dissatisfaction with physicians, lack of personal attention, testimonials about the effectiveness of alternative treatments, and rising health care costs are among the common reasons given by patients who seek unconventional treatments.

KeyTerms

Conventional Western medicine Traditional medical practice based on methods that are tested through rigorous scientific trials.

Allopathic medicine See conventional Western medicine.

Primary care physician A medical practitioner who provides routine treatment of ailments; typically, the patient's first contact for health care.

Osteopath A medical practitioner with specialized training in musculoskeletal problems who uses diagnostic and therapeutic methods of conventional medicine in addition to manipulative measures.

Dentist Practitioner who specializes in diseases of the teeth, gums, and oral cavity.

Oral surgeon A dentist who specializes in surgical procedures of the oral-facial complex.

Orthodontist A dentist who specializes in the correction and prevention of teeth irregularities.

Ophthalmologist Medical specialist concerned with diseases of the eye and prescription of corrective lenses.

Optometrist Health care practitioner who specializes in the prescription and adaptation of lenses.

Physician assistant A health care practitioner trained to treat most standard cases of care.

Nurse Health care practitioner who assists in the diagnosis and treatment of health problems and provides many services to patients in a variety of settings.

Complementary and alternative medicine A branch of medicine concerned with treatments and health care practices not widely taught in medical schools, not generally used in hospitals, and not usually reimbursed by medical insurance companies.

FIGURE 15.2 Life expectancy and physiological age prediction questionnaire.

Name: _____ Date: _____

Course: _____ Section: _____ Gender: _____ Age: _____

Instructions

Circle the points to the correct answer to each question. At the end of each page, obtain a net score for that page. Be completely honest with yourself. Your age prediction is based on your lifestyle habits, should you continue those habits for life. Using this questionnaire, you will learn about factors that you can modify or implement that can add years and health to your life. The scoring system is provided at the end of the questionnaire. Please note that the questionnaire is not a precise scientific instrument, but rather an estimated life expectancy analysis according to the impact of lifestyle factors on health and longevity. This questionnaire is not intended to substitute for advice and tests conducted by medical and health care practitioners.

I. Questionnaire*

1. What is your current health status?
   A. Excellent $\quad$ +2
   B. Good $\quad$ +1
   C. Average $\quad$ 0
   D. Fair $\quad$ −1
   E. Poor $\quad$ −2
   F. Bad $\quad$ −3

2. How many days per week do you accumulate 30 minutes of moderate-intensity physical activity (50 to 60% of heart rate reserve—see Chapter 4)?
   A. 6 to 7 $\quad$ +3
   B. 3 to 5 $\quad$ +1
   C. 1 to 2 $\quad$ 0
   D. Less than once per week $\quad$ −3

3. How often do you participate in a high-intensity cardio-respiratory exercise (over 60% of heart rate reserve) for at least 20 minutes?
   A. 3 or more times per week +2
   B. 2 times per week $\quad$ +1
   C. Once a week $\quad$ −1
   D. Less than once per week $\quad$ −2

4. How often do you perform strength-training exercises per week (a minimum of 8 exercises using 8 to 12 repetitions to near-fatigue on each exercise)?
   A. 1–2 times $\quad$ +2
   B. Less than once or less than 8 exercises with 8 to 12 reps per session $\quad$ 0
   C. Do not strength-train $\quad$ −1

5. How many times per week do you perform flexibility exercises (at least 15 minutes per stretching session)?
   A. 3 or more $\quad$ +1
   B. 1 to 3 times $\quad$ +.5
   C. Less than 1 $\quad$ 0
   D. Do not perform flexibility exercises $\quad$ −.5

6. How many servings of fruits and vegetables do you eat on a daily basis?
   A. 9 or more $\quad$ +3
   B. 6 to 8 $\quad$ +2
   C. 5 $\quad$ +1
   D. 3 to 4 $\quad$ 0
   E. 2 or less $\quad$ −2

7. How many grams of fiber do you consume on an average day?
   A. 25 or over $\quad$ +1
   B. Between 13 and 24 $\quad$ 0
   C. 10 to 12 or don't know $\quad$ −1
   D. Less than 10 $\quad$ −2

8. As a percentage of total calories, what is your average fat intake on a daily basis?
   A. 20% to 30% $\quad$ +1
   B. 30% $\quad$ 0
   C. 30% to 35% or don't know $\quad$ −1
   D. Over 35% $\quad$ −2

9. As a percentage of total calories, what is your average saturated fat intake on a daily basis?
   A. 5% or less $\quad$ +1
   B. More than 5% but less than 10% $\quad$ 0
   C. Don't know $\quad$ −1
   D. Over 10% $\quad$ −2

10. How many servings of red meat (3 to 6 ounces) do you consume on a weekly basis?
    A. 1 or less $\quad$ +1
    B. 2 to 3 $\quad$ 0
    C. 4 to 7 $\quad$ −1
    D. More than 7 $\quad$ −2

Page score: [   ]

(continued)

(Figure 15.2 Life expectancy and physiological age prediction questionnaire—continued)

11. How many servings of fish (3 to 6 ounces) do you consume on a weekly basis?
    A. 2 or more   +1
    B. 1   0
    C. None   −1

12. How many alcoholic drinks (a 12-ounce bottle of beer, a 4-ounce glass of wine, or a 1.5-ounce shot of 80 proof liquor) do you consume per day?
    A. Men 2 or less, women 1 or less   +1
    B. None   0
    C. Men 3–4, women 2–4   −1
    D. 5 or more   −3

13. How many international units of vitamin E do you get from supplements on a daily basis?
    A. 400   +2
    B. Over 200 but less than 400   +1
    C. Between 50 and 200   0
    D. None   −1

14. How many milligrams of vitamin C do you get from food on a daily basis?
    A. Between 250 and 500   +1
    B. Over 90 but less than 250   +.5
    C. Less than 90   −1

15. How many micrograms of selenium do you get on a daily basis (preferably from food)?
    A. Between 100 and 200   +1
    B. Between 50 and 99   +.5
    C. Less than 50   −1

16. How many milligrams of calcium and how many international units of vitamin D do you get from food and supplements on an average day?
    A. Calcium = 1,200, Vitamin D = 400 or more   +1
    B. Calcium = 1,200, Vitamin D = unknown   +.5
    C. Calcium = 800 to 1,200, Vitamin D = less than 400   0
    D. Calcium = less than 800, Vitamin D = less than 400   −1

17. How many times per week do you eat breakfast?
    A. 7   +1
    B. 5 to 6   +.5
    C. 3 to 5   0
    D. Less than 3   −.5

18. How many cigarettes do you smoke each day?
    A. Never smoked cigarettes or more than 15 years since giving up cigarettes   +2
    B. None for 5 to 15 years   +1
    C. None for 1 to 5 years   0
    D. None for 0 to 1 year   −1
    E. Smoker, less than 1 pack per day   −3
    F. Smoker, 1 pack per day   −5
    G. Smoker, up to 2 packs per day   −7
    H. Smoker, more than 2 packs per day   −10

19. Do you use tobacco products other than cigarettes?
    A. Never have   0
    B. Less than once per week   −1
    C. Once per week   −2
    D. 2 to 6 times per week   −3
    E. More than 6 times per week   −5

20. How often are you exposed to secondhand smoke or other environmental pollutants?
    A. Less than 1 hour per month   0
    B. Between 1 and 5 hours per month   −1
    C. Between 5 and 29 hours per month   −2
    D. Daily   −3

21. Do you use addictive drugs, other than tobacco or alcohol?
    A. None   0
    B. 1   −3
    C. 2 or more   −5

22. What is the age of your parents (or how long did they live)?
    A. Both over 76   +3
    B. Only one over 76   +1
    C. Both are still alive and under 76   0
    D. Only one under 76   −1
    E. Neither one lived past 76   −3

23. What is your body composition category (see Table 7.9 on page 184)?
    A. Excellent   +2
    B. Good   +1
    C. Average   0
    D. Overweight   −1
    E. Significantly overweight   −2

24. What is your blood pressure?
    A. 120/80 or less (both numbers)   +2
    B. 120–140 or 80–90 (either number)   −1
    C. Greater than 140/90 (either number)   −3

25. What is your HDL-cholesterol?
    A. Men greater than 45, women over 55   +2
    B. Men 35 to 44, women 45 to 54   0
    C. Don't know   −1
    D. Men less than 35, women below 45   −2

26. What is your LDL-cholesterol?
    A. Less than 130   +2
    B. Don't know   −1
    C. 130 to 159   −1
    D. 160 or higher   −2

27. Do you floss and brush your teeth regularly?
    A. Every day   +.5
    B. 3 to 6 days per week   0
    C. Less than 3 days per week   −.5

28. Are you a diabetic?
    A. No   0
    B. Yes, well-controlled   −1
    C. Yes, poorly or not controlled   −3

29. How often do you sunbathe (tan)?
    A. Not at all   +1
    B. Between 1 and 3 times per year   −.5
    C. More than 3 times per year   −1

30. How often do you wear a seat belt?
    A. All the time   +1
    B. Most of the time   −.5
    C. Less than half the time   −1

Page score: [＿＿＿＿]

(continued)

31. How fast do you drive?
    A. Always at or below
       the speed limit 0
    B. Up to 5 mph over the
       speed limit −.5
    C. Between 5 and 10 mph
       over the speed limit −1
    D. More than 10 mph
       over the speed limit −2

32. Do you drink and drive?
    A. Never 0
    B. Yes (even if only once) −5

33. In terms of your sexual activity:
    A. I am not sexually active
       or I am in a monogamous
       sexual relationship +1
    B. I have more than one
       sexual partner but I always
       practice safer sex −1
    C. I have multiple sexual
       partners and I do not
       practice safer sex
       techniques −3

34. What is your marital status?
    A. Happily married +1
    B. Single and happy 0
    C. Single and unhappy −.5
    D. Divorced −1
    E. Widowed with a belief
       in life hereafter −1
    F. Widowed −2
    G. Married and unhappy −2

35. On the average, how many
    hours of sleep do you get
    each night?
    A. 7 to 8 +1
    B. 7 0
    C. 6 to 7 −1
    D. Less than 6 −2

36. Your stress rating according
    to the Life Experiences Survey
    (see Figure 12.2) is:
    A. Excellent +1
    B. Good 0
    C. Average −.5
    D. Fair −1
    E. Poor −2

37. Your Type A behavior rating is:
    A. Low 0
    B. Medium −1
    C. High −2

38. When under stress (distress),
    how often do you practice
    stress management
    techniques?
    A. Always +1
    B. Most of the time +.5
    C. Not applicable (don't
       suffer from stress) 0
    D. Sometimes −1
    E. Never −2

39. Do you suffer from
    depression?
    A. Not at all 0
    B. Mild depression −1
    C. Severe depression −2

40. How often do you associate
    with people who have a
    positive attitude about life?
    A. Always +.5
    B. Most of the time 0
    C. About half of the time −.5
    D. Less than half the time −1

41. Do you have close family or
    personal relationships whom
    you can trust and rely on for
    help in times of need?
    A. Yes +1
    B. No −1

42. Do you feel loved and can
    you routinely give affection
    and love?
    A. Yes +1
    B. No −1

43. Do you have a good sense
    of humor?
    A. Yes +1
    B. No −1

44. How satisfied are you with
    your school work?
    A. Satisfied +.5
    B. It's okay 0
    C. Not satisfied −.5

45. How do you rate your
    present job satisfaction?
    A. Love it +1
    B. Like it 0
    C. It's okay −.5
    D. Don't like it −1
    E. Hate it −2
    F. Not applicable 0

46. How do you rate yourself
    spiritually?
    A. Very spiritual +1
    B. Spiritual 0
    C. Somewhat spiritual −.5
    D. Not spiritual at all −1

Page score: [   ]

_____

**Net score for
all questions:** [   ]

How To Score

To estimate the total number of years that you will live, (a) determine a net score by totaling the results from all 46 questions, (b) obtain an age change score by multiplying the net score by the age correction factor given below, and (c) add or subtract this number from your base life expectancy age (73 for men and 80 for women—the current life expectancies in the United States). For example, if you are a 20-year-old male and the net score from the answers to all questions was −16, your estimated life expectancy would be 68.2 years (age change score = −16 × .3 = −4.8, life expectancy = 73 − 4.8 = 68.2).

You can also determine your real physiological age by subtracting a positive age-change score or adding a negative age-change score to your current chronological (calendar) age. For instance, in the previous example, the real physiological age would be 24.8 years (20 + 4.8). If the age change score had been +4.8, the real physiological age would have been 16.2 years. Thus, a healthy lifestyle will always make your physiological age younger than your chronological age. Your real physiological age will have much greater significance in middle and older age, when it is not uncommon to see real-age reductions of 10 to 25 years in people who lead healthy lifestyles. Thus a 50-year-old person could easily have a real physiological age of 30.

Age Correction Factor (ACF)*

Age	ACF
≤30	.3
31–40	.4
41–50	.5
51–60	.6
61–70	.6
71–80	.5
81–90	.4
≥91	.3

*Adapted from: M. F. Roizen, *RealAge*, (New York: Cliff Street Books, 1999).

Age Change Score (ACS) = ☐ (net score) × ☐ (ACF) = ☐

Life expectancy

Men = 73 ± ☐ (ACS) = ☐ years

Women = 80 ± ☐ (ACS) = ☐ years

Real physiological Age**

Men = ☐ (your age) ± ☐ (ACS) = ☐ years

Women = ☐ (your age) ± ☐ (ACS) = ☐ years

**Subtract a positive ACS from, or add a negative ACS to, your current age.

conclusion

State your feelings about the experience of taking this questionnaire, analyze your results, and list lifestyle factors that you can work on that will positively affect your health and longevity.

_____

_____

_____

_____

_____

_____

_____

_____

_____

_____

_____

_____

Unconventional medicine is referred to as complementary and alternative medicine because patients use it to either augment their regular medical care or as a replacement for conventional practices. In 1997, over 46 percent of Americans used complementary and alternative medicine services. This figure represented about 629 million appointments with practitioners,[2] thereby surpassing the total number of visits to all U.S. primary care physicians.

The National Center for Complementary and Alternative Medicine (NCCAM), under the National Institutes of Health, was recently established to examine methods of healing that have previously been unexplored by science. The NCCAM defines complementary and alternative medicine as those treatments and health care practices not widely taught in medical schools, not generally used in hospitals, and not usually reimbursed by medical insurance companies. Many physicians, nonetheless, now endorse complementary and alternative treatments, and an ever-increasing number of medical schools are offering courses in this area.

Alternative medicine practices have not gone through the same standard scrutiny as conventional medicine. Nonallopathic treatments are often based on theories that have not been scientifically proven. This does not imply that unconventional medicine practices do not help people. Many people have found relief from ailments or been cured through unconventional treatments. In due time, however, these theories will need to be investigated using scientific trials similar to those in conventional medicine.

Complementary and alternative medicine includes a wide range of healing philosophies, approaches, and therapies. The practices most often associated with **nonallopathic medicine** are **acupuncture, chiropractics, herbal medicine, homeopathy, naturopathic medicine, ayurveda, magnetic therapy**, and **massage therapy**. Each of these practices, some of which are hundreds or thousands of years old, offers a different approach to treatments based on its beliefs about the body.

Many of these practitioners believe that their treatment modality aids the body as it performs its own natural healing process. Because of their approach, alternative treatments usually take longer than conventional allopathic medical care. Nonallopathic treatments are usually less harsh on the patient, and practitioners tend to avoid surgery and extensive use of medications.

Unconventional therapies are frequently viewed as holistic, implying that the practitioner looks at all the dimensions of wellness when evaluating a person's condition. Practitioners often persuade patients to adopt healthier lifestyle habits that not only help to improve current conditions but prevent other ailments as well. Complementary and alternative medicine also allows patients to better understand treatments, and patients are often allowed to administer self-treatment.

Costs for complementary and alternative medicine practices are typically lower than conventional medicine costs. With the exception of acupuncture and chiropractic care, most nonallopathic treatments are not covered by health insurance. Typically, patients pay directly for these services. In 1997, a conservative estimate of $21.2 billion was spent on alternative medical treatments, with at least $12.2 billion paid out-of-pocket.[3] These costs exceeded the out-of-pocket expenses for all hospitalizations in the United States. If you are considering alternative medical therapies, consult with your health care insurance provider to determine which therapies are reimbursable.

Complementary and alternative medicine does have shortcomings. Many of the practitioners do not have the years of education given to conventional medical personnel and often know less about physiological responses that occur in the body. Some practices are completely void of science; hence, the practitioner can rarely explain the specific physiologic benefits of the treatment used. Much of the knowledge is based on experiences with previous patients.

KeyTerms

Unconventional medicine See complementary and alternative medicine.

Nonallopathic medicine See complementary and alternative medicine.

Acupuncture Chinese medical system that requires body piercing with fine needles during therapy to relieve pain and treat ailments and diseases.

Chiropractics Health care system that believes that many diseases and ailments are related to misalignments of the vertebrae and emphasizes the manipulation of the spinal column.

Herbal medicine Unconventional system that uses herbs to treat ailments and disease.

Homeopathy System of treatment based on the use of minute quantities of remedies that in large amounts produce effects similar to the disease being treated.

Naturopathic medicine Unconventional system of medicine that relies exclusively on natural remedies to treat disease and ailments.

Ayurveda Unconventional Hindu system of medicine based on herbs, diet, massage, meditation, and yoga to help the body boost its own natural healing.

Magnetic therapy Unconventional treatment that relies on magnetic energy to promote healing.

Massage therapy The rubbing or kneading of body parts to treat ailments.

The practice of complementary and alternative medicine is not regulated like that of conventional medicine. The training and certification of practitioners, malpractice liability, and evaluation of tests and methods used in treatments are not routinely standardized. Many states, however, license practitioners in the areas of chiropractic services, acupuncture, naturopathy, homeopathy, herbal therapy, and massage therapy. Other therapies, however, are unmonitored.

> **"Natural" does not imply that a product is safe. Many products, including some herbs, can be toxic in large doses.**

Another concern in unconventional medicine is the lack of regulation of natural and herbal products. The word "natural" does not imply that the product is safe. Many products, including some herbs, can be toxic in large doses. Additionally, an estimated 15 million Americans combine high-dose vitamins and/or herbal supplements with prescription drugs (about one-fifth of all prescription users).[4] Such combinations can yield undesirable side effects. Individuals should always let their health care practitioners know which medications and alternative (including vitamin and mineral) supplements are being taken in combination.

Herbal medicine has been around for centuries. Through trial and error, by design, or by accident, people have found that certain plant substances have medicinal properties. Today many of these plant substances have been replaced by products that are safer, more effective, and have fewer negative side effects. Although science has found the mechanisms whereby some herbs work, much work remains to be done.

Many herbs or herbal remedies are not safe for human use and continue to meet resistance from the scientific community. One of the main concerns is that active ingredients in drug therapy must be administered in accurate dosages. With herbal medicine, the potency cannot always be adequately controlled.

Some herbs produce undesirable side effects. For example, Ephedra (ma huang), a popular weight loss and energy supplement, can cause high blood pressure, rapid heart rate, tremor, seizures, headaches, insomnia, stroke, and even death. More than 1,100 ephedra-related adverse effects have been reported, including 10 deaths and 13 permanent disabilities. St. John's wort, commonly taken as an antidepressant, can produce serious interactions with drugs used to treat heart disease. Ginkgo biloba impairs blood clotting, thus it can cause bleeding in people who are also taking regular blood-thinning medication or aspirin therapy. Other herbs like yohimbe, chaparral, comfrey, and jin bu juan have been linked to adverse events.

Increasingly, conventional health care providers can refer you to someone who is familiar with alternative treatments. But you need to be an informed consumer. Ask your primary care physician to obtain valid information regarding the safety and effectiveness of a particular treatment. At times, nonetheless, the medical community resists and rejects unconventional therapies. If your physician is unable or unwilling to provide you with this information, medical, college, or public libraries and popular bookstores are good places to search for this information. You need to educate yourself about the advantages and disadvantages of alternative treatments, risks, side effects, expected results, and length of therapy.

Information on a wide range of medical conditions or specific diseases can also be obtained by calling the National Institutes of Health (NIH) at (301) 496-4000. Ask the operator to direct you to the appropriate NIH office. The NCCAM office also provides a Web site (nccam.nih.gov) with access to over 180,000 bibliographic references to research published on complementary and alternative medicine during the last 35 years.

When selecting a primary care physician or a nonallopathic practitioner, local and state medical boards, other health regulatory boards and agencies, and consumer affairs departments can provide information about a given practitioner's education, accreditation, license, and complaints that may have been filed against this health care provider. Many of the unconventional medical fields also have a national organization that provides guidelines for practitioners and health consumers. These organizations can guide you to the appropriate regulatory agencies within your state where you can obtain information regarding a specific practitioner.

You may also talk to other individuals who have undergone similar therapies and learn about the confidence and competence of the practitioner in question. Keep in mind, however, that patient testimonials do not adequately assess the safety and effectiveness of alternative treatments. Whenever possible, search for results of controlled scientific trials of the therapy in question and use this information in your decision process.

When undergoing any type of treatment or therapy, always discuss this information with all of your health care providers, whether conventional or unconventional. Adequate health care management requires that health care providers be informed of all concurrent therapies, so they will have a complete picture of the treatment plan. Lack of knowledge by one health care provider regarding treatments by another provider can interfere with the healing process or even worsen a given condition.

Millions of Americans have benefited from complementary and alternative medicine practices. You may also benefit from such services, but you need to make careful and educated decisions about the available options. By finding well-trained (and preferably licensed) practitioners, you increase your chances for recovery from ailments and disease.

Quackery and Fraud

The rapid growth of the fitness and wellness industry during the last three decades has spurred the promotion of fraudulent products that deceive consumers into purchasing "miraculous," quick, and easy ways to achieve total well-being. Fraudulent products are easily promoted under the guise of new medical breakthroughs or alternative medicine practices that are all too familiar to the consumer and are readily accepted without scientific proof. **Quackery** and **fraud** have been defined as the conscious promotion of unproven claims for profit.

Today's market is saturated with "special" foods, diets, supplements, pills, cures, equipment, services, beauty aids, books, and videos that promise quick, dramatic results. Advertisements for these products often are based on testimonials, unproven claims, secret research, half-truths, and quick-fix statements that the uneducated consumer wants to hear. In the meantime, the organization or enterprise making the claims stands to make a large profit from the consumers' willingness to pay for astonishing and spectacular solutions to problems related to their unhealthy lifestyle. Not only are consumers wasting time and money that could go toward proven treatments, but they often suffer adverse side effects that, in extreme cases, may even cause death.

Television, magazine, and newspaper advertisements are not necessarily reliable. For instance, one piece of equipment sold through television and newspaper advertisements promised to "bust the gut" through 5 minutes of daily exercise that appeared to target the abdominal muscle group. This piece of equipment consisted of a metal spring attached to the feet on one end and held in the hands on the other end. According to handling and shipping distributors, the equipment was "selling like hotcakes," and companies could barely keep up with consumer demands.

Three problems became apparent to the educated consumer: First, there is no such thing as spot-reducing; therefore, the claims could not be true. Second, 5 minutes of daily exercise burn hardly any calories and, therefore, have no effect on weight loss.

Third, the intended abdominal (gut) muscles were not really involved during the exercise. The exercise engaged mostly the gluteal and lower back muscles. This piece of equipment now can be found at garage sales for about a tenth of its original cost!

Although people in the United States tend to be firm believers in the benefits of physical activity and positive lifestyle habits as a means to promote better health, most do not reap these benefits because they simply do not know how to put into practice a sound fitness and wellness program that will give them the results they want. Unfortunately, many uneducated wellness consumers are targets of deception by organizations that make fraudulent claims for their products.

Deception is not limited to advertisements. Deceit is found all around us. One can find it in newspaper and magazine articles, trade books, radio, and television shows. To make a profit, popular magazines occasionally exaggerate health claims or leave out pertinent information to avoid offending advertisers. Some publishers print books on diets or self-treatment approaches that have no scientific foundation. Consumers should even be cautious about news reports of the latest medical breakthroughs. Reporters have been known to overlook important information or give certain findings greater credence than they deserve.

Precautions must also be taken when seeking health advice on the Internet. The Internet is full of both credible and dubious information. The following tips can help as you conduct a search on the Internet:

- Look for credentials of the person or organization sponsoring the site.

- Check when the site was last updated. Credible sites are updated often.

- Check the appearance of the information on the site. It should be presented in a professional manner. If every sentence ends with an exclamation point, you have a good cause for suspicion.

- Exercise caution if the site's sponsor is trying to sell a product. If so, be leery of opinions posted on the site. They could be biased, given that the company's main objective is to sell a product. Credible companies trying to sell a product on the Internet usually reference their sources of health information and provide additional links that support their product.

KeyTerms

Quackery/Fraud The conscious promotion of unproven claims for profit.

- Compare a site's content to other credible sources. The contents should compare favorably to that of other reputable sites or publications.

- Note the address and contact information for the company. A reliable company will list more than a P.O. box, an 800 number, and the company's e-mail address. When only the latter information is provided, consumers may never be able to locate the company for questions, concerns, or refunds.

- Be on the alert for companies that claim to be innovators while criticizing competitors or the government for being close-minded or trying to keep them from doing business.

- Watch for advertisers that use valid medical terminology in an irrelevant context or use vague pseudomedical jargon to sell their product.

Not all people who promote fraudulent products, however, know they are doing so. Some may be convinced that the product is effective. If you have questions or concerns about a health product, you may write to the National Council Against Health Fraud (NCAHF), P.O. Box 141, Fort Lee, NJ 07021. The purpose of this organization is to provide the consumer with responsible, reliable, evidence-driven health information. The organization also monitors deceitful advertising, investigates complaints, and offers public information regarding fraudulent health claims. You may also report any type of quackery to them on their Web site at http://www.ncahf.org/. The site contains an updated list of reliable and unreliable health Web sites for the consumer.

Other consumer protection organizations offer to follow up on complaints about quackery and fraud. The existence of these organizations, however, should not give the consumer a false sense of security. The overwhelming number of complaints made each year to these organizations makes it impossible for them to follow up on each case individually. The FDA's Center for Drug Evaluation Research, for example, has developed a priority system to determine which health fraud product it should regulate first. Products are rated on how great a risk they pose to the consumer. With this in mind, you can use the following list of organizations to make an educated decision before you spend your money. You can also report consumer fraud to these organizations:

- The Food and Drug Administration (FDA). The FDA regulates safety and labeling of health products and cosmetics. You can search for the office closest to you in the federal government listings (blue pages) of the phone book.

- The Better Business Bureau (BBB). The BBB can tell you whether other customers have lodged complaints about a product, a company, or a salesperson. You can find a listing for the local office in the business section of the phone book or you can check their Web site at http://www.betterbusinessbureau.com/.

- The Consumer Product Safety Commission (CPS). This independent federal regulatory agency targets products that threaten the safety of American families. Unsafe products can be researched and reported on their Web site at http://www.cpsc.gov/.

Another way to get informed before you make your purchase is to seek the advice of a reputable professional. Ask someone who understands the product but does not stand to profit from the transaction. As examples, a physical educator or an exercise physiologist can advise you regarding exercise equipment; a registered dietitian can provide information on nutrition and weight control programs; a physician can offer advice on nutritive supplements. Also, be alert to those who bill themselves as "experts." Look for qualifications, degrees, professional experience, certifications, and reputation.

Keep in mind that if it sounds too good to be true, it probably is. Fraudulent promotions often rely on testimonials or scare tactics and promise their products will cure a long list of unrelated ailments; they use words like quick-fix, time-tested, new-found, miraculous, special, secret, all natural, mail-order only, and money-back guarantee. Deceptive companies move often enough that customers have no way of contacting the company to ask for a reimbursement.

When claims are made, ask where the claims are published. Refereed scientific journals are the most reliable sources of information. When a researcher submits information for publication in a refereed journal, at least two qualified and reputable professionals in the field conduct blind reviews of the manuscript. A blind review means the author does not know who will review the manuscript and the reviewers do not know who submitted the manuscript. Acceptance for publication is based on this input and relevant changes.

HEALTH/FITNESS CLUB MEMBERSHIPS

As you follow a lifetime wellness program, you may want to consider joining a health/fitness facility. Or, if you have mastered the contents of this book and if your choice of fitness activity is one you can pursue on your own (walking, jogging, cycling), you may not need to join a health club. Barring injuries, you may continue your exercise program outside the walls of

Reliable sources of health, fitness, nutrition, and wellness information

Newsletter	Approx. Yearly Issues	Annual Cost
Bottom Line / Personal Health P.O. Box 53408 Boulder, CO 80322-3408	12	$49
Consumer Reports Health Letter P.O. Box 56356 Boulder, CO 80323-2148	12	$24
HealthNews P.O. Box 8963 Waltham, MA 02254-9959	12	$29
Tufts University Diet & Nutrition Letter P.O. Box 57857 Boulder, CO 80322-7857	12	$28
University of California Berkeley *Wellness Letter* P.O. Box 420148 Palm Coast, FL 32142	12	$29

Reliable health web sites

- American Cancer Society
  http://cancer.org/
- American Heart Association
  http://americanheart.org
- Clinical Trials Center
  http://www.med-library.com/medlibrary/
- Department of Health and Human Services
  http://www.healthfinder.gov
- HospitalWeb
  http://neuro-www.mgh.harvard.edu/hospitalweb.shtml
- National Cancer Institute
  http://cancernet.nci.nih.gov/
- National Center for Complementary and Alternative Medicine
  http://nccam.nih.gov/
- The National Library of Medicine
  http://www.nlm.nih.gov/
- The National Institutes of Health
  http://www.nih.gov/
- The Centers for Disease Control
  http://www.cdc.gov/
- The Global Health Network
  http://www.pitt.edu/HOME/GHNet/GHNet.html
- The Medical Matrix
  http://www.medmatrix.org/Index.asp
- The National Council for Reliable Health Information
  http://www.ncahf.org/
- The Annals of Internal Medicine
  http://www.acponline.org/index.html
- The Food and Drug Administration
  http://www.fda.gov/
- WebMD
  http://webmd.com/
- World Health Organization
  http://www.who.ch/

a health club for the rest of your life. You also can conduct strength training and stretching programs in your own home (see Chapters 5 and 6).

To stay up-to-date on fitness and wellness developments, you probably should buy a reputable and updated fitness/wellness book every 4 to 5 years. You might subscribe to a credible health, fitness, nutrition, or wellness newsletter to stay current. You can also surf the World Wide Web, but be sure that the sites you are searching are from credible and reliable organizations.

If you are contemplating membership in a fitness facility, do all of the following:

- Examine all exercise options in your community: health clubs and spas, YMCAs, gyms, colleges, schools, community centers, senior centers, and the like.

- Check to see if the facility's atmosphere is pleasurable and nonthreatening to you. Will you feel comfortable with the instructors and other people who go there? Is it clean and well kept up? If the answer is no, this may not be the right place for you.

- Analyze costs versus facilities, equipment, and programs. Take a look at your personal budget. Will you really use the facility? Will you exercise there regularly? Many people obtain memberships and permit dues to be withdrawn automatically from a local bank account, yet seldom attend the fitness center.

- Find out what types of facilities are available: walking/running track, basketball/tennis/racquetball courts, aerobic exercise room, strength training room, pool, locker rooms, saunas, hot tubs, handicapped access, and so on.

- Check the aerobic and strength-training equipment available. Does the facility have treadmills, bicycle ergometers, stair climbers, cross-country skiing simulators, free weights, strength-training units? Make sure the facilities and equipment meet your activity interests.

- Consider the location. Is the facility close, or do you have to travel several miles to get there? Distance often discourages participation.

- Check on times the facility is accessible. Is it open during your preferred exercise time (for example, early morning or late evening)?

- Work out at the facility several times before becoming a member. Are people standing in line to use the equipment, or is it readily available during your exercise time?

- Inquire about the instructors' qualifications. Do the fitness instructors have college degrees or professional certifications from organizations such as the American College of Sports Medicine (ACSM) or the International Dance Exercise Association (IDEA)? These organizations have rigorous standards to ensure professional preparation and quality of instruction.

- Consider the approach to fitness (including all health-related components of fitness). Is it well-rounded? Do the instructors spend time with members, or do members have to seek them out constantly for help and instruction?

- Ask about supplementary services. Does the facility provide or contract out for regular health and fitness assessments (cardiorespiratory endurance, body composition, blood pressure, blood chemistry analysis)? Are wellness seminars (nutrition, weight control, stress management) offered? Do these have hidden costs?

PURCHASING EXERCISE EQUIPMENT

A final consideration is that of purchasing your own exercise equipment. The first question you need to ask yourself is: Do I really need this piece of equipment? Most people buy on impulse because of television advertisements or because a salesperson convinced them it is a great piece of equipment that will do wonders for their health and fitness. With some creativity, you can implement an excellent and comprehensive exercise program with little, if any, equipment (see Chapters 4, 5, and 6).

Many people buy expensive equipment only to find they really do not enjoy that mode of activity. They do not remain regular users. Stationary bicycles (lower body only) and rowing ergometers were among the most popular pieces of equipment in the 1980s. Most of them now are seldom used and have become "fitness furniture" somewhere in the basement.

Exercise equipment does have its value for people who prefer to exercise indoors, especially during the winter months. It supports some people's motivation and adherence to exercise. The convenience of having equipment at home also allows for flexible scheduling. You can exercise before or after work or while you watch your favorite television show.

If you are going to purchase equipment, the best recommendation is to actually try it out several times before buying it. Ask yourself several questions: Did you enjoy the workout? Is the unit comfortable? Are you too short, tall, or heavy for it? Is it stable, sturdy, and strong? Do you have to assemble the machine? If so, how difficult is it to put together? How durable is it? Ask for references—people or clubs that have used the equipment extensively. Are they satisfied? Have they enjoyed using the equipment? Talk with professionals at colleges, sports medicine clinics, or health clubs.

Another consideration is to look at used units for signs of wear and tear. Quality is important. Cheaper brands may not be durable, so your investment would be wasted.

Finally, watch out for expensive gadgets. Monitors that provide exercise heart rate, work output, caloric expenditure, speed, grade, and distance may help motivate you, but they are expensive, need repairs, and do not enhance the actual fitness benefits of the workout. Look at maintenance costs and check for service personnel in your community.

SELF-EVALUATION AND BEHAVIORAL OBJECTIVES FOR THE FUTURE

The main objective of this book is to provide the information and experiences necessary to implement your personal fitness and wellness program. If you have implemented the programs in this book, including exercise, you should be convinced that a wellness lifestyle is the only way to attain a higher quality of life.

Most people who engage in a personal fitness and wellness program experience this new quality of life after only a few weeks of training and practicing healthy lifestyle patterns. In some instances, however —especially for individuals who have led a poor lifestyle for a long time—a few months may be required to establish positive habits and feelings of well-being. In the end, though, everyone who applies the principles of fitness and wellness will reap the desired benefits.

Self-Evaluation

Throughout this course you have had an opportunity to assess various fitness and wellness components and write behavioral objectives to improve your quality of life. You now should take the time to evaluate how well you have achieved your own objectives. First of all, assess how well you accomplished your goals for the seven dimensions of wellness. Use the form provided in Figure 1.23 (page 28). Second, if time allows and facilities and technicians are available, reassess the health-related components of physical fitness. If you are unable to reassess these components, determine subjectively how well you accomplished your objectives. You will find a self-evaluation form in Figure A.1 of Appendix A.

Behavioral Objectives for the Future

The real challenge will come now that you are about to finish this course: a lifetime commitment to fitness and wellness. Adhering to a program in a structured setting is a lot easier, but from now on you will be on your own. If you have not achieved all of your objectives during this course, or if you need to reach beyond your current achievements, the "Self Evaluation of Wellness Components" provided in Figure 15.3 will help you chart the future. This guide provides a list of various wellness components, each accompanied by a scale from poor to excellent. Using the Wellness Scale, rate yourself for each component according to the following instructions:

1. Indicate with an "I" (I = Initial) the rating from poor to excellent where you stood on each component at the beginning of the semester. For example, if at the start of this course, you rated poor in cardiorespiratory endurance, place an "I" under the poor column for this component.

2. Mark with a "C" (C = Current) a second column (between poor and excellent) to indicate where you stand on each component at the current time. If your level of cardiorespiratory endurance improved to average by the end of the semester, write a "C" under this column. If you were not able to work on a given component, simply make a "C" out of the "I."

3. Select one or two components you intend to work on in the next 2 months. Developing new behavioral patterns takes time, and trying to work on too many components at once most likely will lower your chances for success. Start with components in which you think you will have a high chance for success.

Next, place a "G" (G = Goal) under the intended column (rating) to accomplish by the end of this period. If your goal in the next 2 months is to achieve a good level of cardiorespiratory endurance, place a "G" under the good column for this component in the Wellness Scale.

Use Figure 15.4 to write the goals and behavioral objectives for two components you intend to work on during the next 2 months. As you write and work on these goals and objectives, review the goal setting guidelines provided in Chapter 2, pages 41–43. Using these guidelines will help you design an effective plan of action to reach your goals.

One final assignment that you should complete is to summarize your feelings about your past and present lifestyle, what you have learned in this course, and changes that you were able to successfully implement. Figure 15.5, page 417, can be used for this experience. You are encouraged to keep this figure in a place that you will remember so that you may review it in months and years to come.

THE FITNESS/WELLNESS EXPERIENCE AND A CHALLENGE FOR THE FUTURE

Patty Neavill is a typical example of someone who often tried to change her life but was unable to do so because she did not know how to implement a sound exercise and weight control program. At age 24 and at 240 pounds, she was discouraged with her weight, level of fitness, self-image, and quality of life in general. She had struggled with her weight most of her life. Like thousands of other people, she had made many unsuccessful attempts to lose weight.

Patty put her fears aside and decided to enroll in a fitness course. As part of the course requirement, a battery of fitness tests was administered at the beginning of the semester. Patty's cardiorespiratory fitness and strength ratings were poor, her flexibility classification was average, and her percent body fat was 41.

Following the initial fitness assessment, Patty met with her course instructor, who prescribed an exercise and nutrition program like the one in this book. Patty fully committed to carry out the prescription. She walked or jogged five times a week. She enrolled in a weight training course that met twice a week. Her daily caloric intake was set in the range of 1,500 to 1,700 calories.

Determined to increase her level of activity further, Patty signed up for recreational volleyball and basketball courses. Besides being fun, these classes provided 4 additional hours of activity per week.

She took care to meet the minimum required servings from the basic food groups each day, which contributed about 1,200 calories to her diet. The remainder of the calories came primarily from complex carbohydrates.

At the end of the 16-week semester, Patty's cardiorespiratory fitness, strength, and flexibility ratings had all improved to the good category, she lost 50 pounds, and her percent body fat had decreased to 22.5!

Patty was tall. At 190 pounds, most people would have thought she was too heavy. Her percent body fat, however, was lower than the average for college female physical education major students (about 23 percent body fat).

A thank-you note from Patty to the course instructor at the end of the semester read:

> *Thank you for making me a new person.*
> *I truly appreciate the time you spent with me.*
> *Without your kindness and motivation, I would*
> *have never made it. It is great to be fit and trim.*
> *I've never had this feeling before, and I wish*
> *everyone could feel like this once in their life.*
> *Thank you,*
> *Your trim Patty!*

Patty never had been taught the principles governing a sound weight loss program. In Patty's case, not only did she need this knowledge, but, like most Americans who never have experienced the process of becoming physically fit, she needed to be in a structured exercise setting to truly feel the joy of fitness.

Even more significant, Patty maintained her aerobic and strength-training programs. A year after ending her calorie-restricted diet, her weight increased by 10 pounds, but her body fat decreased from 22.5 to 21.2 percent. As you may recall from Chapter 9, this weight increase is related mostly to changes in lean tissue, lost during the weight-reduction phase.

In spite of only a slight drop in weight during the second year following the calorie-restricted diet, the 2-year follow-up revealed a further decrease in body fat, to 19.5 percent. Patty understood the new quality of life reaped through a sound fitness program, and, at the same time, she finally learned how to apply the principles that regulate weight maintenance.

Prior to her marriage, a young lady who never had been on a jogging program became convinced that aerobic exercise would improve her fitness and help her maintain recommended body weight. Her fiancé believed in fitness and had been jogging regularly for several years. An exercise prescription was written, and they started jogging together.

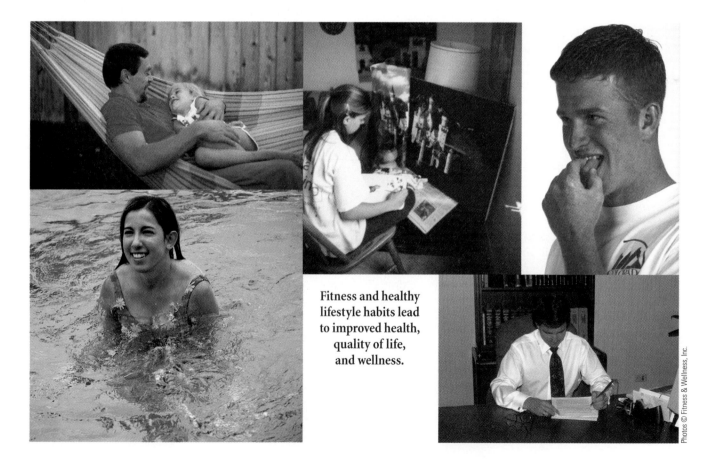

Fitness and healthy lifestyle habits lead to improved health, quality of life, and wellness.

FIGURE 15.3 Self-evaluation of wellness components.

Name: _____ Date: _____

Course: _____ Section: _____ Gender: _____ Age: _____

Wellness Rating

Wellness Components	Poor	Fair	Average	Good	Excellent
Cardiorespiratory Endurance					
Muscular Strength/Endurance					
Muscular Flexibility					
Body Composition					
Nutrition					
Cardiovascular Disease Prevention					
Cancer Prevention					
Stress Control					
Tobacco Use					
Substance Abuse Control*					
Sexuality*					
Accident Prevention and Personal Safety					
Spirituality*					
Health Education					

*These components are personal, and you are not required to reveal this information. If you think that counseling is necessary, you are encouraged to seek professional help.

FIGURE 15.4 Behavioral objectives for the future.

Select two wellness components that you will work on during the next couple of months. Specify your goals and write specific objectives that will lead to the accomplishment of these goals (you may not need six objectives; write only as many as needed).

Goal: _____

Objectives:

1. _____

2. _____

3. _____

4. _____

5. _____

6. _____

Goal: _____

Objectives:

1. _____

2. _____

3. _____

4. _____

5. _____

6. _____

Exercise helped accomplish her goals through her first two pregnancies. The feeling of being physically fit was a reward in itself, but being able to jog 2 consecutive miles was seldom truly enjoyable. With young children at home, the couple was forced to take turns jogging so that one always could be home. Her jogging program consisted of a 20-minute jog: 1 mile out and 1 mile back.

One day 25 minutes went by and she had not returned home. At 30 minutes, there was a knock on the door: "Honey, I feel great, I'll be back in 10 minutes." This same event was repeated at 40 and 50 minutes. That young lady had jogged for a full 60 minutes for the first time in her life, and the experience was genuinely joyful. That day, this lady finally reached "the top of the mountain" and experienced the joy of being physically fit. Jogging became as easy as a "bird in flight." She has not stopped jogging in more than 25 years! It wasn't easy at first, but knowledge, commitment, support, action, and perseverance paid off.

Fitness was also the factor that led to improvements in other wellness components in the lives of this couple (continuing health education, proper nutrition, stress reduction, and chronic disease prevention). Fitness is the daily "bread and butter" that enhances their quality of life. Their children now also follow the parents' active lifestyle. This has prompted the parents to say: "The family that exercises together stays together."

If you have read and successfully completed all of the assignments set out in this book, including a regular exercise program, you should be convinced of the value of exercise and healthy lifestyle habits in achieving a new quality of life.

Perhaps this new quality of life was explained best by the late Dr. George Sheehan, when he wrote:

> For every runner who tours the world running marathons, there are thousands who run to hear the leaves and listen to the rain, and look to the day when it is all suddenly as easy as a bird in flight. For them, sport is not a test but a therapy, not a trial but a reward, not a question but an answer.

The real challenge will come now: a lifetime commitment to fitness and wellness. To make the commitment easier, enjoy yourself and have fun along the way. Implement your program based on your interests and what you enjoy doing most. Then adhering to your new lifestyle will not be difficult.

Your activities over the last few weeks or months may have helped you develop "positive addictions" that will carry on throughout life. If you truly experience the feelings Dr. Sheehan expressed, there will be no looking back. If you don't get there, you won't know what it's like. Fitness and wellness is a process, and you need to put forth a constant and deliberate effort to achieve and maintain a higher quality of life. Improving the quality of your life, and most likely your longevity, is in your hands. Only you can take control of your lifestyle and thereby reap the benefits of wellness.

WEB INTERACTIVE

How Can I Determine an Exercise Program that Meets My Needs?

This site features a general four-part guide to help you determine your appropriate exercise intensity level, its frequency, and the best types of exercises for you based on your goals for weight loss, improving muscle tone, increasing flexibility, and/or overall fitness.

http://kirtland.cc.mi.us/~balbahl/exprog.htm

Getting Started with an Exercise Program

This comprehensive site, from Georgia State University's Department of Kinesiology and Health, features information on the benefits of exercise, how to choose a personal trainer, exercise safety and precautions, and more.

http://www.gsu.edu/~wwwfit/getstart.html

National Center for Complementary and Alternative Medicine

This comprehensive site features information about a variety of complementary therapies geared for consumers, clinical practitioners, and investigators. The site also features a complementary medicine database, clinical trials information, and a list of resources.

http://www.nccam.nih.gov/fi/

INTERACTIVE SITES:

Dr. Koop's Preventionaire

A quick personal information survey to help guide you toward a healthy lifestyle, with information to share with your doctor that will empower you to take control of your own health.

http://www.drkoop.com/wellness/prevention

RealAge

This site features an online personal assessment of a variety of lifestyle behaviors that also suggests behaviors that will enable people to live younger longer.

http://www.realage.com

Lifestyle Behavior Risk Assessment (LiBRA)

This site, sponsored by the Health Education Department of Michigan State University's Olin Health Center, features a comprehensive series of questions on the following subjects: eating habits, exercise habits, stress, preventive health, smoking, sexual health, alcohol. Based on your responses, you will be able to determine your overall health risk for a variety of health conditions.

http://www.approg.cl.msu.edu/olin

n*tes

1. R. J. Donatelle and L. G. Davis, *Access to Health* (Boston: Allyn and Bacon, 2000).
2. D. M. Eisenberg et al., "Trends in Alternative Medicine Use in the United States, 1990–1997," *Journal of the American Medical Association* 280, no. 18 (1998): 1569–1575.
3. See note 2.
4. See note 2.

Suggested Readings

■ Roizen, M. F. *Real Age: Are You As Young As You Can Be?* New York: Cliff Street Books, 1999.

FIGURE 15.5 Wellness lifestyle self-assessment.

I. Explain the exercise program that you implemented in this course. Express your feelings about the outcomes of this program and how well you accomplished your fitness goals.

II. List nutritional or dietary changes that you were able to implement this term and the effects of these changes on your body composition and personal wellness.

(continued)

(Figure 15.5 Wellness lifestyle self-assessment—continued)

III. List other lifestyle changes that you were able to make this term that may decrease your risk for disease. In a few sentences, explain how you feel about these changes and their impact on your overall well-being.

IV. Briefly evaluate this course and its impact on your quality of life. Indicate what you feel will be needed for you to continue to adhere to an active and healthy lifestyle.

Appendix A

Physical Fitness and Wellness Profile

Fill out the following profile as you obtain the results for each fitness and wellness component. Attempt to determine the four fitness components (cardiorespiratory endurance, muscular strength/endurance, muscular flexibility, and body composition) during the first 2 or 3 weeks so you may proceed with your exercise program. After determining each component, discuss with your instructor the objectives to be accomplished and the date of completion.

© 2002 EyeWire Collection/Getty Images

FIGURE A • 1 Personal fitness and wellness profile.

Name: _____ Course: _____ Section: _____ Gender: _____ Age: _____

Item	Pre-Assessment			Objective[a]	Post-Assessment		
	Date	Test Results	Classification		Date	Test Results	Classification
Cardiorespiratory Endurance							
Muscular Strength							
Muscular Flexibility							
Body Composition							
Cardiovascular Risk							
Cancer Risk							
Lung							
Colon-Rectum							
Skin							
Breast[b]							
Cervical[b]							
Endometrial[b]							
Prostate[c]							
Testicular[c]							
Pancreatic							
Kidney & Bladder							
Esophageal & Stomach							
Ovarian[b]							
Thyroid							
Leukemia							
Lymphomas							
Stress							
Life Exp. Survey							
Vulnerability Scale							
Tobacco Use[d]							

INSTRUCTOR'S SIGNATURE: _____ STUDENT'S SIGNATURE: _____

[a] Indicate specific objective and date of completion.
[b] Women only
[c] Men only
[d] For test results indicate type and amount smoked; for classification indicate smoker, ex-smoker, nonsmoker.

Appendix B

Nutritive Value of Selected Foods

© 2002 Chris Cole/Image Bank/Getty Images

Food	Amount	Weight (g)	Calories	Protein (g)	Fat (g)	Sat. Fat (g)	Cholesterol (g)	Carbohydrate (g)	Fiber (g)	Calcium (mg)	Iron (mg)	Sodium (mg)	Vit A (IU)	Thiamin (Vit B₁) (mg)	Riboflavin (Vit B₂) (mg)	Niacin (mg)	Vit C (mg)	Folate (mcg)
Apples, fresh, w/peel, lrg	1 ea	150	88	0.3	1	0.1	0	23	4.1	10	0.3	0	80	0.03	0.02	0.1	9	4.2
Applesauce, swtnd, w/o salt, cnd	1 cup	255	194	0.5	0	0.1	0	51	3.1	10	0.9	8	28	0.03	0.07	0.5	4	1.53
Apricots, pitted, fresh, whole	3 ea	114	55	1.6	0	0	0	13	2.7	16	0.6	1	2978	0.03	0.05	0.7	11	9.8
Apricots, w/skin, in heavy syrup, cnd, whole	½ cup	120	100	0.6	0	0	0	26	1.9	11	0.4	5	1476	0.02	0.03	0.5	4	2.04
Asparagus, spears, ckd w/o salt	4 ea	60	14	1.6	0	0	0	3	1	12	0.4	7	323	0.07	0.08	0.6	6	87.6
Avocado, Calif, fresh	½ ea	120	212	2.5	21	3.1	0	8	5.9	13	1.4	14	734	0.13	0.15	2.3	9	78.6
Bagel, plain, 3½" diameter	1 ea	68	187	7.1	1	0.1	0	36	1.6	50	2.4	363	0	0.37	0.21	3.1	0	59.84
Banana, fresh, med	1 ea	140	129	1.4	1	0.3	0	33	3.4	8	0.4	1	113	0.06	0.14	0.8	13	26.74
Bar, granola, hard	1 ea	24	113	2.4	5	0.6	0	15	1.3	15	0.7	71	36	0.06	0.03	0.4	0	5.52
Beans, black, mature, ckd w/o salt	1 cup	172	227	15.2	1	0.2	0	41	15	46	3.6	2	10	0.42	0.1	0.9	0	255.9
Beans, chickpea/garbanzo, mature, ckd	1 cup	164	269	14.5	4	0.4	0	45	12.5	80	4.7	11	44	0.19	0.1	0.9	2	282.0
Beans, frijoles/refried, cnd	½ cup	145	136	8	2	0.7	0	23	7.7	51	2.4	434	0	0.04	0.02	0.5	9	15.95
Beans, green, snap/string, ckd	½ cup	65	23	1.2	0	0	0	5	2.1	30	0.8	2	433	0.05	0.06	0.4	6	21.64
Beans, kidney, red, mature, cnd	1 cup	185	157	9.7	1	0.1	0	29	11.8	44	2.3	631	0	0.19	0.16	0.8	2	93.61
Beans, lima, fordhook, immature, ckd f/fzn w/o salt, drained	½ cup	85	85	5.2	0	0.1	0	16	4.9	19	1.2	45	162	0.06	0.05	0.9	11	18.02
Beans, mung, mature, sprouted, raw	½ cup	52	16	1.6	0	0	0	3	0.9	7	0.5	3	11	0.04	0.06	0.4	7	31.62
Beans, pinto, mature, ckd w/o salt	1 cup	171	234	14	1	0.2	0	44	14.7	82	4.5	3	3	0.32	0.16	0.7	4	294.1
Beef, chuck arm pot roast, brsd, choice, ¼" trim	3 oz	85	296	22.9	22	8.6	84	0	0	8	2.6	50	0	0.06	0.2	2.7	0	7.65
Beef, corned, cnd	3 oz	85	212	23	13	5.3	73	0	0	10	1.8	855	0	0.02	0.12	2.1	0	7.65
Beef, ground, hamburger patty, brld, well done, 16% fat	3 oz	85	225	24.3	13	5.3	84	0	0	8	2.4	70	0	0.06	0.27	5	0	9.35
Beef, ground, hamburger patty, brld, well done, 18% fat	3 oz	85	238	24	15	5.9	86	0	0	10	2.1	76	0	0.05	0.2	5.1	0	9.35
Beef, liver, fried	3 oz	85	184	22.7	7	2.3	410	7	0	9	5.3	90	30689	0.18	3.52	12.3	20	187
Beef, T-bone steak, brld, choice, ¼" trim	3 oz	85	263	19.7	20	7.7	57	0	0	7	2.3	54	0	0.08	0.18	3.4	0	5.95
Beef, top sirloin steak, lean, brld, choice, ¼" trim	3 oz	85	172	25.8	7	2.6	76	0	0.7	9	2.9	56	0	0.11	0.25	3.6	0	8.5
Beer	12 fl-oz	360	148	1.1	0	0	0	13	0.7	18	0.1	18	0	0.02	0.09	1.6	0	21.6
Beer, light	12 fl-oz	354	99	0.7	0	0	0	5	0	18	0.1	11	0	0.03	0.11	1.4	0	14.51
Beets, cnd, drained, diced	½ cup	80	25	0.7	0	0	0	6	1.4	12	1.5	155	9	0.01	0.03	0.1	3	24.16
Biscuits, homemade	1 ea	35	124	2.5	6	1.5	1	16	0.5	82	1	203	29	0.12	0.11	1	0	21.35
Blueberries, fresh, bilberries	½ cup	73	41	0.5	0	0	0	10	2	4	0.1	4	73	0.04	0.04	0.3	9	4.67
Brandy, 86 proof	1 oz	28	70	0	0	0	0	0	0	0	0	0	0	0	0	0	0	0
Bread, banana, prep f/recipe w/veg shortening	1 pce	50	169	2.2	6	1.5	22	28	0.7	9	0.7	99	46	0.09	0.1	0.7	1	5.5
Bread, cracked wheat	1 pce	25	65	2.2	1	0.2	0	12	1.4	11	0.7	134	0	0.09	0.06	0.9	0	15.25
Bread, French	1 pce	35	96	3.1	1	0.2	0	18	1	26	0.9	213	0	0.18	0.12	1.7	0	33.25
Bread, mixed grain	1 pce	26	65	2.6	1	0.2	0	12	1.7	24	0.9	127	0	0.11	0.09	1.1	0	20.8
Bread, pita pocket, white	1 ea	60	165	5.5	1	0.1	0	33	1.3	52	1.6	322	0	0.36	0.2	2.8	0	57
Bread, pumpernickel	1 pce	32	80	2.8	1	0.1	0	15	2.1	22	0.9	215	0	0.1	0.1	1	0	25.6
Bread, rye	1 pce	25	65	2.1	1	0.2	0	12	1.5	18	0.7	165	2	0.11	0.08	1	0	21.5
Bread, white, f/recipe w/2% milk	1 pce	25	71	2	1	0.3	1	12	0.5	14	0.7	90	20	0.1	0.1	0.9	0	22.75
Bread, whole wheat	1 pce	25	62	2.4	1	0.2	0	12	1.7	18	0.8	132	0	0.09	0.05	1	0	12.5
Broccoli, med stalk, 8" long, ckd w/o add salt	1 ea	140	39	4.2	0	0.1	0	7	4.1	64	1.2	36	1943	0.08	0.16	0.8	104	70
Broccoli, spear, raw, 5" long	1 ea	114	32	3.4	0	0.1	0	6	3.4	55	1	31	1758	0.07	0.14	0.7	106	80.94
Brownie, chocolate, w/walnuts, prep f/rec	1 ea	20	93	1.2	6	1.5	15	10	0.4	11	0.4	69	153	0.03	0.04	0.2	0	5.8
Brussels Sprouts, ckd, drained	½ cup	78	30	2	0	0.1	0	7	2	28	0.9	16	561	0.08	0.06	0.5	48	46.8
Buns, hamburger	1 ea	40	114	3.4	2	0.5	0	20	1.1	56	1.3	224	0	0.19	0.12	1.6	0	38

Food	Amount	Weight (g)	Calories	Protein (g)	Fat (g)	Sat. Fat (g)	Cholesterol (g)	Carbohydrate (g)	Fiber (g)	Calcium (mg)	Iron (mg)	Sodium (mg)	Vit A (IU)	Thiamin (Vit B_1) (mg)	Riboflavin (Vit B_2) (mg)	Niacin (mg)	Vit C (mg)	Folate (mcg)
Buns, hot dog/frankfurter	1 ea	40	114	3.4	2	0.5	0	20	1.1	56	1.3	224	0	0.19	0.12	1.6	0	38
Burger/Patty, vegetarian, Gardenburger, original	1 ea	71	130	8	3	1	11	18	5	84	0	290	50	0.11	0.15	1.1	0	10.08
Burger/Patty, vegetarian, soy	1 ea	71	142	14.9	6	1	0	6	3.3	21	1.5	390	0	0.64	0.43	7.1	0	55.38
Butter, salted	1 Tbs	5	36	0	4	2.5	11	0	0	1	0	41	153	0	0	0	0	0.15
Buttermilk, skim, cultured	1 cup	245	99	8.1	2	1.3	9	12	0	285	0.1	257	81	0.08	0.38	0.1	2	12.25
Cabbage, ckd w/o add salt, drained, shredded	1/2 cup	85	19	0.9	0	0	0	4	2	26	0.1	7	112	0.05	0.05	0.2	17	17
Cabbage, raw, shredded	1/2 cup	45	11	0.6	0	0	0	2	1	21	0.3	8	60	0.02	0.02	0.1	14	19.35
Cake, angel food, cmrcl prep	1 pce	60	155	3.5	0	0.1	0	35	0.9	84	0.3	449	0	0.06	0.29	0.5	1	21
Cake, carrot, w/cream cheese icing	1 pce	96	419	4.4	25	4.7	52	45	1.2	24	1.2	236	3310	0.13	0.15	1	1	11.52
Cake, chocolate, w/chocolate icing, 1/8th	1 pce	69	253	2.8	11	3.3	29	38	1.9	30	1.5	230	59	0.02	0.09	0.4	0	11.73
Cake, devils food, marshmallow iced	1 pce	99	408	3.5	21	5.8	52	52	1.2	47	1.3	338	0	0.04	0.07	0.4	0	12.3
Cake, pound, w/butter	1 pce	30	116	1.7	6	3.5	66	15	0.1	10	0.4	119	182	0.05	0.07	0.3	0	2.11
Cake, white, w/chocolate icing	1 pce	71	259	1.8	8	3.7	13	46	0.8	55	0.5	219	166	0.08	0.69	3.9	0	21
Calamari/Squid, fried, mixed species	1 cup	150	262	26.9	11	2.8	390	12	0	58	1.5	459	52	0.01	0.06	0.2	6	9.5
Candy Bar, Almond Joy, fun size	1½ oz	42	196	1.8	11	7.3	8	24	2	26	0.6	61	5	0.01	0.16	0.5	0	6
Candy Bar, Mars almond	1 ea	50	234	4.1	12	3.6	8	31	1	84	0.6	85	94	0.02	0.13	0.2	0	0.82
Candy Bar, Milky Way, 2.1 oz bar	1 ea	60	254	2.7	10	4.7	8	43	1	78	0.5	144	65	0.02	0.03	0.2	0	1.4
Candy Bar, Special Dark sweet chocolate	1 ea	41	226	2	13	8.3	0	25	2	11	1	3	14	0.01	0.05	0.1	1	2.24
Candy, caramels, plain/chocolate	1 oz	28	107	1.3	2	1.8	2	22	0.3	39	0.1	69	9	0	0.05	0.1	0	
Candy, hard, all flvrs	1 oz	28	110	0	0	0	0	27	0	1	0.1	11	0	0	0	0	0	0
Candy, Kisses, milk chocolate	1 oz	28	144	1.9	9	5.2	6	17	1	53	0.4	23	52	0.02	0.08	0.1	0	
Candy, M & M's peanut chocolate	1 oz	28	144	2.7	7	2.9	3	17	1	28	0.3	13	26	0.03	0.05	1	0	9.8
Candy, M & M's plain chocolate	1 oz	28	138	1.2	6	3.7	4	20	0.7	29	0.3	17	57	0.02	0.06	0.1	0	1.68
Candy, milk chocolate, w/almonds	1 oz	28	147	2.5	10	4.8	5	15	1.7	63	0.5	21	21	0.02	0.12	0.2	0	3.36
Carrots, ckd w/o add salt, drained, slices	1/2 cup	73	33	0.8	0	0	0	8	2.4	23	0.5	48	17924	0.02	0.04	0.4	2	10.15
Carrots, raw, whole, 7½" long	1 ea	81	35	0.8	0	0	0	8	2.4	22	0.4	28	22784	0.08	0.05	0.8	8	11.34
Catsup/Ketchup	1 Tbs	15	16	0.2	0	0	0	4	0.2	3	0.1	178	152	0.01	0.01	0.2	2	2.25
Cauliflower, ckd, drained	1/2 cup	63	14	1.2	0	0	0	3	1.7	10	0.2	9	11	0.03	0.03	0.3	28	27.72
Celery, raw, med stalk, 8" long	1 ea	40	6	0.3	0	0	0	1	0.7	16	0.2	35	54	0.02	0.02	0.1	3	11.2
Cereal, 100% Bran, rte, dry	1/2 cup	33	89	4.1	2	0.3	0	24	9.8	23	4.1	229	0	0.79	0.89	10.5	31	23.43
Cereal, All-Bran, rte, dry	1/4 cup	21	55	2.6	1	0.1	0	16	6.8	74	3.1	43	525	0.27	0.29	3.5	10	63
Cereal, Alpha-Bits, rte, dry	1 cup	28	110	2.2	0	0.1	0	24	1.2	8	2.7	178	1235	0.36	0.42	4.9	0	98.84
Cereal, bran flakes, rte, dry	¾ cup	30	96	2.8	0	0.1	0	24	5.3	17	8.1	220	750	0.38	0.43	5	12	99.9
Cereal, Cheerios	1 cup	23	84	2.4	1	0.3	0	18	2	42	6.2	218	958	0.29	0.33	3.8	6	76.59
Cereal, Chex, corn, rte, dry	1 cup	28	105	2	0	0.1	0	24	0.5	94	8.4	270	0	0.35	0	4.7	6	93.24
Cereal, Chex, wheat, rte, dry	1 cup	46	159	4.8	0	0.2	0	37	5.1	92	13.8	412	0	0.34	0.06	4.6	12	92
Cereal, corn flakes, rte, dry	1 cup	25	91	1.6	0	0.1	0	22	0.7	1	7.8	266	625	0.32	0.35	4.2	14	88.25
Cereal, Corn Pops, rte, dry	1 cup	28	107	1	0	0.1	0	26	0.4	2	1.7	111	700	0.36	0.39	4.7	0	98.84
Cereal, Cream of Wheat, quick, ckd w/water	1 cup	244	132	3.7	0	0.1	0	27	1.2	51	10.5	142	0	0.24	0	1.5	0	109.8
Cereal, Crispy Rice, rte, dry	¾ cup	22	87	1.4	0	0.1	0	19	0.3	4	0.6	161	971	0.41	0.46	5.4	12	108.6
Cereal, Frosted Flakes, rte, dry	1 cup	35	135	1.4	0	0.1	0	32	0.7	1	5.1	226	847	0.42	0.49	5.6	17	105
Cereal, Frosted Mini Wheats, rte, dry	1 cup	55	186	5.2	1	0.2	0	45	5.9	20	15.4	92	0	0.38	0.44	5.4	0	110
Cereal, granola, rte, dry	1/2 cup	57	257	6	10	1.3	0	38	3.6	43	1.8	92	737	0.18	0.06	0.6	0	8.55
Cereal, Grape Nuts, rte, dry	1/2 cup	57	205	6.2	1	0.2	0	46	5	19	15.9	348	1323	0.37	0.42	4.9	12	98.04
Cereal, Honey Bran, rte, dry	1/2 cup	30	102	2.6	1	0.2	0	25	3.3	14	4.8	173	16	0.39	0.45	5.3	16	20.1
Cereal, Life, plain, rte, dry	1 cup	44	167	4.3	2	0.3	0	35	2.8	134	12.3	240	2488	0.55	0.62	7.3	0	146.9
Cereal, Mueslix, five grain muesli, rte, dry	1 cup	82	289	6.2	5	0.7	0	63	5.6	67	8.9	107	107	0.75	0.84	9.8	1	196.8
Cereal, Nutri-Grain, wheat, rte, dry	1 oz	28	101	2.4	0	0.1	0	24	1.8	8	0.8	190	1	0.36	0.42	4.9	15	98.84
Cereal, oatmeal, unsalted, ckd w/water	1/2 cup	120	74	3.1	1	0.2	0	13	2	10	0.8	1	19	0.13	0.02	0.2	0	4.8

Food	Amount	Weight (g)	Calories	Protein (g)	Fat (g)	Sat. Fat (g)	Cholesterol (g)	Carbohydrate (g)	Fiber (g)	Calcium (mg)	Iron (mg)	Sodium (mg)	Vit A (IU)	Thiamin (Vit B₁) (mg)	Riboflavin (Vit B₂) (mg)	Niacin (mg)	Vit C (mg)	Folate (mcg)
Cereal, raisin bran, rte, dry	1 cup	49	155	3.9	1	0.1	0	38	6.4	22	9	299	623	0.31	0.35	4.2	0	82.81
Cereal, Shredded Wheat, sml biscuits, rte, dry	1 cup	19	68	2.1	0	0.1	0	15	1.9	7	0.8	2	0	0.05	0.05	1	0	9.5
Cereal, Smacks, rte, dry	1 cup	37	141	2.4	0	0.4	0	32	1.3	4	2.5	70	1028	0.52	0.59	6.8	21	136.9
Cereal, Special K, rte, dry	1 cup	21	78	4.3	0		0	15	0.7	3	5.9	169	508	0.36	0.4	4.7	10	63
Cereal, Total, wheat, rte, dry	1 cup	33	116	3.3	1	0.2	0	26	2.9	284	19.8	218	1375	1.65	1.87	22.1	66	439.8
Cereal, Wheaties, rte, dry	1 cup	29	106	3.1	1	0.2	0	23	2	53	7.8	215	725	0.36	0.41	4.8	14	96.57
Cheese Puffs/Cheetos	1 oz	28	155	2.1	10	1.8	1	15	0.3	16	0.7	294	74	0.07	0.1	0.9	0	33.6
Cheese Spread, low fat, low sod	1 pce	34	61	8.4	2	1.5	12	1	0	233	0.1	2	92	0.01	0.13	0	0	3.06
Cheese, American, proc, shredded	1 oz	28	105	6.2	9	5.5	26	1	0	172	0.1	401	339	0.01	0.1	0	0	2.18
Cheese, blue	1 oz	28	99	6	8	5.2	21	1	0	148	0.1	391	202	0.01	0.11	0.3	0	10.19
Cheese, cheddar, diced	1 oz	28	113	7	9	5.9	29	0	0	202	0.2	174	297	0.01	0.11	0	0	5.1
Cheese, feta	1 oz	28	74	4	6	4.2	25	1	0	138	0.2	313	125	0.04	0.24	0.3	0	8.96
Cheese, monterey jack, shredded	1 oz	28	105	6.9	8	5.3	25	0	0	209	0.2	150	266	0	0.11	0	0	5.1
Cheese, mozzarella, part skm milk, low moist, shredded	1 oz	28	78	7.7	5	3	15	1	0	205	0.1	148	197	0.01	0.1	0	0	2.77
Cheese, parmesan, grated	1 Tbs	5	23	2.1	2	1	4	0	0	69	0	93	35	0	0.02	0	0	0.4
Cheese, ricotta, part skm	1 oz	28	39	3.2	2	1.4	9	1	0	76	0.1	35	121	0.01	0.05	0	0	3.67
Cheese, Swiss, shredded	1 oz	28	105	8	8	5	26	1	0	269	0	73	237	0.01	0.1	0	0	1.79
Cheesecake	1 pce	85	273	4.7	19	8.4	47	22	0.4	43	0.5	176	465	0.02	0.16	0.2	0	15.3
Cherries, sweet, fresh	10 ea	75	54	0.9	1	0.2	0	12	1.7	11	0.3	0	160	0.04	0.04	0.3	5	3.15
Chicken, broiler/fryer, breast, rstd	1 ea	98	193	29.2	8	2.1	82	0	0	14	1	70	91	0.06	0.12	12.5	0	3.92
Chicken, broiler/fryer, dark meat, w/o skin, rstd	3 oz	85	174	23.3	8	2.3	79	0	0	13	1.1	79	61	0.06	0.19	5.6	0	6.8
Chicken, broiler/fryer, drumstick, rstd	1 ea	52	112	14.1	6	1.6	47	0	0	6	0.7	47	52	0.04	0.11	3.1	0	4.16
Chicken, broiler/fryer, meat only, w/o skin, rstd	3 oz	85	162	24.6	6	1.7	76	0	0	13	1	73	45	0.06	0.15	7.8	0	5.1
Chips, corn	1 oz	28	151	1.8	9	1.3	0	16	1.4	36	0.4	176	26	0.01	0.04	0.3	0	5.6
Chips, tortilla, chili & lime	18 pce	28	110	2	2	0	0	22	2	60	3.6	200	0	0.02	0.05	0.4	0	2.8
Chips, tortilla, plain	1 oz	28	140	2	7	1.4	0	18	1.8	43	0.4	148	55	0.07	0.1	2.3	2	8.71
Cod, batter fried	3½ oz	100	173	17.4	8	1.6	50	7	0.2	29	0.7	91	30	0.02	0.05	2.2	3	6.6
Cod, stmd/poached	3½ oz	100	102	22.4	0	0.1	46	0	0	9	0.3	80	28	0.06	0.04	0.4	2	7.8
Coffee, brewed	¾ cup	180	4	0.2	0	0	0	1	0	4	0.1	4	0	0	0	0.4	0	0.18
Collards, ckd w/o add salt	½ cup	95	25	2	0	0	0	5	2.7	113	0.4	9	2973	0.04	0.1	0.5	17	88.35
Cone, ice cream, wafer/cake type	1 ea	115	480	9.3	8	1.4	0	91	3.4	29	4.1	164	0	0.29	0.41	5.1	0	117.3
Cookie, chocolate chip, prep w/marg f/rec	2 ea	20	98	1.1	6	1.6	6	12	0.6	8	0.5	72	127	0.04	0.04	0.3	0	6.6
Cookie, chocolate sandwich, creme filled	4 ea	40	189	1.9	8	1.5	0	28	1.3	10	1.6	242	1	0.03	0.07	0.8	0	17.2
Cookie, fig bar	4 ea	56	195	2.1	4	0.6	0	40	2.6	36	1.6	196	18	0.09	0.12	1	0	15.12
Cookie, oatmeal raisin, prep f/rec	2 ea	26	113	1.7	4	0.8	9	18	0.8	26	0.7	140	167	0.06	0.04	0.3	0	7.8
Cookie, peanut butter, prep f/rec	2 ea	24	114	2.2	6	1.1	7	14	0.5	9	0.5	124	144	0.05	0.05	0.8	0	13.2
Cookie, shortbread, cmrcl, plain	4 ea	32	161	2	8	2	6	21	0.6	11	0.9	146	28	0.11	0.11	1.1	0	18.88
Cookie, vanilla, wafer type, 12–17% fat	10 ea	40	176	2	6	1.5	20	29	0.8	19	1	125	11	0.11	0.13	1.2	0	20
Coriander, raw	¼ cup	4	1	0.1	0	0	0	0	0.1	4	0.1	1	111	0	0	0	1	0.41
Corn, yellow, vac pack, cnd	½ cup	83	66	2	0	0.1	0	16	1.7	4	0.3	226	200	0.03	0.06	1	7	40.92
Cornbread, prep f/dry mix	1 ea	60	188	4.3	6	1.6	37	29	1.4	44	1.1	467	123	0.15	0.16	1.2	0	33
Cornmeal, yellow, degermed, enrich, dry	½ cup	120	439	10.2	2	0.3	0	93	8.9	6	5	4	496	0.86	0.49	6	0	224.4
Cottage Cheese, 2% fat	½ cup	113	101	15.5	2	1.4	9	4	0	77	0.2	459	79	0.03	0.21	0.2	0	14.8
Cottage Cheese, creamed, sml curd	½ cup	105	109	13.1	5	3	16	3	0	63	0.1	425	171	0.02	0.17	0.1	0	12.81
Crab, blue, cnd, drained	1 cup	135	134	27.7	3	0.3	120	0	0	136	1.1	450	7	0.11	0.11	1.8	4	57.38
Crackers, cheese	10 ea	10	50	1	3	0.9	1	6	0.2	15	0.5	100	16	0.06	0.04	0.5	0	8
Crackers, graham, plain/honey, 2½ square	2 ea	14	59	1	1	0.2	0	11	0.4	3	0.5	85	0	0.03	0.04	0.6	0	8.4
Crackers, matzoh, plain, svg	1 ea	28	111	2.8	0	0.1	0	23	0.8	4	0.9	1	0	0.11	0.08	1.1	0	32.76

Food	Amount	Weight (g)	Calories	Protein (g)	Fat (g)	Sat. Fat (g)	Cholesterol (mg)	Carbohydrate (g)	Fiber (g)	Calcium (mg)	Iron (mg)	Sodium (mg)	Vit A (IU)	Thiamin (Vit B_1) (mg)	Riboflavin (Vit B_2) (mg)	Niacin (mg)	Vit C (mg)	Folate (mcg)
Crackers, rye, wafers	2 ea	14	47	1.3	0	0	0	11	3.2	6	0.8	111	1	0.06	0.04	0.2	0	6.3
Crackers, saltine	1 ea	11	48	1	1	0.3	0	8	0.3	13	0.6	143	0	0.06	0.05	0.6	0	13.64
Crackers, standard, reg, snack type, round	1 ea	3	15	0.2	1	0.1	0	2	0	4	0.1	25	0	0.01	0.01	0.1	0	2.31
Crackers, triscuit	1 ea	5	24	0.5	1	0.2	0	3	0.5		0.2	26						
Crackers, wheat	1 ea	2	9	0.2	0	0.1	0	1	0.1	1	0.1	16	0	0.01	0.01	0.1	0	0.36
Cream Cheese	1 oz	28	98	2.1	10	6.2	31	1	0	22	0.3	83	400	0	0.06	0	0	3.7
Cream, light	1 Tbs	15	29	0.4	3	1.8	10	1	0	14	0	6	95	0	0.02	0	0	0.34
Cream, whipping, heavy	1 Tbs	15	52	0.3	6	3.5	21	0	0	10	0	6	221	0	0.02	0	0	0.56
Croissant, butter	1 ea	57	231	4.7	12	6.6	38	26	1.5	21	1.2	424	424	0.22	0.14	1.2	0	35.34
Cucumber, w/o skin, raw, sliced	½ cup	60	7	0.3	0	0	0	2	0.4	8	0.1	1	44	0.01	0.01	0.1	2	8.4
Dates, fresh, whole	10 ea	83	228	1.6	0	0.2	0	61	6.2	27	1	2	42	0.07	0.08	1.8	0	10.46
Dinner, chicken, cacciatore, w/noodles, low cal, fzn	1 ea	308	311	22.5	10	2.4	59	33	3.4	29	3.2	934	732	0.28	0.4	8	26	32.22
Doughnut, cake	1 ea	47	198	2.3	11	1.7	17	23	0.7	21	0.9	257	27	0.1	0.11	0.9	0	22.09
Doughnut, raised, glazed	1 ea	60	242	3.8	14	3.5	4	27	0.7	26	1.2	205	8	0.22	0.13	1.7	0	25.8
Egg Substitute, Egg Beaters, new	¼ cup	61	30	6	0	0	0	1	0	20	1.1	125	300		0.85		0	32.0
Egg Whites, raw	1 ea	33	16	3.5	0	0	0	0	0	2	0.6	54	0	0	0.15	0	0	0.99
Egg Yolks, raw, lrg	1 ea	17	61	2.8	5	1.6	218	0	0	23	0.6	7	331	0.03	0.11	0	0	24.82
Eggs, hard ckd/bld, lrg	1 ea	50	78	6.3	5	1.6	212	1	0	25	0.6	62	280	0.03	0.26	0	0	22
Eggs, scrambled, plain, lrg	1 ea	64	106	7.1	8	2.4	225	1	0	45	0.8	179	436	0.03	0.28	0.1	0	19.2
Eggs, whole, fried	1 ea	46	92	6.2	7	1.9	211	1	0	25	0.7	162	394	0.03	0.24	0.1	0	17.48
Entree, lasagna, w/meat, prep f/rec	1 pce	220	352	20.7	14	7.2	52	36	2.5	243	2.8	351	902	0.21	0.3	3.8	13	17.82
Entree, macaroni & cheese, prep f/rec w/margarine	½ cup	100	215	8.4	11	4.4	21	20	0.6	181	0.9	543	430	0.1	0.2	0.9	0	5.15
Entree, meatloaf, beef	1 pce	111	232	20.2	14	5.6	107	5	0.2	37	2.1	185	148	0.06	0.28	3.3	1	14.28
Entree, quiche, lorraine	1 pce	242	724	20.5	56	25.9	304	34	1	318	2.6	303	1323	0.36	0.67	2.8	1	26.48
Entree, spaghetti, w/meatballs, prep f/rec	1 cup	248	332	18.6	12	3.3	74	39	7.7	124	3.7	1009	1587	0.25	0.3	4	22	9.99
Entree, spaghetti, w/tomato sauce & cheese, prep f/rec	1 cup	250	260	8.8	9	2	8	37	2.5	80	2.2	955	1075	0.25	0.17	2.2	12	8
Figs, dried, unckd	1 ea	21	54	0.6	0	0	0	14	2.5	30	0.5	2	28	0.01	0.02	0.1	0	1.57
Fish Sticks/Portions, heated f/fzn, 4x1x.5	2 ea	56	152	8.8	7	1.8	63	13	0	11	0.4	326	59	0.07	0.1	1.2	0	10.19
Flour, all purpose, white, bleached, enrich	1 cup	125	455	12.9	1	0.2	0	95	3.4	19	5.8	2	0	0.98	0.62	7.4	0	192.5
Flour, whole wheat	1 cup	120	407	16.4	2	0.4	0	87	14.6	41	4.7	6	0	0.54	0.26	7.6	0	52.8
Frankfurter/Hot Dog, beef & pork, 10 pack	1 ea	57	182	6.4	17	6.1	28	1	0	6	0.7	638	0	0.11	0.07	1.5	0	2.28
Frankfurter/Hot Dog, beef, 8 pack	1 ea	57	180	6.8	16	6.9	35	1	0	11	0.8	585	0	0.03	0.06	1.4	0	2.28
Frankfurter/Hot Dog, turkey	1 ea	45	102	6.4	8	2.7	48	1	0	48	0.8	642	0	0.02	0.08	1.9	0	3.6
Frozen Yogurt, vanilla/strawberry, nonfat, sml scoop	4 oz	113	112	5.6	0	0.1	2	22	1.7	196	0.1	75	7	0.05	0.23	0.1	1	11.99
Fruit Cocktail, in heavy syrup, cnd	1 cup	245	179	1	0	0	0	46	2.5	15	0.7	15	502	0.04	0.05	0.9	5	6.37
Fruit Cocktail, in juice	1 cup	248	114	1.1	0	0	0	29	2.5	20	0.5	10	756	0.03	0.04	0.9	7	6.2
Fruit Punch, prep f/pwd	1 cup	240	89	0	0	0	0	23	0	38	0.1	34	51	0.06	0	0	28	0.24
Fudge, chocolate, prep f/rec	1 oz	28	107	0.5	2	1.4	4	22	0.2	12	0.1	17	53	0	0.02	0	0	0.56
Grapefruit, pink, fresh, 3¾" diameter	½ ea	123	37	0.7	0	0.1	0	9	1.7	14	0.1	0	319	0.04	0.02	0.2	47	15.01
Grapes, tokay/empress/red flame, fresh	10 ea	50	36	0.3	0	0.1	0	9	0.5	6	0.1	1	36	0.05	0.03	0.2	5	1.95
Haddock, fillet, brd, fried	3 oz	85	184	17.1	9	1.9	65	7	0.2	53	1.5	145	69	0.08	0.09	3.7	0	11.6
Halibut, Greenland, fillet, bkd/brld	3 oz	85	203	15.7	15	2.6	50	0	0	3	0.7	88	51	0.06	0.09	1.6	0	0.85
Honey, strained, extracted	1 Tbs	21	64	0.1	0	0	0	17	0	1	0.1	1	0	0	0.01	0	0	0.42
Hot Cocoa/Choc, prep f/rec w/whole milk	1 cup	250	192	9.8	6	3.6	20	29	2	315	1.1	128	515	0.1	0.44	0.4	2	15
Hummos/Hummos, raw	1 cup	246	421	12.1	21	3.1	0	50	12.5	123	3.9	600	62	0.23	0.13	1	19	146.1
Instant Breakfast, prep f/dry mix w/nonfat milk	1 cup	282	216	15.7	1	0.7	9	36	0.2	407	4.8	268	2343	0.4	0.42	5.5	31	118.2

Food	Amount	Weight (g)	Calories	Protein (g)	Fat (g)	Sat. Fat (g)	Cholesterol (g)	Carbohydrate (g)	Fiber (g)	Calcium (mg)	Iron (mg)	Sodium (mg)	Vit A (IU)	Thiamin (Vit B₁) (mg)	Riboflavin (Vit B₂) (mg)	Niacin (mg)	Vit C (mg)	Folate (mcg)
Instant Breakfast, prep f/dry mix w/whole milk	1 cup	281	280	15.4	9	5.4	38	36	0.2	396	4.9	262	2151	0.41	0.47	5.5	31	117.7
Jam/Preserves, pkt	1 ea	14	39	0.1	0	0	0	10	0.2	3	0.1	4	2	0	0	0	1	4.62
Jelly	1 Tbs	18	51	0.1	0	0	0	13	0.2	1	0.5	5	3	0	0.02	0	0	0.18
Juice, apple, unswtnd, cnd/btld	1/2 cup	124	58	0.1	0	0	0	14	0.1	9	0.5	4	1	0.03	0.02	0.1	1	0.12
Juice, cranberry cocktail	1 cup	253	144	0	0	0	0	36	0.3	8	0.4	5	10	0.02	0.02	0.1	90	0.51
Juice, grape, unswtnd, btld/cnd	1/2 cup	127	77	0.7	0	0	0	19	0.1	11	0.3	4	10	0.03	0.05	0.3	0	3.3
Juice, grapefruit, unswtnd, cnd	1/2 cup	124	47	0.6	0	0	0	11	0.1	9	0.2	1	9	0.05	0.02	0.3	36	12.9
Juice, grapefruit, unswtnd, prep f/fzn conc	1 cup	247	101	1.4	0	0	0	24	0.2	20	0.3	2	22	0.1	0.05	0.5	83	8.89
Juice, lemon, fresh	1 Tbs	15	4	0.1	0	0	0	1	0.1	1	0	0	3	0	0	0	7	1.94
Juice, orange, prep f/fzn	1/2 cup	125	56	0.9	0	0	0	13	0.2	11	0.1	1	98	0.1	0.02	0.3	49	54.75
Juice, prune, w/o pulp	1/2 cup	88	60	0.7	0	0	0	14	0.5	2	0.9	4	54				3	
Juice, tomato, w/salt, cnd	1 cup	244	41	1.9	0	0	0	10	1	22	1.4	881	1357	0.11	0.08	1.6	45	48.56
Kale, ckd w/o add salt, drained	1/2 cup	55	15	1.9	0	0	0	3	1.1	40	0.5	13	4070	0.03	0.04	0.3	23	7.32
Kiwifruit/Chinese Gooseberries, fresh, med	1 ea	76	46	0.8	0	0	0	11	2.6	20	0.3	4	133	0.02	0.04	0.4	74	28.88
Lamb, leg, whole, lean, rstd, choice, 1/4" trim	3 oz	85	162	24.1	7	2.3	76	0	0	7	1.8	58	0	0.09	0.25	5.4	0	19.55
Lamb, loin chop, lean, brld, choice, 1/4" trim	3 oz	84	181	25.2	8	2.9	80	0	0	16	1.7	71	0	0.09	0.24	5.8	0	20.16
Lemonade, white, fzn conc	12 oz	340	615	1	0	0.1	0	160	0	24	2.4	14	323	0.09	0.02	0.3	60	34
Lentils, sprouts, stir fried	1 cup	124	125	10.9	1	0.1	0	26	1.4	17	3.8	12	51	0.27	0.33	1.5	16	83.08
Lentils, unsalted, ckd	1 cup	200	232	18	1	0.1	0	40	4.8	38	6.7	1	16	0.34	0.11	2.1	3	361.6
Lettuce, butterhead, Boston/bibb, leaf, raw	2 pce	15	2	0.2	0	0	0	0	15.8	5	0	1	146	0.01	0.15	0	1	11
Lettuce, romaine, raw, chpd	1 cup	55	8	0.9	0	0.2	0	1	0.2	20	0.6	4	1430	0.06	0.06	0.3	13	74.64
Lobster, northern, stmd	1 cup	145	142	29.7	1	0.2	104	2	0.9	88	0.6	551	126	0.01	0.1	1.6	0	16.1
Lunchmeat Spread, liverwurst, cnd	1 oz	28	87	3.6	7	2.5	33	2	0	0	2.3	193	3818	0.05	0.5		1	1.4
Lunchmeat, bologna, beef & pork	1 pce	28	88	3.3	8	3	15	1	0.5	3	0.4	285	0	0.05	0.04	0.7	0	3.99
Lunchmeat, bologna, turkey	2 pce	57	113	7.8	9	2.9	56	1	0	48	0.9	500	0	0.03	0.09		0	
Lunchmeat, roast beef, deli style, pouch	3 oz	85	96	17.2	3	1.1	41	1	0	5	1.6	860	0	0.05	0.04	2	0	
Lunchmeat, turkey breast, rstd, fat free	1 pce	28	24	4.2	0	0.1	9	2	0	3	0.3	334	0	0.03	0.04		0	
Mayonnaise, imit, low cal	1 Tbs	15	35	0.1	3	0.5	4	1	0	1	0	75	0		0	0	0	0
Mayonnaise, soybean oil, w/salt	1 tsp	5	36	0.1	4	0.6	3	0	0	1	0	28	14		0	0	0	0.38
Melon, cantaloupe/musk, med 5" diameter	1/4 ea	239	84	2.1	0	0.2	0	20	1.9	26	0.5	22	7705	0.09	0.05	1.4	101	40.63
Melon, honeydew, fresh, wedge, 1/8 melon	1 pce	129	45	0.6	0	0	0	12	0.8	8	0.1	13	52	0.1	0.02	0.8	32	7.74
Milk Shake, chocolate, fast food	10 fl-oz	340	432	11.6	13	7.9	44	70	2.7	384	1.1	330	316	0.2	0.83	0.5	1	11.9
Milk, evaporated, whole, w/add vit A, cnd	1/2 cup	126	169	8.6	10	5.8	37	13	0	329	0.2	133	500	0.06	0.4	0.2	2	9.95
Milk, low fat, 1%, w/add vit A	1 cup	244	102	8	3	1.6	10	12	0	300	0.1	123	500	0.1	0.41	0.2	2	12.44
Milk, low fat, 2%, chocolate	1 cup	250	179	8	5	3.1	17	26	1.2	284	0.6	150	500	0.09	0.41	0.3	2	12
Milk, low fat, 2%, w/add vit A	1 cup	244	121	8.1	5	2.9	18	12	0	297	0.1	122	500	0.1	0.4	0.2	2	12.44
Milk, nonfat/skim, w/add vit A	1 cup	245	86	8.4	0	0.3	4	12	0	302	0.1	126	500	0.09	0.34	0.2	2	12.74
Milk, whole, 3.3%	1 cup	244	150	8	8	5.1	33	11	0	291	0.1	120	307	0.09	0.4	0.2	2	12.2
Milkshake, strawberry, fast food	10 fl-oz	340	384	11.6	8	5.9	37	64	1.4	384	0.4	282	408	0.15	0.66	0.6	3	10.2
Mixed Vegetables, cnd, drained	1 cup	182	86	4.7	0	0.1	0	17	5.5	49	1.9	271	21198	0.08	0.09	1.1	9	42.95
Muffin, English, plain	1 ea	57	134	4.4	1	0.1	0	26	1.5	99	1.4	264	0	0.25	0.16	2.2	0	46.17
Muffin, English, plain, tstd	1 ea	52	133	4.4	1	0.1	0	26	1.5	98	1.4	262	0	0.2	0.14	2	0	38.48
Muffin, wheat bran, prep f/rec w/whole milk	1 ea	45	130	3.2	6	1.2	16	19	3.2	84	1.9	265	363	0.15	0.2	1.8	4	23.4
Mushrooms, raw, pces/slices	1 cup	35	9	1	0	0	0	1	0.4	2	0.4	1	0	0.03	0.15	1.4	1	4.2
Mustard Greens, ckd w/o add salt, drained	1/2 cup	70	10	1.6	0	0	0	1	1.4	52	0.5	11	2122	0.03	0.04	0.3	18	51.38
Nuts, almonds, dried, unblanched, whole	1/4 cup	36	208	7.7	18	1.4	0	7	4.2	89	1.5	0	0	0.09	0.29	1.4	0	10.44
Nuts, Brazil, dried, shelled, 32 kernels	1 oz	28	184	4	19	4.5	0	4	1.5	49	1	1	4	0.28	0.03	0.5	0	1.12
Nuts, cashews, dry rstd, salted	1 cup	137	786	21	63	12.5	0	45	4.1	62	8.2	877	0	0.27	0.27	1.9	0	94.8
Nuts, coconut, unswtnd, dried	1/2 cup	65	429	4.5	42	37.2	0	16	10.6	17	2.2	24	0	0.04	0.06	0.4	1	5.85

Food	Amount	Weight (g)	Calories	Protein (g)	Fat (g)	Sat. Fat (g)	Cholesterol (g)	Carbohydrate (g)	Fiber (g)	Calcium (mg)	Iron (mg)	Sodium (mg)	Vit A (IU)	Thiamin (Vit B_1) (mg)	Riboflavin (Vit B_2) (mg)	Niacin (mg)	Vit C (mg)	Folate (mcg)
Nuts, peanuts, oil rstd, unsalted, chpd	1 oz	28	163	7.4	14	1.9	0	5	1.9	25	0.5	2	0	0.07	0.03	4	0	35.2
Nuts, pecans, dried, halves	1 oz	28	193	2.6	20	1.7	0	4	2.7	20	0.7	0	22	0.18	0.04	0.3	0	6.16
Nuts, walnuts, black, dried, chpd	1 oz	28	170	6.8	16	1	0	3	1.4	16	0.9	0	83	0.06	0.03	0.2	1	18.34
Oil, canola	1 cup	218	1927	0	218	15.5	0	0	0	0	0	0	0	0	0	0	0	0
Oil, corn	1 Tbs	15	133	0	15	1.9	0	0	0	0	0.1	0	0	0	0	0	0	0
Oil, olive	1 Tbs	15	133	0	15	2	0	0	0	0	0.1	0	0	0	0	0	0	0
Oil, peanut	1 cup	216	1909	0	216	36.5	0	0	0	0	0	0	0	0	0	0	0	0
Oil, safflower, greater than 70% linoleic	1 Tbs	15	133	0	15	0.9	0	0	0	0	0	0	0	0	0	0	0	0
Oil, soybean	1 tsp	5	44	0	5	0.7	0	0	0	0	0	0	0	0	0	0	0	0
Okra, bindi, ckd w/o add salt f/raw, drained, pods	8 ea	85	27	1.6	0	0	0	6	2.1	54	0.4	4	489	0.11	0.05	0.7	14	38.85
Olives, w/o pits, ripe, lrg, cnd	10 ea	44	51	0.4	5	0.6	0	3	1.4	39	1.5	384	177	0	0	0	0	0
Olives, w/o pits, ripe, sml, cnd	10 ea	32	37	0.3	3	0.5	0	2	1	28	1.1	279	129	0	0	0	0	0
Onions, yellow, ckd w/o add salt, drained, chpd	1/2 cup	105	46	1.4	0	0	0	11	1.5	23	0.3	3	0	0.04	0.02	0.2	5	15.75
Oranges, fresh, med	1 ea	180	85	1.7	0	0	0	21	4.3	72	0.2	0	369	0.16	0.07	0.5	96	54.54
Oysters, eastern, brd, fried, med	1 ea	45	89	3.9	6	1.4	36	5	0.1	28	3.1	188	136	0.07	0.09	0.7	2	13.95
Oysters, eastern, raw, wild	1/2 cup	120	82	8.5	3	0.9	64	5	0	54	8	253	120	0.12	0.11	1.7	4	12
Pancake, buckwheat, prep f/incomplete dry mix, 4"	1 ea	27	56	2.1	2	0.5	18	8	0.6	69	0.5	144	63	0.05	0.07	0.4	0	4.59
Pancake, plain, homemade, 4"	1 ea	73	166	4.7	7	1.5	43	21	1.1	160	1.3	320	143	0.15	0.21	1.1	0	27.74
Papaya, fresh, med	1/2 ea	227	89	1.4	1	0.1	0	22	4.1	54	0.2	7	645	0.06	0.07	0.8	140	86.26
Pasta, egg noodles, enrich, ckd	1/2 cup	80	106	3.8	1	0.2	26	20	0.9	10	1.3	6	16	0.15	0.07	1.2	0	51.2
Pasta, macaroni noodles, enrich, ckd	1/2 cup	70	99	3.3	0	0.1	0	20	0.9	5	1	1	0	0.14	0.07	1.2	0	49
Pasta, spaghetti noodles, enrich, salted, ckd	1 cup	140	197	6.7	1	0.1	0	40	2.4	10	2	140	0	0.29	0.14	2.3	0	98
Pasta, spaghetti noodles, whole wheat, ckd	1 cup	125	155	6.7	1	0.1	0	33	5.6	19	1.3	4	0	0.14	0.06	0.9	0	6.25
Pastry, cinnamon danish	1 ea	110	443	7.7	25	6.2	23	49	1.4	78	2.2	408	13	0.33	0.29	3.2	0	68.2
Peaches, fresh, sliced	1/2 cup	85	37	0.6	0	0	0	9	1.7	4	0.1	0	455	0.01	0.03	0.8	6	2.89
Peaches, in heavy syrup, cnd	1/2 cup	96	71	0.4	0	0	0	19	1.5	3	0.3	6	319	0.01	0.02	0.6	3	3.07
Peaches, in juice, cnd, whole	1/2 tsp	77	34	0.5	0	0	0	9	1.7	5	0.2	3	293	0.01	0.01	0.4	3	2.62
Peanut Butter, smooth, salted	1 Tbs	32	190	8.1	16	3.3	0	6	1.9	12	0.6	149	0	0.03	0.07	4.3	0	23.68
Pears, bartlett, fresh, med	1 ea	180	106	0.7	1	0	0	27	4.3	20	0.4	0	36	0.04	0.02	0.2	7	13.14
Pears, in heavy syrup, cnd, halves	1/2 ea	103	76	0.2	0	0	0	20	1.6	5	0.2	5	5	0.01	0.01	0.2	1	1.24
Pears, in juice, cnd, halves	1/2 ea	77	38	0.3	0	0	0	10	1.2	7	0.2	7	5	0.01	0.01	0.2	1	0.92
Peas, cnd, drained	1/2 cup	85	59	3.8	0	0.1	0	11	3.5	17	0.8	214	653	0.1	0.07	0.6	8	37.65
Peas, green, ckd f/fzn w/o add salt, drained	1/2 cup	80	62	4.1	0	0.1	0	11	4.4	19	1.3	70	534	0.23	0.08	1.2	8	46.88
Peppers, bell, green, sweet, raw, med	1 ea	200	54	1.8	0	0.1	0	13	3.6	18	0.9	4	1264	0.13	0.06	1	179	44
Peppers, bell, red, sweet, raw, sml	1 ea	74	20	0.7	0	0.1	0	5	1.5	7	0.3	1	4218	0.05	0.02	0.4	141	16.28
Peppers, bell, yellow, sweet, raw, lrg	1 ea	186	50	1.9	0	0.1	0	12	1.7	20	0.9	4	443	0.05	0.05	1.7	341	48.36
Pickles, dill	1 ea	135	24	0.8	0	0.1	0	6	1.6	12	0.7	1731	444	0.02	0.04	0.1	3	1.35
Pickles, sweet, med	1 ea	35	41	0.1	0	0	0	11	0.4	1	0.2	329	44	0	0.01	0.1	0	0.35
Pie, apple, bkd f/fzn, 1/6th of 8"	1 pce	118	280	2.2	13	4.5	0	40	1.9	13	0.5	314	146	0.03	0.03	0.3	4	25.96
Pie, blueberry, prep f/rec, 1/8th of 9"	1 pce	158	387	4.3	19	4.6	0	53	2.2	11	1.9	292	66	0.24	0.21	1.9	1	36.34
Pie, cherry, prep f/rec, 1/8th of 9"	1 pce	118	319	3.3	14	3.5	0	45	1.8	12	2.2	225	483	0.17	0.15	1.5	0	31.86
Pie, chocolate cream, rts, 1/6th of 8"	1 pce	175	532	4.5	34	8.7	9	59	3.5	63	1.9	238	245	0.06	0.19	1.2	4	22.75
Pie, lemon meringue, rts, 1/6th of 8"	1 pce	140	375	2.1	12	2.5	63	66	1.7	78	0.9	204	242	0.09	0.29	0.9	2	18.2
Pie, pecan, rts, 1/6th of 8"	1 pce	138	552	5.5	26	4.9	44	79	4.8	23	1.4	585	242	0.13	0.17	0.3	1	37.26
Pie, pumpkin, rts, 1/6th of 8"	1 pce	114	239	4.4	11	2	23	31	3.1	68	0.9	321	3915	0.06	0.17	0.2	1	22.8
Pineapple, chunks, fresh	1/2 cup	78	38	0.3	0	0	0	10	0.9	5	0.3	1	18	0.07	0.03	0.3	9	8.27
Pineapple, in heavy syrup, cnd, tidbits	1/2 cup	128	100	0.4	0	0	0	26	1	18	0.5	1	18	0.12	0.03	0.4	12	5.89
Pineapple, in juice, cnd	1/2 cup	125	75	0.5	0	0	0	20	0.9	18	0.3	1	48	0.12	0.02	0.4	9	6
Popcorn, air popped, plain	1 cup	6	23	0.7	0	0	0	5	0.9	1	0.2	0	12	0.01	0.02	0.1	0	1.38

Food	Amount	Weight (g)	Calories	Protein (g)	Fat (g)	Sat. Fat (g)	Cholesterol (g)	Carbohydrate (g)	Fiber (g)	Calcium (mg)	Iron (mg)	Sodium (mg)	Vit A (IU)	Thiamin (Vit B₁) (mg)	Riboflavin (Vit B₂) (mg)	Niacin (mg)	Vit C (mg)	Folate (mcg)
Popcorn, ckd in oil, salted	1 cup	11	55	1	3	0.5	0	6	1.1	1	0.3	97	17	0.01	0.01	0.2	0	1.87
Pork, bacon/cracklings, brld/pan fried/rstd	2 pce	15	86	4.6	7	2.6	13	0	0	2	0.2	239	0	0.1	0.04	1.1	0	0.75
Pork, cured, ham, reg, 11% fat, rstd	3 oz	85	151	19.2	8	2.7	50	0	0	7	1.1	1275	0	0.62	0.28	5.2	0	2.55
Pork, ham, whole, rstd	3 oz	85	232	22.8	15	5.5	80	0	0	12	0.9	51	8	0.54	0.27	3.9	0	8.5
Pork, ribs, spareribs, brsd	3 oz	85	337	24.7	26	9.5	103	0	0	40	1.6	79	8	0.35	0.32	4.7	0	3.4
Potato Chips, plain, salted	10 pce	20	107	1.4	7	2.2	0	11	0.9	5	0.3	119	0	0.03	0.04	0.8	6	9
Potatoes, au gratin, prep w/milk & butter f/dry mix	1 cup	245	228	5.6	10	6.3	37	31	2.2	203	0.8	1076	522	0.05	0.2	2.3	8	16.17
Potatoes, baked, w/flesh & skin, long	1 ea	202	220	4.6	0	0.1	0	51	4.8	20	2.7	16	0	0.22	0.07	3.3	26	22.22
Potatoes, hash browns, prep f/fzn	½ cup	78	170	2.5	9	3.5	0	22	1.6	12	1.2	27	0	0.09	0.02	1.9	5	5.07
Potatoes, mashed, w/whole milk	½ cup	105	81	2	1	0.3	2	18	2.1	27	0.3	318	20	0.09	0.04	1.2	7	8.61
Potatoes, sweet, flesh, bkd in skin, med, peeled	1 ea	146	150	2.5	0	0	0	35	4.4	41	0.7	15	31860	0.11	0.19	0.9	36	33
Pretzels, hard, salted, twisted	1 oz	28	107	2.5	1	0.2	0	22	0.9	10	1.2	480	0	0.13	0.17	1.5	0	47.88
Prunes, dried	5 ea	61	146	1.6	6	1	0	38	4.3	31	1.5	3	1212	0.05	0.1	1.2	2	2.26
Pudding, choc, rte, 5oz can	5 oz	142	189	3.8	6	0.9	4	32	1.4	128	0.7	183	51	0.04	0.22	0.5	3	4.26
Pudding, tapioca, 5oz can	5 oz	142	169	2.8	5	0.8	1	28	0.1	119	0.3	226	0	0.03	0.14	0.4	1	4.26
Pudding, vanilla, 5oz can	5 oz	142	185	3.3	5	0	10	31	0.1	125	0.2	192	30	0.03	0.2	0.4	1	0
Raisins, seedless, unpacked	1 oz	28	84	0.9	1	0	0	22	1.1	14	0.6	3	2	0.04	0.02	0.2	1	0.92
Raspberries, fresh	1 cup	123	60	1.1	1	0	0	14	8.3	27	0.7	0	160	0.04	0.11	1.1	31	31.98
Raspberries, swnd, frzn	1 cup	250	400	10	15	9.1	12	62	5.5	368	3.1	245	400	0.09	0.53	0.8	1	27.5
Rice, brown, ckd	½ cup	96	107	2.5	1	0.2	0	22	1.7	10	0.4	1	0	0.09	0.02	1.5	0	3.84
Rice, white, reg, ckd	½ cup	103	134	2.8	0	0.1	0	29	0.4	10	1.2	3	0	0.17	0.01	1.5	0	59.74
Rice, wild, ckd	½ cup	100	101	4	2	0	0	21	1.8	3	0.6	3	0	0.05	0.09	1.3	0	26
Rolls, hard, white	1 ea	50	146	4.9	2	0.3	0	26	1.1	48	1.6	272	0	0.24	0.17	2.1	0	47.5
Salad Dressing, blue cheese/roquefort	1 Tbs	15	76	0.7	8	1.5	3	1	0	12	0.1	164	32	0	0.02	0.02	0	1.21
Salad Dressing, french	1 Tbs	16	69	0.1	7	1.5	3	3	0	2	0.1	219	208	0	0	0	2	0.67
Salad Dressing, French, low cal	1 Tbs	15	20	0	1	0.1	0	3	0	2	0.1	118	195	0	0	0	3	0.73
Salad Dressing, Italian	1 Tbs	15	70	0.1	7	1.1	0	2	0	2	0	118	12	0	0	0	1	0
Salad Dressing, Italian, diet, 2cal/tsp, cmrcl	1 Tbs	15	16	0	0	0.2	1	1	0	0	0	118	0	0	0	0	0	0
Salad Dressing, ranch	1 Tbs	15	80	0	8	1.2	5	0	0	0	0	105	48	0	0	0	0	0
Salad Dressing, thousand island	1 Tbs	15	57	0.1	5	0.9	4	2	0	2	0.1	150	48	0	0	0	0	0.94
Salad Dressing, thousand island, low cal	1 Tbs	15	24	0.1	2	0.2	2	2	0.2	2	0.1	153	155	0	0	0	0	0.84
Salad, chicken, w/celery	½ cup	78	268	10.6	25	3.1	48	1	0.2	16	0.6	201	200	0.03	0.07	3.3	1	8.46
Salad, pasta, garden primavera, prep f/dry	¾ cup	142	280	8	12	2.5	2	34	2	80	1.8	730	261	0.15	0.17	2	1	8.38
Salad, potato	½ cup	125	179	3.4	10	1.8	85	14	1.6	24	0.8	661	199	0.1	0.07	1.1	12	16.4
Salad, tuna	1 cup	205	383	32.9	19	3.2	27	19	0	35	2	824	0	0.06	0.14	13.7	5	0.56
Salami, beef & pork, dry	1 oz	28	117	6.4	10	3.4	22	1	0	2	0.4	521	0	0.17	0.08	1.4	0	13.09
Salmon, pink, w/bone, cnd, not drained	3 oz	85	118	16.8	5	1.3	47	0	0	181	0.7	471	47	0.02	0.16	5.6	0	4.25
Salmon, sockeye, fillet, bkd/brld	3 oz	85	184	23.2	9	1.6	74	0	0	6	0.5	56	178	0.18	0.15	5.7	0	1.74
Salsa, homemade, Mexican sauce	1 Tbs	15	3	0.1	0	0	0	1	0.2	1	0	1	57	0.01	0	0.1	2	
Sandwich, bacon, lettuce & tomato, on soft white	1 ea	130	323	10.8	18	4.7	22	30	1.7	54	2.1	619	271	0.36	0.2	3.4	12	35.5
Sandwich, egg salad, on soft white	1 ea	111	361	9.1	24	4.2	149	29	1.2	67	2.1	499	239	0.25	0.3	1.9	0	35.39
Sandwich, peanut butter & jam, on soft white, unsalted	1 ea	100	348	11.5	15	3.1	2	46	3	60	2.2	290	2	0.27	0.17	5.3	0	40.04
Sandwich, reuben, grilled	1 ea	237	458	27.6	29	9.8	80	25	2.2	286	4.2	1933	453	0.21	0.34	2.8	13	37.79
Sardines, Atlantic, w/bones, cnd in oil, drained	1 oz	28	58	6.9	3	0.4	40	0	0	107	0.8	141	63	0.02	0.06	1.5	0	3.3
Sauce, soy, made f/soy & wheat	1 Tbs	16	9	1.3	0	0	0	1	0.1	3	0.3	871	0	0.01	0.03	0.4	0	2.56
Sauce, teriyaki, rts	1 Tbs	18	15	1.1	0	0	0	3	0	4	0.3	690	0	0.01	0.01	0.2	0	3.6
Sauerkraut, w/liquid, cnd	½ cup	118	22	1.1	0	0	0	5	2.9	35	1.7	780	21	0.02	0.03	0.2	17	27.97

Food	Amount	Weight (g)	Calories	Protein (g)	Fat (g)	Sat. Fat (g)	Cholesterol (g)	Carbohydrate (g)	Fiber (g)	Calcium (mg)	Iron (mg)	Sodium (mg)	Vit A (IU)	Thiamin (Vit B_1) (mg)	Riboflavin (Vit B_2) (mg)	Niacin (mg)	Vit C (mg)	Folate (mcg)
Sausage, pork, smkd, link	1 ea	68	265	15.1	22	7.7	46	1	0	20	0.8	1020	0	0.48	0.17	3.1	1	3.4
Scallops, brd, fried, mixed species, lrg	2 ea	31	67	5.6	3	0.8	19	3	0	13	0.3	144	23	0.01	0.03	0.5	1	11.47
Seaweed, spirulina, dried	1 cup	119	345	68.4	9	3.2	0	28	4.3	143	33.9	1247	678	2.83	4.37	15.3	12	111.8
Shrimp/Prawns, brd, fried, lrg	7 ea	85	206	18.2	10	1.8	150	10	0.3	57	1.1	292	161	0.11	0.12	2.6	1	6.89
Shrimp/Prawns, ckd, lrg	3 oz	85	84	17.8	1	0.2	166	0	0	33	2.6	190	186	0.03	0.03	2.2	2	2.98
Soda, cola	12 fl-oz	369	151	0	0	0	0	38	0	11	0.1	15	0	0	0	0	0	0
Soda, cola/Coke, diet, w/sacc, low sod	12 fl-oz	340	0	0	0	0	0	0	0	14	0.1	54	0	0	0	0	0	0
Soda, ginger ale	12 fl-oz	366	124	0	0	0	0	32	0	11	0.7	26	0	0	0	0	0	0
Soda, lemon lime	12 fl-oz	340	136	0	0	0	0	35	0	7	0.2	37	0	0	0	0.1	0	0
Soda, root beer	12 fl-oz	340	139	0	0	0	0	36	0	17	0.2	44	0	0	0	0	0	0
Sole/Flounder, fillet, bkd/brld	3 oz	85	99	20.5	1	0.3	58	0	0	15	0.3	89	32	0.07	0.1	1.9	0	7.82
Soup, beef bouillon/broth, cnd, prep w/water	1 cup	240	17	2.7	1	0.3	0	0	0	14	0.4	782	0	0	0.05	1.9	0	4.8
Soup, chicken noodle, prep w/water	1 cup	241	75	4	2	0.7	7	9	0.7	17	0.8	1106	711	0.05	0.06	1.4	0	21.69
Soup, clam chowder, Manhattan, prep f/cnd	1 cup	244	112	12.3	2	0	10	11	3.1	41	1.8	725	2297				4	
Soup, clam chowder, New England, prep w/milk	1 cup	248	164	9.5	7	3	22	17	1.5	186	1.5	992	164	0.07	0.24	1	3	9.67
Soup, cream of chicken, prep w/milk	1 cup	248	191	7.5	11	4.6	27	15	0.2	181	0.7	1047	714	0.07	0.26	0.9	1	7.69
Soup, cream of mushroom, prep w/milk	1 cup	245	201	6	13	5.1	20	15	0.5	176	0.6	906	152	0.08	0.28	0.9	2	9.8
Soup, minestrone, prep w/water	1 cup	241	82	4.3	3	0.6	2	11	1	34	0.9	911	2338	0.05	0.04	0.9	1	36.15
Soup, pea, split, w/ham, prep w/water	1 cup	245	184	10	4	1.7	7	27	2.2	22	2.2	975	431	0.14	0.07	1.4	1	2.45
Soup, tomato, prep w/milk	1 cup	248	161	6.1	6	2.9	17	22	2.7	159	1.8	744	848	0.13	0.25	1.5	68	20.83
Soup, tomato, prep w/water	1 cup	245	86	2.1	2	0.4	0	17	0.5	12	1.8	698	691	0.09	0.05	1.4	67	14.7
Soup, vegetable beef, prep w/water	1 cup	245	78	5.6	2	0.9	5	10	0.5	17	1.1	794	1899	0.04	0.05	1	2	10.54
Soup, vegetable, vegetarian, prep w/water	1 cup	250	75	2.2	2	0.3	0	12	0.5	22	1.1	852	3118	0.05	0.05	0.9	2	11
Sour Cream, cultured	1 Tbs	14	30	0.4	3	1.8	6	1	0	16	0	7	111	0	0.02	0	0	1.51
Spinach, ckd w/o add salt, drained	½ cup	103	24	3.1	0	0	0	4	2.5	140	3.7	72	8436	0.1	0.24	0.5	10	150.1
Spinach, raw, chpd	½ cup	55	12	1.6	0	0	0	2	1.5	54	1.5	43	3693	0.04	0.1	0.4	15	106.9
Spinach, w/o add salt, cnd, drained	½ cup	103	24	2.9	1	0.1	0	4	2.5	131	2.4	28	9039	0.02	0.14	0.4	15	100.7
Squash, acorn, ckd	1 cup	245	83	1.6	0	0	0	22	6.4	64	1.4	7	632	0.25	0.02	1.3	16	27.69
Squash, summer, ckd w/o add salt, drained	½ cup	90	18	0.8	0	0.1	0	4	1.3	24	0.3	1	258	0.04	0.04	0.5	5	18.09
Squash, winter, avg, bkd, mashed	½ cup	103	40	0.9	1	0.1	0	9	2.9	14	0.3	1	3664	0.09	0.02	0.7	10	28.84
Strawberries, fresh, whole	1 cup	149	45	0.9	1	0	0	10	3.4	21	0.6	2	40	0.03	0.1	0.3	84	26.37
Strawberries, slices, swtnd, fzn	1 cup	250	240	1.3	0	0	0	65	4.8	28	1.5	8	60	0.04	0.13	1	104	37.25
Stuffing, bread, prep f/dry mix	½ cup	70	125	2.2	6	1.2	0	15	2	22	0.8	380	219	0.1	0.07	1	0	70.7
Sugar, beet/cane, brown, packed	1 tsp	5	19	0	0	0	0	5	0	4	0.1	2	0	0	0	0	0	0.05
Sugar, white, granulated	1 tsp	4	15	0	0	0	0	4	0	0	0	0	0	0	0	0	0	0
Syrup, maple	1 Tbs	20	52	0	0	0	0	13	0	13	0.2	2	0	0	0	0	0	0
Taco Shells	1 ea	10	47	0.7	2	0.3	0	7	0.7	20	0.2	67	33	0	0	0	0	0
Tangerines/Mandarin oranges, fresh, med	1 ea	116	51	0.7	0	0	0	13	2.7	16	0.1	1	1067	0.12	0.03	0.2	36	23.66
Tea, brewed	¼ cup	180	2	0	0	0	0	1	0	0		5	0	0	0.03		0	9.36
Tempeh	1 cup	166	320	30.8	18	3.7	0	16	9	184	4.5	15	0	0.13	0.59	4.4	0	39.67
Tofu, firm, silken	½ cup	126	78	8.7	3	0.5	0	3	0.1	40	1.3	45	0	0.13	0.05	0.3	0	
Tomatoes, red, ripe, raw, med, whole	1 ea	100	21	0.9	0	0	0	5	1.1	5	0.4	9	623	0.06	0.04	0.6	19	15
Tomatoes, red, ripe, w/o add salt, cnd, in liquid	½ cup	121	23	1.1	0	0	0	5	1.2	36	0.7	179	720	0.05	0.08	0.9	17	9.44
Tortilla/Taco/Tostada Shell, corn	1 ea	148	693	10.7	33	5	0	92	11.1	237	3.7	543	518	0.34	0.08	2	0	8.88
Trout, rainbow, fillet, bkd/brld, wild	3 oz	85	128	19.5	5	1.4	59	0	0	73	0.3	48	42	0.13	0.1	4.9	2	16.15
Tuna, light, cnd in oil, drained	3 oz	85	168	24.8	7	1.3	15	0	0	11	1.2	301	66	0.03	0.1	10.5	0	4.51
Tuna, light, cnd in water, drained	3½ oz	99	115	25.3	1	0.2	30	0	0	11	1.5	335	55	0.03	0.07	13.1	0	3.96
Turkey, average, w/o skin, rstd	3 oz	85	144	24.9	4	1.4	65	0	0	21	1.5	60	0	0.05	0.15	4.6	0	5.95

Food	Amount	Weight (g)	Calories	Protein (g)	Fat (g)	Sat. Fat (g)	Cholesterol (g)	Carbohydrate (g)	Fiber (g)	Calcium (mg)	Iron (mg)	Sodium (mg)	Vit A (IU)	Thiamin (Vit B_1) (mg)	Riboflavin (Vit B_2) (mg)	Niacin (mg)	Vit C (mg)	Folate (mcg)
Turnip Greens, ckd f/fzn, drained	½ cup	73	22	2.4	0	0.1	0	4	2.5	111	1.4	11	5822	0.04	0.05	0.3	16	28.76
Turnips, ckd w/add salt, raw, cubes	½ cup	78	16	0.6	0	0	0	4	1.6	17	0.2	39	0	0.02	0.02	0.2	9	7.18
Veal, loin, brsd	3 oz	85	241	25.7	15	5.7	100	0	0	24	0.9	68	0	0.03	0.26	7.7	0	11.9
Veal, loin, lean, brsd	3 oz	85	192	28.5	8	2.2	106	0	0	27	0.9	71	0	0.04	0.29	8.5	0	12.75
Vinegar, balsamic, 60 grain	1 Tbs	15	21				0	5		13	0.1	3						
Watermelon, fresh, diced	1 cup	160	51	1	1	0.1	0	11	0.8	13	0.3	3	586	0.08	0.08	0.1	15	3.52
Wheat, bulgur, ckd	1 cup	135	112	4.2	0	0.1	0	25	6.1	14	1.3	7	0	0.13	0.03	0.3	0	24.3
Wheat, flakes, rolled, dry	1 cup	30	97	3.5	0	0.1	0	21	4.4	18	1	0	0	0.08	0.04	1.4	0	21.12
Wheat, germ, tstd	1 Tbs	6	23	1.7	1	0.1	0	3	0.8	3	0.5	0	0	0.13	0.03	1.4	0	1.34
Whiskey, 90 proof	2 fl-oz	42	110	0.1	0	0	0	0	0	3	0	0	0	0.1	0.05	0.3	0	0.6
Wine, cooler	4 oz	113	56	0.1	0	0	0	7	0	6	0.3	9	1	0	0	0	2	0.65
Wine, red	⅛ cup	30	22	0.1	0	0	0	1	0	2	0.1	2	0	0.01	0.01	0.1	0	0.12
Wine, Rose	2 fl-oz	59	42	0.1	0	0	0	1	0	5	0.2	3	0	0	0.01	0	0	
Wine, white, med	2 fl-oz	59	40	0.1	0	0	0	0	0	5	0.2	3	0	0	0	0	0	
Yogurt, fruit, low fat, 10g prot/8 oz	1 cup	227	231	9.9	2	1.6	10	43	0	345	0.2	133	104	0.08	0.4	0.2	1	21.11
Yogurt, plain, low fat, 12g prot/8 oz	8 oz	226	143	11.9	4	2.3	14	16	0	413	0.2	159	149	0.1	0.48	0.3	2	25.31
FAST FOOD RESTAURANTS																		
General																		
Burrito, bean	1 ea	166	342	10.8	10	5.3	3	55	6.3	86	3.5	754	254	0.48	0.46	3.1	1	66.4
Chili, con carne	1 cup	255	258	24.8	8	3.5	135	22	4	69	5.2	1015	1675	0.13	1.15	2.5	2	45.9
Cole Slaw, fast food	1 cup	120	178	1.8	13	1.9	6	15	2	41	0.9	324	409	0.05	0.04	0.1	10	46.8
English Muffin, w/butter	1 ea	63	189	4.9	6	2.4	13	30	1.9	103	1.6	386	136	0.25	0.31	2.6	1	56.7
Entree, enchilada, cheese	1 ea	230	451	13.6	27	14.9	62	40		458	1.9	1106	1638	0.12	0.6	2.7	1	92
Hot Dog, plain	1 ea	98	242	10.4	15	5.1	44	18		24	2.3	670	0	0.24	0.27	3.6	0	48.02
Pancake, w/butter & syrup	2 ea	232	520	8.3	14	5.9	58	91		128	2.6	1104	281	0.39	0.56	3.4	3	51.04
Sandwich, chicken, fillet, plain	1 ea	157	444	20.8	25	7.4	52	33	1.2	52	4	826	86	0.28	0.2	5.9	8	86.35
Sundae, hot fudge, fast food	1 ea	164	295	5.9	9	5.2	21	49	0	215	0.6	189	230	0.07	0.31	1.1	2	9.84
Arby's																		
Salad, chef	1 ea	273	136	12.3	6	2.6	84	9		113	3.3	529	3321	0.26	0.25	4.6	35	
Sandwich, beef, Arby Q	1 ea	190	389	17.6	15	5.4	29	48		70	9.2	1268		0.27	0.39	9.2		
Sandwich, beef, French dip & swiss cheese	1 ea	154	369	24.7	16	7.5	58	31	0.9	232	3.6	1237	0	0.18	0.47	7.4	0	16.35
Sandwich, beef 'n cheddar	1 ea	194	508	24.6	26	7.7	52	43		150	6.1	1166		0.42	0.63	9.8	1	
Sandwich, chicken, grilled, deluxe	1 ea	195	365	20	17	3	37	35		59	2.1	764	339	0.27	0.25	11.5	7	
Sandwich, roast beef, regular	1 ea	155	383	22	18	6.9	43	35	1.1	60	4.9	936	0	0.28	0.48	11	1	14
Sauce, Arby's	½ oz	14	15	0.1	0	0	0	3			0.4	113						
Sauce, horsey	½ oz	14	110	0.1	5	1.2	0	3		20		105						
Burger King Corporation																		
Cheeseburger, Whopper	1 ea	294	730	33	46	16	115	46	3	250	4.5	1350	750	0.34	0.48	7	9	
Croissant, w/egg, sausage & cheese	1 ea	110	375	13.8	29	10	162	16	0.6	94	2.2	712	250				0	
Hamburger, Whopper	1 ea	270	640	27	39	11	90	45	3	80	4.5	870	500	0.33	0.41	7	9	
Onion Rings, reg svg	3 ea	30	75	1	3	0.5	0	10	1.5	24	0.3	196	0				0	
Potatoes, french fries, salted, med svg	1 ea	116	370	5	20	5	0	43	3	0	1.1	240	0				4	
Sandwich, chicken, broiler	1 ea	168	373	20.3	20	4.1	54	28	1.4	41	3.7	325	203				4	
Sandwich, fish, big	1 ea	255	700	26	41	6	90	56	3	60	2.7	980	100				1	
Dunkin Donuts, Inc.																		
Croissant, plain	1 ea	18	81	1.2	5	1.2	2	8	0	6	0.5	78	0				0	
Hidden Valley																		
Salad Dressing, ranch, reduced fat & cal	2 Tbs	28	58	0.5	5	0.9	10	2	0	11	0.1	237	15				0	
International Dairy Queen Inc.																		
Frozen Yogurt Cone, med	4 oz	113	148	5.1	1	0.3	3	32	0	143	1	91	0	0.05	0.2		1	
Frozen Yogurt, nonfat	4 oz	113	133	4	4	0		28	0	133	1	93	0				0	

Food	Amount	Weight (g)	Calories	Protein (g)	Fat (g)	Sat. Fat (g)	Cholesterol (g)	Carbohydrate (g)	Fiber (g)	Calcium (mg)	Iron (mg)	Sodium (mg)	Vit A (IU)	Thiamin (Vit B_1) (mg)	Riboflavin (Vit B_2) (mg)	Niacin (mg)	Vit C (mg)	Folate (mcg)
Hamburger, homestyle	1 ea	138	290	17	12	5	45	29	2	60	2.7	630	200	0.29	0.25	3.9	4	
Ice Cream Cone, vanilla, med	1 ea	142	237	5.7	6	4.3	22	38	0	179	1.3	115	538	0.06	0.26	0.1	2	
Milk Shake, vanilla, med	1 ea	397	520	12	14	8	45	88	0.3	400	1.4	230	400	0.12	0.6	0.8	0	
Onion Rings, svg	3 oz	85	241	3.8	12	3	0	29	2.3	15	1.1	135	0	0.09	0.05	0.4	0	
Sandwich, fish, fillet	1 ea	182	396	17.1	17	3.7	48	42	2.1	43	1.9	674	0	0.32	0.24	3.2	0	
Sundae, chocolate, med	1 ea	184	315	6.3	8	4.7	24	56	0	197	1.1	165	590	0.06	0.27	0.3	0	
Jack in the Box																		
Bowl, chicken, teriyaki	1 ea	502	670	26	4	1	15	128	3	100	4.5	1730	6500				24	
Cheeseburger, Jumbo Jack	1 ea	296	640	31	38	15	105	44	2	250	4.5	1340	750	0.44	0.54	2	9	
Hamburger	1 ea	104	250	12	9	3.5	30	30	2	100	3.6	610	0	0.16	0.28	2.1	0	
Hamburger, sourdough, jack	1 ea	233	690	34	45	15	105	37	2	200	4.5	1180	750	0.68	0.5	8.4	9	
Sandwich, chicken, supreme	1 ea	305	830	33	49	7	65	66	3	200	3.6	2140	500	0.49	0.4	13.7	9	
Kentucky Fried Chicken Corporation																		
Chicken, leg, original recipe	1 ea	54	124	11.5	8	1.8	66	4	0	18	0.6	374	89				1	
Chicken, wing, hot & spicy	1 ea	55	210	10	15	4	55	9	1	20	0.7	350	100				1	
Chicken, wing, original recipe	1 ea	45	134	8.6	10	2.4	53	5	0	19	0.3	396	96				1	
Long John Silver's																		
Dinner, fish & fries, batter fried, 2pce	1 ea	261	610	27	37	7.9	60	52		40	1.8	1480		0.38	0.34	8	9	
McDonald's Nutrition Information Center																		
Biscuit, sausage & egg	1 ea	175	541	17.7	36	9.8	241	34	1	98	2.7	1140	295	0.53	0.57	4.1	0	27.73
Cheeseburger	1 ea	115	304	14.3	12	5.7	38	33	1.9	190	2.6	779	285	0.31	0.29	3.6	2	22.37
Cheeseburger, Quarter Pounder	1 ea	186	493	26	28	12.1	88	35	1.9	279	4.2	1200	465	0.37	0.4	6.3	2	31.06
Chicken, nuggets, McNuggets, 4 pce, svg	1 ea	71	190	5.5	11	2.5	40	10	0	9	0.7	340	0	0.08	0.11	5	0	
Danish, apple	1 ea	115	394	3.8	18	5.5	44	56	1.1	88	1.2	318	548	0.33	0.19	2.2	1	
Frozen Yogurt Cone, vanilla, low fat	3 oz	85	142	3.8	4	2.8	19	22	0	94	0.3	71	283	0.46	0.42	5.7	1	
Hamburger, Big Mac	1 ea	204	529	24.6	29	9.4	80	42	2.8	236	4.2	1011	283	0.37	0.3	6.3	3	46.53
Hamburger, Quarter Pounder	1 ea	160	391	21.4	20	7.4	65	34	1.9	140	4.2	763	93	0.5	0.45	3.3	2	25.63
McMuffin, egg	1 ea	138	294	17.2	12	4.6	238	27	1	203	2.7	802	507	0.68	0.33	4.5	1	33.47
McMuffin, sausage	1 ea	135	434	15.7	28	9.6	54	31	1.2	241	2.2	892	241	0.12	0.5	0.3	0	18.95
Milk Shake, vanilla, sml	1 ea	289	355	10.8	9	5.9	39	58	0	345	0.4	246	296	0.14	0.14	1.3	1	
Muffin, apple bran, fat free	1 ea	75	197	3.9	2	0.3	0	40	2	66	0.9	250	0	0.71	0.43	5.6	1	5.03
Pie, apple	1 ea	307	1037	12	52	14	0	136	4	80	4.3	797		0.05	0	1.9	96	33.16
Potatoes, french fries, sml svg	1 ea	68	210	3	10	1.5	0	26	2	9	0.4	135	0	0.08	0.02	0.9	9	25.57
Potatoes, hash browns	1 ea	55	135	1	8	1.6	0	15	1	7	0.4	342	0				9	8.64
Salad, garden, shaker	1 ea	149	100	7	6	3	75	4	2	150	1.1	120	1500				15	
Sandwich, Filet O Fish	1 ea	131	378	13.4	21	3.8	42	35	1.7	126	1.5	731	168	0.29	0.21	2.3	0	26.73
Sauce, sweet & sour, pkt 1	1/6 oz	32	57	0	0	0	0	13	0	2	0.2	160	343	0	0.01	0.1	0	
Pizza Hut, Inc.																		
Pizza, cheese, pan, med, 12"	2 pce	205	495	22.8	21	9.5	47	53	3.8	273	2.8	951	1000	0.57	0.61	5.2	7	
Pizza, cheese, thin n' crispy, med, 12"	2 pce	148	350	18.8	14	6.8	43	36	3.4	247	1.8	911	922	0.39	0.39	4.8	5	
Pizza, pepperoni, pan, 12"	2 pce	211	539	22.4	24	8.1	49	57	4.1	209	3.3	1157	966	0.63	0.49	5.4	8	
Pizza, pepperoni, personal pan	1 ea	255	637	27	28	10	55	69	5	250	4	1339	1164	0.56	0.66	8.2	10	0
Pizza, supreme, pan, med, 12"	2 pce	255	581	28	28	11.2	56	52	5.6	219	4.3	1428	912	0.8	0.79	6	10	
Subway International																		
Sandwich, chicken breast, rstd, on white, 6"	1 ea	246	332	26	6	1	48	41	3	35	3	967	617				15	
Sandwich, Italian bmt, on white, 6"	1 ea	246	445	21	21	8	56	39	3	44	4	1652	753				15	
Sandwich, meatball, on white, 6"	1 ea	260	404	18	16	6	33	44	3	32	4	1035	712				16	
Sandwich, roast beef, deli style	1 ea	180	245	13	4	1	13	38	2	23	3	638	565				14	
Sandwich, tuna, w/lt mayonnaise, on wheat, 6"	1 ea	253	391	19	15	2	32	46	3	38	3	940	729				15	
Sandwich, turkey, on white, 6"	1 ea	232	273	17	4	1	19	40	3	30	4	1391	601				15	

Food	Amount	Weight (g)	Calories	Protein (g)	Fat (g)	Sat. Fat (g)	Cholesterol (g)	Carbohydrate (g)	Fiber (g)	Calcium (mg)	Iron (mg)	Sodium (mg)	Vit A (IU)	Thiamin (Vit B₁) (mg)	Riboflavin (Vit B₂) (mg)	Niacin (mg)	Vit C (mg)	Folate (mcg)
Taco Bell Inc.																		
Burrito, beef, big supreme	1 ea	298	520	24	23	10	55	54	11	150	2.7	1520	3000				5	
Burrito, seven layer	1 ea	234	438	13.2	19	5.8	21	55	10.7	165	3	1058	1240				5	
Burrito, supreme	1 ea	255	440	17	19	8	35	51	10	150	9	1230	2500	0.4	2.1	2.9	5	
Taco	1 ea	83	192	9.6	11	4.3	27	13	3.2	85	1.1	351	532	0.05	0.15	1.3	0	
Taco, soft	1 ea	92	225	9.2	10	4.1	26	12	3.1	82	1.1	337	511	0.39	0.22	2.7	0	
Wendy's Foods International																		
Cheeseburger, w/bacon, jr	1 ea	170	393	20.5	19	7.5	58	35	1.9	171	3.6	895	390	0.31	0.32	6.6	9	28.85
Chicken, nuggets	6 pce	94	292	13.9	20	3.6	37	14	0	24	0.5	589	0	0.15	0.14	9	1	
Frosty, dairy dessert, med	1 ea	298	440	11	11	7	50	73	0	410	1.4	260	1000	0.14	0.62	0.4	0	22.9
Hamburger, bacon classic, big	1 ea	251	517	30.1	26	10.7	88	41	2.4	206	4.5	1298	622	0.4	1.36	5.3	13	
Salad, caesar, w/o dressing, side	1 ea	130	151	12.4	8	3.4	25	9	2	190	1.6	538	2501				22	
Salad, chicken, grilled, w/o dressing	1 ea	338	195	22.1	8	1.7	46	10	4	188	2.1	676	5872				35	
Salad, garden, deluxe, w/o dressing	1 ea	271	110	6.7	6	1	1	10	3.9	189	1.5	319	5883				35	
Salad, taco, w/o chips	1 ea	510	411	28.7	20	10.5	69	31	8.7	403	4.5	1132	2582	0.29	0.5	3.2	28	88.27
Sandwich, chicken, brd	1 ea	208	433	27.4	16	3.1	54	47	1.8	93	2.7	754	217	0.43	0.32	13.3	13	
Sandwich, chicken, club	1 ea	220	483	30.6	20	4.4	64	48	1.9	95	2.9	957	222				14	
Sandwich, chicken, grilled	1 ea	177	283	22.6	7	1.5	61	34	1.8	84	2.7	698	201				9	
CONVENIENCE FOODS & MEALS																		
El Charrito																		
Entree, enchilada, beef, family size, 6 pack	1 ea	200	353	11.8	17	6.5	33	39	5.2	196	2.4	837	1961				3	
Healthy Choice																		
Dinner, fish, herb baked, fzn	1 ea	273	300	14.1	6	1.3	31	48	4.4	35	0.6	424	2650				0	
Dinner, meatloaf, traditional, fzn	1 ea	340	316	15.3	5	2.5	37	52	6.1	48	2.2	459	745				55	
Entree, burrito, chicken, con queso, fzn	1 ea	216	253	10.1	4	1.8	25	43	4.3	29	1.3	426	1084				4	
Entree, lasagna, roma, fzn	1 ea	284	311	19.3	7	2.2	26	44	4.4	111	2.7	430	371	0.22	0.19	1.5	4	
Entree, spaghetti, bolognese, fzn	1 ea	284	280	14	6	2	30	43	5	40	3.6	470	500				15	
Lean Cuisine																		
Entree, chow mein, chicken, w/rice	1 ea	241	198	12.3	5	0.9	33	26	1.9	19	0.3	482	95	0.14	0.16	4.7	6	
Entree, lasagna, w/meat sauce	1 ea	291	270	19	6	2.5	25	34	5	150	1.8	560	500	0.15	0.25	3	12	
Entree, ravioli, cheese	1 ea	241	250	12	8	3	55	32	4	200	1.1	500	750	0.06	0.25	1.2	6	48
Entree, spaghetti, w/meatballs, fzn	1 ea	290	322	19.4	8	2.2	6	43	4.9	102	2.6	502	0					
The Budget Gourmet																		
Dinner, chicken, teriyaki, 3 dish	1 ea	340	360	20	12		55	44		80	1.4	610	1500	0.15	0.34	6	12	
Dinner, veal, parmigiana, 3 dish	1 ea	340	440	26	20		165	39		30	4.5	1160	5000	0.45	0.6	6	6	
Entree, beef, sirloin tips, w/country gravy	1 ea	334	365	18.8	21		47	25		71	0.4	670	882	0.18	0.2	4.7	3	
Entree, linguini, w/shrimp	1 ea	284	330	15	15		75	33		10	3.6	1250	5000	0.3	0.17	3	2	
The Budget Gourmet-Slim Select																		
Entree, stroganoff, beef	1 ea	238	269	17.3	10	0.5	58	28		58	2.6	537	288	0.25	0.33	3.8	9	
Weight Watchers																		
Entree, chow mein, chicken	1 ea	255	200	12	2	0.5	25	34	3	40	0.7	430	1499				36	

This food composition table has been prepared for West-Wadsworth Publishing Company and is copyrighted by ESHA Research in Salem, Oregon—the developer and publisher of the Food Processor®, Genesis® R&D, and the Computer Chef® nutrition software systems. The major sources for the data are from the USDA, supplemented by more than 1200 additional sources of information. Because the list of references is so extensive, it is not provided here, but is available from the publisher.

FIGURE **B.1** Daily nutrient intake.

Name: _____   Date: _____   Course: _____   Section: _____   Gender: _____   Age: _____

Foods	Amount	Calories	Protein (gm)	Fat (total gm)	Sat. Fat (gm)	Chol- esterol (mg)	Carbo- hydrates (gm)	Cal- cium (mg)	Iron (mg)	Sodium (mg)	Vit. A (IU)	Vit. B₁ (mg)	Vit. B₂ (mg)	Niacin (mg)	Vit. C (mg)
Totals															

FIGURE B.2 Daily nutrient intake.

Name: _____ Date: _____ Course: _____ Section: _____ Gender: _____ Age: _____

Day	Calories	Protein (gm)	Fat (gm)	Sat. Fat (gm)	Chol-esterol (mg)	Carbo-hydrates (gm)	Calcium (mg)	Iron (mg)	Sodium (mg)	Vit.A (µg RE)	Thiamin Vit.B_1 (mg)	Riboflavin Vit.B_2 (mg)	Niacin (mg)	Vit.C (mg)
One														
Two														
Three														
Totals														
Average[a]														
Percentages[b]														

Recommended Dietary Allowances*

	Calories	Protein (gm)	Fat (gm)	Sat. Fat (gm)	Chol-esterol (mg)	Carbo-hydrates (gm)	Calcium (mg)	Iron (mg)	Sodium (mg)	Vit.A (µg RE)	Thiamin Vit.B_1 (mg)	Riboflavin Vit.B_2 (mg)	Niacin (mg)	Vit.C (mg)
Men														
14–18 yrs.	See	See below[c]	<30%[e] below[d]	<10%[e]	<300[e]	>58%[e]	1,300	12	2,400[e]	1,000	1.2	1.3	16	75
19–30 yrs.			<30%[e]	<10%[e]	<300[e]	>58%[e]	1,000	10	2,400[e]	1,000	1.2	1.3	16	90
31–50 yrs.			<30%[e]	<10%[e]	<300[e]	>58%[e]	1,000	10	2,400[e]	1,000	1.2	1.3	16	90
51+ yrs.			<30%[e]	<10%[e]	<300[e]	>58%[e]	1,200	10	2,400[e]	1,000	1.2	1.3	16	90
Women														
14–18 yrs.			<30%[e]	<10%[e]	<300[e]	>58%[e]	1,300	15	2,400[e]	800	1.0	1.0	14	65
19–30 yrs.			<30%[e]	<10%[e]	<300[e]	>58%[e]	1,000	15	2,400[e]	800	1.1	1.1	14	75
31–50 yrs.			<30%[e]	<10%[e]	<300[e]	>58%[e]	1,000	15	2,400[e]	800	1.1	1.1	14	75
51+ yrs.			<30%[e]	<10%[e]	<300[e]	>58%[e]	1,200	10	2,400[e]	800	1.1	1.1	14	75
Pregnant			<30%[e]	<10%[e]	<300[e]	>58%[e]	1,200	30	2,400[e]	800	1.4	1.4	18	75
Lactating			<30%[e]	<10%[e]	<300[e]	>58%[e]	1,200	15	2,400[e]	1,300	1.5	1.5	17	95

[a] Divide totals by 3 or number of days assessed.

[b] Percentages: Protein and carbohydrates = multiply average by 4, divide by average calories, and multiply by 100. Fat and saturated fat = multiply average by 9, divide by average calories, and multiply by 100.

[c] Use Table 9.2 (Page 253) for all categories.

[d] Protein intake should be .8 grams per kilogram of body weight. Pregnant women should consume an additional 15 grams of daily protein, and lactating women should have an extra 20 grams.

[e] Based on recommendations by nutrition experts.

SOURCE: Adapted from the National Academy of Sciences, *Recommended Dietary Allowances*, © 1989, National Academy Press, Washington, DC.

FIGURE B.3 Daily nutrient intake form for computer software use.

Name: _____   Date: _____

Gender: ☐ Male ☐ Female ☐ Pregnant ☐ Nursing

Activity: ☐ Sedentary ☐ Lightly active ☐ Moderately active ☐ Very active ☐ Extremely active

Height: ☐ ft ☐ in   Weight: ☐ lbs   Age: ☐

Student ID #: _____   Instructor's Name: _____

Class Days: _____   Class Times: _____

No.	Item	Amount
1		
2		
3		
4		
5		
6		
7		
8		
9		
10		
11		
12		
13		
14		
15		
16		
17		
18		
19		
20		
21		
22		
23		
24		
25		
26		
27		
28		
29		
30		
31		

FIGURE B.3 Daily nutrient intake form for computer software use.

Name: _____ Date: _____

Gender: ☐ Male ☐ Female ☐ Pregnant ☐ Nursing

Activity: ☐ Sedentary ☐ Lightly active ☐ Moderately active ☐ Very active ☐ Extremely active

Height: ___ ft ___ in Weight: ___ lbs Age: ___

Student ID #: _____ Instructor's Name: _____

Class Days: _____ Class Times: _____

No.	Item	Amount
1		
2		
3		
4		
5		
6		
7		
8		
9		
10		
11		
12		
13		
14		
15		
16		
17		
18		
19		
20		
21		
22		
23		
24		
25		
26		
27		
28		
29		
30		
31		

Glossary

A

Acquired immunodeficiency syndrome (AIDS) Any of a number of diseases that arise when the body's immune system is compromised by HIV.

Action stage Stage of change in which people are actively changing a negative behavior or adopting a new, healthy behavior.

Activities of daily living Everyday behaviors that people normally do to function in life (cross the street, carry groceries, lift objects, do laundry, sweep floors).

Acupuncture Chinese medical system that requires body piercing with fine needles during therapy to relieve pain and treat ailments and diseases.

Addiction Compulsive and uncontrollable behavior(s) or use of substance(s).

Adenosine triphosphate (ATP) A high-energy chemical compound that the body uses for immediate energy.

Adequate Intakes (AI) The recommended amount of a nutrient intake when sufficient evidence is not available to calculate the EAR and subsequent RDA.

Adipose tissue Fat cells in the body.

Aerobic Exercise that requires oxygen to produce the necessary energy (ATP) to carry out the activity.

Aerobic dance A series of exercise routines performed to music.

Air displacement Technique to assess body composition by calculating the body volume from the air displaced by an individual sitting inside a small chamber.

Alcohol (ethyl alcohol) A depressant drug that affects the brain and slows down central nervous system activity; has strong addictive properties.

Alcoholism Disease in which an individual loses control over drinking alcoholic beverages.

Allopathic medicine See conventional Western medicine.

Altruism True concern for the welfare of others.

Alveoli Air sacs in the lungs where oxygen is taken up and carbon dioxide (produced by the body) is released from the blood.

Amenorrhea Cessation of regular menstrual flow.

Amino acids Chemical compounds that contain nitrogen, carbon, hydrogen, and oxygen; the basic building blocks the body uses to build different types of protein.

Amotivational syndrome A condition characterized by loss of motivation, dullness, apathy, and lack of interest in the future.

Amphetamine Powerful central nervous system stimulant.

Anabolic steroids Synthetic versions of the male sex hormone testosterone, which promotes muscle development and hypertrophy.

Anaerobic Exercise that does not require oxygen to produce the necessary energy (ATP) to carry out the activity.

Angina pectoris Chest pain associated with coronary heart disease.

Angiogenesis Formation of blood vessels (capillaries).

Angioplasty A procedure in which a balloon-tipped catheter is inserted, then inflated, to widen the inner lumen of one or more arteries.

Anorexia nervosa An eating disorder characterized by self-imposed starvation to lose and maintain very low body weight.

Anthropometric measurement techniques Measurement of body girths at different sites.

Anticoagulant Any substance that inhibits blood clotting.

Antioxidants Compounds such as vitamins C and E, beta-carotene, and selenium that prevent oxygen from combining with other substances in the body to form harmful compounds.

Aquaphobic Having a fear of water.

Arrhythmias Irregular heart rhythms.

Atherosclerosis Fatty cholesterol deposits in the walls of the arteries leading to plaque formation.

Atrophy Decrease in the size of a cell.

Autogenic training Stress management technique using a form of self-suggestion, wherein an individual is able to place him/herself in an autohypnotic state by repeating and concentrating on feelings of heaviness and warmth in the extremities.

Ayurveda Unconventional Hindu system of medicine based on herbs, diet, massage, meditation, and yoga to help the body boost its own natural healing.

B

Ballistic stretching Exercises done with jerky, rapid, bouncy movements.

Basal metabolic rate (BMR) The lowest level of oxygen consumption necessary to sustain life.

Behavior modification The process to permanently change negative behaviors in favor of positive behaviors that will lead to better health and well-being.

Benign Noncancerous.

Bioelectrical impedance Technique to assess body composition by running a weak electrical current through the body.

Biofeedback A stress management technique in which a person learns to reliably influence physiological responses of two kinds: either responses that are not ordinarily under voluntary control or responses that ordinarily are easily regulated but for which regulation has broken down because of trauma or disease.

Blood lipids (fats) Cholesterol and triglycerides.

Blood pressure A measure of the force exerted against the walls of the vessels by the blood flowing through them.

Bod Pod Commercial name of the equipment used for the assessment of body composition through the air displacement technique.

Body composition The fat and nonfat components of the human body; important in assessing recommended body weight.

Body mass index (BMI) A technique to determine thinness and excessive fatness that incorporates height and weight to estimate critical fat values at which the risk for disease increases.

Bradycardia Slower heart rate than normal.

Breathing exercise A stress management technique wherein the individual concentrates on "breathing away" the tension and inhaling fresh air to the entire body.

Bulimia nervosa An eating disorder characterized by a pattern of binge eating and purging in an attempt to lose weight and maintain low body weight.

C

Calorie The amount of heat necessary to raise the temperature of 1 gram of water 1 degree Centigrade; used to measure the energy value of food and cost (energy expenditure) of physical activity.

Cancer Group of diseases characterized by uncontrolled growth and spread of abnormal cells.

Carbohydrate loading Increasing intake of carbohydrates during heavy aerobic training or prior to aerobic endurance events that last longer than 90 minutes.

Carbohydrates A classification of dietary nutrient containing carbon, hydrogen, and oxygen; the major source of energy for the human body.

Capillaries Smallest blood vessels carrying oxygenated blood to body tissues.

Carcinogens Substances that contribute to the formation of cancers.

Carcinoma in situ Encapsulated malignant tumor that has not spread.

Cardiac output Amount of blood pumped by the heart in one minute.

Cardiomyopathy A disease affecting the heart muscle.

Cardiorespiratory endurance The ability of the lungs, heart, and blood vessels to deliver adequate amounts of oxygen to the cells to meet the demands of prolonged physical activity.

Cardiovascular diseases The array of conditions that affect the heart and the blood vessels.

Carotenoids Pigment substances in plants that are often precursors to vitamin A. Over 600 carotenoids are found in nature and about 50 of them are precursors to vitamin A, the most potent one being beta-carotene.

Catecholamines "Fight-or-flight" hormones, including epinephrine and nor-epinephrine.

Cellulite Term frequently used in reference to fat deposits that "bulge out"; these deposits are nothing but enlarged fat cells from excessive accumulation of body fat.

Chiropractics Health care system that believes that many diseases and ailments are related to misalignments of the vertebrae and emphasizes the manipulation of the spinal column.

Chlamydia A sexually transmitted disease, caused by a bacterial infection, that can cause significant damage to the reproductive system.

Cholesterol A waxy substance, technically a steroid alcohol, found only in animal fats and oils; used in making cell membranes, as a building block for some hormones, in the fatty sheath around nerve fibers, and in other necessary substances.

Chronic diseases Illnesses that last a long time.

Chronological age Calendar age.

Chylomicron Triglyceride-transporting molecules.

Circuit training Alternating exercises by performing them in a sequence of three to six or more.

Cirrhosis A disease characterized by scarring of the liver.

Cocaine 2-beta-carbomethoxy-3-betabenozoxytropane, the primary psychoactive ingredient derived from coca plant leaves.

Cold turkey Eliminating a negative behavior all at once.

Complementary and alternative medicine A branch of medicine concerned with treatments and health care practices not widely taught in medical schools, not generally used in hospitals, and not usually reimbursed by medical insurance companies.

Complex carbohydrates Carbohydrates formed by three or more simple sugar molecules linked together; also referred to as "polysaccharides."

Concentric Shortening of a muscle during muscle contraction.

Contemplation stage Stage of change in which people are considering changing behavior in the next 6 months.

Contraindicated exercises Exercises that are not recommended because they may cause injury.

Controlled ballistic stretching Exercises done with slow, short, and sustained movements.

Conventional Western medicine Traditional medical practice based on methods that are tested through rigorous scientific trials.

Cool-down Tapering off an exercise session slowly.

Coronary heart disease (CHD) Condition in which the arteries that supply the heart muscle with oxygen and nutrients are narrowed by fatty deposits, such as cholesterol and triglycerides.

Creatine An organic compound derived from meat, fish, and amino acids that combines with inorganic phosphate to form creatine phosphate.

Creatine phosphate (CP) A high-energy compound that is used by the cells to re-synthesize ATP during all-out activities of very short duration.

Cross-training A combination of aerobic activities that contribute to overall fitness.

Cruciferous vegetables Plants that produce cross-shaped leaves (cauliflower, broccoli, cabbage, Brussels sprouts, and kohlrabi); they seem to have a protective effect against cancer.

Daily Values (DVs) Reference values for nutrients and food components used in food labels.

Dentist Practitioner who specializes in diseases of the teeth, gums, and oral cavity.

Deoxyribonucleic acid (DNA) Genetic substance of which genes are made; molecule that contains cell's genetic code.

Diabetes mellitus A disease in which the body doesn't produce or utilize insulin properly.

Diastolic blood pressure Pressure exerted by blood against walls of arteries during relaxation phase (diastole) of the heart; lower of the two numbers in blood pressure readings.

Dietary fiber A complex carbohydrate in plant foods that is not digested but is essential to the digestion process.

Dietary Reference Intakes (DRIs) A general term that describes four types of nutrient standards that establish adequate amounts and maximum safe nutrient intakes in the diet. These standards are Estimated Average Requirements (EAR), Recommended Dietary Allowances (RDA), Adequate Intakes (AI), and Tolerable Upper Intake Levels (UL).

Disaccharides Simple carbohydrates formed by two monosaccharide units linked together, one of which is glucose. The major disaccharides are sucrose, lactose, and maltose.

Distress Negative stress: Unpleasant or harmful stress, under which health and performance begin to deteriorate.

Dopamine A neurotransmitter that affects emotional, mental, and motor functions.

Dynamic training Strength-training method referring to a muscle contraction with movement.

Dysmenorrhea Painful menstruation.

Eccentric Lengthening of a muscle during muscle contraction.

Ecstasy *See* MDMA.

Elastic elongation Temporary lengthening of soft tissue.

Electrocardiogram (ECG or EKG) A recording of the electrical activity of the heart.

Emotional wellness The ability to understand your own feelings, accept your limitations, and achieve emotional stability.

Endorphins Morphine-like substances released from the pituitary gland (in the brain) during prolonged aerobic exercise; thought to induce feelings of euphoria and natural well-being.

Energy-balancing equation A principle holding that as long as caloric input equals caloric output, the person will not gain or lose weight. If caloric intake exceeds output, the person gains weight; when output exceeds input, the person loses weight.

Environmental wellness The capability to live in a clean and safe environment that is not detrimental to health.

Enzymes Catalysts that facilitate chemical reactions in the body.

Essential fat Minimal amount of body fat needed for normal physiological functions; constitutes about 3 percent of total weight in men and 12 percent in women.

Estimated Average Requirements (EAR) The amount of a nutrient that meets the dietary needs in half the people.

Estrogen Female sex hormone; essential for bone formation and conservation of bone density.

Eustress Positive stress. Health and performance continue to improve, even as stress increases.

Exercise A type of physical activity that requires planned, structured, and repetitive bodily movement with the intent of improving or maintaining one or more components of physical fitness.

Exercise intolerance Inability to function during exercise because of excessive fatigue or extreme feelings of discomfort.

Fast-twitch fibers Muscle fibers with greater anaerobic potential and fast speed of contraction.

Fats Nutrients containing carbon, hydrogen, some oxygen, and sometimes other chemical elements.

Ferritin Iron stored in the body.

Fight or flight Physiological response of the body to stress that prepares the individual to take action by stimulating the vital defense systems.

Fixed resistance Type of exercise in which a constant resistance is moved through a joint's full range of motion.

Flexibility The ability of a joint to move freely through its full range of motion.

Folate One of the B vitamins.

Free weights Barbells and dumbbells.

Frequency How often a person engages in an exercise session.

Functional capacity The ability to perform ordinary and unusual demands of daily living without limitations and excessive fatigue or injury.

Functional independence Ability to carry out activities of daily living without assistance from other individuals.

Genital herpes A sexually transmitted disease caused by a viral infection of the herpes simplex virus Types I and II. The virus can attack different areas of the body, but commonly causes blisters on the genitals.

Genital warts A sexually transmitted disease caused by a viral infection.

Girth measurements Technique to assess body composition by measuring circumferences at specific body sites.

Glucose intolerance A condition characterized by slightly elevated blood glucose levels.

Glycemic index An index that is used to rate the plasma glucose response of carbohydrate-containing foods versus the response produced by the same amount of carbohydrate from a standard source, usually glucose or white bread.

Glycogen Form in which glucose is stored in the body.

Goal The ultimate aim toward which effort is directed.

Gonorrhea Sexually transmitted disease caused by a bacterial infection.

Health A state of complete well-being, and not just the absence of disease or infirmity.

Health fitness standards The lowest fitness requirements for maintaining good health, decreasing the risk for chronic diseases, and lowering the incidence of muscular-skeletal injuries.

Health-related fitness Fitness programs that are prescribed to improve the overall health of the individual.

Healthy life expectancy (HLE) Number of years a person is expected to live in good health. This number is obtained by subtracting ill-health years from the overall life expectancy.

Heart rate reserve (HRR) The difference between the maximal heart rate and the resting heart rate.

Heat cramps Muscle spasms caused by heat-induced changes in electrolyte balance in muscle cells.

Heat exhaustion Heat-related fatigue.

Heat stroke Emergency situation resulting from the body being subjected to high atmospheric temperatures.

Hemoglobin Protein-iron compound in red blood cells that transports oxygen in the blood.

Heroin A potent drug that is a derivative of opium.

Herbal medicine Unconventional system that uses herbs to treat ailments and disease.

High-density lipoproteins (HDLs) Cholesterol-transporting molecules in the blood that help clear cholesterol from the blood; also called "good" cholesterol.

High-impact aerobics Exercises incorporating movements in which both feet are off the ground at the same time momentarily.

Homeopathy System of treatment based on the use of minute quantities of remedies that in large amounts produce effects similar to the disease being treated.

Homocysteine An amino acid that, when allowed to accumulate in the blood, may lead to plaque formation and blockage of arteries.

Human immunodeficiency virus (HIV) Virus that leads to acquired immunodeficiency syndrome (AIDS).

Hydrostatic weighing Underwater technique to assess body composition; considered the most accurate of the body composition assessment techniques.

Hypertension Chronically elevated blood pressure.

Hypertrophy An increase in the size of the cell (for example, muscle hypertrophy).

Hypokinetic diseases "Hypo" denotes "lack of"; therefore, lack of physical activity.

Hypotension Low blood pressure.

Hypothermia A breakdown in the body's ability to generate heat; a drop in body temperature below 95 degrees F.

Imagery Mental visualization of relaxing images and scenes to induce body relaxation in times of stress or as an aid in the treatment of certain medical conditions such as cancer, hypertension, asthma, chronic pain, and obesity.

Insulin Hormone secreted by the pancreas; essential for proper metabolism of blood glucose (sugar) and maintenance of blood glucose level.

Insulin resistance The inability of the cells to respond appropriately to insulin.

Intensity In cardiorespiratory exercise, how hard a person has to exercise to improve or maintain fitness. In flexibility exercises, the degree of stretch.

International unit (IU) Measure of nutrients in foods.

Interval training A series of exercise work bouts (intervals) interspersed with low-intensity or rest intervals.

Isokinetic training Strength-training method in which the speed of the muscle contraction is kept constant because the equipment (machine) provides an accommodating resistance to match the user's force (maximal) through the range of motion.

Isometric training Strength-training method referring to a muscle contraction that produces little or no movement, such as pushing or pulling against an immovable object.

Lactic acid End product of anaerobic glycolysis (metabolism).

Lactovegetarians Vegetarians who eat foods from the milk group.

Lean body mass Body weight without body fat.

Life expectancy Number of years a person is expected to live based on the person's birth year.

Life Experiences Survey A questionnaire used to assess sources of stress in life.

Lipoproteins Lipids covered by proteins, they transport fats in the blood; types are LDL, HDL, and VLDL.

Locus of control The extent to which a person believes he or she can influence the external environment.

Low-density lipoproteins (LDLs) Cholesterol-transporting molecules in the blood that tend to increase blood cholesterol; also called "bad" cholesterol.

Low-impact aerobics Exercises in which at least one foot is in contact with the ground or floor at all times.

Magnetic therapy Unconventional treatment that relies on magnetic energy to promote healing.

Maintenance stage Stage of change in which people maintain behavioral change for up to 5 years.

Malignant Cancerous.

Mammogram Low-dose X rays of the breasts used as a screening technique for the early detection of breast cancer.

Marijuana A psychoactive drug prepared from a mixture of crushed leaves, flowers, small branches, stems, and seeds from the hemp plant Cannabis sativa.

Massage therapy The rubbing or kneading of body parts to treat ailments.

Maximal heart rate (MHR) Highest heart rate for a person, related primarily to age.

Maximal oxygen uptake (VO$_{2max}$) Maximum amount of oxygen the body is able to utilize per minute of physical activity, commonly expressed in ml/kg/min. The best indicator of cardiorespiratory or aerobic fitness.

MDA A hallucinogenic drug that is structurally similar to amphetamines.

MDMA A synthetic hallucinogen drug with a chemical structure that closely resembles MDA and methamphetamine. It is also known as "ecstasy."

Meditation A stress management technique used to gain control over one's attention by clearing the mind and blocking out the stressor(s) responsible for the increased tension.

Mediterranean diet Typical diet of people around the Mediterranean region that focuses on olive oil, red wine, grains, legumes, vegetables, and fruits, with limited amounts of meat, fish, milk, and cheese.

Megadoses For most vitamins, 10 times the RDA or more; for vitamins A and D, 5 and 2 times the RDA, respectively.

Melanoma The most virulent, rapidly spreading form of skin cancer.

Mental wellness A state in which your mind is engaged in lively interaction with the world around you.

MET The rate of resting energy expenditure at rest; MET is the equivalent of 3.5 ml/kg/min.

Metabolic fitness Denotes improvements in the metabolic profile through a moderate-intensity exercise program in spite of little or no improvement in physical fitness standards.

Metabolic profile A measurement to assess risk for diabetes and cardiovascular disease through plasma insulin, glucose, lipid, and lipoprotein levels.

Metabolic syndrome *See* Syndrome X.

Metabolism All energy and material transformations that occur within living cells; necessary to sustain life.

Metastasis The movement of cells from one part of the body to another.

Methamphetamine A more potent form of amphetamine.

Minerals Inorganic elements found in the body and in food; essential for normal body functions.

Mitochondria Structures within the cells where energy transformations take place.

Mode Form of exercise.

Moderate physical activity Activity that uses 150 calories of energy per day, or 1,000 calories per week.

Monogamous A sexual relationship in which two people have sexual relations only with each other.

Monosaccharides The simplest carbohydrates (sugars), formed by five- or six-carbon skeletons. The three most common monosaccharides are glucose, fructose, and galactose.

Morbidity Any condition related to or caused by illness or disease.

Motivation The desire and will to do something.

Motor neurons Nerves connecting the central nervous system to the muscle.

Motor unit The combination of a motor neuron and the muscle fibers that neuron innervates.

Muscular endurance The ability of a muscle to exert submaximal force repeatedly over time.

Muscular strength The ability of a muscle to exert maximum force against resistance (for example, 1 repetition maximum [or 1 RM] of the bench press exercise).

Myocardial infarction Heart attack; damage to or death of an area of the heart muscle as a result of an obstructed artery to that area.

Myocardium Heart muscle.

Naturopathic medicine Unconventional system of medicine that relies exclusively on natural remedies to treat disease and ailments.

Negative resistance The lowering or eccentric phase of a repetition during the performance of a strength-training exercise.

Nicotine Addictive compound found in tobacco leaves.

Nitrosamines Potentially cancer-causing compounds formed when nitrites and nitrates, which are used to prevent the growth of harmful bacteria in processed meats, combine with other chemicals in the stomach.

Nonallopathic medicine *See* Complementary and alternative medicine.

Nonmelanoma skin cancer Cancer that spreads or grows at the original site but does not metastasize to other regions of the body.

Nurse Health care practitioner who assists in the diagnosis and treatment of health problems and provides many services to patients in a variety of settings.

Nutrient density A measure of the amount of nutrients and calories in various foods.

Nutrients Substances found in food that provide energy, regulate metabolism, and help with growth and repair of body tissues.

Nutrition Science that studies the relationship of foods to optimal health and performance.

Obesity An excessive accumulation of body fat, usually at least 30 percent above recommended body weight.

Objectives Steps required to reach a goal.

Occupational wellness The ability to perform one's job skillfully and effectively under conditions that provide personal and team satisfaction and adequately reward each individual.

Olestra Fat substitute made from sugar and fatty acids; provides no calories to the body because it passes through the digestive system without being absorbed.

Oligomenorrhea Irregular menstrual cycles.

Omega-3 fatty acids Polyunsaturated fatty acids found primarily in cold-water seafood, flaxseed, and flaxseed oil; thought to lower blood cholesterol and triglycerides.

Omega-6 fatty acids Polyunsaturated fatty acids found primarily in corn and sunflower oils and most oils in processed foods.

Oncogenes Genes that initiate cell division.

One repetition maximum (1 RM) The maximum amount of resistance an individual is able to lift in a single effort.

Ophthalmologist Medical specialist concerned with diseases of the eye and prescription of corrective lenses.

Opportunistic diseases Diseases that arise in the absence of a healthy immune system, which would fight them off in healthy people.

Optometrist Health care practitioner who specializes in the prescription and adaptation of lenses.

Oral surgeon A dentist who specializes in surgical procedures of the oral-facial complex.

Orthodontist A dentist who specializes in the correction and prevention of teeth irregularities.

Osteopath A medical practitioner with specialized training in musculoskeletal problems who uses diagnostic and therapeutic methods of conventional medicine in addition to manipulative measures.

Osteoporosis Softening, deterioration, or loss of bone mass.

Oxygen free radicals Substances formed during metabolism that attack and damage proteins and lipids, in particular the cell membrane and DNA, leading to diseases such as heart disease, cancer, and emphysema.

Oxygen uptake (VO$_2$) The amount of oxygen used by the human body.

Overload principle Training concept that the demands placed on a system (cardio-respiratory or muscular) must be increased systematically and progressively over time to cause physiological adaptation (development or improvement).

Overweight Excess weight according to a given standard, such as height or recommended percent body fat; less than obese.

Ovolactovegetarians Vegetarians who include eggs and milk products in their diet.

Ovovegetarians Vegetarians who allow eggs in their diet.

Pelvic inflammatory disease (PID) An overall designation referring to the effects of other STDs, primarily chlamydia and gonorrhea.

Percent body fat Proportional amount of fat in the body based on the person's total weight; includes both essential and storage fat.

Peripheral vascular disease Narrowing of the peripheral blood vessels (excludes the cerebral and coronary arteries).

Peristalsis Involuntary muscle contractions of intestinal walls that facilitate excretion of wastes.

Physical activity Bodily movement produced by skeletal muscles; requires expenditure of energy and produces progressive health benefits.

Physical fitness The ability to meet the ordinary as well as the unusual demands of daily life safely and effectively without being overly fatigued and still have energy left for leisure and recreational activities.

Physical fitness standards A fitness level that allows a person to sustain moderate-to-vigorous physical activity without undue fatigue; one's ability to closely maintain this level throughout life.

Physical wellness Good physical fitness and confidence in one's personal ability to take care of health problems.

Physician assistant A health care practitioner trained to treat most standard cases of care.

Physiological age The biological and functional capacity of the body as it should be in relation to the person's maximal potential at any given age of the lifespan.

Phytochemicals Compounds found in fruits and vegetables that block the formation of cancerous tumors and disrupt the progress of cancer.

Plastic elongation Permanent lengthening of soft tissue.

Plyometric exercise Explosive jump training, incorporating speed and strength training to enhance explosiveness.

Plyometric training A form of aerobic exercise that requires forceful jumps or springing off the ground immediately after landing from a previous jump.

Positive resistance The lifting, pushing, or concentric phase of a repetition during the performance of a strength-training exercise.

Prayer Sincere and humble communication with a higher power.

Precontemplation stage Stage of change in which people are unwilling to change behavior.

Preparation stage Stage of change in which people are getting ready to make a change within the next month.

Primary care physician A medical practitioner who provides routine treatment of ailments; typically, the patient's first contact for health care.

Processes of change Actions that help you achieve change in behavior.

Progressive muscle relaxation A stress management technique that uses progressive contraction and relaxation of muscle groups throughout the body.

Progressive resistance training A gradual increase of resistance over a period of time.

Proprioceptive neuromuscular facilitation (PNF) Stretching technique in which muscles are stretched out sequentially with intermittent isometric contractions.

Proteins Complex organic compounds containing nitrogen and formed by combinations of amino acids; the main substances used in the body to build and repair tissues.

Pro-vitamin A compound that can be converted into a vitamin.

Quackery/Fraud The conscious promotion of unproven claims for profit.

Range of motion Entire arc of movement of a given joint.

Rate of perceived exertion (RPE) A perception scale to monitor or interpret the intensity of aerobic exercise.

Recommended body weight Body weight at which there seems to be no harm to human health; healthy weight.

Recommended Dietary Allowances (RDA) The daily amount of a nutrient (statistically determined from the EARs) considered adequate to meet the known nutrient needs of almost 98 percent of all healthy people in the United States.

Recovery time Amount of time the body takes to return to resting levels after exercise.

Registered dietician (RD) A person with a college degree in dietetics who meets all certification and continuing education requirements of the American Dietetic Association or Dietitians of Canada.

Relapse To slip or fall back into unhealthy behavior(s); failure to maintain healthy behaviors.

Repetitions Number of times a given resistance is performed.

Resistance Amount of weight that is lifted.

Resting heart rate (RHR) Heart rate after a person has been sitting quietly for 15–20 minutes.

Resting metabolism Amount of energy (expressed in milliliters of oxygen per minute or in total calories per day) an individual requires during resting conditions to sustain proper body function.

Reverse cholesterol transport A process in which HDL molecules attract cholesterol and carry it to the liver, where it is changed to bile and eventually excreted in the stool.

Ribonucleic acid (RNA) Genetic material that guides the formation of cell proteins.

Risk factors Lifestyle and genetic variables that may lead to disease.

Sedentary A lifestyle characterized by inactivity and a lot of sitting.

Semivegetarians Vegetarians who include milk products, eggs, and fish and poultry in the diet.

Set A fixed number of repetitions. One set of bench presses might be 10 repetitions.

Setpoint Weight control theory that the body has an established weight and strongly attempts to maintain that weight.

Sexually transmitted diseases (STDs) Communicable diseases spread through sexual contact.

Shin splints Injury to the lower leg characterized by pain and irritation in the shin region of the leg.

Side stitch A sharp pain in the side of the abdomen.

Simple carbohydrates Formed by simple or double sugar units with little nutritive value; divided into monosaccharides and disaccharides.

Skill-related fitness Fitness programs that are used to improve athletic ability.

Skinfold thickness Technique to assess body composition by measuring a double thickness of skin at specific body sites.

Slow-sustained stretching Exercises in which the muscles are lengthened gradually through a joint's complete range of motion.

Slow-twitch fibers Muscle fibers with greater aerobic potential and slow speed of contraction.

Social wellness The ability to relate well to others, both within and outside the family unit.

Specificity of training Principle that training must be done with the specific muscle the person is attempting to improve.

Sphygmomanometer Device to measure blood pressure; consists of inflatable bladder contained within a cuff and a manometer (either mercury gravity or aneroid) from which the pressure is read.

Spiritual wellness The sense that life is meaningful, that life has purpose, and that some power brings all humanity together; the ethics, values, and morals that guide us and give meaning and direction to life.

Spot reducing Fallacious theory that exercising a specific body part will result in significant fat reduction in that area.

Step aerobics A form of exercise that combines stepping up and down from a bench with arm movements.

Sterols Derived fats, of which cholesterol is the best-known example.

Storage fat Body fat in excess of essential fat; stored in adipose tissue.

Stress The mental, emotional, and physiological response of the body to any situation that is new, threatening, frightening, or exciting.

Stress electrocardiogram An exercise test during which the workload is gradually increased (until the subject reaches maximal fatigue) with blood pressure and 12-lead electrocardiographic monitoring throughout the test.

Stressor Stress-causing event.

Stretching Moving the joints beyond the accustomed range of motion.

Stroke volume Amount of blood pumped by the heart in one beat.

Structured interview An assessment tool used to determine behavioral patterns that define Type A and B personalities.

Subluxation Partial dislocation of a joint.

Substrate Substance acted upon by an enzyme (examples: carbohydrates and fats).

Sun protection factor (SPF) Degree of protection offered by ingredients in sunscreen lotion; at least SPF 15 is recommended.

Supplements Tablets, pills, capsules, liquids, or powders that contain vitamins, minerals, amino acids, herbs, or fiber that are taken to increase the intake of these nutrients.

Suppressor genes Genes that deactivate the process of cell division.

Syndrome X An array of metabolic abnormalities that contribute to the development of atherosclerosis triggered by insulin resistance. These conditions include low HDL-cholesterol, high triglycerides, high blood pressure, and an increased blood clotting mechanism.

Synergistic action The effect of mixing two or more drugs, which can be much greater than the sum of the same drugs acting by themselves.

Synergy A reaction in which the result is greater than the sum of its two parts.

Syphilis A sexually transmitted disease caused by a bacterial infection.

Systolic blood pressure Pressure exerted by blood against walls of arteries during forceful contraction (systole) of the heart; higher of the two numbers in blood pressure readings.

Tachycardia Faster-than-normal heart rate.

Tar Chemical compound that forms during the burning of tobacco leaves.

Techniques of change Methods or procedures used to aid with each process of change.

Telomerase An enzyme that allows cells to reproduce indefinitely.

Telomeres A strand of molecules at both ends of a chromosome.

Termination/adoption stage Stage of change in which people have eliminated an undesirable behavior or maintained a positive behavior for over 5 years.

Thermogenic response Amount of energy required to digest food.

Transfatty acid Solidified fat formed by adding hydrogen to monounsaturated and polyunsaturated fats to increase shelf life.

Triglycerides Fats formed by glycerol and three fatty acids.

Type A Behavior pattern characteristic of a hard-driving, overambitious, aggressive, at times hostile and overly competitive person.

Type B Behavior pattern characteristic of a calm, casual, relaxed, and easy-going individual.

Type C Behavior pattern of individuals who are just as highly stressed as the Type A but do not seem to be at higher risk for disease than the Type B.

Type I diabetes Insulin-dependent diabetes mellitus (IDDM), a condition in which the pancreas produces little or no insulin. Also known as "juvenile diabetes."

Type II diabetes Non-insulin–dependent diabetes mellitus (NIDDM), a condition in which insulin is not processed properly. Also known as "adult-onset diabetes."

Ultraviolet B rays (UVB) Portion of sunlight that causes sunburn and encourages skin cancers.

Unconventional medicine *See* complementary and alternative medicine.

Underweight Extremely low body weight.

Upper Intake Level (UL) The highest level of nutrient intake that appears safe for most healthy people, beyond which exists an increased risk of adverse effects.

Variable resistance Training using special machines equipped with mechanical devices that provide differing amounts of resistance through the range of motion.

Vegans Vegetarians who eat no animal products at all.

Vegetarians Individuals whose diet is of vegetable or plant origin.

Very low-density lipoproteins (VLDLs) Triglyceride-, cholesterol-, and phospholipid-transporting molecules in the blood that tend to increase blood cholesterol.

Vigorous activity Any activity that requires a MET level equal to or greater than 6 METs (21 ml/kg/min); 1 MET = energy expenditure at rest, 3.5 ml/kg/min.

Vigorous exercise Cardiorespiratory exercise that requires an intensity level above 60 percent of maximal capacity.

Vitamins Organic nutrients essential for normal metabolism, growth, and development of the body.

Waist-to-hip ratio A measurement to assess potential risk for disease based on distribution of body fat.

Warm-up Starting a workout slowly.

Weight-regulating mechanism (WRM) A feature of the hypothalamus of the brain that controls how much the body should weigh.

Wellness The constant and deliberate effort to stay healthy and achieve the highest potential for well-being. It encompasses seven dimensions—physical, emotional, mental, social, environmental, occupational, and spiritual—and integrates them all into a quality life.

Workload Amount or intensity of demands placed on the body during physical activity.

Yoga A school of thought in the Hindu religion that seeks to help the individual attain a higher level of spirituality and peace of mind.

Yo-yo dieting Constantly losing and gaining weight.